MILADY'S
Theory and Practice of
Therapeutic Massage

SECOND EDITION

MARK F. BECK

MILADY PUBLISHING COMPANY
(A Division of Delmar Publishers Inc.)

NOTICE TO THE READER

CREDITS:
Publisher: Catherine Frangie
Developmental Editor: Joseph Miranda
Senior Project Editor: Laura V. Miller
Senior Art/Design Supervisor: Susan C. Mathews
Art Coordinator: Nicole F. Reamer
Production Manager: John Mickelbank

Freelance Project Editor: Dianne DiBlasi
Cover Design by: design M design W
Cover Illustration by Jeanne A. Benas

© 1994 Milady Publishing Company
(A Division of Delmar Publishers Inc.)
3 Columbia Circle, Box 12519
Albany, NY 12212-2519

Printed in the United States of America

Printed and distributed simultaneously in Canada

4 5 6 7 8 9 10 XXX 00 99 98 97 96 95

Library of Congress Cataloging-in-Publication Data

Beck, Mark. F.
    Milady's theory and practice of therapeutic massage / Mark F. Beck. —
    2nd ed.
        p.   cm.
    Includes bibliography and glossary/index.
    Rev. ed. of: The theory and practice of therapeutic massage. ©1988
    ISBN 1-56253-120-4 (textbook)
    1. Massage—Therapeutic use. I. Beck, Mark. The theory and practice of
therapeutic massage. II. Title.
RM721.B42   1994

615.8'22—dc20   93-28234
                                                          CIP

Contents

Preface

Congratulations for choosing to become a student of massage therapy! Massage therapy is a rapidly growing profession with a wide variety of opportunities for the motivated and talented practitioner. A career in massage therapy offers the personal satisfaction of knowing that as a result of the service you provide, your clients feel better and enjoy better quality of life.

Throughout history, hands-on techniques have played an important role in the health practices of every major society. Classical techniques along with advances in the field of massage therapy and soft tissue manipulation offer relief for numerous maladies and painful conditions that result from today's high stress lifestyles.

The future of the massage industry is promising. Massage therapy is widely recognized as an effective means of reducing the incidence of stress-related disorders and as well as relieving soft tissue pain and dysfunction. Massage therapy has become an important and respected part of the allied health industry.

The successful massage practitioner must be proficient in more than just the ability to perform a good massage. A survey conducted in 1990 by Knapp and Associates indicates that the most important treatment goals of massage therapy are therapeutic benefits and health promotion, muscular and general relaxation, education, and body awareness. To achieve these goals, the practitioner needs an understanding of the body and its functions, massage techniques, and therapeutic skills such as assessment, application, and evaluation of those skills.

The survey also indicated that over 85% of massage practitioners who responded were self-employed and that two-thirds worked either out of their homes or out of private offices. This indicates that today's massage practitioner must be self-motivated and have some knowledge of small business practices. Since most therapists work independently, skills in client/therapist relations, communications, and promotions are also important.

This textbook contains the information that addresses these concerns and will provide a strong foundation for a career as a professional massage therapist. **Milady's Theory and Practice of Therapeutic Massage** presents information regarding the structure and function of the body relevant to massage, the basic therapeutic techniques used in massage, considerations for the operation of a successful massage business, and a review of a variety of specialized massage techniques. Mastery of the information contained in this textbook, along with the skills taught at your massage school, are important steps into the interesting, lucrative, satisfying, and challenging career of a massage therapist.

Acknowledgments

We, (the author and Delmar Publishers) wish to express our appreciation to the many professional people who have contributed their valuable time and counsel during the preparation of this text. We would also like to thank the following people for contributing to the chapters dealing with their special areas of expertise:

Susan Beck, whose background in consumer science, experience, and knowledge as a certified massage therapist and instructor added so much to the research and development of materials of interest to the professional massage practitioner.

Richard van Why for his unceasing research into the history of massage and the information he provided for the history chapter.

Doris Dietemann, N.D. and instructor, for her contributions to the chapters concerning posture, draping, and various massage techniques.

Gail A. Drum, R.N. and specialist in patient care, who contributed her valuable knowledge and advice to the chapter on massage in nursing and healthcare.

Joel Gerson, author and educator in the field of esthetics, who contributed to the chapters on skin conditions and face massage.

Pat Archer and Jack Meagher for the material provided in the chapter on sports massage.

The author also expresses a special appreciation to the following individuals:

Bobbi Ray Madry for the opportunity and motivation to become involved in this project.

Bob Rogers for the training that began my journey into the marvelous and rewarding profession of massage.

Patricia J. Benjamin, PhD., Guerneville, CA; Nancy W. Dail, director Downeast School of Massage, Waldoboro, ME; Brett A. Pace, licensed massage therapist/instructor, Core Institute School of Massage Therapy, Tallahassee, FL; William L. Smith, licensed massage therapist, Tallahassee, FL; for their assistance and expertise in reviewing this book.

The multitude of teachers, clients, and students who have enriched my knowledge of the applications and effects of massage.

Natasha, wherever you are, for my first real massage and the advice, "Whenever your back hurts like that, find someone who knows how to do massage."

My wife Susan for the unconditional love and encouragement without which this book would not have become a reality.

MARK F. BECK

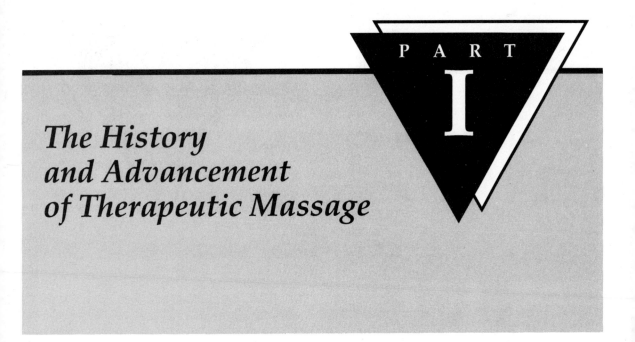

PART
I

The History and Advancement of Therapeutic Massage

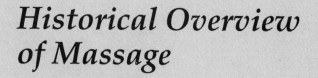

Historical Overview of Massage

1

Learning Objectives

After you have mastered this chapter, you will be able to:

1. Explain why massage is known as one of the earliest remedial practices for the relief of pain and discomfort.

2. Explain why massage is a natural and instinctive remedy for some illnesses and injuries.

3. Explain the use of massage from ancient to modern times as an aid to physiological and psychological well-being.

4. Describe the basic differences in massage systems.

5. Explain why it is important for legitimate practitioners to know massage history.

INTRODUCTION ▼

Massage (muh-**SAHZH**) is defined as the systematic manual or mechanical manipulations of the soft tissues of the body by such movements as rubbing, kneading, pressing, rolling, slapping, and tapping, for therapeutic purposes such as promoting circulation of the blood and lymph, relaxation of muscles, relief from pain, restoration of metabolic balance, and other benefits both physical and mental.

The massage practitioner has been referred to as a massage technician or massotherapist. In the past, a male massage practitioner may have been called a masseur (ma-**SUR**), and a female practitioner a masseuse (ma-**SOOS**). Today, most professionally trained men and women prefer to be called massage practitioners or massage therapists. For practical purposes, **massage practitioner** or **massage therapist** will be the terms used throughout this book.

The origin of the word **massage** can be traced to at least five sources:

The Greek root **masso,** or **massein,** means to touch or to handle but also means to knead or to squeeze.

The Latin root **massa** comes directly from the Greek **masso** and means the same.

The Arabic root **mass'h,** or **mass,** means to press softly.

The Sanskrit word **makeh** also means to press softly.

The modern use of the term **massage** to denote using the hands to apply manipulations of the soft tissues is of fairly recent origin. The term was first used in American and European literature around 1875. In America, the use of the word *massage* was popularized by Douglas Graham from Massachusetts. The term *massage,* as well as the common names for the strokes (effleurage, petrissage, tapotement) and frictions, is generally attributed to a Dutchman, Johan Georg Mezger.

MASSAGE IN ANCIENT TIMES ▼

Even though the term *massage* is fairly new, the practice of various techniques can be traced back to antiquity. Massage is one of the earliest remedial practices of humankind and is said to be the most natural and instinctive means of relieving pain and discomfort. When a person has sore, aching muscles, abdominal pains, a bruise or wound, it is a natural and instinctive impulse to touch, press, and rub that part of the body to obtain relief.

Artifacts have been found in many countries to support the belief that in prehistoric times men and women massaged their muscles and rubbed herbs, oils, and various substances on their bodies as healing and protective agents. According to research reports, in nearly all ancient cultures some form of touch or massage was practiced. In many groups a special person such as a healer,

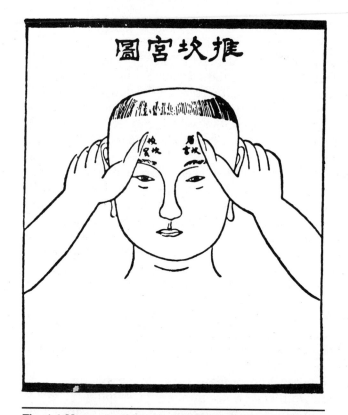

Fig. 1.1 Massage of the forehead. Illustration from the Chinese work *Synopsis of the Technique of Remedial Massage,* 1889. Courtesy New York Public Library picture collection.

spiritual leader, or doctor was selected to administer healing power. These ancient civilizations used therapeutic massage not only as a pain reliever but also to improve their sense of well-being and physical appearance.

Massage has been a major part of medicine for at least five thousand years and important in Western medical traditions for at least three thousand years. Massage was the first and most important of the medical arts and was practiced, developed, and taught primarily by physicians. It has been written about extensively in medical books since 500 B.C. and was a major topic in the first medical texts printed after the discovery of the printing press.

Chinese *Amma* Techniques

In the British Museum, records reveal that as early as 3000 B.C., massage was practiced by the Chinese. *The Cong Fou* of Tao-Tse was one of the ancient Chinese books that described the use of medicinal plants, exercises, and a system of massage for the treatment of disease and the maintenance of health. The Chinese continued to improve their massage techniques through a special procedure they called **amma**. This massage technique was developed over many years of experience in finding the points on the body where various movements such as rubbing, pressing, and manipulations were most effective. Today the use of massage is an integral part of the Chinese health system and is practiced in China's medical clinics and hospitals. A more modern term for Chinese massage is **tui-na,** which literally means **push-pull** (Fig. 1.1).

Japanese *Tsubu* and *Shiatsu*

The practice of the amma method of massage entered Japan around the sixth century A.D. The points of stimulation remained much the same but were called *tsubo*. These points are pressed to effect the circulation of fluids and Ki (life force energy) and stimulate nerves in a finger pressure technique the Japanese called **shiatsu**. This massage method has become quite popular in recent years. Early records show that a book on massage, *The San-Tsai-Tou-Hoei,* was published by the Japanese in the sixteenth century and listed both passive and active massage procedures (Fig. 1.2).

Indian and Hindu Practices

Massage has been practiced on the Indian subcontinent for over three thousand years. Knowledge of massage came to India from

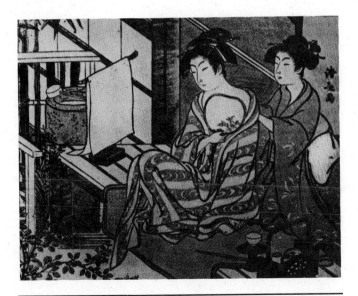

Fig. 1.2 The art of massage was practiced by the Japanese centuries ago. This illustration shows a woman being given a shoulder and back massage by her servant. Louvre collection. Courtesy New York Public Library picture collection.

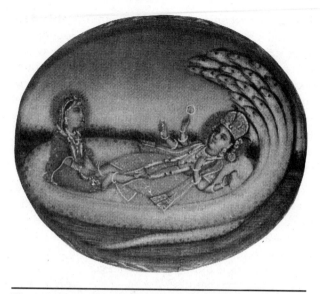

Fig. 1.3 Massage, rubbing, and shampooing were understood and practiced by the Hindus many centuries ago, who recognized their value in diminishing fatigue, inducing sleep, and reducing excess fat. Copyright by the Wellcome Historical Medical Museum. Courtesy New York Public Library picture collection.

the Chinese and was an important part of the Hindu tradition. The *Ayur-Veda* (Art of Life), a sacred book of the Hindus written around 1800 B.C., included massage treatments among its hygienic principles. In writings dating back to 300 B.C., *The Laws of Manu,* or *The Laws of Man* defined the duties of everyday life. These included diet, bathing, exercise, and **tshanpau,** or massage at the bath. **Tshanpau** included kneading the extremities, tapotement, frictioning, anointing with perfumes, and cracking the joints of the fingers, toes, and neck (Fig. 1.3).

Greek Massage and Gymnastics

From the East, the practice of massage spread to Europe and is believed to have flourished well before 300 B.C. The Greeks made gymnastics and the regular use of massage part of their physical fitness rituals. Homer, the Greek poet who wrote the *Iliad* and the *Odyssey* (the story of the Trojan war), in the ninth century B.C., spoke of the use of nutritious foods, exercise, and massage for war heroes to promote healing and relaxation.

The Greek priest-physician **Aesculapius,** who lived in the seventh century B.C., was the first in a long line of physicians and was later worshipped as the god of medicine. He is said to have combined exercise and massage to create gymnastics and founded the first **gymnasium** to treat disease and promote health. The gymnasium and baths became important centers where philosophers and athletes gathered to exercise and discuss ideas. It was a place where the young were educated, soldiers trained, the sick healed. The staff of Aesculapius with its serpents remains today as the symbol of medicine and pharmacy.

Greek women participated in gymnastics and dancing, and used massage as part of their health and beauty regimens. The Greeks referred to exercise as **ascesis,** based on their belief that an **ascete** was a person who exercised his or her body and mind. This was the same principle as today's holistic health concept of the cultivation of total health of body and mind.

The Greek physician Herodicus of the fifth century B.C. prolonged the lives of many of his patients with diet, exercise, and massage using beneficial herbs and oils. Herodotus, the Greek historian of the time, wrote of the benefits of massage. Hippocrates (460-380 B.C.), a pupil of Herodicus and a descendant in the lineage of Aesculapius, later became known as the father of medicine. His code of ethics for physicians, the **Hippocratic Oath,** is still in use today. This oath, which incorporates a code of ethics for physicians and those about to receive medical degrees, binds physicians to honor their teachers, do their best to maintain the health of their patients, honor their patients' secrets, and prescribe no harmful treatment or drug. The Hippocratic Oath can be found in its entirety in most medical dictionaries.

That Hippocrates understood the effects of massage is revealed in one of his descriptions of massage movements. He said, "Hard rubbing binds, much rubbing causes parts to waste, and moderate rubbing makes them grow." This has been interpreted to mean that rubbing can help to bind a joint that is too loose or loosen a joint that is too tight. Vigorous rubbing can tighten and firm, while moderate rubbing tends to build muscle. In his writings, Hippocrates used the word **anatripsis,** which means the art of rubbing a part upward, not downward. He stated that it is necessary to rub the shoulder following reduction of a dislocated shoulder. The advice Hippocrates gave still serves as a valuable guideline for modern practitioners. Hippocrates believed that all physicians should be trained in massage as a method of healing.

Roman Art of Massage and Therapeutic Bathing

The Romans acquired the practice of therapeutic bathing and massage from the Greeks. The Romans built public baths that were available to rich and poor alike. A brisk rubdown with fragrant oils could be enjoyed following the bath. The art of massage was also highly respected as a treatment for weak and diseased conditions and as an aid in removing stiffness and soreness from muscles.

The Romans, as the Greeks before them, used massage as part of their gymnastics. Celsus, who lived during the reign of Emperor

Tiberius (about 42 B.C. to 37 A.D.), was considered to be one of the most eminent of Roman physicians. He wrote extensively on many subjects, including medicine. *De Medicina* deals extensively with prevention and therapeutics using massage, exercise, and bathing. He recommended rubbing the head to relieve headaches and rubbing the limbs to strengthen muscles and to combat paralysis. Massage was used to improve sluggish circulation and internal disorders and to reduce edema. Although circulation of the blood was not completely understood, physicians of the time followed the teaching of Hippocrates and believed that rubbing upward was more effective than rubbing downward.

The Greek physician Claudius Galen (130-200 A.D.), who became physician to the Roman emperor Marcus Aurelius, is said to have discovered that arteries and veins contain blood; however, William Harvey (1578-1657), an English physician, is credited with discovering the circulation of the blood in 1628. Galen was a prolific writer, and his medical texts were the principal ones in use for more than a thousand years. As a physician to gladiators, Galen gained great knowledge of anatomy. His books on hygienic health, exercise, and massage stressed specific exercises for various physical disorders. Greek and Roman philosophers, statesmen, and historians such as Cicero, Pliny, Plutarch, and Plato wrote of the importance of massage and passive and active exercise to the maintenance of a healthy body and mind. Even Julius Gaius Caesar, Roman general and Emperor of Rome (100-44 B.C.), is said to have demanded his daily massage for the relief of neuralgia and prevention of epileptic attacks. Both the Bible and the Koran mention the use of oils and aromatics to lubricate and anoint the skin.

The Decline of Arts and Sciences in the West

With the decline of the Roman Empire, beginning around 180 A.D., the popularity of bathing and massage also declined. According to Richard van Why, "The Roman emperor Constantine (228-337 A.D.) who converted to Christianity, abolished and destroyed the baths and gymnasiums because of widespread abuses of a sexual nature." Oribasius, Antyllus, Caelius Aurelianus, Aetius of Amida, and Paul of Aegina are some of the few medical writers and physicians who lived during the decline of the Roman Empire. They all wrote favorably of the use of massage, exercise, and bathing as therapeutic and conditioning agents.

There is little recorded history of health practices during the Middle Ages (the Dark Ages). This was the period between classical antiquity and the European Renaissance, extending from the downfall of Rome in about 476 to about 1450. The sciences and arts suffered severe setbacks during the Dark Ages. Few medical or historical books were written during this time, and much recorded history was lost. This decline was due in part to wars and to religious superstitions that caused people to fear placing too much importance on the physical self. In Europe in the Middle Ages, the medical institutions abandoned massage in favor of other remedies. Massage was practiced sporadically by laypeople, folk healers, and midwives and was occasionally the object of persecution as a magic cure and the work of Satan.

The Arabic Empire and the Rise of Islam

Beginning in the seventh century, the spread of Islam throughout North Africa, Asia Minor, Mesopotamia, and Persia actually served to preserve much of the Greco-Roman culture. As the Greco-Roman culture fell into decay in the Middle Ages, many of the important teachings of the great physicians and philosophers were carried on by the Persians. The Islamic Persian philosopher/physician **Rhazes,** or **Razi** (860-932 A.D.), was a follower of Hippocrates and Galen and a prolific writer. He wrote several books, the most important of which was an encyclopedia of Arabic, Roman, and Greek medical practices that esteemed the use of exercise, diet, and massage in the treatment of disease and the preservation of health. Another prominent Persian philosopher/physician, Avicenna (980-1037 A.D.), authored what is considered to be the most important single book in medical history. He was an ardent follower of Galen, and the *Canon of Medicine* made numerous references to the use of massage, exercise, and bathing. Eventually these volumes paved the way for the Renaissance as these writings returned to the West by way of trade and conquest.

The Renaissance Revives Interest in Health Practices

The Renaissance (rebirth, 1450-1600) revived interest in the arts and sciences. After a long intellectual slumber, the classical writings of the ancient Greek, Roman, and Persian masters were revived and studied as a basis from which to develop new ideas. Once again, people became interested in the improvement of physical health and appearance. By the second half of the fifteenth century, the printing press had been invented, which led to the publication of many scholarly writings in the arts and sciences. The advancement in the distribution of printed materials also helped stimulate interest in better health practices.

The Growth and Acceptance of Massage as a Healing Aid

By the sixteenth century, medical practitioners began to reinvent and employ massage as part of their healing treatments. Ambroise Pare (1517-1590), a French barber-surgeon, one of the founders of modern surgery and inventor of the ligation of arteries, described in one of his publications the positive effects of massage in the healing process. He classified massage movements as gentle, medium, and vigorous frictions and employed flexion, extension, and circumduction of joints. His concepts were passed down to other French physicians who believed in the value of physical therapeutics. During his lifetime, Pare served as personal physician to four of France's kings. He is credited with restoring the health of Mary, Queen of Scots (1542-1587) by use of massage. Mercurialis (1530-1606), a professor of medicine at the University of Padua, Italy, published a book, *De Arte Gymnastica*, in 1569 on gymnastics and the benefits of massage when integrated into treatments for the body and mind.

The sixteenth, seventeenth and eighteenth centuries witnessed an expansion in all fields of knowledge. Emergent literature from English, French, German, and Italian authors re-established massage as a preferred scientific practice for the maintenance of health and the treatment of disease.

Frictions, manipulations, anointing, bathing, and exercise were regarded as important tools in the medical armament. These subjects were taught in institutions of higher learning to physicians and other practitioners of the healing practices and were based in the sciences of anatomy, physiology, and pathology as they were known in that day and age.

Throughout history a kind of massage or hands-on healing has been practiced by laypeople or commoners. It was often practiced by folk healers and midwives and was passed on as an art and a gift. A body of knowledge was never established, so techniques were lost and rediscovered through the ages (Fig. 1.4).

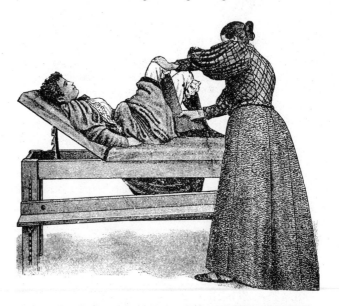

Fig. 1.4 This illustration from a French manual (1898) shows how massage and flexion of the foot and leg are being used to treat a pulled muscle. Courtesy New York Public Library picture collection.

THE DEVELOPMENT OF MODERN MASSAGE TECHNIQUES ▼

In the early part of the nineteenth century, John Grosvenor (1742-1823), a well-respected English surgeon and a practitioner of **chirurgy** (healing with the hands), stressed to his colleagues the value of friction in the relief of stiff joints, gout, and rheumatism. His efforts helped further the belief in massage as an aid to healing.

Per Henrik Ling (1776-1839) of Smaaland, Sweden, a physiologist and fencing master, is known as the father of physical therapy. He systemized and developed movements he found to be beneficial in improving his own physical condition. He called the system of movements **Medical Gymnastics.** He based this system on the developing science of physiology. The Ling System's primary focus was on gymnastics applied to the treatment of disease and consisted of movements classified as active, duplicated, and passive. **Active movements** were performed by the patient and could be referred to as exercise. **Duplicated movements** were performed by the patient in cooperation with the therapist. These correspond to modern-day resistive or assistive exercises. **Passive movements** were performed by the therapist to the patient and would be considered range of motion and massage. In 1813 Ling, established the Royal Swedish Central Institute of Gymnastics, which was chartered and financed by the Swedish government. Ling died in 1839, but his students published his works posthumously. The Ling System, more commonly called Swedish Movements or the Movement Cure, spread throughout Europe and Russia. By 1851 there were thirty-eight institutions for education in the Swedish Movements in Europe, most of them located in Germany. These schools were generally open to learned men. The programs were as long as three years, with classes lasting six to eight hours a day.

Mathias Roth, an English physician, studied under Ling at the Royal Central Institute and in 1851 published the first book in English on the Swedish Movements. He established the first institute in England to teach Swedish Movement Gymnastics and gave private instruction to Charles Fayette Taylor, a New York physician, who in 1858 introduced the methods to the United States. In the United States, the technique became known as **The Swedish Movement Cure.** Charles's brother, George Henry, in the meantime attended the Dr. Sotherberg Institute in Stockholm and completed full training in the Swedish Movements. They both returned to the United States and started an orthopedic practice in New York, where they specialized in the Swedish Movements. Within a year they dissolved their joint practice, but both continued to practice and write about the Swedish Movement Cure. George Henry published the first American textbook on the Swedish Movement Cure in 1860 and established The Improved Movement Cure Institute in New York City. Charles Fayette wrote many articles and published a textbook introducing the Swedish

Movements in 1861. Both brothers practiced and taught the cure until their deaths in 1899. Thus it was the competitive Taylor brothers who introduced the Swedish Movement Cure to the United States and brought massage more into public and medical acceptance.

Modern Massage Terminology

Modern massage terminology is credited to Dr. Johann Mezger (1839-1909) of Holland, who established the practice and art of massage as a scientific subject for physicians in the remedial treatment of disease. He was acknowledged by many of the authors of his day as the founder of scientific massage. Through Dr. Mezger's efforts, massage became recognized as fundamental to rehabilitation in physical therapy. Mezger's preference for the French terminology has remained an influence to this day (thus the use of the terms *effleurage, petrissage, tapotement,* and even *massage*). The word *massage* was not seen or used in the United States until 1874, when Douglas Graham from Boston and Benjamin Lee and Charles Mills from Philadelphia published articles using Mezger's terminology. Dr. Douglas O. Graham, considered by some to be the father of Swedish massage in the United States, was a practitioner and a historian of massage who wrote extensively about the subject for fifty years from 1874 to 1925. He was a founding member of the American Physical Education Association.

By the early part of the nineteenth century, physicians in medical schools in Germany and Scandinavia were including massage in their teachings as a dignified and beneficial asset in the medical field. In 1900, the distinguished German physician Albert J. Hoffa published *Technik Der Massage.* The publication remains one of the most basic books in the field and contains many of the techniques used in Swedish massage.

Throughout Germany, Denmark, Norway, and Sweden, therapeutic exercises, massage, and baths were recommended by physicians for the restoration and maintenance of health. These physicians believed that massage helped the body rid itself of toxins, relieved such ailments as rheumatism, and promoted the healthy functioning of all body systems.

In England in 1894, a group of women formed The Society of Trained Masseuses. By 1920 this society had grown in members and prestige. Later the society became known as the Chartered Society of Massage and Medical Gymnastics; it was registered in 1964 as the Chartered Society of Physiotherapy.

THE DECLINE OF MASSAGE IN THE TWENTIETH CENTURY

The beginning of the twentieth century brought with it a decline in the scientific and medical use of massage. There were several reasons for this decline. The increasing popularity of massage in the nineteenth century precipitated an increase in not only qualified practitioners and schools but also lay practitioners and unscrupulous schools and practitioners.

A special inquiry by the British Medical Association in 1894 revealed numerous abuses in the education and practice of massage practitioners, which dealt a severe blow to the reputation of the profession. The inquiry found many schools using unscrupulous recruitment practices and offering inadequate training. As a result, graduates were unqualified or incompetent and in debt to the school. To repay that debt, students and graduates would work in clinics that would offer poor massage and often became no more than houses of prostitution. Other abuses included false certification and deceptive advertising, in which exorbitant claims were made that were totally unfounded and untrue. The reputation of massage was scandalized among physicians and the general public alike.

Technical innovations also had a detrimental affect on massage. The invention of electricity and various electrical apparatuses, such as the vibrator, greatly affected the use of hands-on therapy in favor of these new electrical modalities. This trend continues to this day.

Technical and intellectual advances in medicine developed new treatment strategies based more on pharmacology and surgical procedures. The old ideas of treating disease through diet, exercise, and bathing gave way to the more sophisticated practices of modern medicine. Physicians no longer learned massage as a part of their training, nor did they employ trained therapists. Massage's place in nursing eroded to no more than the administering of a back rub.

CONTEMPORARY DEVELOPMENTS IN MASSAGE ▼

A number of important developments during the second quarter of the twentieth century continue to influence modern massage.

An Austrian named Emil Vodder developed a method of gentle rhythmical massage along the surface lymphatics that accelerates the functioning of the lymphatic system and effectively treats chronic lymphedema (limf-e-**DEE**-muh) and other diseases of venous or lymph circulation. Today this system is widely known and taught as **Dr. Vodder's Manual Lymph Drainage.**

In the 1940s, a German, Elizabeth Dicke, developed **Bindegewebsmassage,** or **Connective Tissue Massage,** which was later popularized in England by Maria Ebner. Bindegewebsmassage is directed toward the subcutaneous connective tissue and is believed to affect vascular and visceral reflexes related to a variety of pathologies and disabilities. This method continues to be widely employed in many countries for pathologic conditions of circulation or visceral disease.

Dr. James H. Cyriax, an English orthopedic physician, is credited with popularizing **Deep Transverse Friction Massage.** This method broadens the fibrous tissues of muscles, tendons, or ligaments, breaking down unwanted fibrous adhesions and thereby restoring mobility to muscles in a way that cannot be achieved by passive stretching or active exercise. Transverse Friction Massage retains its popularity today in physical therapy and massage therapy regimes as an effective treatment in restoration and rehabilitation of muscle injuries.

Two American physical therapists who have had a major impact on massage therapy in the United States are Gertrude Beard and Frances Tappan. Both have devoted much of their lives to promoting massage as an important part of the healthcare system. Tappan's book, *Healing Massage Techniques* and *Beard's Massage*, remain as standards in the massage industry.

Massage did play an important role immediately following World War I (1914-1918), when it proved beneficial as a restorative treatment in the rehabilitation of injuries. Again in World War II (1939-1945), massage was employed on an even larger scale in the hospitals of the Armed Forces. However, in the years following World War II manual massage played a secondary role in physical therapy as more mechanical and electrical means of stimulation and rehabilitation gained popularity. During the post-war recovery, massage was directed more toward relaxation and athletics and less toward rehabilitation. Most practitioners were employed in athletic clubs or YMCAs or as trainers for athletic teams (Fig. 1.5).

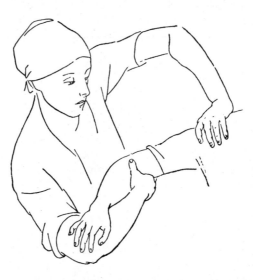

Fig. 1.5 This illustration is from Methuen's book, *What Every Masseuse Should Know,* 1917. Reprinted courtesy of the New York Public Library picture collection.

A Massage Renaissance in the United States

Beginning around 1960, another massage renaissance began to take place in the United States and continues to this day. With the decline of the use of massage in traditional medicine, a surge of interest in the use and value of massage developed in the paraprofessional and lay public. Several factors precipitated this trend. Increased awareness of physical and mental fitness as well as the increasing cost of traditional medicine opened the way for viable alternatives in healthcare. The development of the wellness model, which placed more emphasis on prevention and recognized the importance of controlling stress, advocated the value of massage. The psychological benefits of touch and its proven use in the treatment of pain returned massage to a place of prominence in the healthcare system.

During this time, chiropractic began to receive more recognition. Chiropractic developed in the West when Dr. David Palmer began teaching techniques of directed manual pressure against the bony processes to manipulate the vertebrae of the spine and other articulations of the body. Today, chiropractors use many subtle massage-type techniques and often employ massage practitioners as assistants.

During the 1970s and 1980s, a significant rise in the popularity of massage as well as a number of other forms of bodywork occurred in the United States. Several professional associations and numerous schools emerged to teach and promote a variety of massage disciplines. Massage education was no longer part of university or medical curriculum. Massage training was done largely through private schools or apprenticeships. In the late 1980s, an effort to return massage and bodywork to the mainstream of health and wellness care prompted members from the various disciplines and associations to meet and share their ideas. In 1991, a Federation of Bodywork Organizations was formed to assure equitable recognition of all forms of bodywork in the development of standards and legislation. Recognition for massage therapists in the United States became a reality in 1992, when the first National Certification for Therapeutic Massage and Bodywork exams were administered. With a growing number of states requiring professional licensing and schools and associations developing more sophisticated standards, massage continues to emerge as a recognized and respected allied healthcare profession.

MASSAGE SYSTEMS

The methods of massage generally in use today descend directly from the Swedish, German, French, English, Chinese, and Japanese systems.

1. The Swedish system is based on the Western concepts of anatomy and physiology and employs the traditional manipulative techniques of effleurage, petrissage, vibration, friction, and tapotement. The Swedish system also employs movements that can be slow and gentle, vigorous or bracing, according to the results the practitioner wishes to achieve.
2. The German method combines many of the Swedish movements and emphasizes the use of various kinds of therapeutic baths.

3. The French and English systems also employ many of the Swedish massage movements for body massage. Many excellent facial massage and beauty therapy treatments originated in France and England.

4. Acupressure stems from the Chinese medical practice of acupuncture. It is based on the Traditional Oriental Medical principles for assessing and treating the physical and energetic body and employs various methods of stimulating acupuncture points in order to regulate *chi* (the life force energy). The aim of this method is to achieve therapeutic changes in the person being treated as well as relieve pain, discomfort, or other physiological imbalance.

5. The Japanese system, called **shiatsu,** a finger pressure method, is based on the Oriental concept that the body has a series of energy (*tsubo*) points. When pressure is properly applied to these points, circulation is improved and nerves are stimulated. This system is said to improve body metabolism and to relieve a number of physical disorders.

The following are additional systems that have gained recognition as beneficial forms of massage.

Sports massage refers to a method of massage especially designed to prepare an athlete for an upcoming event and to aid in the body's regenerative and restorative capacities following a rigorous workout or competition. This is achieved through specialized manipulations that stimulate circulation of the blood and lymph. Some sports massage movements are designed to break down lesions and adhesions or reduce fatigue. Sports massage generally follows the Swedish system, with variations of movements applied according to the judgment of the practitioner and the results he or she wants to achieve. Sports teams, especially those in professional baseball, football, basketball, hockey, ice skating, and swimming, often retain a professionally trained massage practitioner. Athletes, dancers, and others who must keep muscles strong and supple are often instructed in automassage (how to massage one's own muscles) and in basic massage on a partner.

Polarity therapy is a method developed by Randolph Stone (1890-1971) using massage manipulations derived from both Eastern and Western practices. Exercises and thinking practices are included to balance the body both physically and energetically.

The Trager method was developed by Dr. Milton Trager. This method uses movement exercises called **mentastics** along with massage-like, gentle shaking of different parts of the body to eliminate and prevent pent-up tensions.

Rolfing is a systematic program developed out of the technique of structural integration by Dr. Ida Rolf. Rolfing aligns the major body segments through manipulation of the fascia (**FAH**-shuh) or the connective tissue.

The method of **reflexology** originated with the Chinese and is based on the idea that stimulation of particular points on the surface of the body has an effect on other areas or organs of the body. Dr. William Fitzgerald is credited with first demonstrating the effects of reflexology in the early 1900s Eunice Ingham worked for Dr. Fitzgerald and later, in the 1930s, she systemized the technique (popular today) that focuses mainly on the hands and feet.

Touch for Health is a simplified form of applied kinesiology (ki-nee-see-**AHL**-o-jee) (principles of anatomy in relation to human movement) developed by Dr. John Thie, D.C. This method involves techniques from both Eastern and Western origins. Its purpose is to relieve stress on muscles and internal organs. There are also a number of styles of bodywork and alternative health-related practices that utilize specialized kinesiology (a form of muscle testing) to derive information about the conditions of the body or how a particular substance or type of treatment might affect it.

The foregoing is a brief list and does not include the great number and forms of massage and bodywork being practiced today. Although there are many excellent massage methods, the Swedish system is still the most widely used and is incorporated into many other procedures. Whatever method the practitioner prefers, it is essential to have a thorough knowledge of all technical movements and their effects on the various body systems. It is important for practitioners to be thoroughly trained in anatomy, physiology, pathology, medical communication, and technique in schools that are licensed or have credentials meeting the professional standards required by state boards and ethical associations. The objectives of all professional practitioners are generally the same: to provide a service that enhances the client's physical health and sense of well-being.

(For a more concise history of massage, the author recommends *The Bodywork Knowledgebase, Lectures on History of Massage* by Richard P. van Why, from which a good portion of this chapter was derived.)

QUESTIONS FOR DISCUSSION AND REVIEW

1. Define the meaning of *massage*.
2. How do we know that ancient civilizations used therapeutic massage and exercise in their social, personal, or religious practices?
3. Why is massage said to be the most natural and instinctive means of relieving pain and discomfort?
4. What did the Chinese call their early massage system?
5. Why did the Greeks and Romans place so much emphasis on exercise and massage?
6. Which Greek physician became known as the father of medicine?
7. Why were the Middle Ages also called the Dark Ages?

8. How did the Arabic Empire and the rise of Islam help preserve the practice of massage?
9. Why was the Renaissance an important turning point for the arts and sciences?
10. How did the invention of the printing press in the fifteenth century help further the practice of massage and therapeutic exercise?
11. What is the basis of Per Henrik Ling's Swedish Movement Cure?
12. Who introduced the Swedish Movement Cure to the United States?
13. What are some of the reasons for the decline of massage at the turn of the twentieth century?
14. Why did the acceptance of massage and therapeutic exercise increase during world wars I and II?
15. Why did manual massage become a secondary treatment following World War II?
16. How has more awareness of health and personal wellness in recent years caused a renewed interest in massage?
17. What is the difference between passive and active exercise?
18. Describe the theory on which the Japanese *shiatsu* system of massage is based.
19. What part does proper exercise and use of massage play in athletics?
20. Of what benefit is the history of therapeutic massage to the student who wishes to pursue a career in the field?
21. Which massage system is the most widely used in general massage?
22. In what way are the Chinese and Japanese systems similar?
23. Why is massage used as a treatment in sports or athletic medicine?

Requirements for the Practice of Therapeutic Massage

Learning Objectives

After you have mastered this chapter, you will be able to:

1. Explain the educational and legal aspects of scope of practice.
2. Explain how state legislation defines the scope of practice of therapeutic massage.
3. Explain why the massage practitioner must be aware of the laws, rules, regulations, restrictions, and obligations governing the practice of therapeutic massage.
4. Explain why it is necessary to obtain a license to practice therapeutic body massage.
5. Explain the difference between certifications and licenses.
6. Give reasons why a license to practice massage might be revoked, canceled, or suspended.

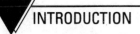

INTRODUCTION

Therapeutic massage is a personal health service employing various soft tissue manipulations for the improvement of the client's health and well-being; therefore, the massage practitioner has an ethical responsibility to the public and to individual clients. In addition to being technically well trained, the practitioner must understand the laws, rules, regulations, limitations, and obligations concerning the practice of massage.

SCOPE OF PRACTICE

In the world of healthcare, practitioners are able to perform certain duties as prescribed by their occupation, their license, and their level of training. For instance, in a healthcare facility, a nurse's aid can attend to a patient's comfort and care, but cannot distribute medications. A licensed practical nurse can distribute specified medications except for narcotics, injections, and IVs. A registered nurse must oversee these distributions and handle the dangerous drugs and injections. The orders for any of these must come from a physician. According to law, only doctors can diagnose illness and other medical conditions and prescribe the medications and course of treatment for those conditions. Each of these practitioners is operating within his or her scope of practice.

Scope of practice defines the rights and activities legally acceptable according to the licenses of a particular occupation or profession. The scope of practice of any licensed occupation is described in the legal description and definitions contained in the licensing regulation. The scope is determined in part by the educational focus of the professional training. Many occupations and professions have national or state regulatory boards that help define and enforce adherence to a scope of practice. National or state boards develop and upgrade professional standards and oversee testing and licensing procedures.

At the time of publication of this text, only nineteen of the fifty-two states have adopted licensing regulations governing the practice of massage. The definition of massage and the educational requirements contained in those regulations define the scope of practice of massage in those states. Whereas there is some basic agreement between those states regarding the need to license massage, there is a vast diversity in defining the purpose, object, procedure, or educational requirements. With only about one third of the states requiring licenses for massage and the lack of a national standard, there is not a clearly defined scope of practice for massage therapy. Regardless of this fact, it is important for massage practitioners to recognize and practice within their legal and professional boundaries and refer clients to appropriately trained and licensed professionals when indicated.

LICENSES: THEY ARE THE LAW

In the United States, laws and regulations for massage may fall under the auspices of the state, the county, the municipality, or may not exist at all. Where massage laws are in effect, massage practitioners must register with the proper authorities and satisfy certain requirements to obtain a license to practice. These requirements may vary depending on the licensing agency and the original motives for instituting the legislation. Many municipalities adopt ordinances to curb unethical practices, misleading advertising, and the use of the term *massage* to conceal questionable or illegal activities, especially prostitution and illicit drug sales and distribution. This type of licensing often requires mug shots, fingerprinting, and criminal record searches and has little regard for massage proficiency. As massage becomes more recognized as a reputable and respected healthcare practice, most of these ordinances are being replaced with licensing laws that contain educational, technical, ethical, and sanitation requirements.

Laws and regulations vary greatly from state to state and city to city. Being licensed in one state does not guarantee that the same license will be valid or recognized in another state. If your license is from a city, you can be guaranteed that the only place that licence is valid is in the city where the license was issued. A practitioner who has a license and wishes to practice in another city or state should contact the proper agency in the area where he or she wishes to practice. Usually the county commissioner's office, the city attorney, or the mayor's office will be able to provide information concerning the regulation of massage. If there is reciprocity between the two licensing agencies, the valid license will be honored; if not, the practitioner should provide proof of ability to meet any requirements and make applications as required.

In the United States a growing number of states are adopting legislation that requires all massage practitioners to obtain and maintain a license. These state laws usually take precedence over city and county laws and are professional licenses wherein the applicant must satisfy an educational requirement as well as pass a written and practical examination before being issued a license to practice massage.

Licensed physical therapists, physicians, registered nurses, osteopaths, chiropractors, athletic trainers, and podiatrists may practice massage as part of their therapeutic treatments. However, these professionals usually obtain a license specifically for the practice of massage when they wish to be known as massage practitioners.

Massage establishments must abide by local laws, rules, and regulations. Where it is required, they must be licensed and employ only licensed practitioners . In addition to massage ordinances and licenses, local business and zoning laws must be followed when setting up a massage business. Most states require massage practitioners to display their licenses at their place of business.

▼ EDUCATIONAL REQUIREMENTS

Educational requirements to enroll in a program of instruction at a certificate-granting school or institute of massage may differ, but generally a high school diploma or equivalency diploma is required. In some states that have massage licensing, a student actively enrolled in a qualified school of massage may work as an apprentice under the supervision of a licensed massage practitioner.

The educational requirements to practice massage or bodywork vary depending on the discipline or techniques and the licensing requirements of the city or state where the practice is located. There are many disciplines or styles of hands-on therapies being practiced. Few of these have clearly defined educational requirements. Professional organizations affiliated with these various disciplines often set educational guidelines that include the length and content of training programs and recognize schools that comply with those guidelines. The American Massage Therapy Association Commision on Massage Training Approval/Accreditation (COMTAA) for example, requires that schools have programs with a minimum of 500 classroom hours of training before they will be considered for approval. Many competent practitioners have received their training through an apprenticeship or by attending workshops and have had no formal schooling.

If a license is required to practice massage, an educational requirement is usually included in the licensing legislation. Without a national standard for massage therapy, educational requirements contained in licensing laws vary widely. City or municipal licenses may contain no educational requirement or may require as much as 1000 hours of training. Of the states that license massage at the time of publication of this text, the educational requirements vary from 250 to 1250 hours of training.

With the development of the National Certification for Therapeutic Massage and Bodywork, the recommended standard educational requirement has been established as the equivalent of 500 hours of training including the subjects of anatomy, physiology, pathology, business practices, massage technique, and ethics.

▼ HEALTH REQUIREMENTS FOR PRACTITIONERS

Since massage is a touch or hands-on profession, the massage practitioner is expected to be physically and mentally fit and be free of any communicable diseases. Some state licensing requirements or employers may request a health certificate or written confirmation from a physician. It is the practitioner's duty to keep himself or herself in top physical condition. Massage is hard work and requires that the practitioner have physical stamina and the ability to concentrate on giving a therapeutic massage.

REASONS LICENSE MAY BE REVOKED, SUSPENDED, OR CANCELED ▼

Because the practice of massage deals with the health and welfare of the public and specifically that of individual clients, the profession must be regulated by the issuance of licenses only to people who have met the requirements to practice. The professional massage practitioner must have integrity, the necessary technical skills, and a willingness to comply with rigid health standards.

The following are grounds on which the practitioner's license may be revoked, canceled, or suspended:

1. Being guilty of fraud or deceit in obtaining a license
2. Having been convicted of a felony
3. Being engaged currently or previously in any act of prostitution
4. Practicing under a false or assumed name
5. Being addicted to narcotics, alcohol, or like substances that interfere with the performance of duties
6. Being willfully negligent in the practice of massage so as to endanger the health of a client
7. Prescribing drugs or medicines (unless you are a licensed physician)
8. Being guilty of fraudulent or deceptive advertising

CERTIFICATION VERSUS LICENSE ▼

A license is issued from a state or municipal regulating agency as a requirement for conducting a business or practicing a trade or profession. A certification, on the other hand, is a document that is awarded in recognition of an accomplishment or achieving or maintaining some kind of standard. A certification may be given for successfully completing a course of study or passing an examination showing a level of proficiency or ability. Certificates are awarded by schools and institutions to show the successful completion of a course of study. Professional organizations have certificates of membership to indicate that the recipient has met the qualifications to become a member. Often those organizations have testing programs that provide recognition of achievements in their chosen professions. Many professions (the massage profession included) have a national certification program whereby proficiency toward a national standard can be achieved and certified. These certifications do lend an air of credibility to a practitioner but do not take the place of a license where a license is required to practice.

▼ QUESTIONS FOR DISCUSSION AND REVIEW

1. Why must the massage practitioner be concerned about the laws, rules, regulations, and obligations pertaining to the practice of therapeutic body massage?
2. What are the legal and educational aspects of scope of practice?
3. Why do laws governing the practice of massage often differ from one state to another?
4. Does having a license in one locale permit a practitioner to practice anywhere? Why?
5. What is the general educational requirement for a license to practice massage?
6. What are the reasons a person would receive a certificate?
7. What are the specific grounds which a practitioner's license may be revoked, canceled, or suspended?

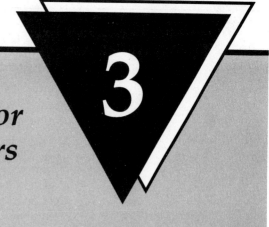

Professional Ethics for Massage Practitioners

Learning Objectives

After you have mastered this chapter, you will be able to:

1. Define the meaning of professional ethics.
2. Explain how the practice of good ethics helps build a successful massage practice.
3. Discuss the importance of good health habits and professional projection.
4. Discuss the importance of human relations and success attitudes.
5. Discuss ways to build a sound business reputation.

▼ INTRODUCTION

Ethics is the study of the standards and philosophy of human conduct and is defined as a system or code of morals of an individual, a group, or a profession. To practice good ethics is to be concerned about the public welfare, the welfare of individual clients, your reputation, and the reputation of the profession you represent. A professional person is one who is engaged in an avocation or occupation requiring some advanced training to gain knowledge and skills. However, without ethics there can be no true professionalism.

Ethical conduct on the part of the practitioner gives the client confidence in the place of business, the services rendered, and the entire industry. A satisfied client is your best means of advertising because his or her good recommendation helps you maintain public confidence and build a sound business following. The business establishment that becomes known for its professional ethics will stay in business longer than one that makes extravagant claims and false promises or that is involved in questionable practices.

▼ PROFESSIONAL ETHICS FOR THE MASSAGE PRACTITIONER

Ethics are standards of acceptable and professional behavior by which a person or business conducts business. The following are business ethics to which you as a massage professional should adhere:

1. Treat all clients with the same fairness and courtesy.
2. Provide the highest quality care for those who seek your professional services.
3. Keep all communications with clients honest and confidential.
4. Set an example of professionalism by your conduct at all times.
5. In no way allow or encourage any kind of sexual activity in your practice. Be respectful of the therapeutic relationship, and maintain appropriate boundaries.
6. Live up to your promises and your obligations.
7. Give efficient service backed by knowledge and skills.
8. Perform only those services for which you are qualified, and refer to appropriate medical personnel when indicated.
9. Respect and cooperate with other ethical healthcare providers to promote health and wellness.
10. Know and obey all laws, rules, and regulations of your city, county, and state pertaining to your work.
11. Strive to improve the credibility of massage as a valuable health service by educating the public and medical community as to its benefits.
12. Be fair and honest in all advertising of services.
13. Communicate in a professional manner on the telephone, in personal conversations, and in letters.

14. Refrain from the use of improper language and any form of gossip.
15. Eliminate prejudice in the profession and do not discriminate against colleagues or clients.
16. Be well organized so that you make the most of your time.
17. Maintain your physical, mental, and emotional well-being so that you are looked on as a credit to your profession.
18. Continue to learn about new developments in your profession by participating in local and national professional associations and pursuing continuing education and training.
19. Keep foremost in your mind that you are a professional person engaged in giving an important and beneficial personal service.
20. Do your utmost to keep your place of business clean, neat, and attractive. Remember that people judge you by first impressions.

PERSONAL HYGIENE AND HEALTH HABITS

To inspire confidence and trust in your clients, you should project a well-groomed, professional appearance at all times. In a personal service business, personal health and good grooming are assets that clients admire and are essential for your protection and that of the client.

Your personal health and grooming habits should include the following:

1. Bathe or shower daily and use a deodorant as necessary.
2. Keep your teeth and gums healthy. Visit your dentist regularly.
3. Use mouthwash and avoid foods that contribute to offensive breath odor.
4. Keep your hair fresh and clean, and wear an appropriate hairstyle. Hair should be worn in a style that you do not have to touch or fuss with during a massage session. In addition, your hair must not touch the client during the session.
5. Avoid strong fragrances such as perfumes, colognes, and lotions.
6. Keep your hands free of blemishes and calluses. Use lotion to keep your hands soft and smooth.
7. Keep your nails clean and filed so they do not extend to the tips of the fingers. Sharp nails should never come in contact with the client's skin. Never wear garish nail polish.
8. If you are a woman, wear appropriate makeup in subdued, flattering colors. Be sure makeup is applied neatly.
9. If you are a man, keep beard or mustache neat and well groomed. If you prefer the clean-shaven look, be sure to shave as often as necessary.
10. Avoid gum chewing or smoking in the presence of clients.

11. Keep your face clean and free of blemishes.
12. Practice all rules of sanitation for the client's and for your own protection.
13. Have a complete physical examination by a physician before beginning work as a massage practitioner. Continue to have checkups, follow your physician's advice, and do all that is possible to maintain optimum health.
14. If you perspire heavily, take precautions so that your perspiration does not drop on your client.
15. Take time for relaxation and physical fitness. Get massages regularly. A regimen of daily exercise is recommended. This may be accomplished by participation in active sports of your choice (swimming, tennis, etc.), working out at the gym, or by devising a set of beneficial exercises you can do at home.
16. Eat a well-balanced, nutritious diet. Maintain your normal weight for your height and bone structure. You should not be extremely overweight or extremely underweight. If you have a weight problem, follow your physician's advice on how to attain your most healthful weight.
17. Be aware of good posture when walking, standing, sitting, and working. Poor posture habits such as slouching contribute to fatigue, foot problems, and strain to your back and neck.
18. Wear the appropriate clothing for your profession. Clothing should be loose enough to allow for optimal movement. It should be free of accessories that might catch on the massage table or touch the client when you are performing the massage (such as a long chain, necklace or tie, a wide belt, or long sleeves). Consider clothing that allows your body heat to escape. Clothing items made of natural fibers such as cotton are good. Clothing made of synthetic fabrics holds the heat of your body and will be uncomfortable for the physical exertion of this profession.

▼ HUMAN RELATIONSHIPS

In addition to gaining the necessary technical skills as a professional massage practitioner, you must be able to understand your client's needs. This is the basis of all good human relations. A pleasant voice, good manners, cheerfulness, patience, tact, loyalty, empathy, and interest in the client's welfare are some of the desirable traits that help build the client's confidence in you and your place of business.

It is important to be able to interact with people without becoming too familiar. Often clients will confide their personal feelings, and they trust you not to betray their confidence. This is where the art of listening is an invaluable asset. Listen with empathy, change the subject when necessary (tactfully), and never betray the client's confidence in you.

Respect the therapeutic relationship between client and practitioner and refrain from crossing sexual boundaries. Know the difference between sensuality and sexuality, intimacy and touch. In the United States, most situations involving touch between adults are sexual in nature. Since massage involves touch and nudity, it is not uncommon for sexual feelings to arise in the client or the practitioner. It is essential for the practitioner to be clear regarding ethical boundaries and act appropriately to avoid sexual interactions, which may have disastrous personal or professional consequences.

The following rules for good human relations will help you interact successfully with people from all walks of life:

Tact: Tact is your ability to deal with a client who is overly critical, finds fault, and is hard to please. It may be that he or she just wants attention. Tact helps you deal with this client in an impersonal but understanding manner. To be tactful is to avoid what is offensive or disturbing and to do what is most considerate for all concerned. For example, you might discover that a client needs medical care and you feel you should suggest that he or she see a physician. You must approach the problem with the utmost tact and diplomacy.

Cheerfulness: A cheerful attitude and a pleasant facial expression will go a long way toward putting a client at ease.

Patience: Patience is the ability to be tolerant under stressful or undesirable conditions. Your patience and understanding will be the best medicine when you deal with people who are ill, handicapped, or in pain. Patience helps you change negative feelings to more positive ones.

Honesty: To be honest does not mean that you must be brutally frank with a client. You can answer questions in a factual but tactful manner. For example, if a client has unrealistic expectations regarding the benefits of a treatment, you can discuss what can or cannot be accomplished in a sincere, conscientious manner.

Intuition: Intuition is your ability to have insight into people's feelings. When you genuinely like people, it is easier to show sympathy and understanding for their problems. People will often confide in you when their intuition tells them you are trustworthy. In turn, your own intuition will help you avoid embarrassing situations and involving yourself in problems you cannot solve. Remember, the primary reason your clients come to you is for relaxation. Keep conversations to a minimum to allow the client maximum relaxation.

Sense of humor: It is important to have a sense of humor, especially when dealing with difficult people or situations. A good sense of humor helps you remain optimistic, courteous, and in control.

Maturity: Maturity is not so much a matter of how old you are, but what you have gained from your life experience. Maturity is the quality of being reliable, responsible, self-disciplined, and well adjusted.

Self-esteem: Self-esteem is projected by your attitudes about yourself and your profession. If you respect yourself and your profession, you will be respected by others.

Self-motivation: Self-motivation is your ability to set positive goals and put forth the energy and effort required to achieve those goals. It means making sacrifices when necessary to save time and money and to achieve your goals.

▼ BUILDING A PROFESSIONAL IMAGE

If you want to be successful in business, you must prepare for success. Preparation, planning, and performance are the assets that help you do your job in the most professional manner. You should take every opportunity to pursue new avenues of knowledge. Attend professional seminars, read trade journals and other publications relating to your business, and become active in associations where you can exchange ideas with other dedicated people.

Your business image is important and should be built on good service and truth in advertising. A reliable reputation is particularly important in the personal service business because you are dealing with the health and well-being of individuals. Consistently high standards and good service are the foundations on which successful businesses are built.

▼ YOUR BUSINESS NAME

Using appropriate wording in your business name in advertising will help you establish a good reputation. You can see how the name "Smitty's Massage Parlour" or "Smith Massage Clinic" can totally change how your business is perceived by potential clients.

Some massage professionals, especially those entering a new community, may feel they need to state in their advertising that only therapeutic and proper massage is given. Keeping regular business hours, rather than late-night hours, also improves your reputation.

Another point to remember is that using proper draping techniques to ensure your client's privacy is very important in building a good reputation. Word of mouth is the massage professional's best advertising. Satisfied clients will spread the message that you work in a professional manner.

▼ QUESTIONS FOR DISCUSSION AND REVIEW

1. Why is it important to have a code of ethics for your business?
2. Why is a satisfied client your best means of advertising?
3. Why do successful business managers prefer employees who are concerned with personal and professional ethics?

4. Why is it necessary for the massage practitioner to have strict personal hygiene and health habits?
5. What is meant by professional projection in attitude and appearance?
6. How do you define human relations as applied to working with or serving others?
7. Why is the practice of human relations so important to the massage practitioner?
8. When building your business (practice) image, how can you be sure the public gets the right message?

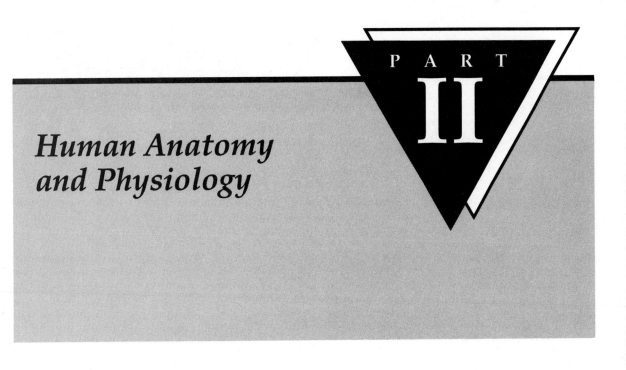

Human Anatomy and Physiology

PART

II

Overview

4

Learning Objectives

After you have mastered this chapter, you will be able to:

1. Explain the meanings of the important terms indicated in bold ace listed in this chapter.
2. Explain why a massage therapist should have a good understanding of anatomy, physiology, and pathology.
3. Explain the physiological and psychological affects of stress and pain and the role of massage therapy in the management of stress and pain.
4. Describe the healing functions of the body in terms of inflammation and tissue repair.
5. Describe the wellness model and how massage may be a part of that model.
6. Be able to derive the meaning of medical terms by breaking the terms into their parts and defining the parts.

INTRODUCTION ▼

An elementary knowledge of histology, anatomy, physiology, and pathology is necessary in mastering the theory and practice of therapeutic massage. The massage practitioner should study the structures and functions of the human body in order to know when, where, and how to apply massage movements for the most beneficial results. This knowledge enables the practitioner to adjust the massage treatment to the needs of the individual and to anticipate results.

DEFINITION OF ANATOMY AND PHYSIOLOGY ▼

Anatomy is the science of morphology or structure of an organism or body. Physiology concerns the normal functions performed by the various systems of the body. Anatomy and physiology are interrelated in that the structures are associated with their functions. Structure and function are dependent on the interaction of the organism's parts, and each part has a role in the operation of the whole.

Anatomy (uh-**NAT**-o-mee) is defined as the study of the gross structure of the body or the study of an organism and the interrelations of its parts. For example, when we describe the skeleton or other anatomic parts of the body, naming the parts and how they relate to one another, we are describing anatomy.

Physiology (fiz-ee-**AH**-lo-jee) is the science and study of the vital processes, mechanisms, and functions of an organ or system of organs. When we describe how the organs or parts of the body function and how their functions relate to one another, we are speaking of physiology.

Histology (his-**TAHL**-o-jee) is a form of microscopic anatomy. It is the branch of biology concerned with the microscopic structure of tissues of a living organism. All living structures are composed of cells and intercellular materials that are organized to form the various tissues, organs, and systems of the body.

Pathology (pa-**THAL**-o-jee) is the study of the structural and functional changes caused by disease.

RELATIONSHIP OF ANATOMY AND PHYSIOLOGY TO MASSAGE AND BODYWORK ▼

Therapeutic massage is applied to and directly affects the structures and the functions of the human organism. Massage has direct affects such as increased local circulation of venous (**VEE**-nuhs) blood and lymph (**LIMF**), stretching of muscle tissue, and loosening of adhesions and scar tissue. Massage has indirect affects of increased circulation to the muscles and internal organs, reduced blood pressure, and general relaxation of tense muscles. Massage has reflex effects such as reduced heart rate and slower, deeper breathing.

An important purpose of massage and bodywork is to promote beneficial and functional improvement in the recipient's body. The more understanding therapists have of the human body and how it functions, the better they will be able to direct their treatment to produce desired affects. A working knowledge of anatomy and physiology gives therapists a basis from which they can plan effective treatments and discuss those applications with other healthcare professionals. As therapists continue to develop therapeutic skills by learning more effective methods of bodywork, a thorough knowledge and understanding of anatomy and physiology becomes essential.

▼ PHYSIOLOGICAL CHANGES DURING DISEASE

Physiologically the body strives to maintain the delicate balance in its internal environment. Changes in the stresses posed by the external environment constantly force the body to compensate to maintain that delicate internal balance called **homeostasis** (ho-mee-o-**STAY**-sis). When the body's homeostasis is disturbed, the person may experience symptoms of disease.

Signs and Symptoms of Disease

Disease is an abnormal and unhealthy state of all or part of the body wherein it is not capable of carrying on its normal function. Diseases generally have symptoms and signs. A **symptom** is caused by the disease and is perceived by the victim, such as dizziness, chills, nausea, or pain. A symptom is a clear message to the individual that something is wrong. **Signs** of a disease are observable indications such as abnormal pulse rate, fever, abnormal skin color, or physical irregularities. When signs and symptoms of disease appear, it is advisable to seek help from proper medical authorities. Symptoms and signs, along with medical examinations, medical histories, and laboratory tests, are the bases for proper diagnosis and treatment of most disease conditions.

There are many possible direct causes for disease, including disease-producing organisms, trauma, environmental agents, malnutrition, degenerative processes, and stress. Other conditions that may be a predisposing factor include age, working or living conditions, sex, and heredity.

Stress

Stress is any psychological or physical situation or condition that causes tension or strain. Stress can be any element or situation that requires our body or mind to compensate in order to maintain the delicate internal balance and harmony. Stress may affect individuals differently. What is extremely stressful to one person may not affect another at all. However, if too many stressful conditions occur without an affective method to manage or cope with them, the health of the individual will suffer. Regardless of the source or nature of the stress, the physiological reaction of the body is essentially the same.

Stress is most notably associated with the adrenal glands and their secretion of the "fight or flight" hormones. The principal and most understood adrenal hormones are **adrenaline** (uh-**DREN**-uh-lin) and **cortisol** (**KAUR**-ti-zol). When we encounter high levels of stress, the adrenal secretions give us a physical and mental boost that heightens our senses, sharpens our reflexes, and prepares our muscles for maximum exertion. The adrenal glands by no means work alone. In conjunction with the pituitary (pi-**TOO**-i-tar-ee) and the hypothalamus (high-po-**THAL**-uh-muhs), they affect the function of most of the internal systems. Muscle tone increases, blood pressure rises, and breathing deepens. Blood is directed toward the skeletal muscles and nervous system and away from the digestive organs. Digestion virtually stops. Glycogen, glucose, and oxygen-carrying red blood cells are mobilized. Blood-coagulating chemicals are added to the blood, and the kidneys retain fluids in case of injury and bleeding. Cortisol promotes the breakdown of the body's proteins to form glucose and acts as an anti-inflammatory and anti-allergenic.

These biochemical effects are essential in emergency, fight or flight situations; however, if the dosage of these hormones is sustained over a long period of time, as it would be with long-term stress, the consequences can be devastating. The ongoing anti-inflammatory effect of cortisol, for example, would inhibit the natural inflammatory response to injury. The body's healing process of flooding the injured area with wound-healing leukocytes, nutrients, fibroblasts, and oxygen would be interfered with and eventually decrease the body's ability to resist infection of all kinds. Continued secretion of adrenaline would eventually exhaust not only the adrenal glands but, because of its effect on the sympathetic nervous system, would have the same effect on the organs as severe loss of sleep—exhaustion! Other effects of sustained levels of these hormones include gastric ulcers, high blood pressure, depressed immune system function, atherosclerosis (ath-eer-o-skler-**O**-sis) and, finally, death.

Stress in and of itself is not the problem. Life is inherently stressful. When effectively worked with, stress tends to strengthen our physical, mental, and emotional resolve. However, when we load ourselves with unrelenting, inescapable, and overburdening stress, it becomes unhealthy and even deadly.

Pain

Pain is one of the body's primary sensations, along with touch, pressure, hot, and cold. Its function is primarily protective in that it warns of tissue damage or destruction somewhere in the body.

Pain is the result of stimulation to specialized nerve ends located near the surface of the body, in the covering of the bones, in the arterial and intestinal walls, and, to a lesser extent, in the deeper organs, muscles, and viscera (**VIS**-er-uh).

There are two responses to pain; psychological and physical. The physical response to pain is very similar to the body's response to stress. Blood pressure and pulse increase, and blood flow is shifted from the intestines and brain to the muscles as mental alertness intensifies, readying the body for a fight or flight. The physical experience of pain also informs about the location, intensity, and duration of the pain.

The individual's psychological and emotional reaction to pain varies depending on many factors, such as previous experience with pain, training in coping with pain, anxiety, tension, and fatigue. The fear and anxiety associated with pain can be more debilitating than the actual pain.

Pain-Spasm-Pain Cycle

A painful syndrome of interest to the massage therapist is the **pain-spasm-pain cycle** associated with muscle spasms. The cycle may start with a rather minor injury such as a bruise or muscle strain that in itself has little affect on the function of the organism. The natural reflex reaction to the tissue damage and pain is a contraction of the muscles that surround the injury, which acts to support and protect the damaged tissue. The contracted muscles constrict the blood vessel and capillaries in the muscles, inhibiting blood flow to the area (a condition known as **ischemia** [is-**KEE**-mee-uh]). At the same time the metabolic activity of the contracting muscles increase, consuming more energy. Oxygen and nutrients are burned, producing increased amounts of metabolic wastes. The available oxygen is quickly burned, and the amounts of lactic acid and other toxins collect in the tissues. Soon **ischemic pain** appears, which is often more intense than the pain from the original injury. The reflex reaction to the ischemic pain is identical to the response to the original injury. It is easy to see how this can become a vicious cycle that can perpetuate itself and continue long after the original injury heals.

The Role of Therapeutic Massage in Stress, Pain, and the Pain-Spasm-Pain Cycle

Therapeutic massage combines the power of sensitive touch with the knowledge of anatomy and physiology to become a valuable tool in relieving the psychological and physical suffering of stress and pain. Skillfully applied massage provides pleasurable stimulation which is carried to the brain on thicker, faster, more numerous nerve fibers that actually override or drown out the pain signals. Even though the diversion is temporary, it gives the individual a chance to relax and disassociate with the noxious stimulus, possi-

bly long enough to shut down the fight or flight reaction. Psychologically, the reassuring touch of the therapist helps relieve anxiety
and fear. The individual in many cases is able to regain some sense
of control over the situation. Physically, as soothing, pleasant
sensations flood the brain, adrenal secretions subside, breathing
slows and deepens, blood pressure lowers, pulse rate slows, and
the body relaxes and begins to recuperate.

In the case of the pain-spasm-pain cycle where pain is intensified
because of ischemia, skillfully applied massage therapy is very
effective in breaking the cycle, relieving the pain, and restoring
mobility. Sen-sitive touch can divert some attention away from the
acute intensity of the pain. By gentle palpation, the actual source of
the pain can be isolated and differentiated from the contracted and
ischemic areas around it. By massaging the contracted ischemic
tissues, chronic spasms can be relieved and circulation restored. As
oxygen and nutrients flood the area and lactic acid and other
irritants are removed, the pain disappears and mobility is restored.

Even though massage is an effective tool in controlling pain, it
must be remembered that pain is an indication of tissue damage or
nerve irritation. Generally the more severe the pain the more severe
the tissue damage. Acute or severe pain is a warning that something
is physically wrong and should be checked by a physician. If
massage is used as an aid for controlling pain, the attending
physician should be advised. If massage increases the overall level
of pain, it should be discontinued. Please note that some massage
techniques can be uncomfortable as they are being applied; however, the discomfort should not be so intense that it hurts the client
or lingers beyond the direct application of the manipulation.

Infection

The most common cause of disease in humans is the invasion of the
body by disease-producing **micro-organisms** such as bacteria,
viruses, fungi, or protozoa. If micro-organisms enter the body in
sufficient numbers to multiply and become harmful and are capable of destroying healthy tissue, the body reacts by developing
an **infection.** If the invading organisms are confined to a small area,
the condition is considered a local infection. If, however, the
organisms spread through the body, the condition is termed a
systemic infection.

Massage should not be applied in cases of systemic infection or
to the site of local infection.

HEALING MECHANISMS OF THE BODY ▼

Inflammation

If invading micro-organisms cause any destruction of tissue, inflammation occurs. Inflammation will also result from physical

injury such as a sprain or blow, excessive heat, cold or radiation, or physical irritants such as splinters, stings, and chemical exposure where tissue is damaged.

When tissue is damaged, substances are released that cause dramatic secondary reactions that are collectively called **inflammation.** Inflammation is a protective tissue response that is characterized by swelling, redness, heat, and pain. Blood vessels in the area of the damaged tissues dilate, increasing blood flow to the area and causing the redness and heat. Capillary walls become more permeable, allowing large quantities of blood plasma and white blood cells to enter the tissue spaces and resulting in the swelling. The swelling puts pressure on local nerve endings, causing pain. Increased numbers of white blood cells, called leukocytes, flood the area to engulf and digest the invading organisms and the damaged tissue debris.

Sometimes toxic bacteria or the reaction between the invading organisms and the white blood cells release a substance into the blood stream that affects the body's heat-regulating system. The resulting elevated body temperature is called a **fever.** Fever is a warning sign that usually accompanies infectious diseases or infected burns and cuts. In cases of sudden onset or high fever (above 102 degrees), a physician should be consulted. In some ways fever, if it is not extremely high, is a natural protective device. Fever increases the metabolic rate and the production of the immune substances that battle the invading organisms. The increased temperature itself destroys certain organisms. At the same time the discomfort and weakness that accompany fever will cause the patient to rest, thereby conserving energy to battle the infection. Extreme or prolonged fever may be dangerous or even fatal. Prolonged fever will cause dehydration, so fluids must be replaced. Fevers above 106 to 108 degrees may cause damage to the tissues of the kidneys, liver, or other organs or may cause irreparable brain damage, possibly resulting in death.

Massage of inflamed tissue or while fever is present is also contraindicated.

Tissue Repair

The degree of tissue repair varies depending on the location and type of tissue and the nature of the damage or injury. Skin and surface tissues undergo a great deal of wear and tear and are easily and quickly repaired. Bone and ligaments repair much more slowly and may require immobilization. Muscle and tendons repair with noticeable scaring and weakness. Neurons of the central nervous system injured by trauma or infection do not repair at all.

Injury or wound healing and repair will only take place when infection-causing bacteria have been destroyed. Escaping fluid from the damaged tissues and capillaries will fill the wound and coagulate, forming a clot to seal the wound. Connective tissue cells called fibroblasts migrate to the area and produce connective tissue fibers that begin to span the wound, providing a structure for regenerating vascular and epithelial tissue. When the wound is healed, this formation of fibrous connective tissue is called scar tissue. If the wound is small, the damage is completely and quickly restored to normal. If, however, the wound is large, measures must be taken to bring the wound surfaces close together in order to prevent the formation of excessive scar tissue.

Properly applied tissue stretching and friction massage will minimize the formation of scar tissue and adhesions resulting from tissue trauma.

THE WELLNESS MODEL

Wellness is a concept in which a person takes personal responsibility for his or her state of health. It is a preventive plan wherein a person makes an effort to recognize conditions, situations, and practices that may be threatening or detrimental to his or her health and takes steps to change or eliminate that process in order to live a more healthful life. Wellness involves taking an active role in being healthy, and adopting practices that enhance health such as a low-fat, high-fiber diet, exercise, a balance between work and play, and a positive mental and spiritual attitude. Wellness also means reducing health risks and eliminating practices that add stressful dangers to our life styles.

Wellness takes into consideration more than our state of physical health. Wellness is often represented as an equilateral triangle with the sides depicting body, mind, and spirit or physical, psychological/mental, and attitude/emotional. When all three aspects are healthy and in balance, optimum wellness is experienced. A wellness-oriented person strives to attain a healthy balance between these three (Fig. 4.1).

Health might be gauged on a scale that ranges from minus five to zero to plus five. Minus five equates with severe illness combined with a poor attitude. Zero is OK, (that is there is no perceivable sickness). Five equates with optimum health and vitality. The great majority of our society hovers between minus –3 and 2. A wellness-oriented individual would strive to maintain his or her health rating above a plus 3 on the scale (Fig. 4.2).

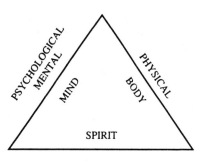

Fig. 4.1

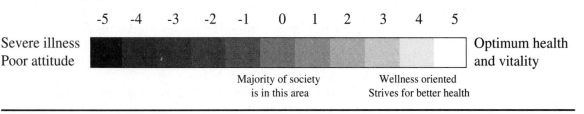

Fig. 4.2

▼ MEDICAL AND ANATOMICAL TERMINOLOGY

Any profession or trade uses a language or vocabulary that is specific or peculiar to the practices, equipment, and processes of that system. Massage and bodywork is no different. Most of the terminology related to massage is derived from the healthcare and medical field.

Anatomical and medical terminology refers to the vocabulary or jargon commonly used by health professionals when communicating to one another concerning conditions of patients, descriptions of procedures, and anatomical structures. It is important for massage therapists to have an understanding of the body's structure and function. Therefore, becoming familiar with the related terminology is essential. By having an understanding of how medical terms are constructed, the massage therapist will be less intimidated by the long words, be better able to communicate with other health professionals, and (by speaking their language), be better respected and accepted by the medical community.

The history of medical terminology goes back nearly 2000 years to the time when Western civilization first began systematically studying the human body. Since the languages of these first researchers were Greek and Latin, these became and remain the basic language for medical terminology.

Composition of Medical Terminology

In medical terminology, big words are compound words constructed of root words (or stems), prefixes, and suffixes. There are many terms that are constructed from relatively few word parts.

The stem, or root word, generally indicates the body part or structure involved. Occasionally two or more stems will be combined to show relation or position (for example, cardiopulmonary). When stems are combined, a single-letter syllable is often used to create what is called a combining form. This is a word root plus a vowel that is used with another word root to form a compound word. A combining form is usually an (o) or an (i).

A prefix is one or more syllables added in front of the stem to further its meaning. A suffix likewise is added to the end of the word. Suffixes often denote a diagnosis, symptom, or surgical procedure or identify a word as a noun or adjective.

Anatomical terms often include more than one word. Generally the first word acts as an adjective and will indicate the region or location of the structure. The second word is the noun and names the structure (for example, femoral artery, thoracic duct).

By breaking the terms into their parts, the logical meaning can be derived.

Following is a list of prefixes, suffixes, and stem words along with their meanings. As you study the following chapters, be aware of anatomical and medical terms and decipher their meaning by examining the parts. During discussions with peers and other healthcare practitioners, use proper terminology and make note of unfamiliar terms. Examine them and determine their meaning by breaking them apart and defining their parts. Practice and become familiar with the language. When in doubt, always keep a medical dictionary available. When a term is used that you do not understand, check your dictionary.

Alphabetical Listing of Common Word Elements Used to Construct Medical Terms

Prefixes

Word Part	Definition	Example
a-	absent, without, away from	abacterial
ab-	away from	abduction
ad-	to, toward	adduction
ambi-	both	ambidextrous
a-; an-	without	atypical
ant-	against	antibody, antidote
ante-	before	anterior
bi-	two	biceps
bio-	life	biology
carcin-	cancer	carcinogenic
circum-	around	circumvent
co-	with, together	cooperate
contra-	against, counter to	contraindicate
de-	down, from	descend
di-	two	dissect
dis-	apart, away from	dislocate
dors-	back	dorsal
dys-	abnormal, impaired	dysfunction
e-	out, from	emetic
ect-	outside, without	ectoplasm
end-(o)	inside, within	endoderm
epi-	upon, over, in addition	epimysium
ex-	out of	exit, excrete
extra-	beyond, outside of, in addition	extracellular
flex-	bent	flexion
front-	front, forehead	frontalis
hemi-	half	hemiplegic
hetero-	the other	heterosexual
hom-	common, same	homogenous
hydro-	denoting water	hydrotherapy
hyper-	above, extreme	hypertensive
hypo-	under, below	hypodermic
in-	within, into, not, negative	internal, inept
infra-	beneath	infraspinatus

intra-	inside	intravenous
leuk-(o)	white	leukocyte
macr-	large, long	macrophage
mal-	abnormal, bad	malpractice
medi-	middle, midline	medial
mega-	large, extreme	megadose
micr-(o)	small	microscope
mon-(o)	one, single	monolith
multi-	many, multiple	multiply
narc-	stupor, numbness	narcotic
ne-(o)	new	neophyte, neonatal
nutri-	nourish	nutrition
para-	next to, resembling, beside,	paralysis, paraplegic
path-	pertaining to disease	pathology
per-	through	perforate
peri-	around	periosteum
poly-	many, much	polyunsaturated
post-	after, later in time	posthumous
pre-, pro-	before in time	previous
pseud-(o)	false	pseudonym
quad-	four	quadriplegic
re-	back, again	repeat, review
retro-	backward	retrofit
sub-	under, below	subscapularis
super-	above, in addition	superior
supra-	over, above, upper	supraspinatus
syn-	together, along with	synergist
tri-	three	triceps
uni-	single, one	unilateral

Suffixes

-al; -ar	pertaining to an area	femoral, clavicular
-ase	denoting an enzyme	lactase
-algia	painful condition	neuralgia
-desis	a binding	tenodesis
-ectomy	surgical removal of body part	tonsillectomy
-gram	a record	sonogram
-graph	write, draw, record	electrocardiograph
-ia	a noun ending of a condition	leukemia
-ic	a noun/adjective ending	pelvic, hypodermic
-ist	one who does	artist, antagonist
-itis	inflammation	arthritis
-oid	resembling	styliod, lipoid
-ology	study of, science of	biology
-oma	tumor	carcinoma
-ostomy	forming an opening	colostomy
-otomy	excision, cutting into	lobotomy

-pathic	diseased	psychopathic
-phobia	morbid fear of	claustrophobia
-tomy	surgical procedure	colostomy

Common Word Roots Or Stems

aur	ear	auricular
arth(ro)	joint	arthritis
brachi	arm	brachialis
cardi	heart	cardiac
cephal	head	brachiocephalic
cerebr(o)	brain	cerebrospinalis
cervic	neck	cervix, cervical
chondr(o)	cartilage	osteochondritis
cost	rib	intercostal
crani	skull	cranial
cyt	cell	leukocyte
dent	teeth	dentine, dental
derm	skin	subdermal
fibr	fiber	fibrositis
gastr(o)	stomach	gastritis
gyn	woman	gynecology
hem	blood	hematoma
hepat	liver	hepatitis
hist	tissue	histology
labi	lip	quadratus labii
my(o)	muscle	myology
nephr(o)	kidney	nephritis
neur(o)	nerve	neurology
ocul	eye	ocular
oss, ost(e)	bone	osteoblast
phleb	vein	phlebitis
pneum	lung	pneumonia
pod	foot	podiatrist
psych	mind	psychologist
pulmo	lung	cardiopulmonary
therm	heat	thermometer
vas	vessel	vascular

QUESTIONS FOR DISCUSSION AND REVIEW

1. What is anatomy?
2. What is physiology?
3. What is histology?
4. What is pathology?
5. Define *disease*.
6. Differentiate between a sign and a symptom of a disease.
7. What is the physiological reaction to stress?

8. What is the physical reaction of the body to pain?
9. Describe what is meant by the pain-spasm-pain cycle.
10. Describe the role of the massage therapist in breaking the pain-spasm-pain cycle.
11. Explain the difference between infection and inflammation.
12. What are the four principal signs and symptoms of inflammation?
13. What is fever?
14. When does fever become dangerous?
15. How are medical terms constructed?
16. What do the parts of a medical term generally indicate?

Human Anatomy and Physiology

5

Learning Objectives

After you have mastered this chapter, you will be able to:

1. Demonstrate knowledge of basic human anatomy and physiology as a requisite in mastering the theory and practice of therapeutic body massage.

2. Name the anatomical planes, regions, and cavities and parts of the body.

3. Name the ten most important body systems.

4. Explain the structures and functions of the various body systems.

▼ INTRODUCTION

An elementary knowledge of anatomy and physiology is necessary in mastering the theory and practice of therapeutic body massage. To obtain the most beneficial results, the practitioner who knows the principles of anatomy and physiology is better able to adjust the massage treatment to the needs of the client and to control results.

Anatomy (a-**NAT**-o-mee) is the science of **morphology** (morf-**AL**-o-jee) or structure of an organism or body. **Physiology** (fiz-ee-**OL**-o-jee) concerns the normal functions performed by the various systems of the body. **Histology** (his-**TOL**-o-jee) is a form of microscopic anatomy. It is the branch of biology concerned with the microscopic structure of tissues of a living organism. All living structures are composed of cells and intercellular materials that are organized to form the various systems of the body.

▼ LEVELS OF COMPLEXITY OF LIVING MATTER

All substances are made of subatomic particles that form **atoms.** Atoms are arranged in specific patterns and structures called **molecules.** Molecules are arranged in such a way as to produce compounds and matter. Within the human organism the basic unit of structure and function is the **cell.** Cells are organized into layers or groups called **tissues.** Groups of tissues form complex structures that perform certain functions. These structures called **organs** are arranged in **organ systems.** Organ systems are arranged to form an organism. The human body is the organism we study in relation to therapeutic massage (Fig. 5.1).

Cells

All living matter is composed of **protoplasm** (**PRO**-to-plazm), a colorless, jelly-like substance in which food elements, such as protein, fats, carbohydrates, mineral salts, and water, are present. Cells are the basic functional units of all living matter of animals, plants, and bacteria. Living cells differ from one another in size, shape, structure, and function. In the human body cells are highly specialized to perform such vital functions as movement, digestion, thought, and reproduction.

The principal parts of a cell are the **cytoplasm** (**SIGH**-to-plazm), **centrosome** (**SEN**-tro-sohm), **nucleus,** and **cell membrane.** A thin cell membrane or wall permits soluble substances such as nutrients and waste products to enter and leave the protoplasm. Near the center of the cell is a nucleus (dense protoplasm). Outside the nucleus are the cytoplasm (less dense protoplasm) and a centrosome (Fig. 5.2).

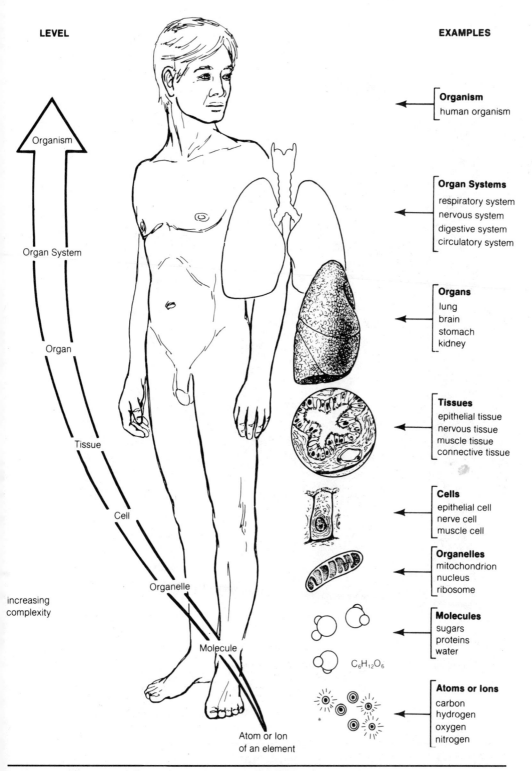

LEVEL

EXAMPLES

Organism
human organism

Organ Systems
respiratory system
nervous system
digestive system
circulatory system

Organs
lung
brain
stomach
kidney

Tissues
epithelial tissue
nervous tissue
muscle tissue
connective tissue

Cells
epithelial cell
nerve cell
muscle cell

Organelles
mitochondrion
nucleus
ribosome

Molecules
sugars
proteins
water

$C_6H_{12}O_6$

Atoms or Ions
carbon
hydrogen
oxygen
nitrogen

Organism

Organ System

Organ

Tissue

Cell

Organelle

increasing
complexity

Molecule

Atom or Ion
of an element

Fig. 5.1 Levels of complexity of the human organism.

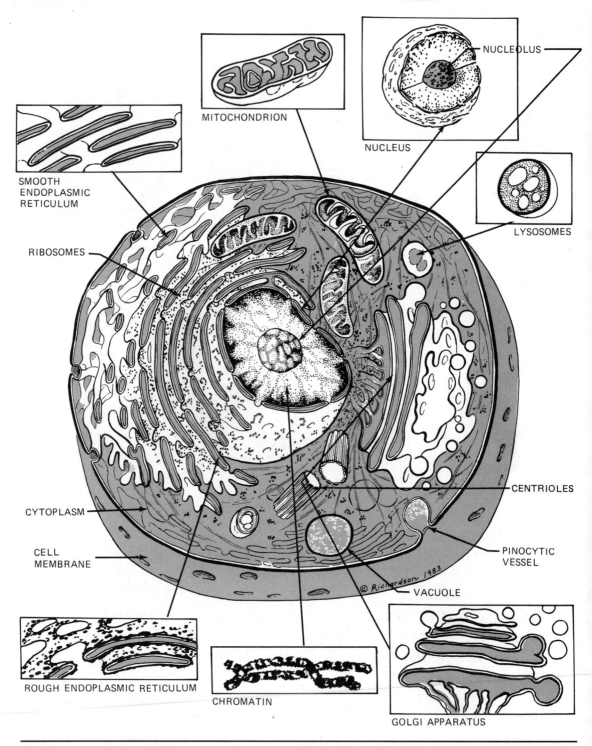

SMOOTH
ENDOPLASMIC
RETICULUM

MITOCHONDRION

NUCLEOLUS

NUCLEUS

LYSOSOMES

RIBOSOMES

CYTOPLASM

CELL
MEMBRANE

CENTRIOLES

PINOCYTIC
VESSEL

VACUOLE

© Richardson 1983

ROUGH ENDOPLASMIC RETICULUM

CHROMATIN

GOLGI APPARATUS

Fig. 5.2 Structure of a typical animal cell.

Structure of the Cell

The protoplasm of the cell contains the structures shown in Fig. 5.2.

The cytoplasm contains a network of various membranes that mark off several distinct parts called **cytoplasmic organelles.** Organelles perform specific functions necessary for cell survival. (See Table 5.1.) The centrosome and nucleus control cell reproduction. As long as the cell receives an adequate supply of food, oxygen, and water, eliminates waste products, and is surrounded by a favorable environment (proper temperature, and the absence of waste products, toxins, and pressure), it will continue to grow and function. When these requirements are not provided, the cell will stop growing and will eventually die.

Cell Division

The human body is composed of more than 100 trillion cells, which develop from a single cell, the fertilized ovum (egg). During the early developmental stages, the repeated division of the ovum results in many specialized cells that differ from one another in composition and function. This process is **differentiation** (dif-er-en-shee-**A**-shun).

After the tissues and organs of the organism have developed, growth and maintenance of the various tissues are carried on through cell division. As a cell matures and is nourished, it grows in size and eventually divides into two smaller daughter (like) cells. This form of cell division, called **mitosis** (migh-**TO**-sis), produces new cells.

In the human body, some cells reproduce continually, some occasionally, and some not at all. For example, skin and intestinal lining cells are exposed to continuous wear and tear and reproduce continually throughout life. Most body cells are capable of growth and self-repair during their life cycle. However, delicate nerve cells in the central nervous system are incapable of self-repair after injury or destruction and disease.

From the time the cell forms until it reproduces is the life cycle of a cell. In the human body, when a cell reaches maturity, reproduction takes place by indirect division or **mitosis,** in which a series of changes occurs in the nucleus before the entire cell divides in half.

Mitosis is accomplished in five stages: interphase, prophase, metaphase, anaphase, and telophase.

1. **Interphase:** This is a normal state of the cell during which most of the cellular work and growth are done. During interphase, chromosomes exist in thin threads. It is during mitosis that the chromosomes assume the twin helical (rod-like) structure.
2. **Prophase:** Prophase occurs when the chromosomes, composed of DNA (deoxyribonucleic acid), which houses the genes, become larger and more defined. They can be seen within the cell duplicated in two coiled strands called

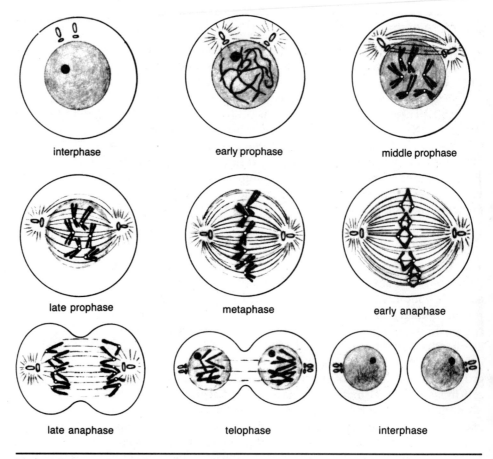

interphase   early prophase   middle prophase

late prophase   metaphase   early anaphase

late anaphase   telophase   interphase

Fig. 5.3 Stages of mitosis in animal cells.

chromatids (**KRO**-muh-tids) During the last part of the prophase, the nuclear membrane disappears.

3. **Metaphase:** During metaphase, the chromosomes arrange themselves in a plane called the equatorial plane. The nuclear membrane and the nucleolus are absent.

4. **Anaphase:** During anaphase, the chromatids are separated and are again called chromosomes.

5. **Telophase:** This is the stage when the chromosomes reach the centrioles (small bodies) and begin to uncoil. The cytoplasm divides into two parts or two cells (Fig. 5.3).

Direct division of a cell, **amitosis** (a-mi-**TO**-sis), is the method of reproduction in which the nucleus and cytoplasm divide by simple construction without the duplicating of chromosomes.

Cellular Activity

The activity of cells may be divided into three categories: vegetative, growth and reproduction, and specialized.

TABLE 5.1 STRUCTURE AND FUNCTION OF CELLULAR ORGANELLES ▼

An organelle is a discreet structure within a cell, having specialized functions, identifying molecular structures, and a distinctive chemical composition.

ORGANELLE	STRUCTURE	FUNCTION
Cell membrane	A thin covering of the outer surface of the cytoplasm composed of protein and lipid molecules.	Transports materials between the outside and inside of the cell. Helps to control cell activity and contains cellular material.
Centrosome	A nonmembranous structure near the nucleus—two rod-shaped centrioles.	Divides into two parts during mitosis and moves to the opposite poles of the dividing cell.
Chromatin	Network of fibers composed of protein and DNA that form the chromosomes.	Contains the genes by which hereditary characteristics are transmitted and determined.
Endoplasmic reticulum	Network of sacs and canals.	There are two varieties: a smooth type that produces lipid and a rough type that produces protein. Synthesizes protein for cell utilization and transport.
Fibrils and microtubules	Minute rods and tubules.	Support the cytoplasm and contribute to movement of substances within the cytoplasm.
Golgi apparatus	Composed of flattened membranes and small vesicles.	Collects the products of cell synthesis, synthesizes carbohydrates, holds protein molecules for secretion.
Lysosome	Membraneous structure containing hydrolytic enzymes.	Digests foreign substances.
Mitochondria	Shape varies according to function, but all exhibit a double membrane with the inner membrane lifted into folds.	Contains enzymes for releasing energy and converting it to useful forms for cell operation.
Nuclear membrane	The covering structure of the nucleus that separates the nucleus and the cytoplasm.	Controls passage of substances between the nucleus and the cytoplasm.
Nucleolus	A dense body composed mainly of protein with some RNA molecules, and found in the nucleus of most cells.	Forms ribosomes.
Nucleus	Protein-coated hereditary material (DNA) containing chromosomes that transmit heredity.	Supervises all cell activity.
Ribosome	Minute particle or granule composed of RNA and protein molecules.	Synthesizes proteins.
Vacuole	Membrane-lined containers.	Involved in rapid ejection of fluids or introduction of substances.

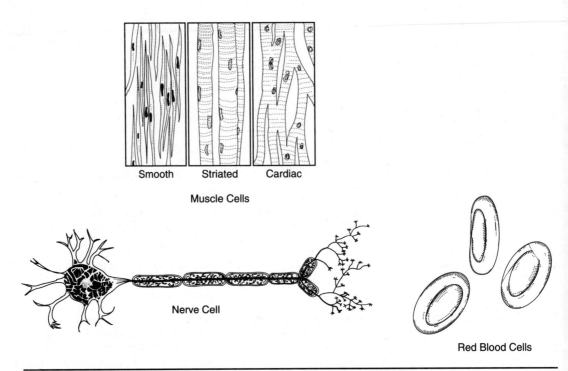

Fig. 5.4 Variations in specialized cells.

1. **Vegetative:** Vegetative activities include maintenance of the cell such as absorption, assimilation, and excretion of waste products.
2. **Growth and reproduction:** Growth involves the development of additional structural materials. Reproduction is the process of mitosis or indirect division of cells. The centriole and nucleus play important roles in this process.
3. **Specialized activities:** Because of cell differentiation, different cells perform different functions. For example, muscle cells exhibit contractility. Epithelial cells secrete and absorb. Nerve cells transmit nerve impulses. The cell is usually in the vegetative state, and then as time passes it either grows and reproduces or undergoes regression (atrophy) and finally dies (Fig. 5.4).

Metabolism

As the basic units of life, cells perform individually much like small factories. All chemical reactions within a cell that transform food for cell growth and operation are broadly termed **cellular metabolism.** Metabolism is the complex chemical and physical process that takes place in living organisms whereby the cells are nourished and carry out their various activities. Different kinds of cells perform specialized metabolic processes; however, all cells perform basic reactions that include the building up or breaking down of proteins, carbohydrates, fats, and other nutrients. There are two phases of metabolism: anabolism and catabolism. **Anabolism** (a-**NAB**-a-lizm) is the process of building up of larger molecules from smaller ones. This process requires energy because it is the constructive phase of cellular metabolism during which time substances needed for cell growth and repair are manufactured. **Catabolism** (ka-TAB-o-lizm) is the breaking down of larger substances or molecules into smaller ones. This process releases energy that may be stored by special molecules to be used for other reactions, such as muscle contraction or heat production.

Anabolism and catabolism are carried out simultaneously and continuously in the cells. Their activities are closely regulated so that the breaking-down or energy-releasing reactions are balanced with building-up or energy-using reactions. Therefore, homeostasis (the maintenance of normal, internal stability in an organism) is maintained.

ENZYMES ▼

Enzymes are protein substances that act as organic catalysts to initiate, accelerate, or control specific chemical reactions in the metabolic process, while they themselves remain unchanged. The reaction promoted by a particular enzyme is very specific. Therefore, because cellular metabolism includes hundreds of different chemical reactions, there are hundreds of different kinds of enzymes.

Enzymes are involved in the process of releasing energy from nutrients, principally from carbohydrates, fats, and proteins. Energy is the capacity to produce change in matter or to do work. During the digestive process, carbohydrates are broken down into simple sugars (glucose), fats are split into fatty acids, and proteins are converted into amino acids. These materials are absorbed by the blood and transported to the cells of the body, where they become the fuel for cell metabolism. As they are further broken down into other compounds, energy is released. Some of this energy is in the form of heat, while some is used to carry on the various cellular functions or to promote further cellular metabolism. Some energy may be stored in a special molecule called **adenosine** (a-**DEN**-o-seen) **triphosphate (ATP).** ATP stores the energy until it is released for muscular and other cellular activity.

TISSUES ▼

The basic unit of tissue is the cell. Tissues are collections of similar cells that carry out specific functions of the body. Tissues comprise all body organs and are subdivided into five main categories:
1. Epithelial tissue
2. Connective tissue

3. Muscular tissue
4. Nervous tissue
5. Liquid tissue.

The human body develops from a single cell. By the second week of growth of a human fetus (the embryonic stage), distinct layers of cells develop. The innermost layer of cells is called the **endoderm,** the middle layer is the **mesoderm,** and the outermost layer is called the **ectoderm.** These layers form the primary germ layer, which in turn forms all tissues and organs of the body.

The endodermal (inner layer) cells produce the epithelial linings of the respiratory and digestive tracts as well as linings of the urethra and urinary bladder. The mesodermal (middle layer) cells develop into all types of muscle, bone, blood, blood vessel tissues, various connective tissues, lymph, and the linings of all body cavities as well as the kidneys and the reproductive organs. The ectodermal (outer layer) cells form the glands of the skin, linings of the mouth, the anal canal, the epidermis, hair, nails, and the nervous system.

Epithelial Tissue

Epithelial tissue is a thin protective layer or covering that functions in the process of absorption, excretion, secretion, and protection. There are various classifications of epithelial tissue named according to the shape or number of layers of cells. Epithelial cells are classified by shape as **squamous** (SKWA-muhs) (flat), **cuboidal** (small cube shape), and **columnar** (tall or rectangular). These cells are also classified according to arrangement. For example, a simple squamous arrangement is one cell thick, the stratified squamous arrangement is several cells thick, and the transitional squamous is an arrangement of several layers of cells that are flat and closely packed.

Epithelial tissue covers all the surfaces of the body both inside and out. It forms the skin, the covering of the organs, and the inner lining of all the hollow organs. It also makes up the major tissue of the glands. Because epithelial tissue acts as a surface covering or a lining, it always has a free surface that is exposed to outside influences, whereas the other surface is well anchored in the connective tissue from which it derives nourishment (Fig. 5.5).

Membranes

Membranes are structures closely associated with epithelial tissue. There are two main categories of membranes: epithelial membranes and fibrous connective tissue membranes. **Epithelial membranes** have their outer surface faced with epithelium. They are further divided into two main subgroups: mucous membranes and serous membranes. **Mucous membranes** produce a thick, sticky substance that acts as a protectant and lubricant. Mucous mem-

Simple squamous

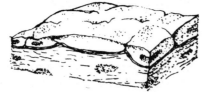

1. *Simple squamous:* found in protective layers of tissue.

Stratified squamous

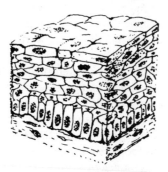

2. *Stratified squamous:* Found in vocal chords, intestines, and like organs.

Simple columnar

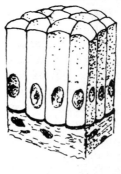

3. *Simple columnar:* Found in the stomach and bowels.

Cuboidal

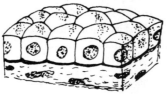

4. *Cuboidal:* Found in lining of ducts and pigmented layer of the retina of the eye.

Transitional squamous

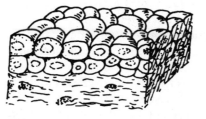

5. *Transitional squamous:* Found in the lining of the urinary bladder and kidney.

Fig. 5.5 Types of epithelial tissue.

branes line the surfaces of the digestive and upper respiratory tracts. In some instances their secretions contain a high number of enzymes that perform specific actions, such as digestion.

Serous membranes produce a more watery substance that also acts as a lubricant. Serous membranes line the body cavities and sometimes form the outermost surface of the organs contained in those cavities. The covering of the serous membranes in the body cavities is a special epithelial tissue called the **mesothelium** (mez-o-**THEE**-lee-um). This is a smooth covering that allows the movements of the organs to take place with little or no friction. Three major serous membranes are the pleura that encase the lungs, the pericardium around the heart, and peritoneum that lines the abdominal cavity.

The second category of membrane is the **connective tissue membranes.** These include the **fascial membranes,** which serve to anchor and support the organs and the skeletal membranes that cover bones and cartilage. **Superficial fascia** refers to the connecting layer between the skin and those structures underlying the skin. **Fascia** is the fibrous tissue between muscle bundles or forming the sheath around muscles or other structures that support nerves and blood vessels. **Deep fascia** refers to fibrous tissue sheaths, containing little or no fat, that penetrate deep into the body separating major muscle groups and anchoring them to the bones. Blood vessels, nerves, and the spinal cord are all covered by fascia.

Skeletal membrane covers bones and cartilage. The membrane covering bone is the **periosteum** (per-ee-**OS**-tee-um). The membrane covering cartilage is the **perichondrium** (per-i-**KON**-dree-um). Cavities and capsules in and around joints are lined with a connective tissue membrane called **synovial membrane,** which secretes synovium, or synovial fluid, an agent that acts as lubricant between the ends of bones and in spaces of great activity and friction. There are many other membranes in the body. All of them can be classified as either epithelial or connective (Fig. 5.6).

Connective Tissue

Connective tissue binds structures together, provides support and protection, and serves as a framework. There is an abundance of intercellular substance (matrix) in connective tissue, consisting of fibers and thick, gel-like fluid.

The loose connective tissue, or **areolar** (a-**REE**-o-lar) **tissue,** binds the skin to the underlying tissues and fills the spaces between the muscles. This is the tissue that lies beneath most layers of epithelium. It is rich in blood vessels and provides nourishment to the epithelial tissues. **Adipose tissue** is areolar tissue that has an abundance of fat-containing cells. Adipose tissue acts as a protection against heat loss and stores energy in the form of fat molecules. It is found in abundance in certain abdominal membranes, and around the surface of the heart, between the muscles, around the kidneys, and just beneath the skin.

Reticular tissue resembles fine fibers when viewed under a microscope. These fibers form the framework of the liver and lymphoid organs. **Fibrous connective tissue** is composed of collagen (albuminoid substance) and elastic fibers that are closely arranged to form tendons and ligaments. **Tendons** or **sinews** are white, glistening cords or bands that serve to attach muscle to bone. **Ligaments** are tough, fibrous bands that connect bones to bones or support viscera.

Cartilage

Fibrocartilage is found between the vertebrae and in the pubic symphysis where strong support and minimal-range movement are required. In dense fibrous connective tissue, repair to damaged tissue is slower due to poor blood supply.

Hyaline (**HIGH**-a-lin) a type of cartilage that contains little fibrous tissue and is made up of cells embedded in a somewhat

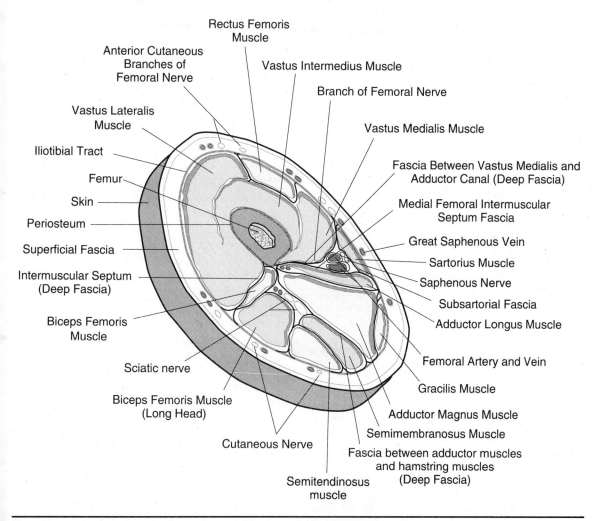

Fig. 5.6 Planes of fascia form compartments—cross section of the thigh.

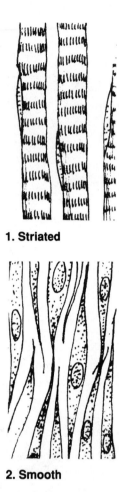

1. Striated

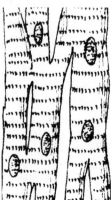

2. Smooth

3. Cardiac

Fig. 5.7 Types of muscle tissue.

translucent matrix, as found in the nose and trachea and on the end of bones and in movable joints.

Elastic cartilage is the most resilient of cartilages and is found in the external ear, the larynx, and like structures.

Bone Tissue

Bone or osseous (bone-like) tissue is connective tissue in which the intercellular substance is rendered hard by being impregnated with mineral salts, chiefly calcium phosphate and calcium carbonate. Compact, dense material forms the dense, outer layer of a long bone, while cancellous (porous) material forms the bone's inner tissue. Dentine, the substance beneath the enamel of the teeth, closely resembles bone but is harder and denser. Unlike bone, dentine contains no distinct cells or blood vessels.

Muscle Tissue

The main function of muscle tissue fibers is to contract their elongated cells, which pulls attached ends closer together, causing a body part to move. The three types of muscle tissue are skeletal muscle tissue, smooth muscle tissue, and cardiac muscle tissue.

Skeletal muscles are usually attached to bone or other muscle by way of tendons and can be controlled by conscious effort. These are called **voluntary muscles.** Skeletal muscles are responsible for moving the limbs of the body, facial expression, speaking, and other voluntary movements. Voluntary muscle cells appear long and thread-like under a microscope and have alternating light and dark cross-markings called **striations** (strigh-A-shuns). Muscles containing striations are called **striated muscles.**

Smooth muscle tissue lacks striations (nonstriated) and cannot usually be stimulated to contract by conscious effort. Muscle contractions generally result from involuntary nerve or gland activity. Smooth muscle tissue is found in the hollow organs of the stomach, small intestine, colon, bladder, and the blood vessels. Nonstriated muscle is responsible for the movement of food through the digestive tract, the constriction of blood vessels, and the emptying of the bladder.

Cardiac muscle tissue occurs only in the heart. It is controlled involuntarily and can continue to function without being directly stimulated by nerve impulses. Cardiac tissue is responsible for pumping blood through the heart into the blood vessels.

Nerve Tissue

Nervous or **nerve tissue** is composed of **neurons** (**NOOR**-ons) (nerve cells). Nerves act as channels for the transmission of messages to and from the various parts of the body, such as sensory nerves in the skin and organs of hearing, taste, smell, and sight. Nervous tissue initiates, controls, and coordinates the body's adaptation to its surroundings. Neurons (nerve cells) are linked together to form nerve pathways.

Liquid Tissue

Liquid tissue is represented by blood and lymph. Blood is a fluid tissue that circulates throughout the body and from which the body cells obtain nutrients and by which waste products are removed. Lymph is derived from the blood and tissue fluid and is collected into the lymphatic vessels along with metabolic waste and toxins. Lymphoid tissue found in the lymph nodes (small, compact, knot-like structures) and in the adenoids, thymus, tonsils, and spleen is important in the production of antibodies. According to some sources, liquid tissue is considered to be connective tissue.

Types of Muscle Tissue

1. **Striated:** Cylindrical fibers in voluntary muscle
2. **Smooth:** Smooth fibers without striations found in involuntary muscles
3. **Cardiac (striated):** Cardiac muscles found exclusively in the heart (Fig. 5.7)

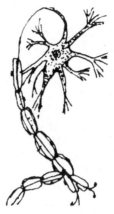

1. Nervous tissue proper

Types of Tissue

1. **Nervous tissue proper:** Neurons consisting of the cell body and nerve fibers
2. **Neuroglia:** Supportive tissue of the central nervous system
3. **Dentine:** Hard, dense, calcareous tissue forming the body of a tooth beneath the enamel
4. **Hemopoietic:** Tissue found in bone marrow and the vascular system
5. **Bone:** Tissue found in all bones of the skeleton
6. **Lymphoid:** Tissue found in lymph nodes and other compact structures such as the tonsils and adenoids (Fig. 5.8)

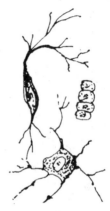

2. Neuroglia

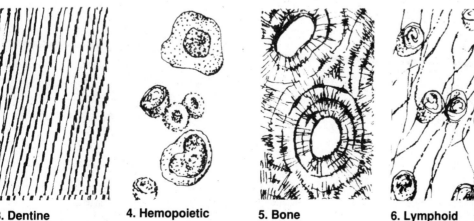

3. Dentine   **4. Hemopoietic**   **5. Bone**   **6. Lymphoid**

Fig. 5.8 Types of tissue.

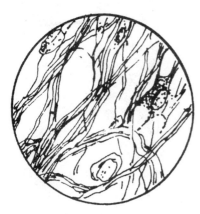

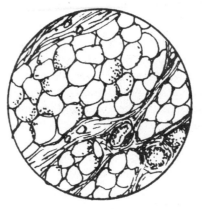

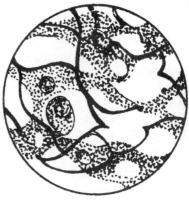

Areolar: Fibroelastic tissue.

Adipose: Tissue containing fat cells.

Reticular: Provides framework for organs such as the liver and spleen.

Fig. 5.9 Loose connective tissue.

Loose Connective Tissue

1. Areolar: Fibroelastic Tissue
2. Adipose: Tissue containing fat cells
3. Reticular: Provides framework of liver and other lymphoid organs (Fig. 5.9)

Cartilage

1. Hyaline: Fundamental type of cartilage consisting of fine white fibers
2. Fibrous: Characterized by callagenous fiber in the matrix
3. Elastic: Characerized by elastic fibiers in the matrix (Fig. 5.10)

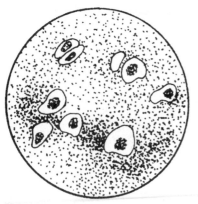

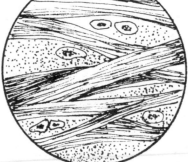

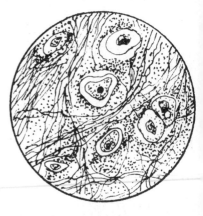

Hyaline: Fundamental type of cartilage consisting of fine white fibers.

Fibrous: Characterized by collagenous fibers in the matrix.

Elastic: Characterized by elastic fibers in the matrix.

Fig. 5.10 Cartilage.

SECTION QUESTIONS FOR DISCUSSION AND REVIEW

1. Why is the cell called the basic unit of all living matter?
2. Name the four principal parts of a cell.
3. Which parts of the cell control reproduction?
4. What conditions are required for a cell to grow and function?
5. By what process does cell reproduction occur in human tissue?
6. Name the five phases of cell mitosis.
7. Name the two phases of metabolism.
8. Explain anabolism.
9. Explain catabolism.
10. What are enzymes and what is their function?
11. Of what substances are tissues composed?
12. Name the five main categories of tissues.
13. What do the terms *endoderm*, *mesoderm*, and *ectoderm* refer to?
14. Where is epithelial tissue found and what is its function?
15. Name the two main types of membranes.
16. What is the main function of connective tissue?
17. What is the main function of areolar (loose) tissue?
18. What is adipose tissue?
19. Name the three types of cartilage.
20. What makes bone tissue hard?
21. What is dentine?
22. Name the three types of muscle tissue.
23. What is the difference between striated and smooth muscle tissue?
24. In what part of the body is cardiac muscle tissue found?
25. What is the main function of nervous tissue proper?
26. Where is liquid tissue found?

▼ THE ANATOMICAL POSITION OF THE BODY

When studying anatomy, it is helpful to know the anatomical terms that designate specific regions of the body. These terms refer to the body as seen in the **anatomic position,** which shows a figure standing upright with the palms of the hands facing forward.

Anatomists divide the body with three imaginary planes called the sagittal (vertical), the coronal (frontal), and the transverse (horizontal) planes.

1. The **sagittal (SAJ**-i-tal) **plane** divides the body into left and right parts by an imaginary line running vertically down the body. *Midsagittal* refers to the plane that divides the body or an organ into right and left halves.
2. The **coronal (KOR**-on-al) **plane** is an imaginary line that divides the body into the anterior (front) or ventral half of the body and the posterior (back) or dorsal half of the body.
3. The **transverse plane** is an imaginary line that divides the body horizontally into an upper and lower portion. A transverse section cuts through a body part perpendicular to the long axis of the body part (Fig. 5.11).

Anatomical Terms and Meanings

TERM	MEANING
1. Cranial or superior aspect	Situated higher, toward the crown of the head
2. Caudal or inferior aspect	Situated lower, farther from the crown of the head
3. Anterior or ventral aspect	Situated before or in front of
4. Posterior or dorsal aspect	Situated behind or in back of
5. Transverse plane	Division of the body at the mid-section into an upper and lower half. Transverse section refers to a plane through a body part per-pendicular to the axis, which is the vertical center line around which the body parts are arranged.
6. Sagittal plane	Vertical plane or section dividing the body into right and left sides. A midsagittal section divides the body into equal left and right halves.
7. Coronal plane	Pertaining to the coronal suture of the skull. The frontal plane or section passes through the long axis of the body, dividing it into front and back halves.
8. Medial aspect	Pertaining to the middle or center, nearer to the midline
9. Lateral aspect	On the side, farther from the midline or center
10. Distal aspect	Farthest point from the origin of a structure or point of attachment. Relatively farther from the median, trunk, or center.
11. Proximal	Nearest the origin of a structure or point of attachment. Relatively nearer to the trunk or median.

BODY CAVITIES AND ORGANS ▼

Once you know the body planes, it is easier to remember where body cavities and organs are located. There are two groups of body cavities: the dorsal or posterior cavities and the ventral or anterior cavities. The **dorsal cavities** contain the brain and spinal cord, with the skull forming the **cranial cavity** and the vertebrae forming the

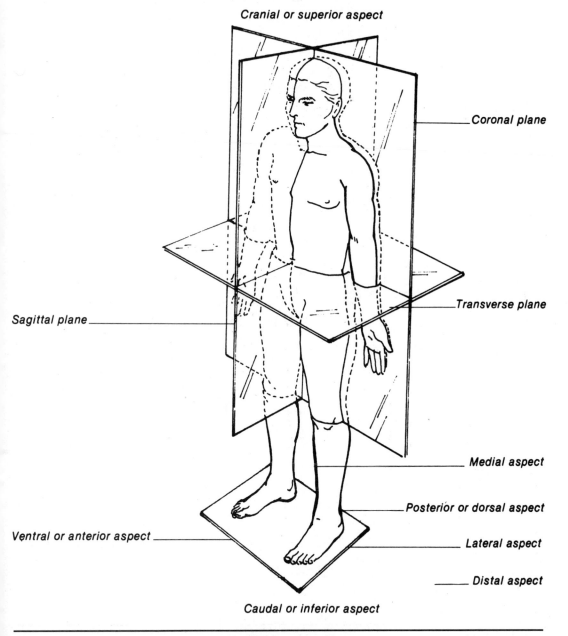

Cranial or superior aspect

Coronal plane

Transverse plane

Sagittal plane

Medial aspect

Posterior or dorsal aspect

Ventral or anterior aspect

Lateral aspect

Distal aspect

Caudal or inferior aspect

Fig. 5.11 Planes of the body in terms of location and position.

vertebral or spinal cavity. The ventral cavities are the thoracic cavity and abdominal cavities. The thoracic cavity is subdivided into the pericardial cavity, which contains the heart, and the pleural cavities, which contain the lungs. The abdominal cavity is situated below the diaphragm and contains the liver, stomach, spleen, pancreas, small and large intestines. The pelvic cavity is actually the lower third of the abdominal cavity and contains the bladder, rectum, and some of the reproductive organs (Fig. 5.12).

Body Cavities

1. Cranial cavity (dorsal)
2. Spinal cavity (dorsal)
3. Thoracic cavity (ventral)
4. Abdominal cavity (ventral)
5. Pelvic cavity (ventral)

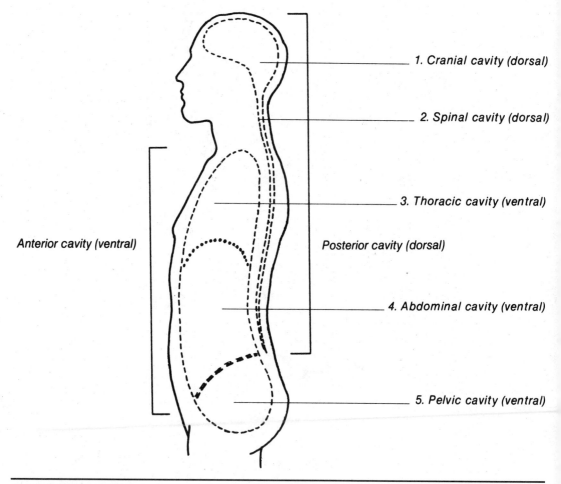

Fig. 5.12 Body cavities.

THE REGIONS OF THE HUMAN BODY ▼

Knowing the regions of the body helps us pinpoint a particular area of the body. For example, the pectoral muscle is located in the pectoral or chest region. The brachial nerve is located in the brachial region. The lower back is the lumbar region. Study the illustrations of regions of the body until you can locate each region and name the parts of the body associated with each region.

Anterior View of the Human Body Regions

1. **Frontal:** Region of the head
2. **Temporal:** Region of the temples
3. **Cervical:** Region of the neck
4. **Deltoid:** Region of the shoulder joint and deltoid muscle
5. **Axillary:** Region of the armpit
6. **Brachial:** Region between the elbow and shoulder
7. **Hypochondrium:** Region of the abdomen lateral to the epigastric region
8. **Umbilical:** Region of the navel (umbilicus). The middle of the three median abdominal regions, below the epigastric region and above the pubic region
9. **Hypogastric:** Region under the stomach and inferior to the umbilical region
10. **Patellar:** Region of the knees and kneecap
11. **Femoral:** Region of the femur or thigh
12. **Inguinal:** Region of the groin
13. **Epigastric:** Region of the abdomen
14. **Pectoral:** Region of the breast and chest (Fig. 5.13)

Posterior View of the Human Body Regions

1. **Parietal:** Region of the head, posterior to the frontal region and anterior to the occipital region
2. **Mastoid:** Region of the temporal bone behind the ear.
3. **Cervical:** Region of the neck
4. **Scapular:** Region of the back of the shoulder or shoulder blade
5. **Lumbar:** Region of the lower back
6. **Gluteal:** Region of muscles of the buttocks
7. **Popliteal:** A diamond-shaped area behind the knee joint (Fig. 5.14)

THE STRUCTURE OF THE HUMAN BODY ▼

The main anatomical parts of the body are:
1. The head
2. The spine
3. The trunk
4. The extremities.

The head is subdivided into:

1. **The cranium:** The upper portion of the head housing the brain
2. **The face:** The front and lower part of the skull including the eyes, nose, and mouth.

The spine is a column of bones that supports the head and trunk of the body and protects the spinal cord.

The trunk is subdivided into:

1. **The thorax or chest:** The upper part of the trunk containing the ribs, lungs, heart, esophagus (food tube), and part of the trachea or windpipe
2. **The abdomen:** Situated below the diaphragm containing the stomach, intestines, liver, and kidneys. The diaphragm is a

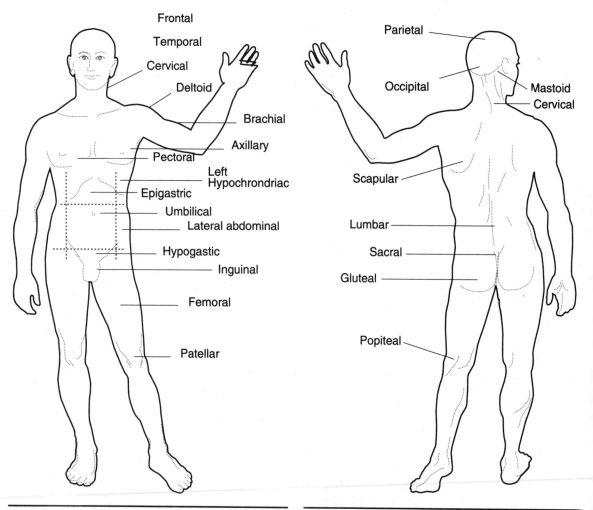

Fig. 5.13 Regions of the body, anterior view. Areas or regions of the body have been identified and named to aid in locating and describing the location of anatomical structures and conditions.

Fig. 5.14 Regions of the body, posterior view. Regions of the body are generally named for underlying bones, joints, muscles, or other anatomical structures in the immediate area.

muscular partition located between the thoracic cavity and the abdominal cavity. It is the main muscle associated with breath-ing. The pelvic cavity is located below the abdomen and contains the bladder, reproductive organs, lower bowel, and rectum.

The extremities include:

1. **The upper limbs:** The shoulder, arm, wrist, and hand
2. **The lower limbs:** The hip, thigh, leg, ankle, and foot.

Body Organs

Body organs are structures containing two or more different tissues that combine to accomplish a definite function. Among the important organs of the body are the brain, heart, lungs, kidneys, liver, sense organs, organs of digestion, organs of reproduction, and the skin.

Organ Systems

When a number of organs work together to perform a bodily function, they comprise an **organ system.** Systems carry on specific functions but are not independent units. All of the body organ systems cooperate for a common purpose, namely the maintenance or function of the entire organism.

The human body is composed of the following ten important organ systems:

1. Integumentary system (skin)
2. Skeletal system
3. Muscular system
4. Circulatory system (blood vascular and lymph vascular)
5. Nervous system
6. Endocrine system
7. Digestive system
8. Respiratory system
9. Excretory system (including urinary system)
10. Reproductive system.

The Integumentary System

The skin is the largest organ of the body. It is often referred to as the outer covering or the integumentary (in-teg-you-**MEN**-ta-ree) system. The skin's functions include protection, heat regulation, secretion and excretion, sensation, absorption, and respiration.

The Skeletal System

The skeletal system is the structure and hard framework on which the other body systems depend for support and protection. The skeletal system is the physical foundation of the body. It is composed of differently shaped bones united by movable and immovable joints. The main function of the skeletal system is to serve as a means of protection, support, and attachment for muscles of locomotion.

The Muscular System

The muscular system is made up of voluntary and involuntary muscles that are necessary for movement of the parts of the body. The muscular system covers and shapes the skeleton. Practically every contraction and movement of the body is due to the action of the muscles. The obvious movements of the arms and hands, the contraction of the heart and stomach, and the changes in facial expression are the direct result of muscular activity.

The Circulatory System (Blood Vascular and Lymph Vascular)

The circulatory (vascular) system controls the circulation of blood and lymph throughout the body. It consists of two divisions: the blood vascular system and the lymph vascular system. The blood vascular system includes the heart and blood vessels (arteries, veins, and capillaries). The pumping action of the heart distributes the vital fluids through the blood vessels to all parts of the body. The blood acts as a two-way carrier of supplies, bringing oxygen and food materials to the cells and taking away waste products and secretions from the tissues.

The lymph (a clear, yellow fluid) bathes all cells and assists in the exchange of supplies required by the cells and carries waste and impurities away from the environment of the cells. The lymph vascular system consists of lymph, lymph nodes, and lymph vessels (lymphatics) through which the lymph circulates. The lymph system also includes the spleen, thymus, tonsils, and adenoids.

The Nervous System

The nervous or neurological system controls and coordinates all the body systems, helping them to work efficiently and harmoniously. The neurological system includes all the nerves of the body, spinal cord, and the brain. It is a highly developed and sensitive organization of nerve tissues. Through the nervous system the individual is made aware of his or her existence and relationship to the outside world. Nerves, branching out from the brain and spinal cord, coordinate all voluntary and involuntary functions of the body.

The Endocrine System

The endocrine system represents a group of specialized organs or glands capable of manufacturing secretions called **hormones** that affect many functions of the body including growth, reproduction, and health. The endocrine glands, such as the pituitary and thyroid, secrete hormones into the blood to regulate the processes of growth and metabolism. Reproduction is made possible by the sex glands and their secretions.

The Digestive System

The digestive system consists of all the structures involved in the process of digestion including the mouth, stomach, intestines, salivary, and gastric glands. The intestines are part of a continuous tube about thirty feet in length. The function of digestion is to break down complex food substances into simple materials fit to be absorbed and used by the body cells. Various digestive glands including the salivary glands, pancreas, and liver, along with glands in the stomach and small intestine, form and discharge enzymes that act on food in the process of digestion.

The Respiratory System

The respiratory system includes the lungs, air passages, nose, mouth, pharynx, trachea, and bronchial tubes, which lead to the lungs. The blood, as it passes through the lungs, is purified by the removal of carbon dioxide and the intake of oxygen.

The Excretory System

The excretory system includes the skin, kidneys, bladder, liver, lungs, and large intestines, which eliminate waste products from the body. The skin (integumentary system) gives off perspiration. The lungs exhale carbon dioxide gas, the kidneys excrete urine, and the large intestine discharges digestive refuse from the body. The liver produces bile and urea, which contains certain waste products.

The Reproductive System

The reproductive system is the system whose function it is to ensure continuance of the species by the reproduction of other human beings. In the female, the ovaries discharge an ovum or egg cell that appears prior to menstruation. The testes in the male manufacture sperm cells. The union of the ovum with sperm results in fertilization and conception.

In the following sections of this chapter, each organ system will be discussed in more detail.

SECTION QUESTIONS FOR DISCUSSION AND REVIEW

1. What is anatomic position?
2. What are three anatomical planes of the body?
3. Why is it important to know the anatomical position and the planes and regions of the human body?
4. Name the subdivisions of the ventral and dorsal cavities and the major organs found in each.
5. What are the four main anatomical parts of the body and the structures found in each?
6. Name the ten important organ systems of the body.

▼ REVIEW

I. Match each term in the left column with the correct definition in the right column.

_____ **1.** superior   **a.** farthest from center

_____ **2.** inferior   **b.** pertaining to the middle

_____ **3.** anterior   **c.** dividing front and back

_____ **4.** posterior   **d.** toward the side

_____ **5.** transverse plane   **e.** dividing left and right

_____ **6.** sagittal plane   **f.** closer to the origin

_____ **7.** cronal plane   **g.** toward the top

_____ **8.** medial   **h.** dividing upper and lower

_____ **9.** lateral   **i.** toward the front

_____ **10.** distal   **j.** toward the feet

_____ **11.** proximal   **k.** toward the back

II. Match each term in the left column with the correct definition in the right column.

_____ **1.** cervical   **a.** region of the groin

_____ **2.** axillary   **b.** side of the cranium

_____ **3.** femoral   **c.** region of the armpit

_____ **4.** lumbar   **d.** behind the knee

_____ **5.** inguinal   **e.** inferior to the umbilical region

_____ **6.** popliteal   **f.** region of the neck

_____ **7.** gluteal   **g.** region of the lower back

_____ **8.** parietal   **h.** between the shoulder and elbow

_____ **9.** hypogastric   **i.** region of the thigh

_____ **10.** brachial   **j.** region of the buttocks

SYSTEM ONE: THE INTEGUMENTARY SYSTEM—THE SKIN

The word **integument** means covering or skin. The skin is the largest organ of the body and serves as an interface with the environment and protection for the body.

The principal functions of the skin are:

1. **Protection:** The skin protects the body from injury and bacterial invasion.
2. **Heat regulation:** The healthy body maintains a constant internal temperature of about 98.6° F (37°C). As changes occur in the outside temperature, the blood and sweat glands of the skin make the necessary adjustments in their functions.
3. **Secretion and excretion:** By means of its sweat (sudoriferous) and oil (sebaceous) glands, the skin acts both as a secretory and an excretory organ. The sudoriferous (sweat) glands excrete (eliminate) perspiration, which is waste matter. The sebaceous (oil) glands secrete (produce and release) sebum, which is a lubricant. The skin is about 50 to 70 percent moisture. Sebum (oil) coats the surface of the skin and helps to maintain its moisture level. The sebum level slows down evaporation of moisture and keeps excess water from penetrating the skin.
4. **Sensation:** The papillary layer of the dermis provides the body with a sense of touch. Nerves supplying the skin register basic types of sensations, such as heat, cold, pain, pressure, and touch. Nerve endings are most abundant in the fingertips. Complex sensations, such as the feelings of vibration, seem to depend on a combination of these nerve endings.
5. **Absorption:** The skin has limited powers of absorption through its pores. Some cosmetics, chemicals, and drugs can be absorbed in small amounts.
6. **Respiration:** The skin breathes through its pores much as the body breathes through its lungs, but on a much smaller scale. Oxygen is taken in and carbon dioxide is discharged.

The Structure of the Skin

The structure of the skin contains two clearly defined divisions: the **epidermis** (cuticle or scarf), which is the outermost layer, and the **dermis** (corium or true skin), which is the deeper layer that extends to form the subcutaneous tissue.

Although the epidermis comprises almost a solid sheet of cells, the dermis is a more semisolid mixture of fibers, water, and a gel called "ground" substance. There are three kinds of fibers that intermingle with the cells of the dermis: collagen, reticulum, and elastin. Collagen makes up about 70 percent of the dry weight of the skin and gives it strength, form, and flexibility. Reticulum fibers form a fine branching pattern in connective tissue that helps to link the bundles of collagen fibers. Collagen contains a protein called elastin that has elastic properties and helps to give the skin its resiliency. The dermis contains an elastic network of cells through which are distributed nerves, blood and lymph vessels, and sweat and oil glands (Figs. 5.15 and 5.16).

The Dermis

The papillary layer of the skin (directly beneath the epidermis) contains the papillae, the cone-like projections made of fine strands of elastic tissue that extend upward into the epidermis. Some of the papillae contain looped capillaries; others contain terminations of nerve fibers called **tactile corpuscles.**

The **reticular layer** of the skin contains fat cells, blood and lymph vessels, sweat and oil glands, hair follicles, and nerve endings.

The **subcutaneous** (sub-kyou-**TAY**-nee-us) **tissue** (subcutis) is regarded as a continuation of the dermis. It varies in thickness according to the age, sex, and general health of the individual. Fatty (adipose) tissue gives smoothness and contour to the body, provides a reservoir for fuel and energy, and serves as a protective cushion for the upper skin layers.

The Epidermis

The **stratum granulosum** (gran-you-**LO**-sum) (granular layer of the skin) consists of cells that look like granules. These cells are almost dead and undergo a change into a horny substance called keratin.

The **stratum** or **malpighian** (mal-**PIG**-ee-an) layer (also called stratum mucosum) consists of cells containing **melanin** (**MEL**-a-nin) (coloring matter) of the skin. Melanin helps to protect the sensitive cells from the action of strong light rays.

The **stratum germinativum** (jer-mi-na-**TEE**-vum) is the deepest layer of the epidermis comprising a single layer of cells that are well nourished by the dermis. These cells undergo mitosis, pushing other cells closer to the body surface. This layer also contains melanocytes that produce the pigment melanin.

The skin varies in thickness, being thinnest on the eyelids and thickest on the palms of the hands and soles of the feet. Continued pressure over any part of the skin will cause it to thicken and may produce a **callus.**

Nutrition And The Skin

Blood and lymph supply nutrients to the skin. As much as one half of the total blood supply of the body is distributed to the skin. Blood and lymph, as they circulate through the skin, contribute certain materials for growth, nourishment, and repair of skin, hair, and nails. In the subcutaneous tissue are found networks of arteries and lymphatics, which send their smaller branches to hair papillae, hair follicles, and the glands of the skin. Capillaries are quite numerous in the skin.

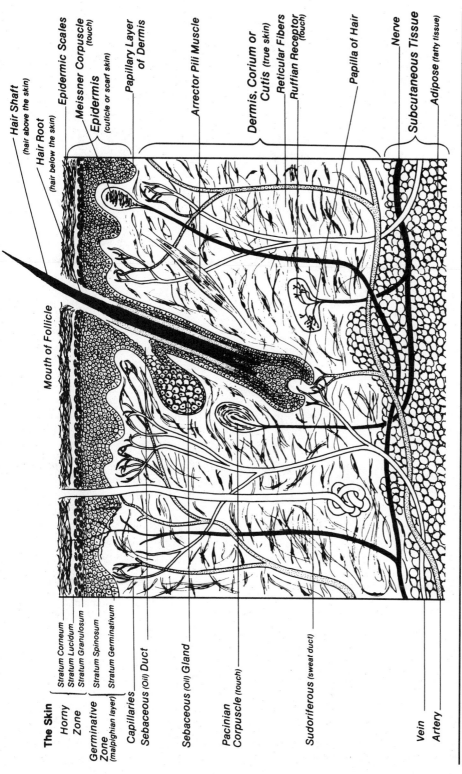

Fig. 5.15 The integumentary system (showing skin and hair).

*1 Square Inch
(6.452 Sq. cm)
of Skin Contains*

65 hairs

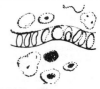

9,500,000 cells

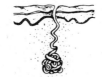

95-100 sebaceous glands

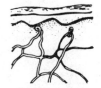

*19 yards (17 meters) of blood
vessels*

650 sweat glands

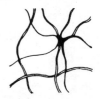

78 yards (70 meters) of nerves

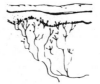

78 sensory apparatuses for heat

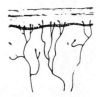

*19,500 sensory cells at the ends
of nerve fibers*

*1,3000 nerve endings to record
pain*

*160-165 pressure apparatuses for
the perception of tactile stimuli*

13 sensory apparatuses for cold

Fig. 5.16 Structures in the skin.

Aging Skin

As people age, the collagen network of the skin tends to lose its elasticity, causing the skin to become less firm and supple. With age, the deeper or dermal layer of the skin undergoes changes. The skin may become thinner, drier, and more prone to growths. It may become lined and crepey. Swelling (edema) of tissues may appear around and under the eyes. Pliability of the skin depends on elasticity of the fibers of the dermis. For example, after expansion healthy skin will regain its former shape almost immediately.

Structural Changes of The Skin

Because the skin is the covering of the entire body, its condition must be taken into consideration before massage treatment is given. The skin may be sensitive to touch or it may show signs of damage due to disease or injury. The massage practitioner must be aware of any skin condition that may require the attention of the client's physician. Freckles, birthmarks (port-wine stains), and the like present no problem; however, a lesion or any discontinuity of tissue should be reported to the client and referred to a physician before receiving a massage.

Healthy skin is slightly moist, soft, flexible, and possesses a slightly acid reaction. The texture of skin revealed by feel and appearance should be smooth and fine grained. The color of the skin depends partly on the blood supply but more on the coloring matter melanin. Skin pigment varies in different people and is determined by genetics. Regardless of native pigmentation, healthy skin is of good color. An overly pale, ashy, reddish, or yellow cast to the skin may indicate health problems.

Massage benefits the skin by improving circulation of the blood, which carries nutrients to the cells.

The Appendages Associated With The Skin

Glands of the Skin

The skin contains two types of duct glands (exocrine glands) that extract materials from the blood to form new substances. These are the **sudoriferous** (soo-du-RIF-er-us) (sweat) glands and **sebaceous** (see-**BAY**-shus) (oil) glands. Sweat glands are under the control of the autonomic nervous system and are located in the dermis. They consist of a coiled base or fundas and a tube-like duct that terminates at the surface of the skin to form a sweat pore. Practically all parts of the body are supplied with sweat glands, but they are more abundant in the armpits, soles of the feet, palms of the hands, and forehead. The activity of the sweat glands is greatly increased by heat, exercise, and mental excitement (Figs. 5.17 to 5.19).

The sudoriferous glands respond to elevated body temperatures resulting from environmental conditions or physical activity. The

Connective tissue
Sebaceous cells

Fig. 5.17 Sebaceous (oil) gland.

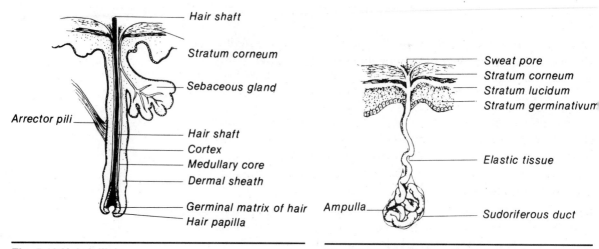

Fig. 5.18 Hair follicle.

Fig. 5.19 Sudoriferous (sweat) gland.

tubular extensions of these glands open at the body surface as a pore. Fluid secreted by the eccrine glands is mostly water and contains some bodily wastes, such as urea and uric acid. Therefore, the skin acts in some degree as an organ of excretion.

The Hair and Nails

Hair and nails are appendages of the skin. They are composed of hard keratin, a protein which in its soft form is found in skin. Hard keratin, as found in hair, has a sulfur content of 4 to 8 percent and a lower moisture and fat content than soft keratin and is particularly tough, elastic material. It forms continuous sheets (fingernails) or long endless fibers (hair). Soft keratin contains about 2 percent sulfur, 50 percent moisture, and a small percentage of fats. In the epidermis keratin occurs as flattened cells or dry scales (Fig. 5.20).

Hair grows over the entire body, with the exception of the palms of the hands, soles of the feet, some areas of the genitalia, the mucous membranes of the lips, the nipples, the navel, and the

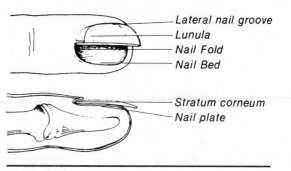

Fig. 5.20 Fingernail.

eyelids. The heavier concentration of hair is on the head, under the armpits, on and around the genitals, and on the arms and legs. An individual's genes strongly influence the distribution of hair, its thickness, quality, color, and rate of growth, and whether it is curly or straight.

Each hair develops from a tube-like depression (hair follicle) that extends through the epidermis, into and often through the dermis, and into the subcutaneous layer. As epidermal cells at the base of the follicle are nourished by the blood supply, they divide and push up through the hair follicle, die, and keratinize, becoming a shaft of hair.

Associated with hair follicles are sebaceous (oil) glands, and arrector pili (a-**REK**-tor **PIGH**-ligh) muscles. The arrector pili muscles are fanlike muscles connected with the base of the follicle and positioned in such a way that they contract in reaction to cold or emotional stimuli. This reaction often results in a condition called **goose bumps** because the skin appears bumpy, like that of a plucked goose.

Lesions of The Skin

A lesion is a structural change in the tissues caused by injury or disease. There are three types: primary, secondary, and tertiary. The massage practitioner is concerned with primary and secondary lesions only. Knowing how to identify the principal skin lesions helps the practitioner to avoid affected areas. The client should be advised to seek medical attention.

Definitions Pertaining to Primary Lesions

Bulla: A blister containing a watery fluid, similar to a vesicle, but larger

Macule: A small, discolored spot or patch on the surface of the skin, neither raised nor sunken, as freckles

Papule: A small, elevated pimple in the skin, containing fluid, but which may develop pus

Pustule: An elevation of the skin having an inflamed base, containing pus

Tubercle: A solid lump larger than a papule. It projects above the surface or lies within or under the skin. It varies in size from a pea to a hickory nut.

Tumor: An external swelling, varying in size, shape, and color

Vesicle: A blister with clear fluid in it, vesicles lie within or just beneath the epidermis (example: Poison ivy produces small vesicles.)

Wheal: An itchy, swollen lesion that lasts only a few hours (Examples: hives, or the bite of an insect, such as a mosquito)

Definitions Pertaining to Secondary Lesions

The secondary skin lesions are those in the skin that develop in the later stages of disease.

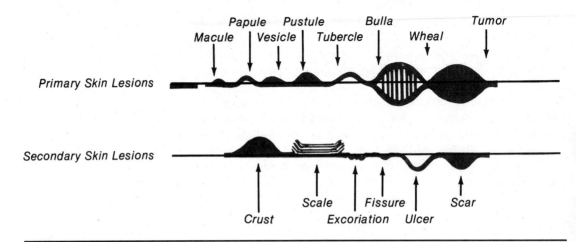

Fig. 5.21 Skin lesions.

Crust: An accumulation of serum and pus, mixed perhaps with epidermal material (example: the scab on a sore)

Excoriation: A skin sore or abrasion produced by scratching or scraping (example: a raw surface due to the loss of the superficial skin after an injury)

Fissure: A crack in the skin penetrating into the derma, as in the case of chapped hands or lips

Scale: An accumulation of epidermal flakes, dry or greasy (example: abnormal or excessive dandruff)

Scar (cicatrix) (**SICK**-ay-trix): Likely to form after the healing of an injury or skin condition that has penetrated the dermal layer.

Stain: An abnormal discoloration remaining after the disappearance of moles, freckles, or liver spots, sometimes apparent after certain diseases

Ulcer: An open lesion on the skin or mucous membrane of the body, accompanied by pus and loss of skin depth (Fig. 5.21).

Disorders of the Skin

Problem, Blemished Skin

The massage practitioner need not be concerned about diagnosis or treatment of skin disorders, but he or she should be able to recognize some of the more common conditions in order to explain to the client why massage should or should not be given. The practitioner can suggest or recommend that the client see a dermatologist for skin conditions that are contraindications for massage.

Blackheads (comedones) are small masses of hardened, discolored sebum that appear most frequently on the face, shoulders, chest, and back. Blackheads are often accompanied by pimples during adolescence and are primarily due to overstimulated sebaceous glands. Proper cleansing of the skin will help to reduce the skin's oiliness. Any case of excessive pimples or blackheads should be treated by a dermatologist.

Massage should not be given over areas where these skin conditions are more severe. However, stimulation of blood circulation is beneficial and massage, exercise, and proper diet will, in most cases, improve these conditions.

Dermatitis (der-ma-**TIE**-tis) is an inflammatory condition of the skin. The lesions come in various forms, such as vesicles or papules.

Eczema (ek-ze-muh), an inflammation of the skin, either acute or chronic in nature, can appear in many forms of dry or moist lesions. The term **eczema** is applied to any number of surface lesions. It is usually a red, blistered, oozing area that itches painfully. Eczema may be the result of some type of allergy or internal disorder and should be referred to a physician for treatment.

Psoriasis (so-**RYE**-a-sis) is a common chronic, inflammatory skin disease whose cause is unknown. It is usually found on the scalp, elbows, knees, chest, and lower back, but rarely on the face. The lesions are round dry patches covered with coarse, silvery scales. If irritated, bleeding points occur. Although not contagious, psoriasis can be spread by irritation. Massage over such a condition should be avoided.

Occupational disorders refer to abnormal conditions resulting from contact with chemicals. Some individuals may develop allergies to ingredients in some substances with which they work. An example is often seen when a cosmetologist is allergic to hair tints.

A client may have a condition of the skin known as **staphylodermatitis,** an inflammation caused by staphylococci, bacteria that are generally found in milk and other dairy products. Massage should not be given when the skin is inflamed. The client should have the condition diagnosed by a physician.

A **bruise** is a superficial injury (contusion) generally caused by a blow or impact with some object; while not breaking the skin, it causes a reddish-blue or purple discoloration. Severe bruises should be avoided during massage.

Acne is a chronic inflammatory disorder of the skin, usually related to hormonal changes and overactive sebaceous glands during adolescence. Common acne is also known as **acne simplex** or **acne vulgaris.** Although acne generally starts at the onset of puberty, it also afflicts adult men and women.

Modern studies show that acne is often due to heredity, but the condition can be aggravated by emotional stress and environmental factors. A well-balanced diet, drinking plenty of water, and developing healthful personal hygiene are recommended. Acne may be present on the back, chest, and shoulders. Acne may be accompanied by blackheads, pustules, and pimples that are red, swollen, and contain pus. In more advanced cases of acne, cysts (which are red, swollen lumps beneath the surface of the skin) may appear. Massage should be avoided when severe acne is present. If an area with moderate acne is massaged, any excess oil should be removed with alchohol.

Seborrhea (seb-o-**REE**-uh) is a skin condition caused by over activity and excessive secretion of the sebaceous glands. An oily or shiny condition of the nose, forehead, or scalp indicates the presence of seborrhea. It is readily detected on the scalp by the unusual amount of oil on the hair. Seborrhea is often the basis of an acne condition. Massage should not be given over infected areas.

Rosacea (ro-**ZAY**-shee-uh) is associated with excessive oiliness of the skin and a chronic inflammatory condition of the cheeks and nose. It is characterized by redness owing to dilation of blood vessels and the formation of papules and pustules. The skin becomes coarse, and the pores enlarged. Rosacea is usually caused by an inability to digest certain foods and intolerance to strong beverages. It may also be caused by overexposure to extreme climate, faulty elimination, and hyperacidity. Massage is not given over affected areas.

A **steatoma** (stee-uh-**TOE**-muh) or **sebaceous cyst** is a subcutaneous tumor of the sebaceous glands that contains sebum. It usually appears as a small growth on the scalp, neck, or back. A steatoma is sometimes called a **wen.** Massage is not given over the affected area.

Asteatosis (as-tee-uh-**TOE**-sis) is a condition of dry, scaly skin, characterized by absolute or partial deficiency of sebum, usually due to aging or bodily disorders. In local conditions, such as scaling of the hands, it may be caused by alkalis in soaps and similar products. When the skin is unbroken, a mild lubricant may be massaged into the skin.

A **furuncle** (**FYOU**-rung-kl), or boil, is caused by bacteria that enter the skin through the hair follicles. It is a subcutaneous abscess that fills with pus. A boil can be painful if neglected and should be treated by a physician.

Serious Skin Conditions

The massage practitioner should not attempt to diagnose any kind of bump, lesion, ulceration, or discoloration as skin cancer but should be able to recognize serious skin disorders and suggest that the client seek medical attention without delay.

Skin Cancer

There are three kinds of skin cancer. The least malignant and most common is called **basal cell carcinoma.** This type of cancer is characterized by light or pearly nodules and visible blood vessels.

Squamous cell carcinoma is different in appearance from the basal type; it consists of scaly, red papules. Blood vessels are not visible. This cancer is more serious than the basal cell carcinoma.

The most serious skin cancer is the **malignant melanoma.** This cancer is characterized by dark (brown, black, or discolored) patches on the skin.

A **tumor** is an abnormal growth of swollen tissue that can be located on any part of the body. Some tumors are benign (mild in character) and are not likely to recur after removal, which means they are not harmful. Some tumors are malignant and are more serious, as they can recur after removal. Tumors are removed by surgery, X-ray, or chemical treatments.

Venereal Diseases

Venereal diseases are those diseases associated with the sexual organs and are characterized by sores and rashes on the skin. Venereal diseases can become latent and appear at a later time. This can be dangerous because the affected person may not seek treatment. Venereal diseases can also affect unborn children.

Syphillis (**SIF**-i-lis) is a serious disease that is transmitted by sexual contact with an infected person. When a sore first appears, especially one that is hard and ulcerated (with a hole in the center), a physician should be consulted. Without treatment the sore may go away only to appear later in the form of a rash. This is called **secondary syphillis,** which can cause degeneration of various parts of the body, ultimately causing death.

Gonorrhea (gon-o-**REE**-uh) is a more common disease than syphillis and is characterized by a discharge and burning sensation when urinating. Women may show no symptoms. If left untreated, harmful bacteria can enter the bloodstream.

Herpes

Herpes (**HER**-peez) generally affects the mouth, skin, and other parts of the face (commonly called **cold sores** and **fever blisters**). Herpes virus can cause a variety of diseases known for their persistence in a latent state and recurrence at regular intervals. The virus usually enters the body through the mucous membranes.

Herpes simplex is generally defined as a recurrent spreading cutaneous infection. Examples are **herpes facialia** (herpes simplex), a type of herpes that affects the lips, mouth, pharynx, or parts of the face. **Herpes progenitalis** is a type of herpes simplex in which vesicles occur on the genitalia.

AIDS

Just a decade ago AIDS (acquired immune deficiency syndrome) was unheard of, but the disease has spread at an alarming rate since the early 1980s. The World Health Organization has reported that AIDS has become an international concern. AIDS is caused by a virus that is linked to the viral family that causes leukemia (a cancer of the blood). The virus breaks down the body's immune system, which produces antibodies and cells that destroy harmful bacteria. When the body loses its natural resistance, it is unable to combat various infections.

There is a great deal of controversy about how AIDS is spread, but intensive research has revealed that it is not spread by casual contact such as being in the same room with an AIDS patient or by just touching a person. The disease is most often transmitted by sexual activity, by blood transfusions, and by the use of contaminated needles, and it can be transmitted to an unborn child through the placenta.

Progress is being made in the prevention and treatment of AIDS by screening tests and by educating the public about the seriousness of the disease.

Allergies

An **allergy** is a sensitivity that certain persons develop to normally harmless substances. Contact with certain types of cosmetics, medicines, and hair preparations or consumption of certain foods may bring about an itching skin eruption, accompanied by redness, swelling, blisters, oozing, and scaling. Many allergies are accompanied by headaches, congestion, or emotional inconsistency.

Millions of people suffer from various forms of allergies. Allergic dermatitis (eczema), one of the more common allergies, can be caused by a number of different factors: food, substances in the air, or materials the victim uses. Many objects, including necklaces, rings, hairpins, and bracelets, contain metals (such as nickel) that cause dermatitis. Hair dyes, makeup, and chemicals are a few of the substances to which some people are allergic.

Pigmentations of the Skin

Changes in skin color may be observed in various skin disorders and in many systemic disorders. Certain drugs taken internally can affect pigmentation. Foods eaten in excess can affect the skin. The carotene in carrots is an example. A suntan is an example of external changes in the pigmentation of the skin. The fairer the skin, the easier it is to sunburn and the more difficult it may be to acquire an even suntan.

Generally, a skin that tans easily will not be sensitive to massage. However, when skin has been overexposed, it may become sensitive. When there is sunburn or peeling due to sunburn, massage may be painful.

Lentigines (len-TIJ-i-neez), or freckles, are small yellowish to brownish color spots on parts exposed to sunlight and air.

Stains are abnormal brown skin patches, having circular and irregular shape. Their permanent color is due to the presence of blood pigment. They occur during aging, after certain diseases, and after the disappearance of moles, freckles, and liver spots. The cause of these stains is unknown.

Chloasma (klo-AZ-muh) is characterized by increased deposits of pigment in the skin. It is found mainly on the forehead, nose, and cheeks. Chloasma is also called **moth patches** or **liver spots**.

A **naevus** is commonly known as a birthmark. It is a small or large discoloration of the skin due to pigmentation or dilated capillaries and is present on the skin at birth. Generally, such colored spots or areas are not affected by massage.

Leucoderma (loo-ko-**DER**-muh)are abnormal light patches of skin, due to congenital defective pigmentations. **Vitiligo** (vit-i-**LYE**-go)is an acquired condition of leucoderma that affects skin or hair.

Albinism (**AL**-bin-izm)is a congenital absence of melanin pigment in the body that affects the color of the skin, hair, and eyes. In albinos the hair is silky and white, and the skin is pinkish white and will not tan.

A **keratoma** (ker-a-**TOE**-muh), or callus, is a superficial, thickened patch of epidermis caused by friction on the hands and feet. This condition is usually treated by a chiropodist.

Color changes of the skin, such as a crack on the skin, a type of thickening, or any discoloration ranging from shades of red to brown and purple to almost black, may be danger signals and should be examined by a dermatologist.

SECTION QUESTIONS FOR DISCUSSION AND REVIEW ▼

1. Define skin as the integumentary system.
2. Name the major functions of the skin.
3. Name the two main layers of the skin.
4. Name the layers of the epidermis.
5. Name two forms of keratin and where they are found in most abundance.
6. What is subcutaneous tissue?
7. How does the skin receive its color?
8. Name the layers of the dermis.
9. What is a gland?
10. Name the two major glands found in the skin and give the function of each.
11. Define the following: sebum, pore, duct.
12. Name the appendages of the skin.
13. What is a lesion?
14. What kind of skin condition is called an occupational disorder?
15. Why is it important for the massage practitioner to observe a client's skin condition?

SYSTEM TWO: THE SKELETAL SYSTEM

The skeletal system is the bony framework of the body. It is composed of bones, cartilage, and ligaments. The skeletal system has five main functions:

1. To offer a framework that supports body structures and gives shape to the body
2. To protect delicate internal organs and tissues
3. To provide attachments for muscles and act as levers in conjunction with muscles to produce movement
4. To manufacture blood cells in the red bone marrow
5. To store minerals such as calcium phosphate, calcium carbonate, magnesium, and sodium.

Composition of Bones

Other than dentine, the dense hard tissue covering the teeth, bone is the hardest structure of the body. Despite its solid and inert appearance, bone is a complex and ever-changing organ. Bone is composed of about one third animal matter and two thirds mineral or earthy matter. The animal (organic) matter consists of bone cells, (osteocytes), blood vessels, connective tissues, and marrow. The mineral (inorganic) matter consists mainly of calcium phosphate and calcium carbonate.

Bone Forms or Shapes

There are several forms or shapes of bones found in the human body, namely:

- Flat bones, such as those in the skull
- Long bones, such as those in the legs and arms
- Short bones, such as those in the fingers and toes
- Irregular bones, such as the vertebrae (spine) (Fig. 5.22).

Shapes of Bones

A typical long bone has enlarged areas on the ends, called the **epiphysis** (e-**PIF**-i-sis), which articulate with other bones. The end surface of the epiphysis is covered with a layer of hyaline cartilage called **articular cartilage.** The articular cartilage provides a smooth shock-absorbing surface where two bones meet to form a joint. The shaft of the bone between the epiphysis is the **diaphysis** (die-**AF**-i-sis).

Except for articular cartilage, the bone is covered by the **periosteum** (per-ee-**OS**-tee-um). The periosteum is a fibrous membrane whose function is to protect the bone and serve as an attachment of all tendons and ligaments. It contains an abundance of nerves, blood, and lymph vessels and is essential to bone nutrition and repair. Beneath the periosteum the walls of the diaphysis are composed of **compact bone tissue**. Compact bone tissue forms the hard bone found in the shafts of long bones and along the outside of flat bones. This bone tissue is strong and rigid.

The inner portion of the bone is made up mostly of **spongy bone,** which consists of irregularly shaped spaces defined by thin, bony plates. This provides a lightweight yet surprisingly strong interior structure to the bones. The spongy bone tissue in the flat bones and at the ends of the long bones is filled with red bone marrow and is the site of production for blood cells. The **medullary cavity** is a hollow chamber formed in the shaft of long bones that is filled with yellow bone marrow.

Marrow is the connective tissue filling the cavities of bones. Its function is largely concerned with the formation of red and white blood cells. There are two types of bone marrow, **red** and **yellow** marrow. Red bone marrow functions in the production of red and white blood cells and platelets. It occupies nearly all the bone cavities of the newborn; however, in the adult it is found in the bone

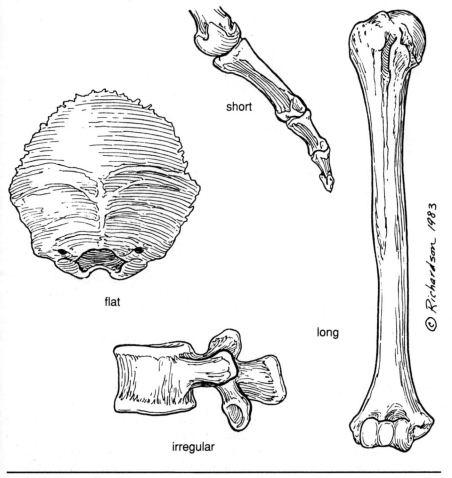

short

flat

irregular

long

© Richardson 1983

Fig. 5.22 Bone shapes.

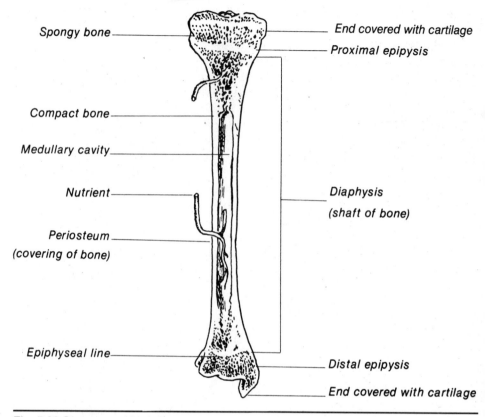

Spongy bone

End covered with cartilage

Proximal epipysis

Compact bone

Medullary cavity

Nutrient

Periosteum
(covering of bone)

Diaphysis
(shaft of bone)

Epiphyseal line

Distal epipysis

End covered with cartilage

Fig. 5.23 Structure of long bone.

spaces of the skull, ribs, sternum, vertebrae, and pelvis. Yellow marrow is the result of inactive blood-producing cells filling with fatty material and is located in the medullary cavities of the long bones (Fig. 5.23).

Bone Nutrition

Bone receives its nourishment through a highly organized system of blood vessels (capillaries) that make their way through the periosteum into the interior of bones. Bone marrow also aids in the nutrition of bone. For proper growth and hardening of bony structures, the diet should contain an adequate amount of calcium, phosphorous, and vitamin D.

▼ THE SKELETON AS A WHOLE

The skeleton is divided into two main parts; the **axial skeleton** and the **appendicular skeleton.** The bones of the skull, thorax, vertebral column and the hyoid bone comprise the axial skeleton (Fig. 5.24). The appendicular skeleton is made up of bones of the shoulder, upper extremities, hips, and lower extremities. The name **appen-**

dicular identifies these parts as appendages or extensions of the axis or axial skeleton.

In the human adult, the skeleton consists of 206 bones, distributed as follows:

The Axial Skeleton

Cranium (8)   Forms a protective structure for the
                                       brain

  frontal (1)
  parietal (2)
  occipital (1)
  temporal (2)
  sphenoid (1)
  ethmoid (1)

Face (14)   Forms the structure of the eyes, nose,
                                       cheeks, mouth, and jaws

  maxilla (2)
  palatine (2)
  zygomatic (2)
  lacrimal (2)
  nasal (2)
  vomer (1)
  interior nasal concha (2)
  mandible (1)

Ear (6)   Forms the internal structure of the
                                       ears

  malleus (2)
  incus (2)
  stapes (2)

Hyoid bone (1)   Supports the base of the tongue

Vertebrae (26)   Form the spinal column which
                                       supports the head and trunk and
                                       protects the spinal cord

                                       Provide attachment for the ribs

  cervical vertebra (7)
  thoracic vertebra (12)
  lumbar vertebra (5)
  sacrum (1)
  coccyx (1)

Thoracic Cage (25)

  ribs (costals) (24)   Form a protective cage for the lungs
                                       and heart
  sternum (1)   Serves as an attachment for the ribs at
                                       the front of the chest

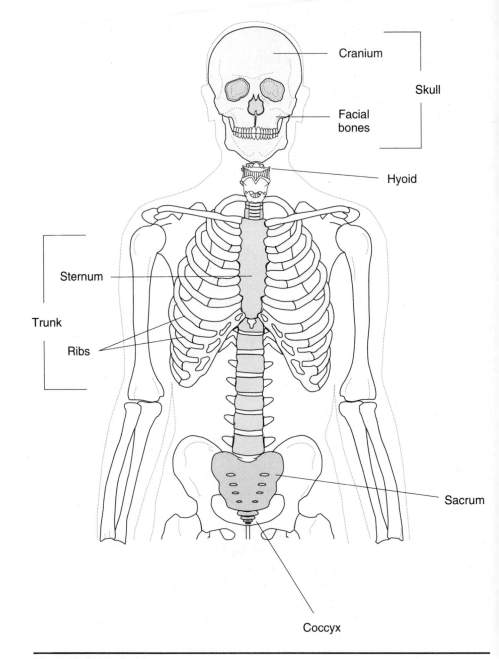

Fig. 5.24 *Axial skeleton.*

The Appendicular Skeleton
Upper extremities (64)

scapula (2)	ulna (2)	metacarpals (10)
clavicle (2)	radius (2)	phalanges (28)
humerus (2)	carpals (16)	

Lower extremities (62)

pelvic bones (fusion of three bones) (2)	patella (2)	tarsals (14)
	fibula (2)	metatarsals (10)
femur (2)	tibia (2)	phalanges (28)

The form or outline of the bones must be carefully followed and the limitations of the range of movements be considered when practicing massage therapy. Knowing the names of bones serves as a guide in recalling the names of related structures connected with the body part being massaged (Figs. 5.25 to 5.29, pages 91 to 96).

Joints

The bones of the skeleton are connected at different parts of their surfaces. Such connections are called **joints** or **articulations.**

Joints are classified according to the amount of motion they permit.

Synarthrotic (SIN-ar-thro-tic) **joints** such as those in the skull, are immovable.

Amphiarthrotic (AM-fee-ar-thro-tic) **joints** have limited motion. Examples are the symphysis pubis and sacroiliac joints.

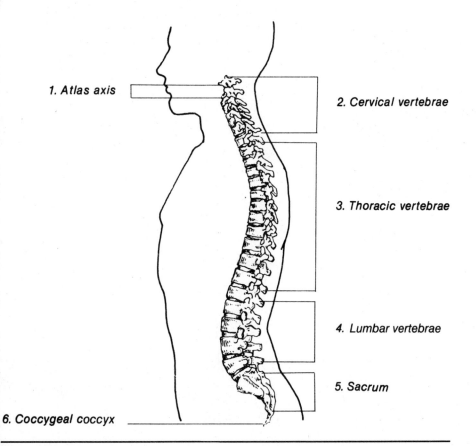

1. Atlas axis

2. Cervical vertebrae

3. Thoracic vertebrae

4. Lumbar vertebrae

5. Sacrum

6. Coccygeal coccyx

Fig. 5.25 Vertebral column.

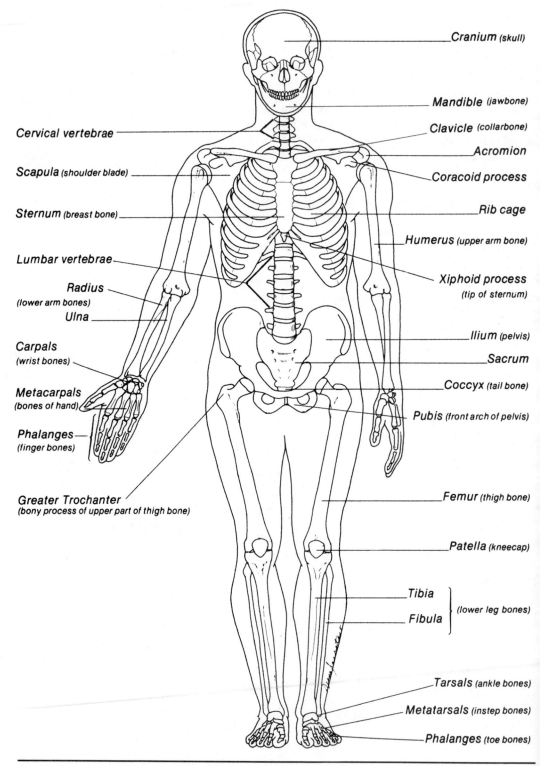

Cranium (skull)

Mandible (jawbone)

Cervical vertebrae

Clavicle (collarbone)

Acromion

Scapula (shoulder blade)

Coracoid process

Sternum (breast bone)

Rib cage

Humerus (upper arm bone)

Lumbar vertebrae

Xiphoid process
(tip of sternum)

Radius
(lower arm bones)

Ulna

Ilium (pelvis)

Carpals
(wrist bones)

Sacrum

Coccyx (tail bone)

Metacarpals
(bones of hand)

Pubis (front arch of pelvis)

Phalanges
(finger bones)

Greater Trochanter
(bony process of upper part of thigh bone)

Femur (thigh bone)

Patella (kneecap)

Tibia

Fibula

(lower leg bones)

Tarsals (ankle bones)

Metatarsals (instep bones)

Phalanges (toe bones)

Fig. 5.26 Skeletal system, anterior view.

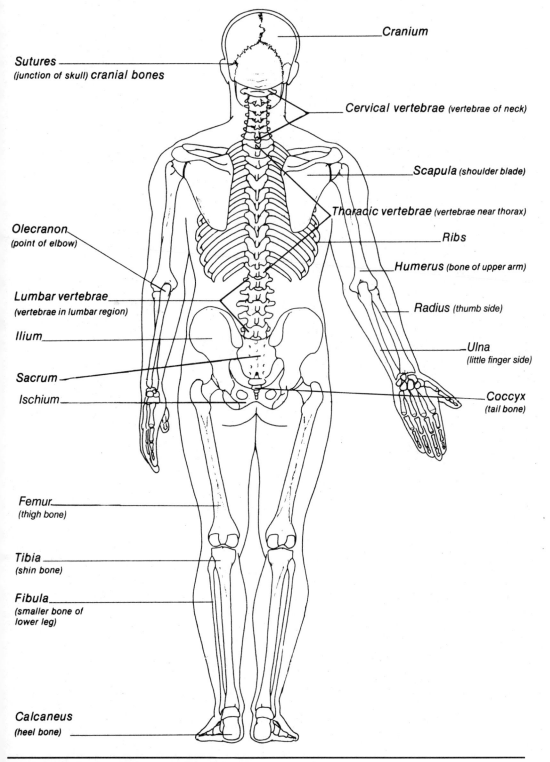

Cranium

Sutures
(junction of skull) *cranial bones*

Cervical vertebrae (vertebrae of neck)

Scapula (shoulder blade)

Thoracic vertebrae (vertebrae near thorax)

Olecranon
(point of elbow)

Ribs

Humerus (bone of upper arm)

Radius (thumb side)

Lumbar vertebrae
(vertebrae in lumbar region)

Ilium

Ulna
(little finger side)

Sacrum

Ischium

Coccyx
(tail bone)

Femur
(thigh bone)

Tibia
(shin bone)

Fibula
(smaller bone of
lower leg)

Calcaneus
(heel bone)

Fig. 5.27 Skeletal system, posterior view.

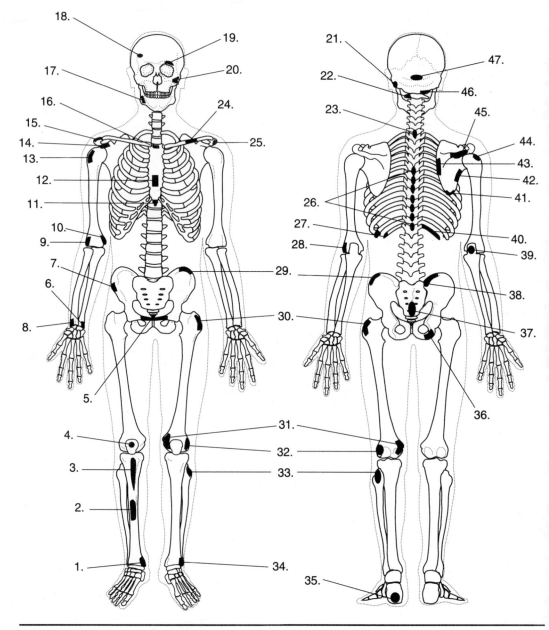

Fig. 5.28 Major bony landmarks on the body.

Labels for Bony Landmarks (Fig. 5.28)

1. Medial malleolus; Inside or medial "ankle bone."
2. Shaft of the tibia; "shin bone."
3. Tuberosity of the tibia; Prominent bump inferior to the patella.
4. Patella; "knee cap."
5. Pubic arch; The middle is the pubic symphysis, the lateral portion (about one and one-half inch to each side of the symphysis) is the ramus of the pubic bone.
6. Pisiform bone; first prominent bone in the heel of the hand.
7. ASIS; Anterior Superior Iliac Spine, pointed bone at the front of the hip.
8. Styloid process of the radius; Lateral process at the distal end of the radius.
9. Lateral epicondyle of the humerus; Bump on outside of elbow at the end of the humerus. Attachment of many of the wrist extensor muscles.
10. Medial epicondyle of the humerus; Bump on inside of elbow at the end of the humerus. Attachment of many of the wrist flexor muscles.
11. Xiphoid process; point at the inferior end of the sternum.
12. Sternum; Breastbone, between ribs on the front of the chest.
13. Bicipital groove; Groove between the greater and lesser tuberosity of the humerus, location of the tendon of the long head of the biceps muscle.
14. Corticoid process.
15. A.C. joint; Joint between the acromion process of the scapula and the clavicle.
16. Sternal notch; Hollow just superior to the sternum and between the heads of the clavicles.
17. Ramus of the mandible; Point at the angle of the jaw bone.
18. Frontal eminence; Slight rise between eyebrow and hairline.
19. Supra-orbital ridge; Upper part of eye socket, under the eyebrow.
20. Zygomatic bone; "Cheek bone."
21. Mastoid process; Bony point behind lower portion of the ear.
22. Transverse process of first cervical vertebra; Just below and deeper than mastoid process.
23. Spinous process of the seventh cervical vertebra; Topmost of the palpable spinous processes.
24. Clavicle; Collar bone.
25. Acromion process; Lateral point of the spine of the scapula.
26. Spinous processes of the vertebra.
27. Ends of the floating ribs.
28. Lateral epicondyle of the humerus; Refer to #9.
29. Crest of the ilium; The "hip bone," also called the iliac crest.
30. Greater trochanter of the femur; Bony knob at the top of the leg bone.
31. Medial epicondyle of the femur; Bony enlargement on the inside of the knee.
32. Lateral epicondyle of the femur; Bony enlargement of the outside of the knee.
33. Head of the fibula; Bump on the outside of the leg just below the knee.
34. Lateral malleolus; Outside or lateral ankle bone, distal end of the fibula.
35. Calcaneus; "Heel bone."
36. Ischial tuberosity; "Sit bone."
37. Distal end of sacrum; Prominent bone at upper end of gluteal crease. (Coccyx or tail bone is located deep between the buttocks.)
38. Posterior superior iliac spine; Bony prominence of the low back at the posterior end of the iliac crest.
39. Olecranon process; Point of the elbow at the proximal end of the ulna.
40. Twelfth rib; Last rib.
41. Inferior angle of the scapula; Lower tip of the scapula.
42. Axillary border of the scapula; Lateral edge of the scapula from the inferior angle to the "arm pit."
43. Vertebral border of the scapula; Medial edge of the scapula nearest the spine.
44. Greater tuberosity of the humerus; Proximal prominence of the humerus.
45. Spine of the scapula; Bony ridge on the posterior scapula.
46. Occipital ridge; Lowest palpable bony ridge on the posterior skull.
47. Occipital protuberance; Small bump on the posterior skull.

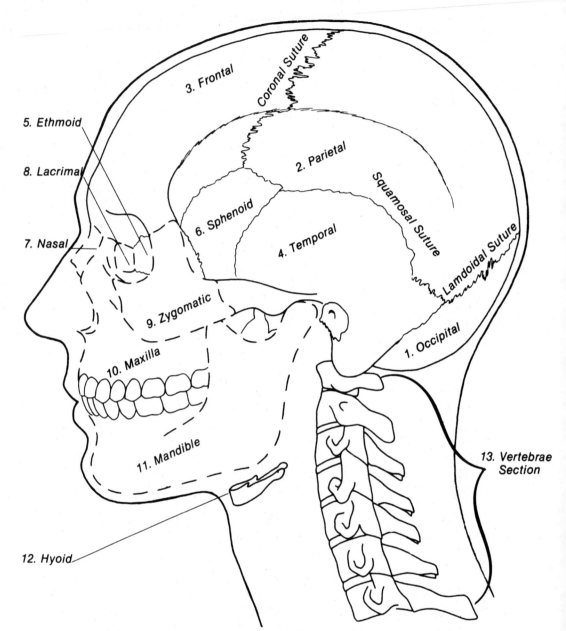

1. Base of skull. 2. Large part of upper and side walls of cranium. 3. Forms forehead, nasal cavity and orbits.
4. Forms sides and base of cranium. 5. Supports nasal cavity and helps to form orbits. 6. Forms anterior part of base of cranium. 7. A pair of bones forming the bridge of the nose. 8. A pair of bones making up part of the orbit at the inner angle of the eye. 9. Bone which helps to form the cheek. 10. Bone of the upper jaw. 11. Bone forming the lower jaw.
12. Bone located between the mandible and the larynx. 13. Smallest vertebrae of the spinal column; forming the framework of the neck.

Fig. 5.29 Cranium, neck, and face bones.

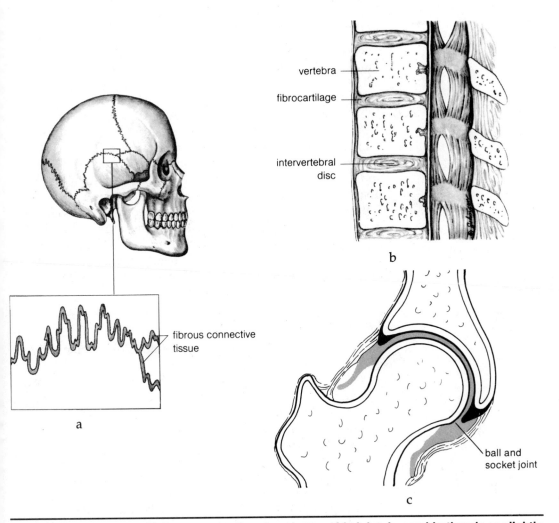

vertebra

fibrocartilage

intervertebral
disc

b

fibrous connective
tissue

a

ball and
socket joint

c

Fig. 5.30 Classification of joints: a. synarthrosis or immovable joint; b. amphiarthrosis or slightly movable joint; c. diarthrosis or freely movable joint.

Diarthrotic (DIE-ar-thro-tic) joints are freely movable. The articulating ends of the bones that meet at these joints are covered with hyaline cartilage called **articular cartilage.** A strong fibrous **joint capsule** surrounds the joint and is firmly attached to both bones. The outside of the capsule is constructed of ligaments that attach the bones, while the inner surface or the lining of the capsule consists of **synovial membrane,** which secretes **synovial fluid** that lubricates the joint surfaces. Diarthrotic joints have a variety of shapes and are capable of several kinds of movements: pivot movement, as in turning the head; saddle movement, as in the thumb; ball and socket movement, as in the hip; and hinge movement, as in the knees (Fig. 5.30).

Cartilage and Ligaments

Cartilage (also called **gristle**) is a firm and tough, elastic substance, similar to bone but without its mineral content. It serves the following purposes:

1. To cushion the bones at the joints
2. To prevent jarring between bones in motion, as in walking
3. To give shape to external features, such as the nose and ears.

Ligaments are bands or sheets of fibrous tissue that connect bone to bone and help to support the bones at the joints, as in the wrist and ankle. The **synovial fluid** is the lubricating fluid whose function is to prevent friction at the joints.

Bursae (BER-see), are fibrous sacks lined with synovial membrane and lubricated with synovial fluid. The purpose of the bursae is to function as a slippery cushion in areas where pressure is exerted, such as between bones and overlying muscle, tendons, or skin. Injury to bursae can cause inflammation and swelling and is called **bursitis** (ber-**SIGH**-tis).

Types of Movable Joints

The various types of movable joints found in the human body are classified as follows:

- Pivot joints have an extension on one bone that rotates in relation to the bone it articulates with, such as in the neck between the atlas and the axis.
- Hinge joints only move through one plane such as in the elbow, knees, and two distal joints of the fingers.
- Ball and socket joints permit the greatest range of movement. A bone with a ball-shaped head articulates in a socket-shaped depression such as in the hips and shoulders.
- Gliding joints have nearly flat surfaces that glide across one another, such as in the spine or hand.
- Saddle joints involve bones with concave articulating surfaces such as in the thumb (Fig. 5.31).

Words That Describe Bone Structures

Condyle (**KON**-dil)	A rounded knuckle-like prominence, usually at a point of articulation
Crest	A ridge
Foramen (**FO**-ray-mun)	A hole
Fossa (**FOS**-uh)	A depression or hollow
Head	A rounded articulating process at the end of a bone
Line	A less prominent ridge of a bone than a crest

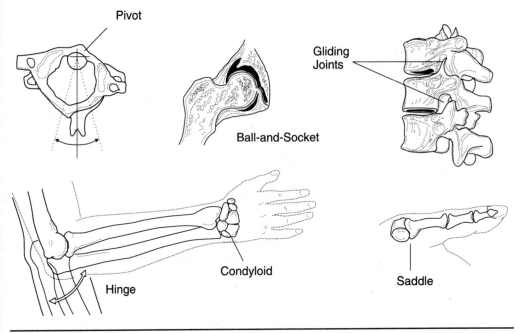

Fig. 5.31 Types of movable joints.

Meatus (**MEE**-ay-tus)	A tube-like passage
Process	A bone prominence or projection
Sinus or antrum	A cavity within a bone
Spine	A sharp, slender projection
Trochanter (**TRO**-kan-tur)	A large process for muscle attachment
Tubercle (**TEW**-bur-kul)	A small, rounded process
Tuberosity	A large, rounded process

Skeletal and Joint Disorders

Fractures

A fracture is a break or rupture in a bone. There are several types of fractures classified according to the severity of the injury: simple or closed, compound or open, greenstick, commuted, and spiral (Fig. 5.32).

Dislocation

A dislocation occurs when a bone is displaced within a joint. This is usually due to a traumatic injury that stretches or tears the ligaments around the joint and requires **reduction** (realigning the bones) and rest while the ligaments heal.

Sprain

A sprain is an injury to a joint that results in the stretching or tearing of the ligaments but is not severe enough to cause a dislocation. Sprains are classified according to their severity.

Class I sprain: There is a stretch in the ligament, some discomfort, and minimal loss of function.

Class II sprain: The ligament is torn with some loss of function. There may or may not be a discoloration due to tissue damage and bleeding.

Class III sprain: This is the most severe, where the ligaments are torn, and there is internal bleeding and severe loss of function.

All classes of strain cause swelling and require rest and support while the tissues heal.

Arthritis

Arthritis is an inflammatory condition of the joints often accompanied by pain and changes of bone structure. There are many kinds of arthritis; the most common are rheumatoid arthritis, osteoarthritis and gouty arthritis.

Rheumatoid arthritis is a chronic inflammatory disease and is the most serious and crippling form of arthritis. It is a systemic

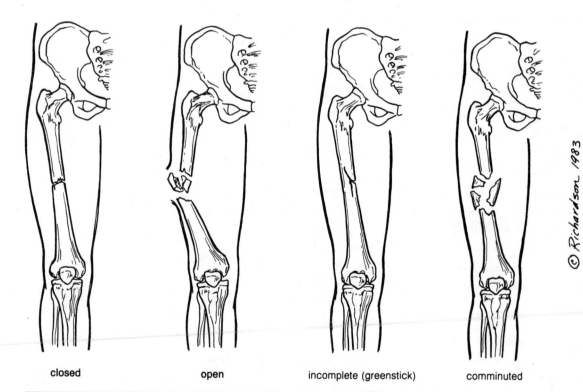

© Richardson 1983

closed   open   incomplete (greenstick)   comminuted

Fig. 5.32 Types of fractures.

disease, often affecting a number of joints, that first affects the synovial membrane that lines the joints. The joints become swollen, hot, and red. The inflammation causes the articular cartilage to erode and the joints to calcify and eventually become immovable. Its cause is unknown, but treatments are available to slow the progress and reduce the discomfort.

Osteoarthritis is a chronic disease that accompanies aging. It usually affects joints that have experienced a great deal of wear and tear or trauma. The knees, hips and spine are common sites for this degenerative disease, which erodes the articular cartilage and results in abnormal bone thickening and progressive joint immobility. There is no cure for osteoarthritis, but medication, exercise, and massage help to relieve pain and maintain mobility. Surgery is sometimes indicated to remove **spurs** or replace affected joints.

Gouty arthritis, also referred to as **gout,** usually affects the feet, especially the metatarsophalangeal joint of the large toe. High levels of uric acid in the blood produce uric acid crystals that deposit in the joint of the large toe resulting in pain and inflammation, and making walking difficult.

Bursitis

Bursitis is an inflammation of the small fluid-filled sacs (bursae) located near the joints that reduce the friction of overlying structures during movement. Bursitis is a painful condition that results from repeated irritation or trauma. The most common site of bursitis is the subdeltiod bursae of the shoulder, but it can develop at any joint. Pain from an acute case of bursitis drastically limits joint mobility. After the inflammation resides, mobility remains limited because of pain and contracted muscles. Mild exercise, range of motion, and massage are very effective for restoring mobility.

Osteoporosis

Osteoporosis (**OS**-tee-o-pour-**O**-sis) literally means increased porosity of the bones. Increased reabsorption of calcium into the blood stream causes a thinning of bone tissue, leaving it more fragile and prone to fracture (especially where bones are weight bearing, such as in the spine and pelvis). When severe osteoporosis is present, the massage therapist must be very cautious to prevent injury.

Spinal curvature

The healthy adult spine has a double S curve. The cervical and lumbar portions of the spine are concave and have a normal lordodic curve. The thoracic portion of the spine is convex and has a normal kyphotic curve. These curvatures provide flexibility, strength, shock absorption, and balance. Sometimes abnormal curvatures develop in the spine.

Scoliosis is a lateral curvature of the spine.

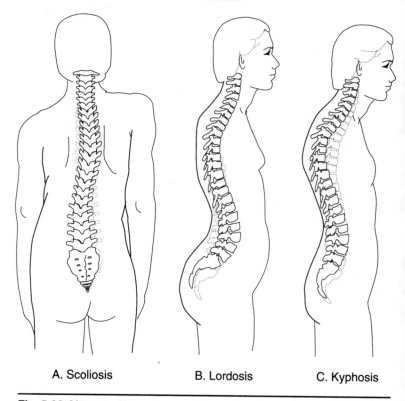

A. Scoliosis   B. Lordosis   C. Kyphosis

Fig. 5.33 Abnormal curvature of the spine: (a) scoliosis, (b) lordosis, (c) kyphosis.

Lordosis is an exaggerated concave curve most commonly found in the lumbar spine.

Kyphosis is an abnormally exaggerated convex curve of the thoracic spine. Occasionally the cervical spine will have a kyphotic curve.

These abnormal curves may develop because of a congenital defect, habitually poor body mechanics, or aging. Regardless of their origin, these abnormal conditions cause tremendous biomechanical stress on the body. Massage and exercise, while not offering a cure for these conditions, are very effective in counteracting the stress and pain associated with these abnormalities (Fig. 5.33).

▼ SECTION QUESTIONS FOR DISCUSSION AND REVIEW

1. What structures make up the skeletal system?
2. Name five functions of bones.
3. Name the organic and inorganic matter found in bones.
4. Name two types of bone tissue and indicate where they are found.
5. Which covering protects the bone?
6. How are the bones nourished?

7. Name the various shapes of bones found in the body. Give an example of each.
8. Name two kinds of marrow and where each is found.
9. What is the function of red bone marrow?
10. What are the two main parts of the skeleton?
11. Name three classifications of joints and differentiate between them.
12. Which structure cushions the bones at the joints?
13. Which structure connects and supports the bones at the joints?
14. Which fluid lubricates the joints?
15. About how many bones are found in the human body?
16. Why must the skeletal system be considered in the practice of massage therapy?
17. List five types of movable joints and give an example of each.
18. What is a fracture?
19. What is a sprain? Describe the difference between the three classes of sprains.
20. What is arthritis? What are the three most common types of arthritis?
21. What is osteoporosis? What precautions must be observed when massaging a person with osteoporosis?
22. Describe three abnormal curves of the spine.

REVIEW ▼

MATCHING TEST I

Insert the letter of the proper term in front of each definition.

_____	1. Upper arm	a. Femur
_____	2. Wrist bones	b. Tarsus
_____	3. Ankle bones	c. Scapula
_____	4. Toe or finger bones	d. Tibia
_____	5. Palm bones	e. Phalanges
_____	6. Spinal column	f. Vertebrae
_____	7. Collar bone	g. Carpals
_____	8. Shoulder blade	h. Metacarpals
_____	9. Thigh bone	i. Humerus
_____	10. Shin bone	j. Clavicle

TRUE OR FALSE TEST

Carefully read each statement and decide if it is true or false; draw a circle around the letter T or F.

1. T F   The hyoid bone supports the base of the ear.

2. T F   The metatarsus and metacarpus are different bones.

3. T F The patella forms the front of the knee joint.

4. T F The upper limbs are attached to the pelvis.

5. T F The clavicle and scapula serve as an attachment for the lower limbs.

6. T F The femur is found in the thigh.

7. T F The ulna and radius are found in the forearm.

8. T F The lungs and heart are found in the thorax.

9. T F The vertebrae provide an attachment for the ribs.

10. T F The pelvis is known as the kneecap.

MATCHING II

Match the definition in the right column with the correct word in the left column.

_____ **1.** crest   **a.** rounded prominence at a joint

_____ **2.** head   **b.** a hole

_____ **3.** spine   **c.** a ridge

_____ **4.** tuberosity   **d.** a hollow or depression

_____ **5.** foramen   **e.** articulating end of a bone

_____ **6.** condyle   **f.** less prominent ridge on a bone

_____ **7.** fossa   **g.** bony prominence

_____ **8.** trochanter   **h.** sharp, slender projection

_____ **9.** line   **i.** larger process for muscle attachment

_____ **10.** process   **j.** large rounded process

SYSTEM THREE: THE MUSCULAR SYSTEM

Muscle is the main organ of the muscular system. Muscle is made of specialized cells or fibers that have the unique ability to change their length. The action of muscle cells produce nearly all the movement of the body. Muscle movement is responsible for locomotion and all motor functions. It is responsible for breathing, moving fluids such as blood and urine, as well as moving food through the digestive system. By their action on the fascia, tendons, ligaments, and bones, muscles also provide the stability to support the body in an erect and weight-bearing posture.

The muscular system shapes and supports the skeleton. Depending on a person's physical development, muscles comprise approximately 40 to 60 percent of the total body weight. The skeletal muscular system consists of over 600 muscles, large and small.

Metabolically, muscles use the majority of food and oxygen we consume to produce energy for movement and heat that our body uses for heat regulation. The muscular system relies on the skeletal, nervous, digestive, and respiratory systems for its activities.

Our stiff, sore, achy, tired, tense, injured, and overworked muscles benefit immensely from massage. Massage has a profound effect not only on the common soft tissue dysfunctions of muscles such as strains and spasms, but also on the activity of the blood, lymph, and nerves associated with the muscles of the body. The effects and benefits of massage on muscles and other systems will be addressed in chapter 6.

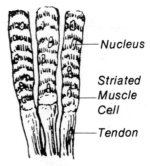

Nucleus

Striated Muscle Cell

Tendon

Striated (Striped) Muscle Cells

Types of Muscles

There are three types of muscular tissue:

1. Voluntary, striated, or skeletal muscles are controlled by the will.
2. Involuntary or nonstriated muscles function without the action of the will.
3. Heart or cardiac muscle is found only in the heart, and is not duplicated anywhere else in the body (Fig. 5.34).

Skeletal (striated) muscles or **voluntary** muscles are put into action by conscious will. They are governed by the central nervous system and appear striated or striped under the microscope. They make up the fleshy areas of the body, are attached to the skeleton, and are in turn fastened to the bones, skin, or other muscles.

Smooth (visceral or involuntary) muscles function without the action of the will. They are controlled by the autonomic nervous system. Smooth muscle consists of spindle-shaped non-striated cells that overlap at the ends, often forming fibrous bands, such as those found in the walls of the stomach, intestines, and blood vessels. Smooth muscle does not attach to bone, is rather slow acting, can maintain a contraction for a long time, and does not fatigue easily.

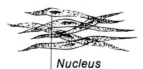

Nucleus

Non-Striated (Smooth) Muscle Cells

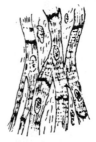

Cardiac (Heart) Muscle Cells

Fig. 5.34 Types of muscle.

Cardiac (heart) muscle is found in the heart. It is composed of cells that are as distinctly striated as the cells of skeletal muscle. Cardiac muscle cells are quadrangular, joined end to end, and grouped in bundles supported by a framework of connective tissue.

Characteristics of Muscles

The characteristics that enable muscles to perform their functions of contraction and movement are irritability, contractility, and elasticity. **Irritability** or excitability is the capacity of muscles to receive and react to stimuli, whether mechanical (massage), electrical (currents), thermal (heat), chemical (acid or salt), or impulses of nervous origin.

Muscle also has **contractility,** which is the ability to contract or shorten and thereby exert force. When cardiac muscle contracts, it reduces the area in the chambers of the heart, causing a pumping action. Likewise, when smooth muscle contracts, the diameter of the related organ decreases. If a skeletal muscle is attached to a pair of articulating bones, when the muscle contracts the attachments are drawn closer together, resulting in movement of the bones.

Muscle has **elasticity,** which is the ability to return to its original shape after being stretched. **Extensibility** is the ability of the muscle to stretch.

Structure of Skeletal Muscles

Massage primarily is performed on and affects the skeletal muscles. Therefore the remainder of this chapter will focus on skeletal muscles.

Skeletal muscles contain several tissues, including muscle tissue, blood and other fluids, nerve tissue, and a variety of connective tissues. The structure of skeletal muscle is unique with its arrangement of contractile fibers aligned and supported in such a way that by contracting, they exert a force on the bony levers of the skeleton, producing movement.

Muscle Tissue

Muscle tissue consists of contractile fibrous tissue arranged in separate parallel bundles (fascicles), which in turn consist of a number of parallel muscle fibers that are held in place by an extensive and intricate connective tissue system. The connective tissue supports the muscle fibers in such a way that when the fibers contract, a force is exerted on whatever structure the muscle is attached to, causing movement.

Muscle tissue is also supplied with a vast network of blood and lymph vessels and capillaries and nerve fibers. The blood supplies the oxygen and nutrients that are essential to carry on the intense metabolic activity as well as carry away the wastes and byproducts of muscle activity. The nerves not only provide the motor impulses to the muscles from the central nervous system (CNS) but also supply the CNS with a variety of sensory information from sensory nerve ends located in the skin, muscles, tendons, and joints.

Connective Tissue

Connective tissues form a continuous net-like framework throughout the body. Connective tissue consists largely of a fluid matrix (ground substance) and collagen fibers that support, bind, and connect the wide range of body structures. Depending on its consistency and the varying proportions of fluid to fibers, a wide array of connective tissues are formed. Some examples are the fluid intercellular environment, the superficial connective tissue just below the skin, the fascia of the muscles, the tendons and ligaments, the tough cartilage, and even bone.

The muscular system is a highly organized system of compartmentalized contractile fibrous tissues that work together to produce movement. The contractile tissue is organized and supported by an intricate network of connective tissue. Connective tissue organizes muscles into functional groups, surrounds each individual muscle, extends inward throughout the muscle creating muscle bundles, and eventually surrounds each muscle fiber. Connective tissue creates a supporting structure for the intricate network of blood vessels and nerves. The connective tissue projects beyond the ends of the muscle to become tendons or flat tendonous sheaths (aponeuroses) which connect the muscles to other structures. Aponeuroses may attach muscles to other muscles or the skin, while tendons intertwine with the fibrous coverings of bones (periosteum). Other connective tissue binds and supports the organs and structures in their proper place and forms anchors for lymph and blood vessels and nerves, holding them in their proper place among the organs, muscles, and bones.

The superficial fascia is situated just below the skin and covers the entire muscular system. The fascia penetrates to the bone (deep fascia), separating muscle groups and covering individual muscles, holding them in their relative positions and at the same time allowing them to move somewhat independently. The layer of connective tissue that closely covers an individual muscle is the **epimysium** (ep-i-**MI**-mee-um). The **perimysium** (**PAR**-a-**MI**-see-um) extends inward from the epimysium and separates the muscle into bundles of muscle fibers or **fascicles** (**FAS**-i-kls) Within the fascicle, each muscle fiber has a delicate connective tissue covering called the **endomysium.**

The connective tissue organizes the muscle fibers and connects the muscle to tendons, tendons to bones, and even bones to bone. Without this complicated system of connecting sheets, hinges, and ropes that transfers, the action of the muscle fibers to the levers of the skeleton, motion and postural stability would not be possible (Fig. 5.35).

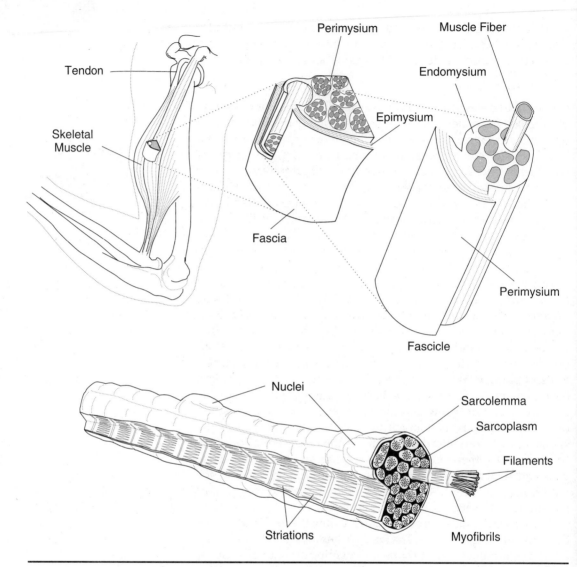

Fig. 5.35 Structure of skeletal muscle.

Muscle Cells or Fibers

The **muscle fiber** or muscle cell is the functional contractile unit of muscle tissue. The muscle cells are long, cylindrical, worm-like structures that usually extend the entire length of the muscle. The muscle cell has a connective tissue covering (endomysium (**EN**-do-**MI**-see-um)) that maintains its parallel position with other cells. Toward the end of the fiber the covering is continuous with tendon fibers that eventually become tendons and attach to the bones.

Beneath the layer of connective tissue is a cell membrane (sarcolemma). Within the **sarcolemma** (**SAR**-ko-**LEM**-uh) the muscle cell is highly organized. Each muscle fiber contains from several hundred to several thousand parallel **myofibrils** (my-o-**FYE**-brils) depending on the size of the muscle fiber. Each myofibril contains thousands of **actin** and **myosin** filaments. These filaments are arranged in organized segments (sarcomeres) that give skeletal muscle the striped or striated appearance for which it is named. It is the interaction between the actin and myosin filaments that gives muscle its unique contractile ability.

The thinner actin filaments are arranged so that one end of the filament is anchored in a transverse Z line while the other end extends outward into the sarcomere. The thicker myosin filaments are stacked to intersperse with the ends of the actin filaments. The Z lines seem to extend across the myofibril, aligning the sarcomeres and the filaments to cause the striated appearance.

When the muscle is at rest, the free ends of the actin slightly overlap. When the muscle is stretched, the actin filaments slide apart along the myosin filaments as the Z lines move further apart. When the muscle contracts, the actin filaments overlap, pulling the Z lines closer together until, under complete muscle contraction, the ends of the myosin are compressed into the transverse structures of the Z lines.

Extending inward from the cell membrane in the area of the transverse Z lines that anchor the actin filaments is an intricate system of **transverse tubules** that contain extracellular fluid. These tubules play an important role in the transmission of the stimulus of muscle contraction. The **sarcoplasmic reticulum** is a network of membranous channels within the muscle cell that surrounds each filament and is closely associated with the transverse tubules. When an impulse is transmitted through the cell membrane and transverse tubules, the sarcoplasmic reticulum releases calcium ions. In the high concentrations of calcium ions in the sarcoplasm (intercellular fluid of the muscle cells) the actin filaments are drawn across the myosin filaments resulting in the shortening of the cell and contraction of the muscle (Figs. 5.36 and 5.37).

Neuromuscular Connection

Nearly every muscle fiber is connected to a branch of a motor neuron. The site where the muscle fiber and nerve fiber meet is called the **neuromuscular junction** or **myoneural junction**. There are a few specialized muscle cells called **spindle cells** that have both sensory and motor functions and are essential for muscle control and coordination. (More about these later in this chapter.) Although a muscle fiber has only one nerve fiber connection, a motor nerve may have many branches and therefore connect to several muscle fibers. A motor neuron and all the muscle fibers that it controls constitute a **motor unit.**. When a motor nerve transmits a stimulus, ALL the muscle fibers connected by its many branches contract simultaneously. Generally, in small muscles that provide intricate movements (i.e., muscles that control speech or eye

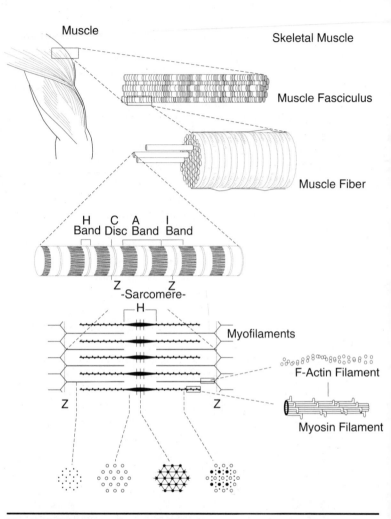

Fig. 5.36 Structure of muscle fibers.

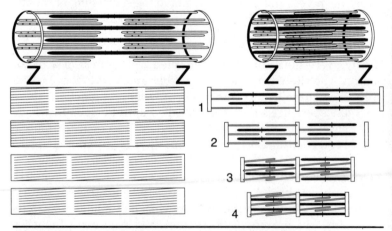

Fig. 5.37 Model of muscle contraction. As actin filaments are pulled across myosin fila-ments, the Z lines are pulled closer together and the overall length of the cell shortens.

movement) the motor units may include as few as two or three muscle fibers, whereas larger muscles that provide less intricate movements (i.e., the vastus muscles or gastrocnemeus) may have several hundred muscle fibers in a single motor unit. Motor units tend to overlap with the muscle fibers of adjacent motor units interspersed among one another. This allows muscle units to support each other and provides for smooth, integrated movement. (Fig. 5.38)

Skeletal Muscle Contraction

Muscle has the unique ability to change chemical energy into mechanical energy or movement. When a nerve impulse travels from the brain or spinal cord through the motor neuron and reaches the end of the nerve fiber, a chemical **neurotransmitter** called **acetylcholine** (as-e-til-**KOE**-leen) is released and bridges the gap between the nerve end and muscle fiber. The acetylcholine affects the muscle fiber membrane and causes an impulse much like a nerve impulse that immediately travels the length of and throughout the muscle fiber. The impulse is transmitted through the

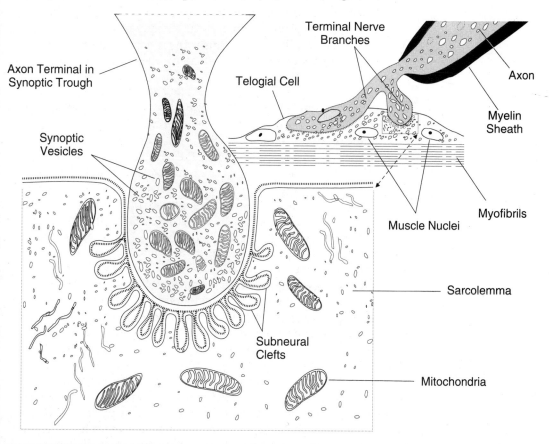

Fig. 5.38 Myoneural junction.

transverse tubules of the muscle fiber, where it contacts the sarco-plasmic reticulum, causing it to release a flood of calcium ions. The calcium ions bond to the actin filaments, which initiates a bridging action and causes the actin and myosin filaments to merge, short-ening the fiber and contracting the muscle. The sliding mechanism between the actin and myosin filaments involves complex chemi-cal, mechanical, and molecular activity that is beyond the scope of this text. All of this mechanical activity requires energy.

The Energy Source for Muscle Activity

The energy for muscle contraction comes from the breakdown of the **adenosine triphosphate (ATP)** molecule. When a muscle con-tracts, an enzyme causes one of the phosphates to split from the ATP molecule, releasing energy and forming **adenosine diphos-phate (ADP)**. There is only enough ATP stored in the muscle cells to sustain a contraction for a few seconds. Fortunately, within a fraction of a second ADP is reconstituted into ATP in one of several ways.

Another cellular substance that has a high-energy phosphate bond is **creatine phosphate**. Even though the energy stored in creatine phosphate cannot be used directly by the muscle, when it contacts ADP, the energy causes the rebonding of the phosphate ion, producing ATP. Unfortunately, the combined amounts of creatine phosphate and ATP available in the cell are still sufficient to sustain a contraction for only a few seconds.

Most of the energy to reconstitute ADP is the result of cellular respiration. **Aerobic cellular respiration** takes place in the cells' mitochondria. Aerobic respiration is responsible for the majority of the sustained energy supply for the constant replenishing of ATP. Most of the food we eat, by the time it goes through the digestive process and is transported to the cells, has been converted to glucose. As the glucose is transported through the cell to the mitochondria, it is converted to pyruvic acid. In the mitochondria a complex metabolic process known as the Krebs cycle or the citric acid cycle takes place, resulting in the production of carbon dioxide, water, and energy in the form of heat and the synthesis of ATP.

The oxygen required to carry on aerobic respiration is carried to the cells from the lungs in the blood by the red blood cells. The amount of oxygen taken in and the rate that it can be delivered to the mitochondria of the cells determines how much ATP can be reconstituted and therefore how much a muscle can do.

When the oxygen available for aerobic respiration is depleted, anaerobic respiration takes place. In **Anaerobic respiration** (in the absence of oxygen), glucose is broken down, releasing enough energy to synthesize some ATP and producing pyruvic acid, which is converted to lactic acid. The lactic acid is carried by the blood stream to the liver, where it is converted back to glucose (ATP is required for this conversion).

During light or moderate activity, the lungs and circulatory system are able to supply the skeletal muscles adequate amounts of oxygen to carry on aerobic respiration. However, after just a few minutes of strenuous output, the pulse and respiration rate increase. As the strenuous activity continues, the circulatory and respiratory systems cannot supply enough oxygen to the muscles, which forces them to rely on the less efficient anaerobic respiration. Anaerobic respiration produces pyruvic and then lactic acid. As lactic acid accumulates, the person develops **oxygen debt.** After the strenuous activity ceases, the heavy breathing and accelerated heart rate continue until the oxygen debt is paid off, and then normal breathing and pulse resume. It is probably this build-up of lactic acid that accounts for the burning sensation in straining muscles and the next-day muscle aches from straining muscles beyond their aerobic abilities.

Muscle Fatigue

If rapid or prolonged muscle contractions continue to the point that oxygen debt becomes extreme, the muscle will cease to respond. This condition is **muscle fatigue.** Muscle fatigue results either because the circulation of blood cannot keep pace with the demand for oxygen or because the waste products accumulate faster than they can be removed, affecting the muscle's ability to respond to nerve impulses.

Muscle Tone

Muscle tone is a type of muscle contraction that is present in healthy muscles even when they are at rest. A muscle possesses tone if it is firm and responds promptly to stimulation under normal conditions. Lack of tone is evidenced by a condition of flaccidness. Exercise and massage help to improve muscle tone.

Muscle Insertion and Origin

As explained earlier, the connective tissue surrounding the muscle fibers extends beyond the ends of the fibers to become the fibrous, rather inelastic, tendons that anchor the ends of the muscle. The arrangement of muscle fibers and tendons varies according to muscle function and location. Some muscles form cord-like tendons at either end of the muscle belly such as the biceps. Other muscles have their attachments spread over a broad area such as the deltoid and trapezius.

The structures to which the tendons attach determine the action that the contracting muscles produce. Skeletal muscles, as their name implies, have at least one end of the muscle that is attached to bone. The end of the muscle is anchored to a relatively immovable section of the skeleton called the **origin** of the muscle. The **origin** of a muscle is generally located more proximal or nearer the center of the body.

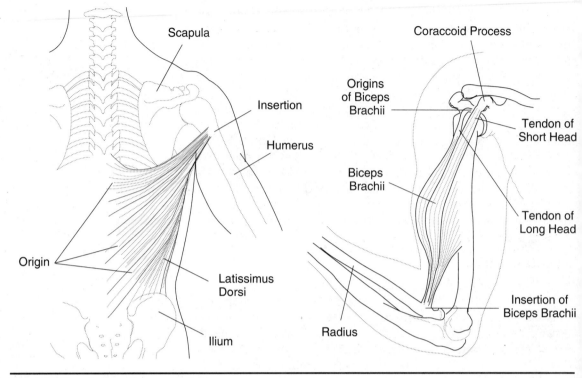

Fig. 5.39 Muscle insertion and origin.

The other end of the muscle attaches either to a bone, the deeper structures of the skin or other muscles and creates the action of the structure. The term applied to the more mobile attachment is the **insertion** of the muscle. The **insertion** of a muscle is generally attached to the more distal aspect of an appendage. In some movements, the roles of insertion and origin of a muscle can be reversed. The action of a muscle contraction can be derived from the knowledge of its insertion and origin (Fig. 5.39).

Isometric and Isotonic Contractions

When a muscle contracts and the ends of the muscle do not move or the body part that the muscle affects does not move, the contraction is an **isometric** contraction. When a person strains to move a heavy object that does not budge, the muscle effort is isometric. In the muscles that stabilize our bodies in an upright posture, most contractions are continuous and isometric.

When a muscle contracts and the distance between the ends of the muscle changes, it is an **isotonic** contraction. When the distance between the ends of a contracting muscle decreases, the isotonic contraction is said to be **concentric.** When the distance between the ends of a contracting muscle increases, the isotonic contraction is said to be **eccentric.** When you do a push-up, as you push up, the loaded muscles are shortening and the contraction is concentric. As you lower yourself to the floor, the loaded muscles are getting longer and the contraction is eccentric. In both directions, the contractions are isotonic.

Muscle Interaction

In some ways the muscular system could be considered as one continuous muscle that covers the entire body and is divided into various chambers by an intricate system of connective tissue. This muscle is controlled by a vast network of neuromuscular units that coordinate their activities through the central nervous system to produce smooth, coordinated, graceful movements.

The classic approach has been to study the effect of the individual muscles on joint action. But this is not physiologic. Normal muscle action is the patterned response of groups of muscles. Muscles have anatomic individuality, but they do not have functional individuality. (See K. Little, Toward More Effective Manipulative Management of Chronic Myofascial Strain and Stress Syndromes, in *The Journal of the American Osteopathic Association*, 68:675,685, March 1969.)

Individual muscles, because of their specific attachments when contracted, result in a specific action. However, muscles never work alone. When an isolated and specific action occurs, the muscle responsible for that action is the **prime mover** (sometimes referred to as the **agonist**). When the prime mover contracts, there is a muscle that causes the opposite action. That opposing muscle is referred to as the **antagonist.** For instance, when the elbow is flexed with the hand in the supine position, the prime mover is the biceps. The opposite action would be to extend the arm. The muscle responsible for arm extension is the triceps, so the antagonist is the triceps. It is clear from this example that when the prime mover contracts and shortens, the antagonist must extend. Most movement, however, is not that simple and even when considering just one joint, several muscles may be involved. Muscles that assist the prime mover are called **synergists** (SIN-er-jists).

In observing the dynamics of movement, there are three components of motion: flexion/extension, abduction/adduction, and rotation. Most joints in the body function in at least two of these components, and many articulations involve all three. A muscle that acts across a joint will have a primary function in one of the three components of motion, but the same muscle may have a secondary or even a tertiary action depending on the mobility of the joint. For instance, in Fig. 5.40, the primary function of the biceps is to flex the elbow; however, a secondary function of the biceps is to assist in supination of the forearm and a minor, tertiary function of the short head of the biceps is to flex the shoulder (Figs. 5.40 to 5.44, pages 116 to 119).

Table 5.2, which begins on page 124, gives a comprehensive view of the location, and action, of muscles.

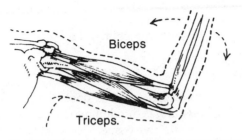

Antagonist muscles. During elbow flexion, the triceps relax while the biceps contract. For extension, the biceps relax while the triceps contract.

Biceps

Triceps.

Fig. 5.40 Muscle interaction.

ACTION		MOVEMENT

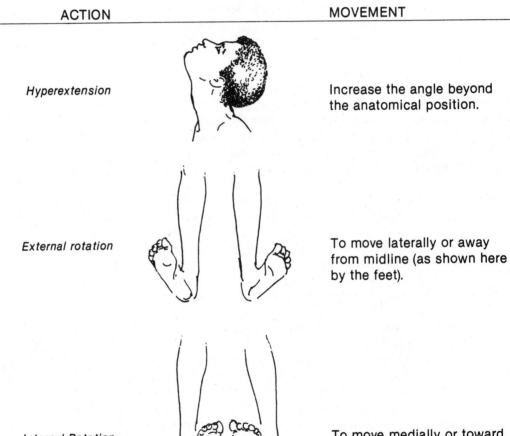

Hyperextension — Increase the angle beyond the anatomical position.

External rotation — To move laterally or away from midline (as shown here by the feet).

Internal Rotation — To move medially or toward the midline.

Fig. 5.41 Motion in diarthrotic joints.

ACTION	MOVEMENT

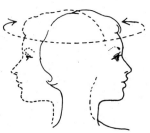

Rotation — To revolve a part about the longitudinal axis.

Dorsiflexion — To move the foot upward.

Eversion — To turn the plantar surface away from the midline.

Inversion — To turn the plantar surface toward the midline.

Plantar flexion — To move the foot downward (extension).

Fig. 5.42 Motion in diarthrotic joints, continued.

ACTION	MOVEMENT

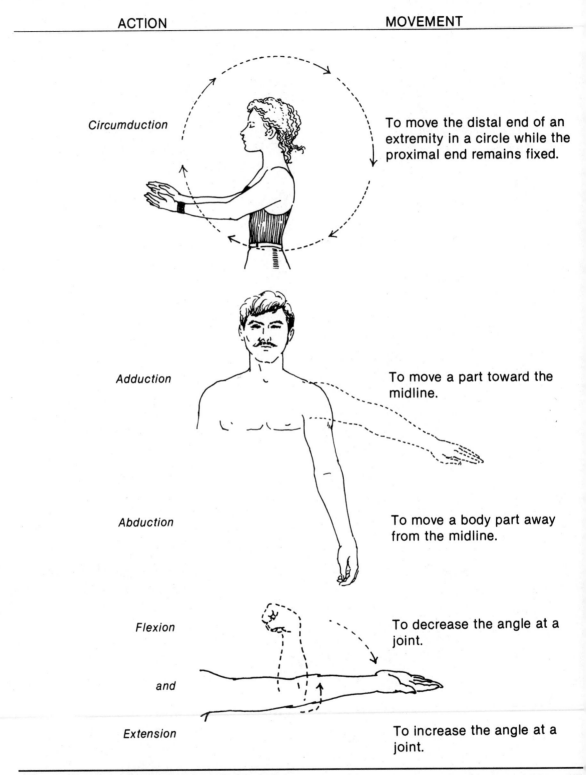

Circumduction

To move the distal end of an extremity in a circle while the proximal end remains fixed.

Adduction

To move a part toward the midline.

Abduction

To move a body part away from the midline.

Flexion

To decrease the angle at a joint.

and

Extension

To increase the angle at a joint.

Fig. 5.43 Motion in diarthrotic joints, continued.

ACTION	MOVEMENT

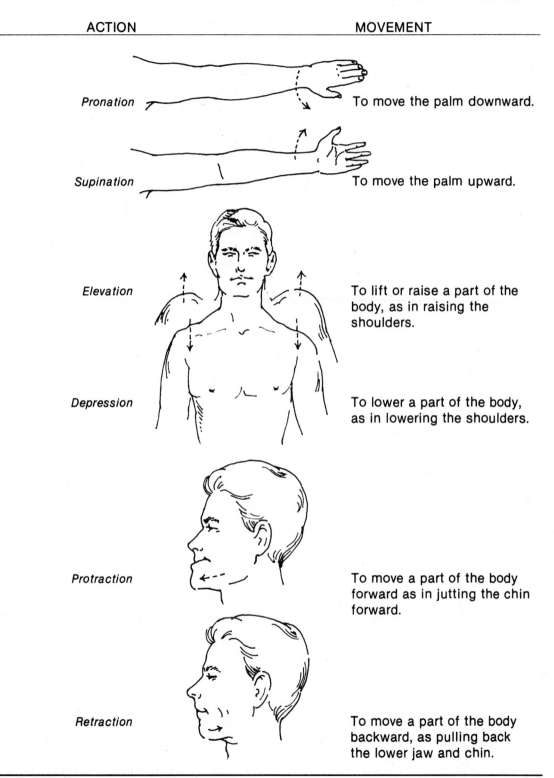

Pronation — To move the palm downward.

Supination — To move the palm upward.

Elevation — To lift or raise a part of the body, as in raising the shoulders.

Depression — To lower a part of the body, as in lowering the shoulders.

Protraction — To move a part of the body forward as in jutting the chin forward.

Retraction — To move a part of the body backward, as pulling back the lower jaw and chin.

Fig. 5.44 Motion in diarthrotic joints, continued.

Terms to Remember

A review of the following words will be helpful in understanding the meaning of technical terms when studying the muscular system (Figs. 5.45 and 5.46, pages 121 to 122).

Anterior: Before, or in front of
Posterior: Behind, or in back of
Superior: Situated above
Inferior: Situated lower
Anguli: At an angle
Levator: That which lifts
Dorsal: Behind, or in back of
Medial: Pertaining to the middle or center
Dilator: That which expands or enlarges
Depressor: That which presses or draws down
Proximal: Nearer to the center or medial line
Distal: Farther from the center or medial line

Common Dysfunctions and Diseases of the Muscular System

Muscle Spasms

Muscle spasms are the most common muscle dysfunction. A spasm is a sudden involuntary contraction of a muscle or a group of muscles that usually occurs when the nerve(s) supplying the muscle(s) is irritated. Spasms vary both in duration and intensity and may affect any muscle tissue (voluntary, involuntary, or cardiac). Some common examples of muscle spasms are hiccups, tics and twitches in the face, torticollis (**TOR**-ti-koll-is), charley-horses, convulsions, and muscle "splinting" associated with injuries. Spasms may occur as a result of injury, disease, or emotional stress (stuttering). Usually spasms cease when their cause is corrected.

Muscle Strains

Muscle strains (also called torn or pulled muscles) are the most common injury to muscle. There are three degrees or grades of muscle strain.

Grade I is an overstretching of a few of the muscle fibers with a minimal tearing of the fibers. There is some pain but no loss of function and no palpable or visual indications.

Grade II involves a partial tear of between 10 and 50 percent of the muscle fibers. There is considerable pain and some loss of function. There is a palpable thickening of the muscle tissue and may be some tissue bleeding.

Grade III is the most severe injury with between 50 and 100 percent muscle tearing. There is a palpable depression and/or bunching of the muscle with severe pain and total or near total loss of muscle function.

Muscle strains may occur in different sites in the muscle. The majority of the strains (80 percent) occur in the muscle belly or at the

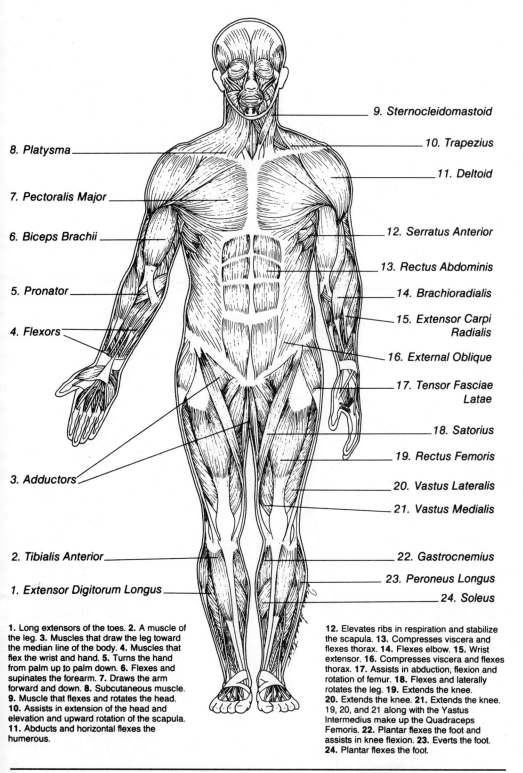

9. Sternocleidomastoid

10. Trapezius

11. Deltoid

8. Platysma

7. Pectoralis Major

6. Biceps Brachii

12. Serratus Anterior

13. Rectus Abdominis

14. Brachioradialis

5. Pronator

15. Extensor Carpi Radialis

4. Flexors

16. External Oblique

17. Tensor Fasciae Latae

18. Satorius

19. Rectus Femoris

20. Vastus Lateralis

21. Vastus Medialis

3. Adductors

2. Tibialis Anterior

22. Gastrocnemius

23. Peroneus Longus

1. Extensor Digitorum Longus

24. Soleus

1. Long extensors of the toes. 2. A muscle of the leg. 3. Muscles that draw the leg toward the median line of the body. 4. Muscles that flex the wrist and hand. 5. Turns the hand from palm up to palm down. 6. Flexes and supinates the forearm. 7. Draws the arm forward and down. 8. Subcutaneous muscle. 9. Muscle that flexes and rotates the head. 10. Assists in extension of the head and elevation and upward rotation of the scapula. 11. Abducts and horizontal flexes the humerous.

12. Elevates ribs in respiration and stabilize the scapula. 13. Compresses viscera and flexes thorax. 14. Flexes elbow. 15. Wrist extensor. 16. Compresses viscera and flexes thorax. 17. Assists in abduction, flexion and rotation of femur. 18. Flexes and laterally rotates the leg. 19. Extends the knee. 20. Extends the knee. 21. Extends the knee. 19, 20, and 21 along with the Yastus Intermedius make up the Quadraceps Femoris. 22. Plantar flexes the foot and assists in knee flexion. 23. Everts the foot. 24. Plantar flexes the foot.

Fig. 5.45 The muscular system, anterior view.

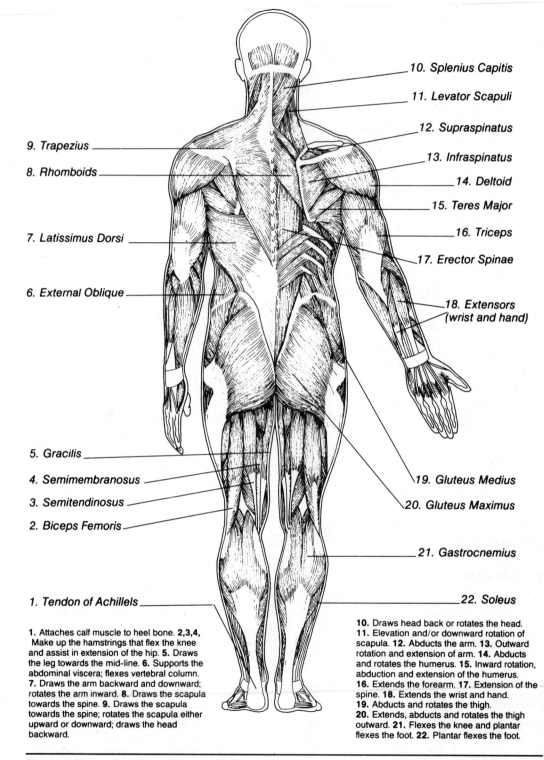

10. Splenius Capitis

11. Levator Scapuli

12. Supraspinatus

13. Infraspinatus

14. Deltoid

15. Teres Major

16. Triceps

17. Erector Spinae

18. Extensors (wrist and hand)

9. Trapezius

8. Rhomboids

7. Latissimus Dorsi

6. External Oblique

5. Gracilis

4. Semimembranosus

3. Semitendinosus

2. Biceps Femoris

1. Tendon of Achillels

19. Gluteus Medius

20. Gluteus Maximus

21. Gastrocnemius

22. Soleus

1. Attaches calf muscle to heel bone. 2,3,4, Make up the hamstrings that flex the knee and assist in extension of the hip. 5. Draws the leg towards the mid-line. 6. Supports the abdominal viscera; flexes vertebral column. 7. Draws the arm backward and downward; rotates the arm inward. 8. Draws the scapula towards the spine. 9. Draws the scapula towards the spine; rotates the scapula either upward or downward; draws the head backward.

10. Draws head back or rotates the head. 11. Elevation and/or downward rotation of scapula. 12. Abducts the arm. 13. Outward rotation and extension of arm. 14. Abducts and rotates the humerus. 15. Inward rotation, abduction and extension of the humerus. 16. Extends the forearm. 17. Extension of the spine. 18. Extends the wrist and hand. 19. Abducts and rotates the thigh. 20. Extends, abducts and rotates the thigh outward. 21. Flexes the knee and plantar flexes the foot. 22. Plantar flexes the foot.

Fig. 5.46 The muscular system, posterior view.

junction between the muscle and the tendon (musculo-tendinous junction). Other less common sites are at the insertion or the origin or in the tendon of the muscle.

Hypertrophy

Muscle hypertrophy is an enlargement of the breadth of a muscle as a result of repeated forceful muscle activity. Most of the hypertrophy is due to the increase in the size of the muscle fibers rather than an increase in the number of muscle fibers. As a result of the increased size, the power of the muscle increases as well as the metabolic support system (i.e., increased blood supply, sarcoplasm, ATP, mitochondria, etc.). It is also likely that the number of actin/myosin filaments and number of fibrils in the muscle fiber increase; however, this has not been substantiated.

Athrophy

Muscle atrophy is the reverse of hypertrophy and is the result of muscle disuse. If a muscle cannot be contracted or is only contracted very weakly, the muscle tissue will rapidly degenerate and begin to waste away. The number and size of the capillaries supplying the muscle decrease as well as the sarcoplasm and its constituents (mitochondria, sarcoplasmic reticulum, glycogen, ATP, etc.). The size of the fibrils and the actin/myosin filaments is reduced as is the power of the muscle. If the nerve supply to the muscle is interfered with, paralysis results and muscle atrophy progresses rapidly. If atrophy continues over an extended period of time, the contractile tissue will continue to degenerate until it is replaced with connective tissue and rehabilitation becomes all but impossible.

Fibrosis and Myofibrositis

Fibrosis refers to the formation of fibrous tissue.

Myofibrosis is the process where muscle tissue is being replaced by fibrous connective tissue. Fibrositis and myofibrositis are inflammatory conditions of the white fibrous tissue, especially the fascial tissues of the muscular system, that cause pain and stiffness. These conditions are often referred to as muscular rheumatism.

Dystrophy

Muscular dystrophy refers to a group of related diseases that seem to be genetically inherited and that cause a progressive degeneration of the voluntary muscular system. With muscular dystrophy, the contractile fibers of the muscles are gradually replaced by fat and connective tissue until those muscles become virtually useless. All the visible effects of muscular dystrophy seem to be in the muscles. It rarely causes pain, and the intellect is not affected. Exercise and massage are helpful in prolonging muscular ability and maintaining flexibility.

▼ TABLE 5.2 LOCATION AND ACTION OF MUSCLES

MUSCLES OF THE UPPER EXTREMITIES
Muscles that Act on and Support the Scapula

MUSCLE	ORIGIN	INSERTION	ACTION	INNERVATION	PALPATION
Trapezius					
Upper	Occiput and ligamentum nuchae of cervical spine	Lateral one third of clavicle and acromian	Elevation and upward rotation of scapula	Cranial XI, Spinal Accessory	From below occiput to acromion
Middle	Spinous process C7–T5	Spine of the scapula	Pulls scapula medially	C3–4	From spinous process T1–5 to acromian
Lower	Spinous process T5–T12	Spine of the scapula	Depression and upward rotation of scapula	C3–4	From spinous process T5–12 to spine of scapula
Rhomboid					
Major	Spinous process T2–5	Lower two thirds of vertebral border of scapula	Retracts and rotates scapula downward	C5, Dorsal scapular	Under Trapezius along vertebral border of scapula
Minor	Spinous process C7–T1	Vertebral border at root of the spine of the scapula	Same as Rhomboid major	C5, Dorsal scapular	Just superior to Rhomboid major, hard to palpate
Levator Scapulae	Transverse process C1-4	Superior third of vertebral border of scapula	Elevation of scapula and moves neck laterally	C3-5	Anterior to upper Trapezius, hard to palpate
Pectoralis Minor	Anterior ribs 3, 4, 5	Coracoid process	Forward rotation and depression of scapula	C8–T1, Medial pectoral	Under Pectoralis major in axillary space, hard to palpate
Serratus Anterior	Anterior ribs 1–8	Anterior aspect of vertebral border of scapula	Stabilization, upward rotation and protraction of the scapula	C5, 6, 7, Posterior thoracic	Lateral ribs below axilla

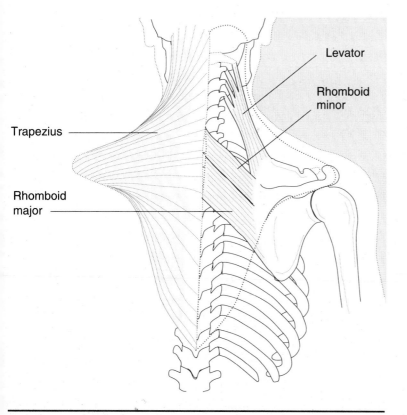

Fig. T5-2.1 Posterior upper thorax; Trapezius m. One side is cut away to show rhomboids and levator.

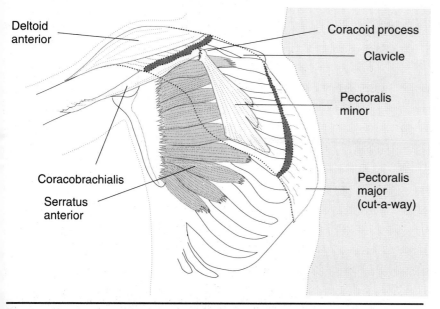

Fig. T5-2.2 Anterior lateral upper thorax (pectoralis major cut away); serratus anterior and pectoralis minor.

MUSCLES OF THE UPPER EXTREMITIES *(continued)*

Muscles that Act on the Upper Arm

MUSCLE	ORIGIN	INSERTION	ACTION	INNERVATION	PALPATION
Pectoralis Major					
Clavicular	Medial half of clavicle, clavicular head	Lateral ridge of bicipital groove distal to Pectoralis major sternal insertion	Adduction, horizontal adduction, medial rotation and flexion of humerus	C5, 6, 7, Lateral pectoral	Anterior of axilla
Sternal	Sternum, costal cartilage of ribs 1–6	Lateral ridge of bicipital groove proximal to Pectoralis major clavicular insertion	Same as Clavicular plus extension of humerus from flexed position	C8, T1, Lateral and medial pectoral	Anterior of axilla
Coracobrachialis	Coracoid process of scapula	Middle of medial humerus	Flexion and adduction of humerus	C6, 7, Musculocutaneous	Hard to palpate
Deltoid					
Anterior	Lateral third of clavicle	Deltoid tuberosity of humerus	Flexion, horizontal adduction, medial rotation	C5, 6 Axillary nerve	This is the rounded shoulder muscle. The anterior in front, the middle lateral to and the posterior in the back of the shoulder joint.
Middle	Acromion and lateral spine of the scapula	Deltoid tuberosity of humerus	Abduction to 90 degrees	C5, 6 Axillary nerve	
Posterior	Lower lip of the spine of the scapula	Deltoid tuberosity of humerus	Extension, horizontal abduction, lateral rotation	C5, 6 Axillary nerve	
Supraspinatus	Supraspinous fossa of scapula	Top of greater tubricle of the humerus	Initiates abduction of the humerus	C5, Suprascapular nerve	Above spine of scapula near acromian
Infraspinatus	Infraspinous fossa of scapula	Greater tubricle of humerus	Lateral rotation of humerus	C5, 6, Suprascapular nerve	Below the spine of the scapula
Subscapularis	Anterior surface of the scapula	Lesser tubricle of the humerus	Medial rotation of humerus	C6, 7 Subscapular nerve	Hard to palpate
Teres Minor	Upper axillary border of scapula	Greater tubricle of humerus	Lateral rotation of humerus	C5, Axillary nerve	Below Posterior deltoid and above Teres major
Teres Major	Lateral border, inferior angle of scapula	Medial ridge of bicipital groove of humerus	Extension, adduction, medial rotation of humerus	C6, 7, Subscapular nerve	With Latissimus dorsi forms posterior border of axilla
Latissimus Dorsi	Thoracolumbar aponerosis from T7 to illiac crest, lower ribs, inferior angle of scapula	Bicipital groove of humerus	Extension, adduction, medial rotation of humerus	C6, 7, 8, Thoracodorsal nerve	Large muscle forming posterior axilla and extending down toward posterior ribs

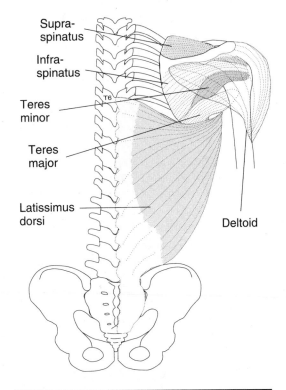

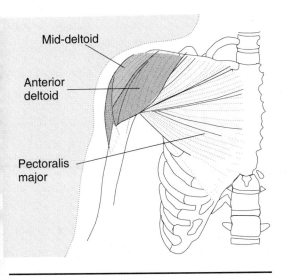

Fig. T5-2.3 Anterior shoulder; pectoralis major, anterior and mid deltoid, overlay or cut away to show coricobrachialis.

Fig. T5-2.4 Posterior shoulder; supra and infraspinatus, posterior deltoid, teres major and minor, latissimus dorsi.

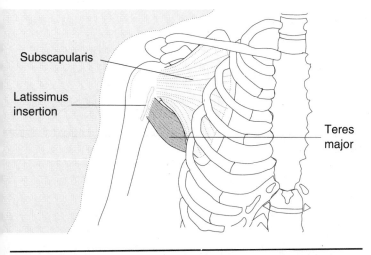

Fig. T5-2.5 Anterior shoulder cutaway shows subscapularis muscle and teres major and latissimus dorsi insertion.

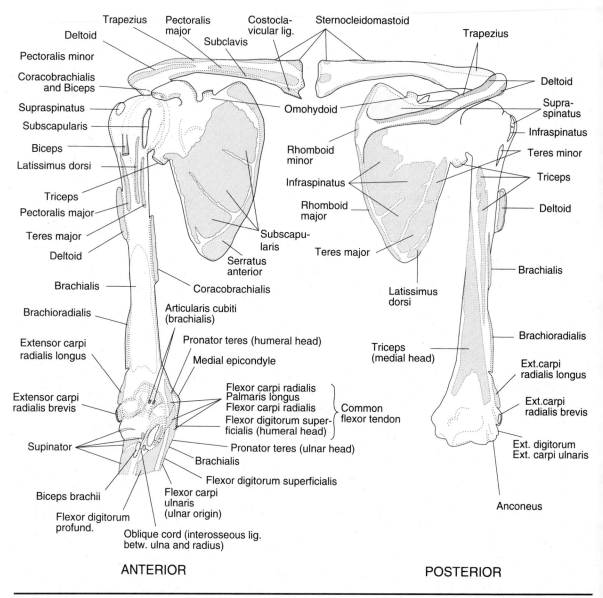

Trapezius
Pectoralis major
Costoclavicular lig.
Subclavis
Sternocleidomastoid
Trapezius
Deltoid
Pectoralis minor
Coracobrachialis and Biceps
Supraspinatus
Subscapularis
Biceps
Latissimus dorsi
Triceps
Pectoralis major
Teres major
Deltoid
Brachialis
Brachioradialis
Extensor carpi radialis longus
Extensor carpi radialis brevis
Supinator
Biceps brachii
Flexor digitorum profund.
Oblique cord (interosseous lig. betw. ulna and radius)
Omohydoid
Rhomboid minor
Infraspinatus
Rhomboid major
Subscapularis
Serratus anterior
Coracobrachialis
Articularis cubiti (brachialis)
Pronator teres (humeral head)
Medial epicondyle
Flexor carpi radialis
Palmaris longus
Flexor carpi radialis
Flexor digitorum superficialis (humeral head)
Common flexor tendon
Pronator teres (ulnar head)
Brachialis
Flexor digitorum superficialis
Flexor carpi ulnaris (ulnar origin)
Deltoid
Supraspinatus
Infraspinatus
Teres minor
Triceps
Deltoid
Teres major
Latissimus dorsi
Brachialis
Triceps (medial head)
Brachioradialis
Ext. carpi radialis longus
Ext. carpi radialis brevis
Ext. digitorum
Ext. carpi ulnaris
Anconeus

ANTERIOR

POSTERIOR

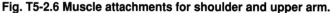

Fig. T5-2.6 Muscle attachments for shoulder and upper arm.

MUSCLES OF THE UPPER EXTREMITIES *(continued)*
Muscles that Act on the Forearm

MUSCLE	ORIGIN	INSERTION	ACTION	INNERVATION	PALPATION
Biceps Brachii					
Short Head	Coracoid process of the scapula	Posterioir portion of the tuberosity of the radius	Flexion of arm and forearm, supinates hand	C5, 6 Musculocutaneous	Anterior surface of humerus
Long Head	Tubricle at top of the glenoid fossa on scapula	Posterior portion of the tuberosity of the radius	Flexion of the elbow, supinates hand	C5, 6, Musculocutaneous	Anterior surface of humerus
Brachialis	Distal half of anterior aspect of the humerus	Tuberosity of the ulna	Flexion of the elbow	C5, 6, Musculocutaneous and C7, 8, Radial nerve	Medial to Biceps on distal anterior humerus
Brachioradialis	Lateral supracondylar ridge of humerus	Styloid process of radius	Flexion of the elbow	C5, 6, Radial nerve	Top of upper foreearm when elbow is flexed
Triceps Brachii					
Long Head	Infraglenoid tuberosity of the scapula	Olecranon process of ulna	Extension of the elbow	C7, 8, Radial nerve	Posterior aspect of humerus
Lateral Head	Proximal half of posterior humerus	Olecranon process of ulna	Extension of the elbow	C7, 8, Radial nerve	Posterior aspect of humerus
Medial Head	Distal two-thirds of posterior humerus	Olecranon process of ulna	Extension of the elbow	C7, 8, Radial nerve	Posterior aspect of humerus
Anconeus	Lateral epicondyle of humerus	Olecranon process of ulna	Extension of the elbow	C7, 8, Radial nerve	Hard to palpate
Pronator Teres	Just proximal to medial epicondyle of humerus	Midlateral surface of radius	Pronates the hand, assists in elbow flexion	C6, 7, Median nerve	In resisted pronation, medial anterior proximal forearm.
Pronator Quadratus	Distal one-fourth of anterior ulna	Distal one-fourth of lateroanteriour radius	Pronates the hand	C8, T1, Median nerve	Cannot palpate
Supinator	Lateral epicondyle, radial collateral and annular ligament and the ridge of the ulna just below the radial notch	Lateral surface of the proximal third of radius	Assists Biceps to supinate hand and forearm	C6, Deep Radial nerve	Deep to Bracioradialis on proximal forearm. Hard to palpate

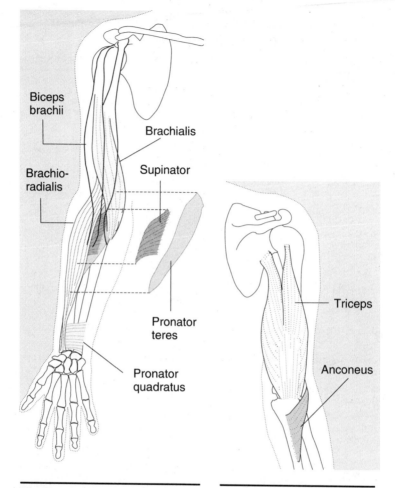

Biceps
brachii

Brachialis

Supinator

Brachio-
radialis

Pronator
teres

Pronator
quadratus

Triceps

Anconeus

Fig. T5-2.7 Anterior arm; biceps brachii, brachialis, brachio-radialis, supinator, pronators.

Fig. T5-2.8 Posterior arm; triceps and anconeus.

MUSCLES OF THE UPPER EXTREMITIES *(continued)*
Muscles that Act on the Wrist and Hand

MUSCLE	ORIGIN	INSERTION	ACTION	INNERVATION	PALPATION
Flexor Carpi Radialis	Medial epicondyle of the humerus	Base of the second and third metacarpals	Flexion, abduction of wrist	C6, 7, Median	Anterior surface of forearm. Tendon prominent on radial side of Palmaris longus tendon at the wrist.
Flexor Carpi Ulnaris					
Humeral head	Medial epicondyle of humerus	Pisiform, hamate and base of fifth metacarpal	Flexion, abduction of wrist	C7, 8, T1, Ulnar	Muscle on proximal half of medial forearm. Tendon on medial anterior wrist proximal to pisiform bone.
Ulnar head	Proximal two-thirds of posterior ulna and olecranon	Common insertion with Humeral head	Flexion, abduction of wrist	C7, 8, T1, Ulnar	
Palmaris Longus	Medial epicondyle of humerus	Palmar aponeurosis	Flexion of wrist	C7, 8, Median	Tendon palpated in middle of anterior wrist
Extensor Carpi Radialis Longus	Distal third of supracondylar ridge of humerus	Dorsal surface of base of second metacarpal	Extension, abduction of wrist	C6, 7, Radial	Next to Brachioradials on dorsal surface of forearm
Extensor Carpi Radialis Brevis	Lateral epicondyle of humerus	Dorsal surface of base of third metacarpal	Extension of wrist	C6, 7, 8, Radial	Next to Extensor carpi radialis longus. Hard to differentiate
Extensor Carpi Ulnaris	Lateral epicondyle of humerus and by aponeurosis from proximal posterior ulna	Lateral dorsal side of base of fifth metacarpal	Extension and abduction of wrist	C6, 7, 8, Deep radial	Ulnar border of dorsal forearm. Tendon on dorsal wrist near ulnar styloid.

(continued)

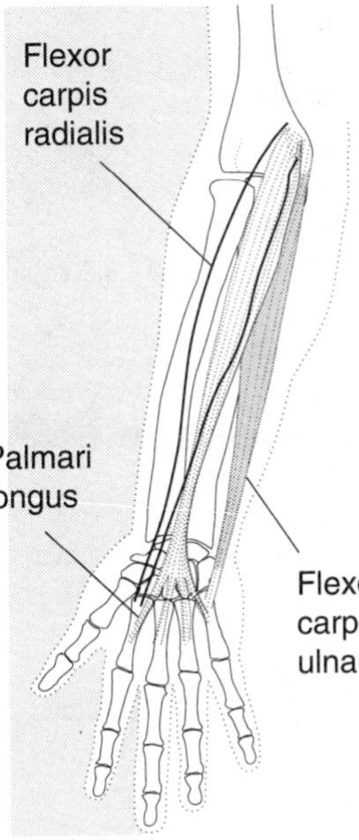

Fig. T5-2.9 Anterior forearm; flexor carpi radialis and ulnaris and palmaris longus.

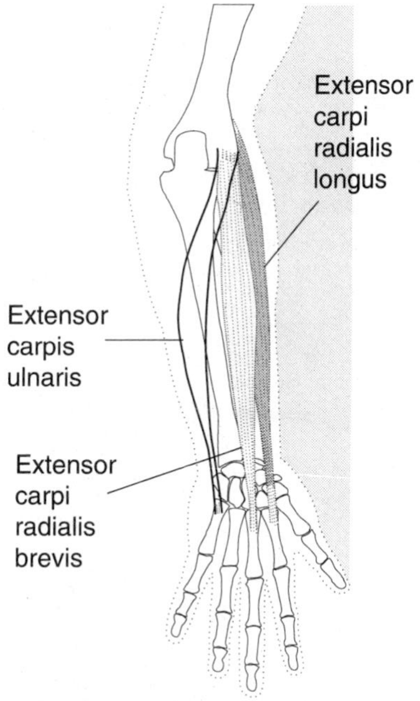

Fig. T5-2.10 Posterior forearm; extensor carpi radialis longus and brevis, extensor carpi ulnaris.

MUSCLES OF THE UPPER EXTREMITIES (continued)
Muscles that Act on the Fingers

MUSCLE	ORIGIN	INSERTION	ACTION	INNERVATION	PALPATION
Flexor Digitorum Superficialis		By four tendons to the sides of the middle phalanges of digits 2–5	Initial action flexes middle phalanx of digits 2–5. Continued action flexes proximal phalnx of digits 2–5 and wrist	C7, 8, T1, Median	Muscle is hard to palpate. Tendon is prominent on ulnar side of wrist between Palmaris longus and Flexor carpi ulnaris tendons.
Humeral head	Medial epicondyle of humerus and ulnar collateral ligament				
Ulnar head	Medial side of coronoid process of ulna				
Radial head	Oblique line of the radius				
Flexor Digitorum Profundus	Proximal three-fourths of anterior and medial ulna and interosseus membrane	By tendons to anterior bases of distal phalanges 2–5	Initially flexes distal phalanges 2–5. Continued action assists flexion of middle, proximal phalanges and wrist.	Digit 2–3; C8, T1, Median Digit 4–5; C7, 8, Ulnar	Muscle lies deep and hard to palpate. Tendons pass through split tendons of Superficialis tendons and can be palpated on anterior surdace of middle phalanges
Flexor Digiti Minimi	Hamate bone and flexor retinaculum	Base of proximal phalanx of little finger	Flexes metacarpo-phalangeal joint of little finger	C8, T1, Ulnar	Palmar surface of 5th metacarpal
Extensor Digitorum	Lateral epicondyle of humerus	By four tendons to digits 2–5. To the forsal base of the middle and distal phalanges	Extension of MP joints and with Lumbricals and interossei extends PIP and DIP joints	C6, 7, 8, Radial	Prominent tendons on back of hand
Extensor Indicis	Distal third of posterior ulna and interosseus membrane	Extensor expansion of index finger with Extensor digitorum tendon	Extension of index finger at PIP and DIP joints with Lumbricals and interosei and extends MP joint.	C6, 7, 8, Radial	Dorsal surface of distal forearm. Tendon prominent of dorsal hand when pointing index finger.
Extensor Digiti Minimi	Lateral epicondyle of humerus	Extensor expansion of little finger with Extensor digitorum tendon	Extension of MP joint and with Lumbricals and interossei extends PIP and DIP joints	C6, 7, 8, Radial	Adjacent to Extensor digitrum. Hard to palpate
Abductor Digiti Minimi	Tendon of Flexor carpi ulnaris and pisiform	Ulnar side of prox-imal phalanx of little finger	Abduction of little finger at MP joint	C8, T1, Ulnar	Ulnar border of fifth metacarpal
Opponens Digiti Minimi	Hook of the Hamate and flxor retinaculum	Ulnar side of fourth metacarpal	Oppostition of the fifth metacarpal	C8, T1, Ulnar	Hard to palpate
Palmar interossei			Adducts thumb, index finger, ring finger and little finger toward axial line of hand through third finger. Assists Lumbricals in MP flexion and DIP and PIP extension		
First	Ulnar side of first metacarpal	Ulnar side of prox-imal phalanx of first digit		C8, T1, Ulnar	Cannot palpate
Second	Ulnar side of second metacarpal	Ulnar side of proximal phalanx of second digit			
Third	Radial side of fourth metacarpal	Radial side of proximal phalanx of fourth digit			

MUSCLES OF THE UPPER EXTREMITIES (continued)
Muscles that Act on the Fingers

MUSCLE	ORIGIN	INSERTION	ACTION	INNERVATION	PALPATION
Fourth	Radial side of fifth metacarpal	Radial side of proximal phalanx of fifth digit			
Dorsal interossei	Adjacent surfaces of all metacarpal bones	Extensor expansion and proximal bases of digits two, three and four.	Abduction of index, middle and ring fingers. Assists lumbrical in MP flexion and DIP and PIP extension	C8, T1, Ulnar	Between metacarpals of dorsal surface of hand
Lumbricals	Flexor digitorum tendons at level of metacarpals	Radial side of extensor expansion at proximal phalanx of digits 2, 3, 4 and 5	Flexion of MP joints and extension of DIP and PIP joints	Digits 2 and 3, C6, 7, Median. Digits 4 & 5, 7 & 8, Ulnar	Hard to palpate

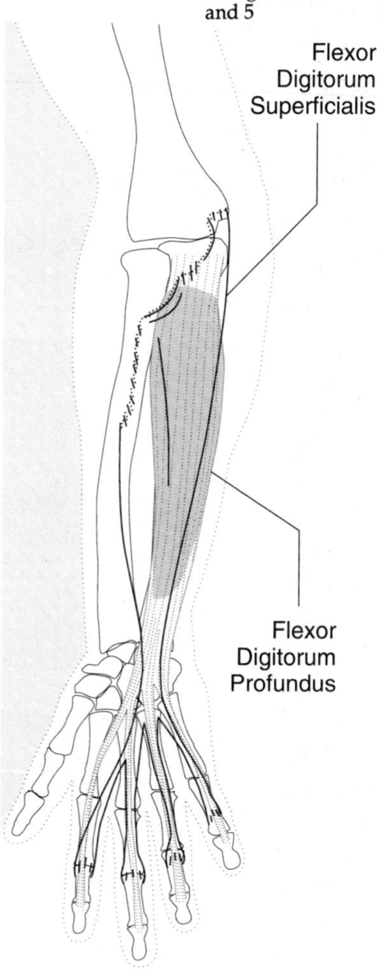

Fig. T5-2.11 Anterior forearm and hand; flexor digitorum profundus and superficialis.

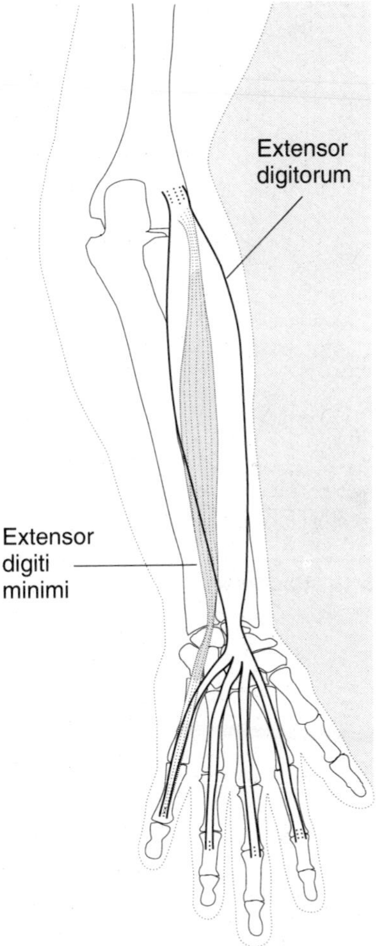

Fig. T5-2.12 Posterior forearm and hand; extensor digitorum, extensor indicus and extensor digiti minimi.

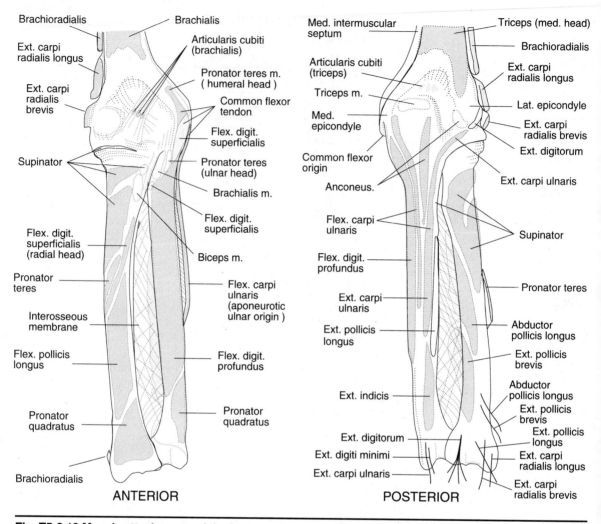

Brachioradialis

Brachialis

Articularis cubiti (brachialis)

Ext. carpi radialis longus

Pronator teres m. (humeral head)

Ext. carpi radialis brevis

Common flexor tendon

Flex. digit. superficialis

Supinator

Pronator teres (ulnar head)

Brachialis m.

Flex. digit. superficialis

Flex. digit. superficialis (radial head)

Pronator teres (ulnar head)

Biceps m.

Pronator teres

Flex. carpi ulnaris (aponeurotic ulnar origin)

Interosseous membrane

Flex. pollicis longus

Flex. digit. profundus

Pronator quadratus

Pronator quadratus

Brachioradialis

ANTERIOR

Med. intermuscular septum

Triceps (med. head)

Brachioradialis

Articularis cubiti (triceps)

Ext. carpi radialis longus

Triceps m.

Lat. epicondyle

Med. epicondyle

Ext. carpi radialis brevis

Common flexor origin

Ext. digitorum

Anconeus.

Ext. carpi ulnaris

Flex. carpi ulnaris

Supinator

Flex. digit. profundus

Pronator teres

Ext. carpi ulnaris

Abductor pollicis longus

Ext. pollicis longus

Ext. pollicis brevis

Abductor pollicis longus

Ext. indicis

Ext. pollicis brevis

Ext. pollicis longus

Ext. digitorum

Ext. carpi radialis longus

Ext. digiti minimi

Ext. carpi radialis brevis

Ext. carpi ulnaris

POSTERIOR

Fig. T5-2.13 Muscle attachments of the lower arm.

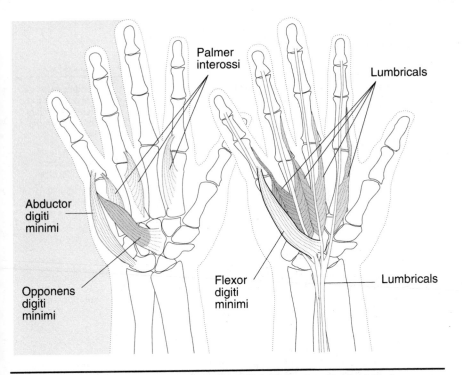

Fig. T5-2.14 Anterior hand; flexor digiti minimi, abductor digiti minimi, opponens digiti minimi, palmar interossi, and lumbricals.

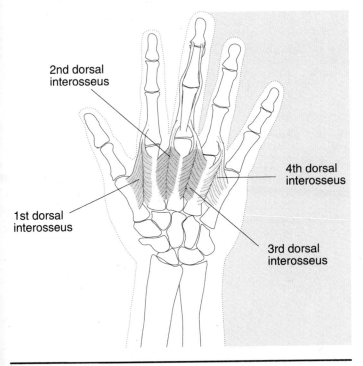

Fig. T5-2.15 Posterior hand; dorsal interossi.

MUSCLES OF THE UPPER EXTREMITIES *(continued)*
Muscles that Act on the Thumb

MUSCLE	ORIGIN	INSERTION	ACTION	INNERVATION	PALPATION
Abductor Pollicis Longus	Middle third of posterior surface of ulna, radius and interosseus	Base of radial side of first metacarpal	Abduction and extension of carpometacarpal joint of thumb	C7, 8, Radial	Tendon palpated just anterior to Extensor pollicis longus on radial side of wrist.
Abductor Pollicis Brevis	Flexor retinaculum, trapezium and scaphoid	Radial side of proximal phalanx of thumb	Abduction of the thumb	C8, T1, Median	Radial side of palmar surface of 1st metacarpal
Adductor Pollicis Transverse Head	Palmar surface of third metacarpal	Ulnar side of base of the first phalax of the thumb	Adduction of the thumb	C8, T1, Deep branch of ulnar	Palmar surface of thumb web space
Oblique Head	Capate bone and base of 2nd and 3rd metacarpals				
Flexor Pollicis Longus	Anterior surface of middle radius and adjacent interosseus membrane	Base of palmar surface of distal phalanx of thumb	Initial action flexes distal joint of thumb. Continued action assists flexion of two proximal joints	C8, T1, Palmar interosseus branch of Median nerve	Tendon palpated of radial side of anterior wrist
Flexor Pollicis Brevis Superficial Head	Flexor Retinaculum and trapezium bone	Radial side of proximal phalanx of thumb and extensor expansion	Flexion of proximal phalanx and assists with opposition of thumb	C6, 7, 8, Median	Considered to be #1 Palmar interossei muscle. Along with Abductor pollicis brevis and Opponens pollicis make up the thenar eminence
Deep Head	Trapezoid and capitate bones			C8, T1, Ulnar	
Extensor Pollicis Longus	Middle third of posterior surface of ulna and interosseus membrane	Base of dorsal surface of distal phalanx of thumb	Extends distal phalanx of thumb. Assists extension of proximal phalanx of thumb and wrist and abduction of wrist	C7, 8, Deep radial	Tendon palpated on radial side of first metacarpal on resisted extension just posterior to Extensor pollicis brevis tendon.
Extensor Pollicis Brevis	Posterior surface of radius and interosseus membrane distal to origin of Abductor pollicis longus	Dorsal surface of proximal phalanx of thumb	Extends proximal phalanx of thumb. Assists in abduction of first metacarpal and wrist	C78, 8, Deep radial	Tendon palpated on radial side of first metacarpal on resisted extension just anterior to Extensor pollicis longus tendon.
Opponens Pollicis	Flexor retinaculum and trapezium bone	Entire radial side of first metacarpal	Opposition of thumb	C6, 7, 8, T1, Median and Ulnar	Part of thenar eminence. Along 1st metacarpal

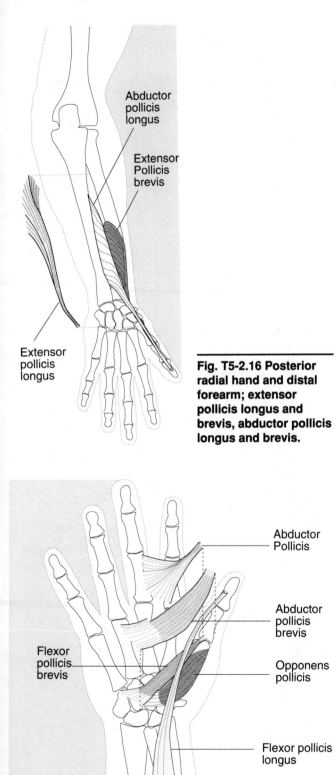

Abductor
pollicis
longus

Extensor
Pollicis
brevis

Extensor
pollicis
longus

Fig. T5-2.16 Posterior radial hand and distal forearm; extensor pollicis longus and brevis, abductor pollicis longus and brevis.

Abductor
Pollicis

Abductor
pollicis
brevis

Opponens
pollicis

Flexor
pollicis
brevis

Flexor pollicis
longus

Fig. T5-2.17 Anterior hand and distal forearm; Adductor pollicis, Flexor Pollicis Longus and Brevis, and Opponens Pollicis.

MUSCLES OF THE LOWER EXTREMITIES
Muscles that Act on the Thigh

MUSCLE	ORIGIN	INSERTION	ACTION	INNERVATION	PALPATION
Psoas Major	Anterior surfaces of transverse processes and sides of bodies and discs of all lumbar vertebrae	Lesser trochanter of the femur	With fixed origin; Flexes thigh. With fixed insertion; Bilaterally Flexes hip, unilaterally, assists lateral flexion of spine.	L2, 3, Lumbar plexus	Deep in abdomen and just above unguinal crease. Hard to palpate
Iliacus	Superior two-thirds of illiac fossa and illiac crest	With Psoas major at lesser trochanter of the femur	Same as Psoas major. Assists in abduction and lateral rotation of hip.	L2, 3, 4, Femoral	Difficult to palpate.
Gluteus Maximus	Posterior gluteal line of ilium and adja-cent iliac crest, the posterior inferior surface of the sacrum and lateral surface of coccyx.	Iliotibial tract of Fascia lata and fluteal tuberosity of femur	Extends and laterally rotates thigh, Supports extended knee	L5, S1, 2, Inferior gluteal	Posterior surface of buttock
Gluteus Medius	Iliac crest and external surface of ilium	Lateral surface of greater trochanter of the femur	Abducts thigh. Anterior fibers rotate hip medially	L4, 5, S1, Superior gluteal	Lateral surface of hip between greater trochanter and iliac crest
Gluteus Minimus	External surface of ilium inferior to Fluteus medius muscle and margin of greater sciatic notch. Anterior portion of iliac spine and ASIS	Anterior border of the greater trochanter of femur	Abducts and medially rotates hip	L4, 5, S1, Superior gluteal	Under Gluteus medius
Tensor Fascia Latae		Iliotibial tract of fascia lata	Abducts and medial rotates thigh. Maintains extension of knee	L4, 5, S1, Superior gluteal	Below anterior iliac spine
Pectineus	Superior ramus of anterior pubis	Between lesser trochanter and linea aspera on posterior femur	Adducts, flexes and medially rotates thigh	L2, 3, 4, Femoral and obtruator	Uppermost of medial thigh muscles, just superior to Adductor longus
Adductor Brevis	Outer surface of the inferior ramus of the pubis	Proximal half of the linea aspera to the lesser trochanter on posterior femur	Adduction, flexion and medial rotation of thigh	L3, 4, Obturator	Deep to Pectineus and Adductor longus. Hard to palpate
Adductor Longus	At the crest of pubis adjacent to pubic symphysis.	Middle one-third of medial lip of linea aspera	Adduction, flexion and medial rotation of thigh	L3, 4, Obturator	Groin muscle just below pubis
Adductor Magnus	Inferior public ramus, ischial ramus and ischial tuberosity	The linea aspera, medial epicondylic ridge and adductor tuberble of the medial femoral condyle	Powerful adduction. Anterior fibers flexion and medial rotation, posterior fibers extension and lateral rotation	L2, 3, 4, Obturator, L4, 5, S1, Sciatic	Medial surface of thigh

MUSCLES OF THE LOWER EXTREMITIES (continued)
Muscles that Act on the Thigh & Lateral Rotaters

MUSCLE	ORIGIN	INSERTION	ACTION	INNERVATION	PALPATION
Gracilis	Inferior half of symphysis pubis and inferior ramus of pubis	The pes anserine. Medial surface of tibia inferior to medial tibial condyle	Adducts thigh, flexion and medial rotation of knee	L3, 4, Obturator	Medial thigh below pubis
Sartorius	Anterior superior iliac spine and iliac notch just inferior of spine	Proximal medial surface of tibia. Pes ancerine	Flexes, laterally rotates and abducts thigh. Assists with flexion and medal rotation of knee	L2, 3, Femoral	Just below ASIS and diagonally across thigh.
Piriformis	Anterior sacrum, greater sciatic notch and anterior portion of the sacrotuberous ligament	Superior edge of greater trochanter of the femur	Lateral rotation of the thigh	L5, S1, Sacral plexus	Cannot palpate
Gemellus Superior	Outer surface of ischial spine	Medial surface of the posterior greater trochanter of the femur	Lateral rotation of the thigh	L5, S1, Sacral plexus	Cannot palpate
Obturator Internus	Ramus of the ischium, inner surface of the ilium and superior and inferior ramus of pubis	Medial surface of the posterior greater trochanter of the femur	Lateral rotation of the thigh	L5, S1, Sacral plexus	Cannot palpate
Gemellus Inferior	Ischial tuberosity	Medial surface of the posterior greater trochanter of the femur	Lateral rotation of the thigh	L5, S1, Sacral plexus	Cannot palpate
Obturator Externus	Pubis and ischium around medial side of obturator foramen	The fossa of the greater trochanter of the femur	Lateral rotation of the thigh	L3, 4, Obturator	Cannot palpate
Quadratus Femoris	Ischial tuberosity	Just distal to the greater trochantic crest	Lateral rotation of the thigh	L5, S1, Sacral plexus	Cannot palpate

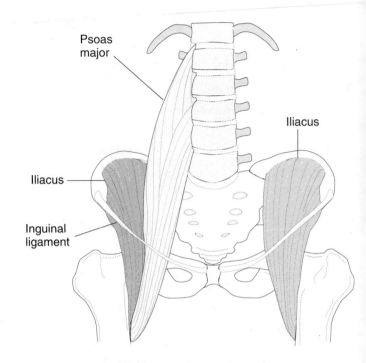

Fig. T5-2.18 Illiacus and psoas.

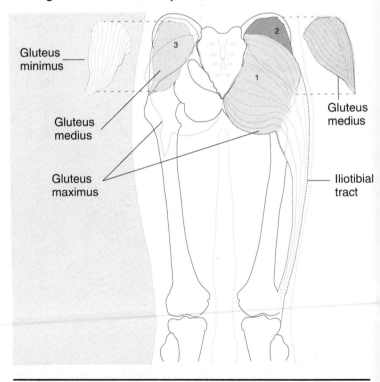

Fig. T5-2.19 Gluteus maximus, gluteus medius, and gluteus minimus.

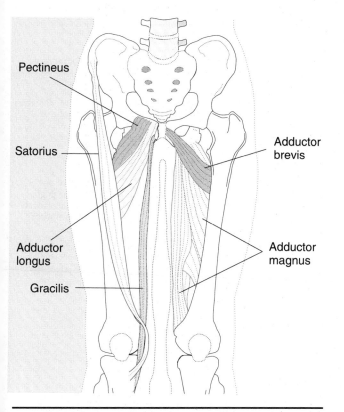

Fig. T5-2.20 Pectineus, adductor magnus, adductor longus, adductor brevis, gracilus, sartorius.

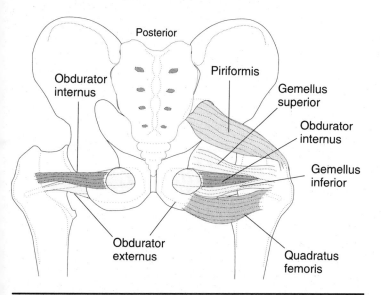

Fig. T5-2.21 Deep rotators; piriformis, gemellus superior, obturator internus, gemellus inferior, obturator externus, and quadratus femoris.

MUSCLES OF THE LOWER EXTREMITIES *(continued)*
Muscles that Act on the Lower Leg

MUSCLE	ORIGIN	INSERTION	ACTION	INNERVATION	PALPATION
Hamstrings					
Biceps Femoris	Ischial tuberosity and sacrotuberous ligament	Lateral side of the head of the fibula and the lateral condyle of the tibia	Both heads; flex and laterally rotate the leg.	L5, S1, 2, Sciatic, tibial division	Muscle on posterior surface of thigh. Tendon on lateral side of posterior knee
Long Head					
Short Head	Lateral lip of the linea aspera		Long head; extends and assists in lateral rotation of the hip	L5, S1, 2, Sciatic, peronial division	
Semitendinouis	Iscial tuberosity	Proximal part of medial surface of the tibia. Pes anserine	Extends the thigh. Flexes and medially rotates the knee	L5, S1, 2, Sciatic, tibial division	Muscle on posterior surface of thigh. Tendon on medial side of posterior knee
Semimembranosus	Iscial tuberosity	Posteromedial aspect of medial condyle of the tibia	Extends the thigh. Flexes and medially rotates the knee	L5, S1, 2, Sciatic, tibial division	Muscle on posterior surface of thigh. Tendon deep and hard to palpate.
Quadriceps Femoris					
Rectus Femoris	Anterior inferior iliac spine and the groove above the acetabulum	Via quadriceps expansion and patella through patellar ligament to tuberosity of tibia	Extends the leg at the knee	L2, 3, 4, Femoral	Anterior surface of thigh
Vastus Lateralis	Anterior and inferior border of greater trochanter, proximal one-half of lateral linea aspera	Via quadriceps expansion and patella through patellar ligament to tuberosity of tibia	Extends the leg at the knee	L2, 3, 4, Femoral	Anteriolateral surface of thigh
Vastus Intermedius	Anterior and lateral surfaces of proximal two-thirds of femur	Via quadriceps expansion and patella through patellar ligament to tuberosity of tibia	Extends the leg at the knee	L2, 3, 4, Femoral	Deep to rectus femoris. Hard to paplate
Vastus Medialis	Medial lip of linea aspera and posterior femur	Via quadriceps expanion and patella through patellar ligament to tuberosity of tibia	Extends the leg at the knee	L2, 3, 4, Femoral	Medial surface of distal two-thirds of anterior thigh

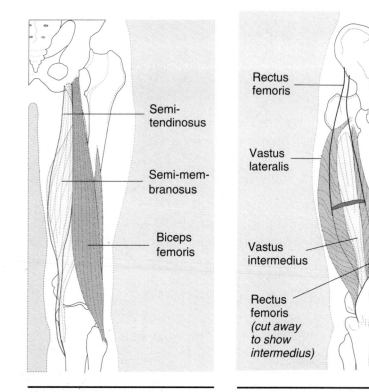

Semi-
tendinosus

Semi-mem-
branosus

Biceps
femoris

**Fig. T5-2.22 Posterior thigh;
hamstrings; biceps femoris,
semitendenosis,
semimembranosis.**

Rectus
femoris

Vastus
lateralis

Vastus
medialis

Vastus
intermedius

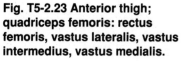

Rectus
femoris
*(cut away
to show
intermedius)*

**Fig. T5-2.23 Anterior thigh;
quadriceps femoris: rectus
femoris, vastus lateralis, vastus
intermedius, vastus medialis.**

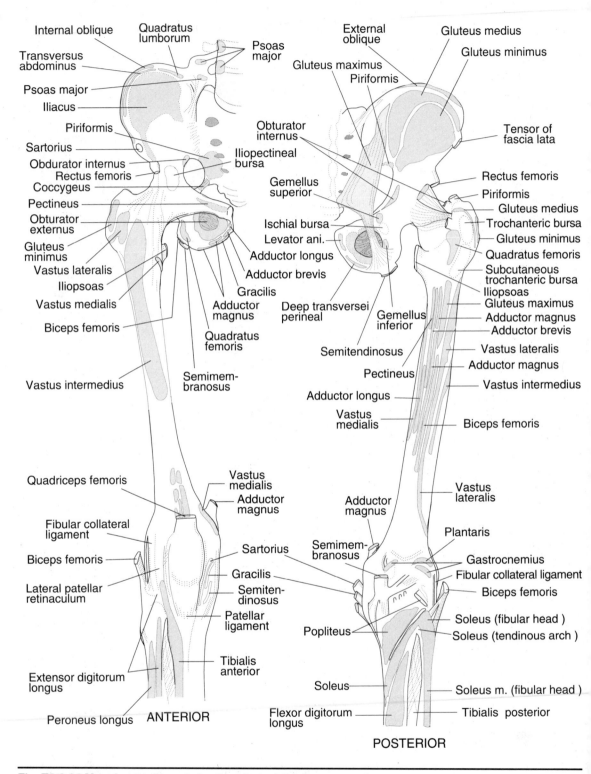

Internal oblique
Quadratus lumborum
Transversus abdominus
Psoas major
Psoas major
Iliacus
Piriformis
Sartorius
Obdurator internus
Rectus femoris
Coccygeus
Pectineus
Obturator externus
Gluteus minimus
Vastus lateralis
Iliopsoas
Vastus medialis
Biceps femoris
Vastus intermedius
Iliopectineal bursa
Obturator internus
Gemellus superior
Ischial bursa
Levator ani.
Adductor longus
Adductor brevis
Gracilis
Adductor magnus
Quadratus femoris
Semimembranosus
Deep transversei perineal
Gemellus inferior
Semitendinosus
Pectineus
Adductor longus
Vastus medialis

External oblique
Gluteus medius
Gluteus minimus
Gluteus maximus
Piriformis
Tensor of fascia lata
Rectus femoris
Piriformis
Gluteus medius
Trochanteric bursa
Gluteus minimus
Quadratus femoris
Subcutaneous trochanteric bursa
Iliopsoas
Gluteus maximus
Adductor magnus
Adductor brevis
Vastus lateralis
Adductor magnus
Vastus intermedius
Biceps femoris

Quadriceps femoris
Vastus medialis
Adductor magnus
Fibular collateral ligament
Biceps femoris
Lateral patellar retinaculum
Sartorius
Gracilis
Semitendinosus
Patellar ligament
Extensor digitorum longus
Tibialis anterior
Peroneus longus
ANTERIOR

Adductor magnus
Semimembranosus
Vastus lateralis
Plantaris
Gastrocnemius
Fibular collateral ligament
Biceps femoris
Soleus (fibular head)
Soleus (tendinous arch)
Popliteus
Soleus
Soleus m. (fibular head)
Flexor digitorum longus
Tibialis posterior
POSTERIOR

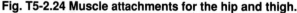

Fig. T5-2.24 Muscle attachments for the hip and thigh.

MUSCLES OF THE LOWER EXTREMITIES (continued)
Muscles that Act on the Foot

MUSCLE	ORIGIN	INSERTION	ACTION	INNERVATION	PALPATION
Popliteus	Lateral condyle of femur	Posterior surface of proximal tibia	Initiates leg flexion by unlocking the knee	L4, 5, S1, Tibial	Cannot palpate
Tibialis Anterior	Lateral condyle and proximal one-half of tibia, interosseus membrane	Medial and plantar surface of medial cuneiform and base of first metatarsal	Dorsalflexion of ankle and inversion of foot	L4, 5, Deep Peroneal	Lateroanterior surface of tibia. Tendon palpated on anterior ankle medial to Extensor hallucis longus M.
Peroneus Tertius	Distal one-third of anterior fibula	Base of fifth metatarsal	Dorsalflexion of the ankle, eversion of foot	L4, 5, S1, Deep Peroneal	Tendon just lateral to tendon of Extensor digitorum
Extensor Digitorum Longus	Lateral condyle of tibia and proximal three-fourths of the anterior fibula	By four tendons to the dorsal surfaces of the second and third phalanges of the four lateral toes	Extension of four lateral toes and dorsalflexion of ankle	L4, 5, S1, Deep Peroneal	Four tendons on dorsum of foot
Extensor Hallucis Longus	Middle two quarters of anterior fibula and interosseus membrane	Base of distal phalanx of large toe	Extends large toe, dorsalflexes ankle and inversion of foot	L4, 5, S1, Deep Peroneal	Tendon on anterior ankle and dorsum of large toe
Gastrocnemius					
Medial Head	Posterior surface of medial condyle of the femur	Middle of posterior surface of the calcaneus via the achilles tendon	Plantarflexes the ankle or assists flexion of the knee	S1, 2, Tibial	Major muscle of posterior calf
Lateral Head	Posterior surface of the lateral condyle of femur				
Plantaris	Distal lateral suprocondylar line of the femur	Posterior surface of the calcaneus via the achilles tendon	Plantarflexes the ankle or assists flexion of the knee	L4, 5, S1, Tibial	Hard to palpate
Soleus	Head and proximal one-third of posterior fibula and middle border and soleal line of tibia	Middle of posterior surface of the calcaneus via the achilles tendon	Plantarflexes the ankle	L5, S1, 2, Tibial	Lateral surface of lower leg below Gastrocnemeus
Flexor Digitorum Longus	Middle one-third of posterior surface of tibia	By four tendons to the plantar surface of the distal phalanges of the four lateral toes	Flexes the four lateral toes. Assists in plantarflexion and inversion of the foot	L5, S1, 2, Tibial	Tendon palpated posterior and inferior to medial malleolus with Posterior tibialis and Flexor digitorum longus
Flexor Hallucis Longus	Distal two-thirds of posterior fibula and adjacent interosseus membrane	Base of plantar surface distal phalanx of large toes	Flexes large toe. Assists plantar-flexion and inversion of foot	L5, S1, 2, Tibial	Tendon palpated posterior and inferior to medial malleolus with Posterior tibialis and Flexor digitorum longus
Tibialis Posterior	Middle third of posterior tibia, proximal two-thirds of medial fibula and interosseus membrane	Plantar surfaces of navalcular, cuboid, 2nd and 3rd and 4th metatarsals.	Inversion of foot. Assists in plantarflexion of ankle	L5, S1, 2, Tibial	Tendon palpated posterior and inferior to medial malleolus with Flexor hallucis longus and Flexor digitorum longus

MUSCLES OF THE LOWER EXTREMITIES (continued)

Muscles that Act on the Foot (continued)

MUSCLE	ORIGIN	INSERTION	ACTION	INNERVATION	PALPATION
Peroneus Longus	Head and proximal two-thirds of lateral surface of fibula and lateral condyle of tibia	Plantar surface of medial cuneiform and base of first metatarsal	Eversion of foot. Assists plantar flexion of ankle	L4, 5, S1, Superficial Peroneal	Proximal half of lateral surface of lower leg
Peroneus Brevis	Distal two-thirds of lateral surface of fibula	Lateral surface of base of fifth metatarsal	Eversion of foot. Assists plantar flexion of ankle	L4, 5, S1, Superficial Peroneal	Posterior and inferior to lateral malleolus with tendon of Peroneus longus

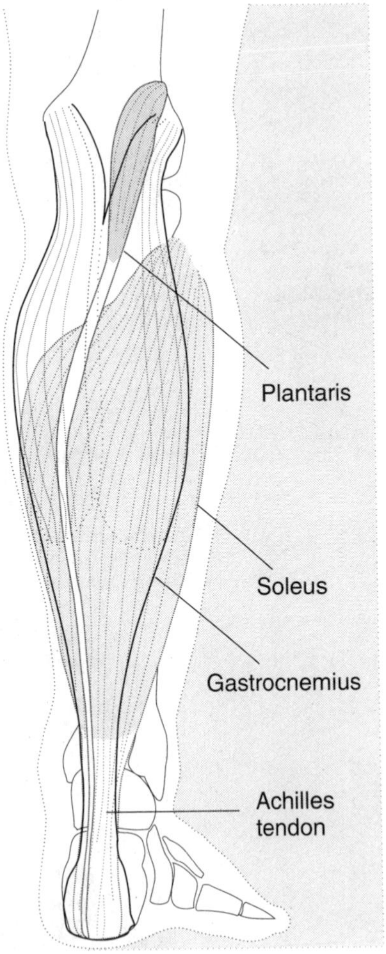

Fig. T5-2.25 Posterior leg; gastrocnemius, soleus, popliteus, plantaris.

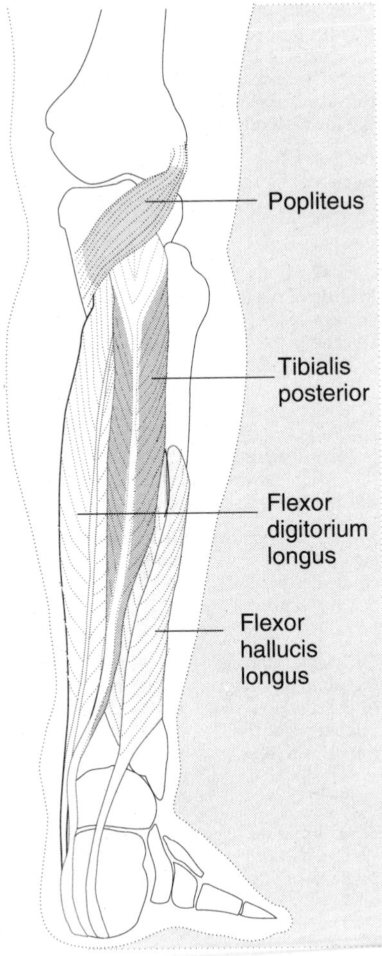

Fig. T5-2.26 Posterior leg (deep); posterior tibialis, flexor digitorum, flexor hallicis.

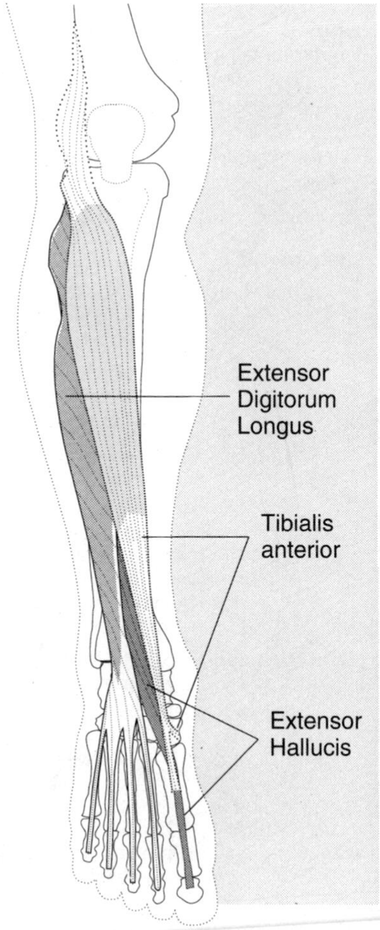

Fig. T5-2.27 Anterior leg; tibialis anterior, extensor digitorum, extensor hallicis.

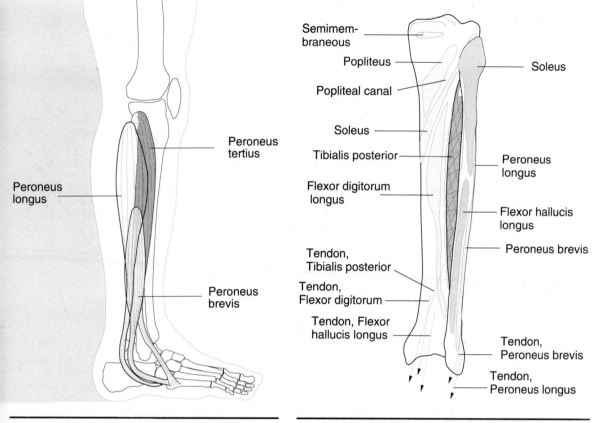

Fig. T5-2.28 Lateral leg; peroneus tertius, peroneus longus, peroneus brevis.

Fig. T5-2.29 Muscle attachments for the lower leg.

MUSCLES THAT ACT ON THE ABDOMEN

MUSCLE	ORIGIN	INSERTION	ACTION	INNERVATION	PALPATION
Rectus Abdominis	Crest of the pubis and pubic symphysis	Xiphiod process and costal cartilage of 5th, 6th and 7th ribs	Flexion of trunk. Tenses abdominal wall and compresses contents	T5–12, Intercostal, Iliohypogastric, Ilio-inguinal	Anterior abdomen from pubis to sternum
External Oblique	External surface of eight lower ribs	Abdominal aponeurosis to linea alba and iliac crest	Bilaterally; Same as above. Unilaterally; Lateral flexion and rotation to opposite side	T8–12, Intercostal, Iliohypogastric, Ilio-inguinal	Lateral surfaces of abdomen
Internal Oblique	Inguinal ligament, Iliac crest and Thoracolumbar fascia	Abdominal aponeurosis, linea alba, and costal cartilages of four lower ribs	Bilaterally; Same as above Unilaterally; Lateral flexion and rotation to same side	T8–12, Intercostal, Iliohypogastric, Ilio-inguinal	Deep to External Oblique Cannot palpate
Transverse Abdominis	Inguinal ligament, Iliac crest and Thoracolumbar fascia and lower six ribs	Abdominal aponeurosis to linea alba and iliac crest	Tenses abdominal wall and compresses contents	T7–12, Intercostal, Ilio-hypergastric, Ilio-inguinal	Cannot palpate

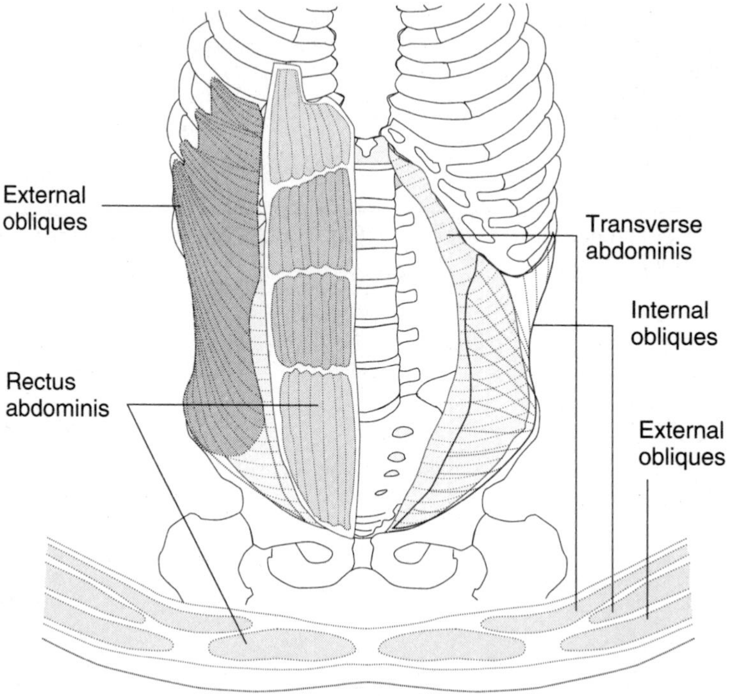

Fig. T5-2.30 Abdominal area: external obliques, internal obliques, transverse abdominis, rectus abdominis.

MUSCLES OF RESPIRATION

MUSCLE	ORIGIN	INSERTION	ACTION	INNERVATION	PALPATION
Diaphragm	The xiphoid process, six lower ribs and costal cartilages, lifaments, bodies and transverse processes of upper lumbar vertebrae	Central tendon of the Diaphragm, a strong aponeurosis with no bony attachment.	Main muscle of repiration, contracts during inspiration increasing thoracic volume. Sparates abdominal and throcic cavities	C3, 4, 5, Phrenic	Cannot palpate. Action can be observed on abdomen during respiration.
Intercostals					
External	Inferior margin of the rib above	Superior margin of the rib below. Fibers angle 45% lateral to medial.	Pull ribs together and elevates ribs during inhalation.	T1–12, Intercostal	External palpated between ribs. Internal and innermost too deep to palpate.
Internal	Inferior margin of the rib above	Superior margin of the rib below. Fibers angle 45% medial to lateral.	External and internal intercostal muscles are situated perpendicular to each other.		
Innermost	Sternum and inferior margin of lower ribs	Inner surface of the ventral ribs			
Serratus Posterior Superior	Spinous process C7–T2, ligamentum nuchae C6–T1 supraspinous ligament	Posterior superior surfaces of ribs 2–5	Raises ribs during deep inhalation.	T1–4, Intercostal	Cannot palpate
Serratus Posterior Inferior	Spinous process T11–L3, supraspinous ligament	Inferior borders of ribs 8–12	Pulls ribs outward and down, opposes diaphragm	T9–12, Intercostal	Cannot palpate

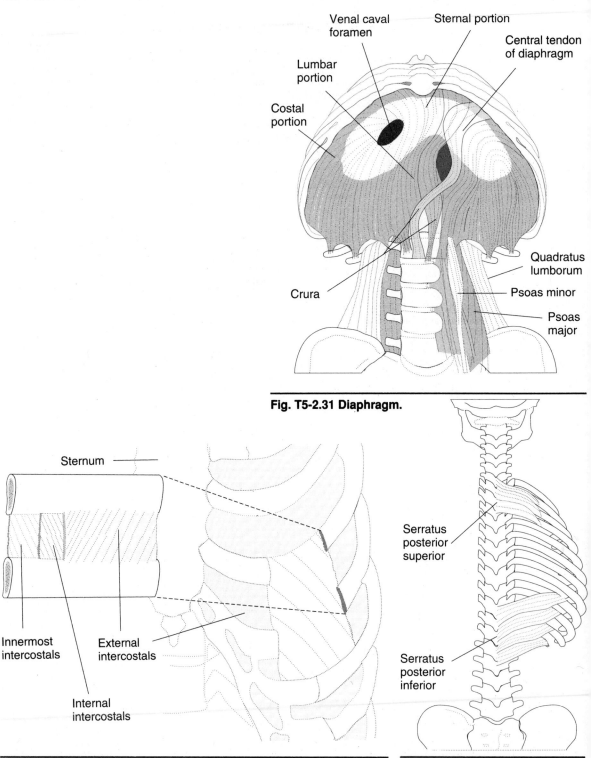

Fig. T5-2.31 Diaphragm.

Fig. T5-2.32 Intercostals.

Fig. T5-2.33 Serratus posterior superior, serratus posterior inferior.

MUSCLES THAT ACT ON THE SPINE

MUSCLE	ORIGIN	INSERTION	ACTION	INNERVATION	PALPATION
Quadratus Lumborum	Posterior iliac crest	Transverse process of L1–4 and inferior border of 12th rib	Lateral flexion of spine or raises hip	T12, L1, 2, 3, Lumbar plexus	Deep to Thoracolumbar sheath. Hard to palpate
Intertransversarii	Transverse processes of cervical, lumbar and T10–12 vertebra	Transverse process of vertebra directly above origin	Lateral flexion and stabilization of spine	Posterior branches of adjacent spinal nerves	Cannot palpate
Interspinales	In pairs between spinous process of cervical lumbar and T1–2 and T11–12 vertebra	Spinous process of vertebra directly above origin	Extension and stabilization of spine	Posterior branches of adjacent spinal nerves	Cannot palpate
Rotatores	Transverse process of each vertebra	Lamina of vertebra directly above	Extension, rotation to opposite side and stabilization of spine	Posterior branches of adjacent spinal nerves	Cannot palpate
Multifidus	Transverse process of C4–L5, PSIS and posterior sacrum	Spans 2–4 vertebra. Inserts on spinous process	Extension, rotation to opposite side and stabilization of spine	Posterior branches of adjacent spinal nerves	Cannot palpate
Semispinalis			Bilaterally; Extension		
Capitis	Transverse process C4–T7	Occipital bone between inferior and superior nuchal lines	Unilaterally, Rotation to opposite side. Stabilization of spine	Posterior branches of adjacent spinal nerves	Cannot palpate
Cervicis	Transverse processes of T1–6	Spinous processes C2–5			
Thoracis	Transverse processes T6–12	Spinous process C6–T8			
Spinalis			Bilaterally; Extension of spine.	Posterior branches of adjacent spinal nerves	Cannot palpate
Capitis	Inseparable from Semispinalis	Same as Semispinalis	Unilaterally, Lateral flexion of the spine		
Cervicis	Ligamentum nuchae	Spinous processes C2–4			
Thoracis	Spinous processes T10–L2	Spinous processes T4–8	Stabilization of spine		
Longissimus			Bi-laterally, Extension of spine.	Posterior branches of adjacent spinal nerves	Deep to Thoracolumbar fascia, latissamus dorsi and trapezeus muscles on either side of spine. Hard to palpate.
Capitis	Articular processes C4–7, Transverse processes T1–4	Posterior surface of mastoid process	Uni-laterally; Lateral flexion of the spine.		
Cervicis	Transverse processes T1–5	Transverse processes C2–6	Stabilization of spine		
Thoracis	Thoracolumbar fascia, transverse process of lumbar vertebra	Transverse processes T1–12 and posterior surface of lower ten ribs			

MUSCLES THAT ACT ON THE NECK

MUSCLE	ORIGIN	INSERTION	ACTION	INNERVATION	PALPATION
Iliocostalis Lumborum	Common origin by broad tendon arising from spinous process T12–L5, medial lip of iliac crest and medial and lateral crest of the sacrum	Inferior borders of posterior angle of ribs. 7–12	Bilaterally; Extension of spine Unilaterally; Lateral flexion of the spine. Stabilization of spine	Posterior branches of adjacent spinal nerves	Deep to thoracolumbar fascia, Latissamus dorsi and Trapezius muscles on either side of spine. Hard to palpate.
Thoracis	Upper borders of posterior angles of ribs 7–12	Transverse process of C7 and angles of ribs 1–6.			
Cervicis	Posterior angles of ribs 3–6	Transverse processes C4—6			
Splienius Capitis	Lower one half of ligamentum nuchae, spinous process C7–T4	Mastoid process and lateral one-third of occiput	Bilaterally; Extension of neck Unilaterally; Rotation of head to same side	Posterior braches of cervical nerves	On posterior neck between Trapezius and Sternocleido-mastoid. Hard to palpate
Cervicis	Spinous process T3–6	Transverse process C1–3			
Sternocleido-mastoid	Sternal head: Superior aspect of manibrium. Clavicular head: Medial one third of clavical	Mastoid process	Bilaterally; Flexion of neck. Unilaterally; Rotation of head to opposite side, lateral flexion	Accessory nerve and C2, 3.	Anterio-lateral aspect of neck, diagonally from origin to insertion.
Scalenus					
Anterior	Anterior tubricles of transverse processes C3–6	Anterior superior aspect of 1st rib	Bilateraly; Raise rib cage in deep inhalation, neck flexion Unilaterally; Lateral flexion of neck, assists in neck rotation to opposite side	C6, 7, 8	Lateral aspect of lower neck poster-ior to Sternocleido-mastoid muscle from anterior aspect of 1st rib to trans-verse process of cervical vertebra, Hard to palpate
Medial	Posterior tubricles of transvers processes C2–7	Lateral anterior aspect of 1st rib			
Posterior	Posterior tubricles of transvers processes C5–7	Lateral anterior aspect of 2nd rib			
Rectus Capitis					
Anterior	Anterior surface and transverse process of C1	Basil surface of occiput anterior to foramen magnum	Neck flexion, rotation to same side	Suboccipital	Cannot palapte
Lateralis	Transverse process of C1	Basil surface of occiput lateral to foramen magnum	Lateral flexion of head	C1	Cannot palapte
Posterior Minor	Posterior arch of C1 spinous process of C2	Medial segment of inferior nuchal line of occiput	Neck, head extension	Occipital	Deep to Trapezius and Semi spinalis. Hard to palpate.
Posterior Major	Spinous process of C2	Inferior nuchal line of occiput lateral to RCP minor attachment	Head extension, and lateral flexion	Occipital	Cannot palpate

MUSCLES THAT ACT ON THE NECK *(continued)*

MUSCLE	ORIGIN	INSERTION	ACTION	INNERVATION	PALPATION
Obliquus Capitis					
Superior	Superior aspect of transverse process of C1	Between inferior and superior nuchal lines of occiput	Head extension, rotation to same side	Occipital	Cannot palpate
Inferior	Spinous process C2	Posterior aspect of transverse process of C1	Rotation to same side	Occipital	Cannot palpate
Longus Colli	Anterior tubricles C3–5, Anterior vertebral bodies C5–T3	Anterior surface of vertebral bodies of C1–4, Anterior tubricals C5–6	Head flexion, lateral flexion and rotation to same side	C1–4	Cannot palpate
Longus Capitis	Anterior tubricals of transverse process C3–6	Inferior surface of occiput	Flexion of head	C1–3	Cannot palpate

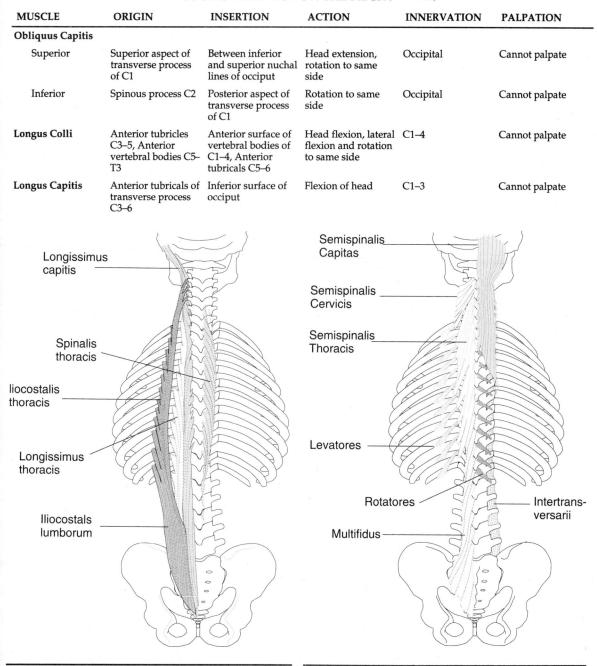

Fig. T5-2.34 Illiocostalis group.

Longissimus capitis

Spinalis thoracis

Iliocostals thoracis

Longissimus thoracis

Iliocostals lumborum

Fig. T5-2.35a Semispinalis group.

Semispinalis Capitas

Semispinalis Cervicis

Semispinalis Thoracis

Levatores

Rotatores

Intertrans-versarii

Multifidus

(cont.)

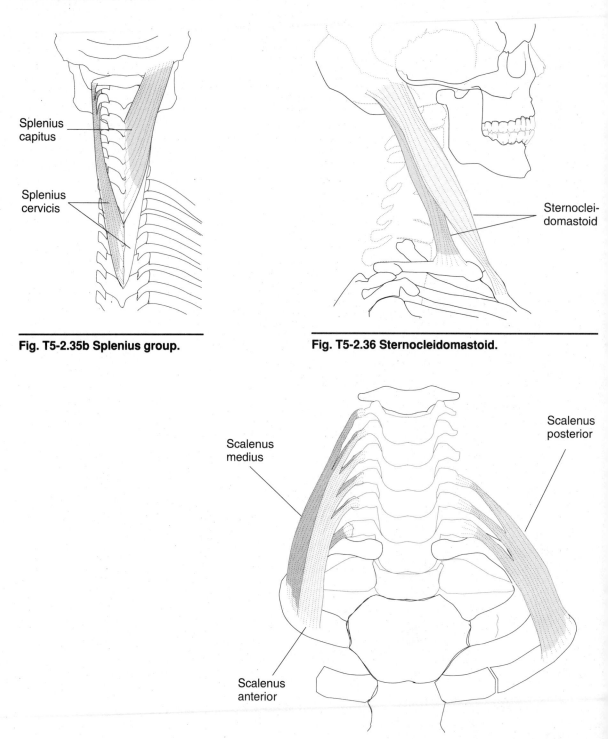

Splenius
capitus

Splenius
cervicis

Fig. T5-2.35b Splenius group.

Sternoclei-
domastoid

Fig. T5-2.36 Sternocleidomastoid.

Scalenus
medius

Scalenus
posterior

Scalenus
anterior

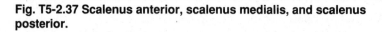

Fig. T5-2.37 Scalenus anterior, scalenus medialis, and scalenus posterior.

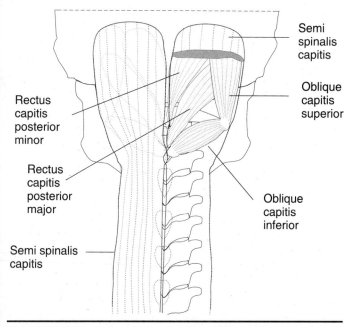

Semi spinalis capitis

Oblique capitis superior

Rectus capitis posterior minor

Rectus capitis posterior major

Oblique capitis inferior

Semi spinalis capitis

Fig. T5-2.38 Posterior neck; rectus capitis posterior major and minor, obliques capitis superior and inferior.

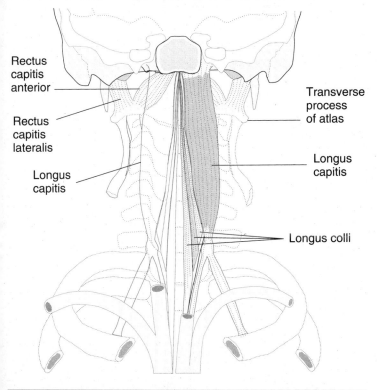

Rectus capitis anterior

Rectus capitis lateralis

Longus capitis

Transverse process of atlas

Longus capitis

Longus colli

Fig. T5-2.39 Anterior neck (deep): rectus capitus anterior and rectus capitus transverse, longus colli and longus capitis.

MUSCLES THAT ACT ON THE HYOID

MUSCLE	ORIGIN	INSERTION	ACTION	INNERVATION	PALPATION
Infrahyoid Muscles					
Sterno-hyoid	Top of sternum and medial end of clavicle	Inferior body of hyoid	Depresses hyoid	C1, 2, 3	Lower anterior neck between SCM and trachea
Sterno-thyroid	Top of sternum and costal cartilage of 1st rib	Thyroid cartilage	Depresses thyroid cartilage	C1, 2, 3	Lower anterior neck between SCM and trachea
Thyro-hyoid	Thyroid cartilage	Inferior body of hyoid	Depressed hyoid or raises thyroid cartilage	C1, 2, 3	Below hyoid, lateral to Sternohyoid. Hard to differentiate and palpate
Omo-hyoid	Superior border of scapula and by tendon to clavicle	Inferior body of hyoid	Depresses hyoid		
Suprahyoid Muscles					
Glenio-hyoid	Mandible under chin	Body of hyoid, superior aspect	Elevates hyoid or depresses mandible	C1, 2	Deep to Mylohyoid, cannot palpate
Myo-hyoid	Mandible from ramus to under chin	Body of hyoid, superior aspect	Elevates hyoid or depresses mandible	Cranial V, Trigeminal	Deep muscle sheath under chin
Stylo-hyoid	Styloid process of temporal bone	Body of hyoid, superior aspect	Elevates hyoid or moves hyoid posteriorly	Cranial VII, Facial	Between hyoid and ramus along with Posterior digastric
Digastric					
Ant. belly	Mandible under chin	By tendon to body of hyoid, superior aspect	Elevates hyoid or depresses mandible	Cranial V, Trigeminal	From hyoid the point of chin
Post. belly	Mastoid process			Cranial VII facial	Between hyoid to ramus of mandible along with Stylo-hyoid muscle

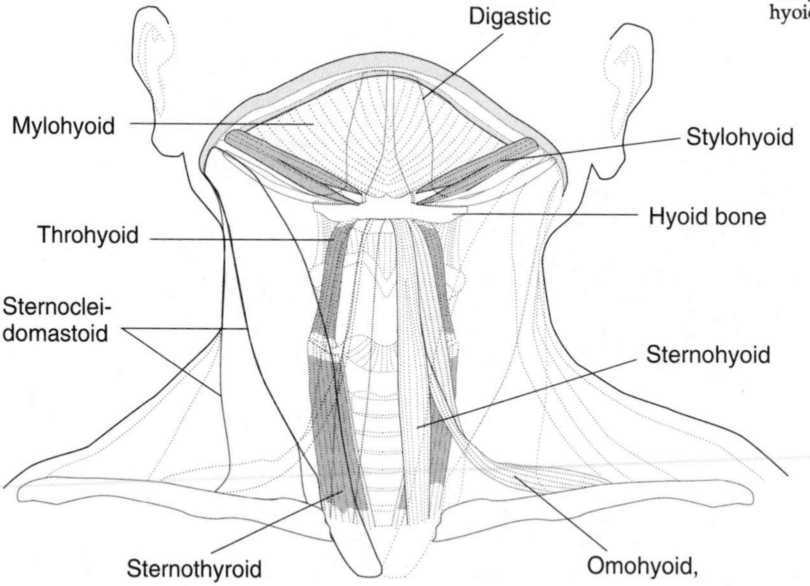

Fig. T5-2.40 Anterior neck; hyoid muscles.

MUSCLES OF MASTICATION

MUSCLE	ORIGIN	INSERTION	ACTION	INNERVATION	PALPATION
Masseter	Zygomatic arch	Lateral surface of ramus of the mandible	Closes jaw	Cranial V, Trigeminal	Lateral jaw, over molars
Temporalis	Temporal bone	Coronoid process and ramus of mandible	Closes and retracts jaw	Cranial V, Trigeminal	Lateral surface of temple area
Buccinator	Maxilla and mandible	Angle of mouth, blending with Obicularis oris	Holds cheeks near teeth postioning food for chewing	Cranial VII, Facial	Cheeks
Internal Pterygoid	Medial surface of pterygoid plate of sphenoid	Medial surface of ramus of the mandible	Closes jaw, Unilaterally; moves jaw to opposite side	Cranial V, Trigeminal	Hard to palpate
External Pterygoid	Lateral surface of pterygoid plate of sphenoid	Anterior surface of condyle of mandible and TMJ capsule	Protrudes lower jaw	Cranial V, Trigeminal	Cannot palpate

MUSCLES OF EXPRESSION

MUSCLE	ORIGIN	INSERTION	ACTION	INNERVATION	PALPATION
Epicranius					
Occipitalis	Posterior occiput above occipital ridge	Epicranial aponeurosis or the Galea aponeurotica	Draws Epicranius towards posterior	Posterior auricular and small occipital	Back of head above occipital ridge
Frontalis	Blended into Procerus, corrugator and Obicularis oculi	Epicranial aponeurosis or the Galea aponeurotica	Rasies eyebrow and wrinkles the forehead	Cranial VII, Facial	Forehead, above eyebrows
Corrugator	Meidal aspect of supraorbital ridge	Deep surface of skin in midle of supra-orbital arch	Draws eyebrows together	Cranial VII, Facial	Under medial eyebrow
Procerus	Fascua over upper nasil cartilage and lower nasil bone	Deep surface of skin between eyebrows	Draws nose up causing wrinkles across nose	Cranial VII, Facial	Bridge of nose
Orbicularis Oculi	Medial palpebral ligament to maxilla, nasil bone, nasil part of frontal bone	Fibers surround eye, and blend with adjacent muscles	Closes the eye	Cranial VII, Facial	Eyelid and surrounding eye
Nasalis	Maxilla above incisors	Blends into procerus	Compresses nostrils	Cranial VII, Facial	Side of nose
Dialator Naris	Greater ala cartilage	Point of the nose	Expands opening of nostril	Cranial VII, Facial	Cannot palpate
Quadratus Labii Superioris	Lower margin of orbit, frontal process of maxilla	Blends into Obicularis oris on upper lip	Raises upper lip	Cranial VII, Facial	Above upper lip, next to nose
Zygomaticus					
Major	Zygomatic bone	Blends into Obicularis oris muscle at upper angle of mouth	Draws angle of mouth back and up	Cranial VII, Facial	Below zygomatic arch when smiling
Minor	Continuous from inferior border of Obicularis occuli	Blends into Obicularis oris on upper lip	Raises upper lip	Cranial VII, Facial	Hard to differentiate from Quadratus labii

MUSCLES OF EXPRESSION *(continued)*

MUSCLE	ORIGIN	INSERTION	ACTION	INNERVATION	PALPATION
Obicularis Oris	From numerous adjacent muscles surrounding mouth	Lips, external skin around mouth and mucous membrane adjacent to the lips inside of mouth	Closes and protrudes lips	Cranial VII, Facial	The lips
Risorius	Fascia over Masseter	Blends into Obicularis oris and skin at corner of the mouth	Draws angle of mouth back	Cranial VII, Facial	On cheek near corner of mouth, Hard to palpate
Depressor Anguli Oris	Anterior inferior surface of mandible	Blends into Obicularis oris and skin at corner of the mouth	Draws angle of mouth down	Cranial VII, Facial	On chin below corner of mouth
Depressor Labii Inferioris	Anterior inferior surface of mandible	Blends into Obicularis oris and skin on lower lip of the mouth	Depresses lower lip	Cranial VII, Facial	On chin below lower lip
Mentalis	Mandible below incisors	Deep skin at point of chin	Raises chin and protrudes lower lip as if pouting	Cranial VII, Facial	The chin
Platisma	Superficial fascia of upper thorax and anteriolateral aspect of neck	Blends into muscles of angle of mouth and chin	Depresses angle of mouth and wrinkles skin of neck	Cranial VII, Facial	Anterio-lateral aspect of neck. Thin muscle and hard to palpate
Auricularis Anterior Superior Posterior	Temporal bone	Deep skin around ear	Raises and moves ear	Cranial VII, Facial	In front, above and behind ear. Small muscles, hard to palpate

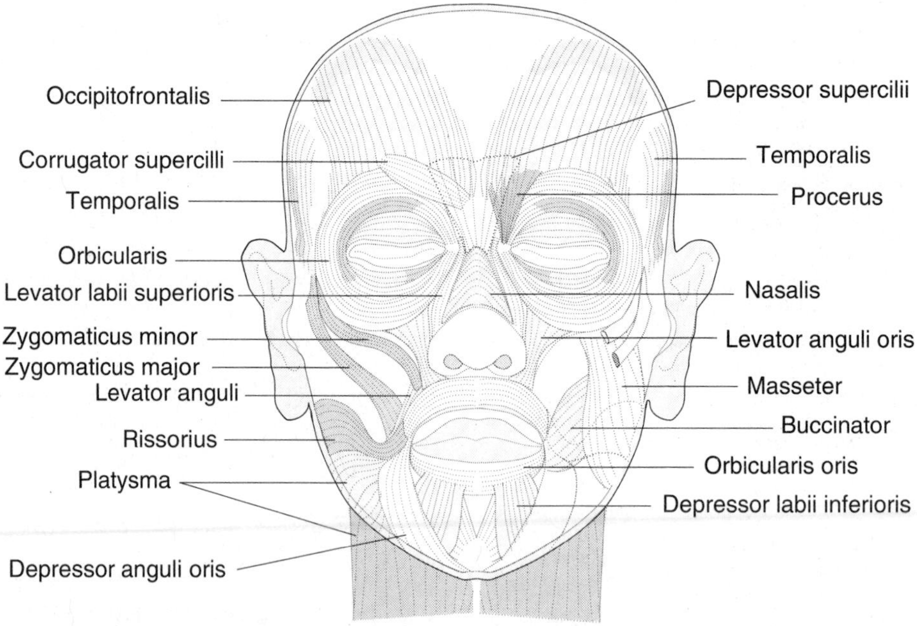

Fig. T5-2.41 Facial muscles.

MUSCLES THAT ACT ON THE EYE

MUSCLE	ORIGIN	INSERTION	ACTION	INNERVATION	PALPATION
Levator Palpebrea Superioris	Common tendonous ring surrounding optic nerve near optic foramen	Upper eye lid	Opens the eye	Cranial III, Oculomotor	Cannot palpate
Superior Oblique	Common tendonous ring surrounding optic via a tendon in superior orbit	Posterior lateral aspect of eyeball	Turns eye out and down	Cranial IV, Trochlear	Cannot palpate
Superior Rectus	Common tendonous ring surrounding optic nerve near optic foramen	Anterior superior aspect of eyeball	Rotates eye up	Cranial III, Oculomotor	Cannot palpate
Lateral Rectus	Common tendonous ring surrounding optic nerve near optic foramen	Anterior lateral aspect of eyeball	Rotates eye laterally	Cranial VI, Abducens	Cannot palpate
Inferior Rectus	Common tendonous ring surrounding optic nerve near optic foramen	Anterior inferior aspect of eyeball	Rotates eye down	Cranial III, Oculomotor	Cannot palpate
Medial Rectus	Common tendonous ring surrounding optic nerve near optic foramen	Anterior medial aspect of eye	Rotates eye medially	Cranial III, Oculomotor	Cannot palpate
Inferior Oblique	Orbital surface of maxilla	Posterior lateral aspect of eyeball	Rotates eye up and out	Cranial III, Oculomotor	Cannot palpate

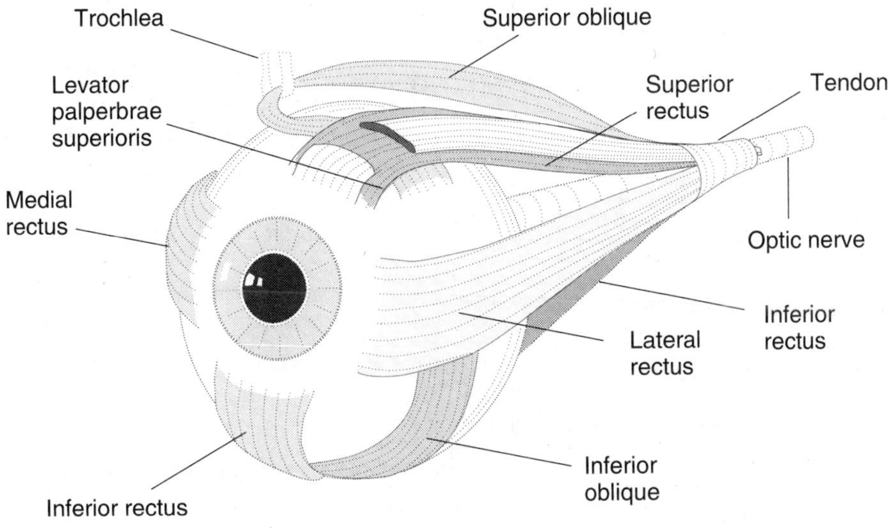

Fig. T5-2.42 Muscles of the eye.

▼ REVIEW

Muscles of the Head and Face

MATCHING TEST I

Insert the letter of the proper term in front of each definition.

_____ **1.** Move ears a. Orbicularis oculi

_____ **2.** Move scalp b. Orbicularis oris

_____ **3.** Opens eye c. Auricularis

_____ **4.** Presses lips together d. Masseter

_____ **5.** Raises lower jaw e. Epicranius

TRUE OR FALSE TEST I

Carefully read each statement and decide if it is true or false; draw a circle around the letter T or F.

1. T F Obliquus inferior and superior muscles do not rotate the eyeball.

2. T F Only the temporalis muscle moves the lower jaw.

3. T F The levator palpebrae superioris muscle opens the eye.

4. T F The epicranius is also known as the occipito-frontalis muscle.

5. T F The corrugator muscle controls the movement of the mouth.

Muscles of the Neck and Chest

MATCHING TEST II

Insert the letter of the proper term in front of each definition.

_____ **1.** Rotates cranium a. Intercostals

_____ **2.** Draws head backward b. Longus colli

_____ **3.** Rotates spine c. Obliquus capitis inferior

_____ **4.** Muscle of respiration d. Obliquus capitis superior

_____ **5.** Raises ribs in breathing e. Diaphragm

TRUE OR FALSE TEST II

Carefully read each statement and decide if it is true or false; draw a circle around the letter T or F.

1. T F Several muscles depress the jaw and raise the hyoid bone.

2. T F The sternocleidomastoid is the only muscle which bends the head forward and sideways.

3. T F The platysma muscle does not draw down the corners of the mouth.

4. T F The pectoralis major and minor muscles control the movement of the arm and shoulder.

5. T F Several groups of muscles raise the ribs in breathing.

Muscles of the Abdomen and Back

MATCHING TEST III

Insert the letter of the proper term in front of each definition.

_____ 1. Flexes trunk   a. Rectus abdominis

_____ 2. Keeps spine erect   b. Quadratus lumborum

_____ 3. Draws head backward   c. Sacrospinalis

_____ 4. Draws arm backward   d. Trapezius

_____ 5. Compresses abdomen   e. Latissimus dorsi

TRUE OR FALSE TEST III

Carefully read each statement and decide if it is true or false; draw a circle around the letter T or F.

1. T F The obliquus externus abdominis is an external muscle of the abdomen and back.

2. T F Only one muscle compresses the abdomen and bends the chest.

3. T F The infraspinatus and supra-spinatus muscles control the movement of the arm.

4. T F The gluteus medius muscle extends the hip joint.

5. T F The spine is kept erect with the aid of the sacrospinalis and multifidus muscles.

Muscles of the Arms and Hands

MATCHING TEST IV

Insert the letter of the proper term in front of each definition.

_____ 1. Flexes hand   a. Brachialis

_____ 2. Flexes forearm   b. Triceps brachialis

_____ 3. Flexes arm   c. Interossei

_____ 4. Separates fingers   d. Deltoid

_____ 5. Extends forearm   e. Palmaris longus

TRUE OR FALSE TEST IV

Carefully read each statement and decide if it is true or false; draw a circle around the letter T or F.

1. T F The movement of the thumb is controlled by one muscle.
2. T F The biceps brachii muscle draws the palm downward.
3. T F The brachioradialis muscle draws the palm upward.
4. T F Quick, short movements of the fingers are produced by the lumbricales muscles.
5. T F The subscapularis muscle rotates the humerus inward.

Muscles of the Legs and Feet

MATCHING TEST V

Insert the letter of the proper term in front of each definition.

_____ 1. Flexes leg   a. Flexor digitorum
_____ 2. Extends leg   b. Biceps femoris
_____ 3. Flexes hip   c. Rectus femoris
_____ 4. Extends foot   d. Pectineus
_____ 5. Flexes toes   e. Soleus

TRUE OR FALSE TEST V

Carefully read each statement and decide if it is true or false; draw a circle around the letter T or F.

1. T F The sartorius muscle bends the thigh and leg.
2. T F The movement of the big toe is controlled by the extensor hallucis longus muscle.
3. T F The extensor digitorum brevis muscle does not extend the four inner toes.
4. T F The soleus and gastrocnemius muscles both extend the foot.
5. T F The gracilis adducts femur and flexes knee joint.

SECTION QUESTIONS FOR DISCUSSION AND REVIEW ▼

1. What is the structure and function of muscles?
2. Approximately how many muscles are there in the human body?
3. Name three types of muscular tissue and give examples of where they are found.
4. What is the difference between voluntary and involuntary muscles?
5. Which characteristics enable muscles to produce movements?
6. What are skeletal muscles?
7. What is the functional unit of skeletal muscle?
8. What structures cause the striated appearance of voluntary muscles?
9. What tissues are found in muscle?
10. To which structures are skeletal muscles attached?
11. What is the origin of a muscle? Give an example.
12. What is the insertion of a muscle? Give an example.
13. Which structure attaches the muscle to the bone?
14. What is the function of fibrous connective tissue in muscle?
15. What is fascia?
16. Name and locate the three connective tissue layers of muscle.
17. What is meant by the term *motor unit*?
18. What is acetylcholine? Where is it found? What does it do?
19. What molecular structure provides the energy for muscle contraction?
20. What is the relationship between oxygen debt and muscle fatigue?
21. When does a muscle have tone?
22. When does a muscle lack tone?
23. Why is it important for the massage practitioner to understand how muscles function?
24. What is meant by extensibility of muscle?
25. Explain the difference between isometric and isotonic muscle contractions.
26. Explain the difference between eccentric and concentric contractions. What do they have in common?
27. To what does the term *agonist* or *prime mover* refer?
28. When flexing the elbow, would the triceps be the prime mover or the antagonist?
29. What are the three components of motion?
30. Do diarthrotic joints remain motionless or are they capable of free movement?
31. Describe three degrees of muscle strain.
32. What is muscle atrophy?
33. What joints have limited motion?
34. Are synarthrotic joints movable or immovable?

SYSTEM FOUR: THE CIRCULATORY SYSTEM

The vascular or circulatory system controls the circulation of the blood and lymph throughout the body by means of the heart, blood, and lymph vessels. The primary function of the circulatory system is to supply body cells with nutrient materials and carry away waste products.

There are two divisions to the vascular system:

1. The **blood-vascular system** or **cardiovascular system** includes the blood, heart, and blood vessels (arteries, capillaries, and veins).
2. The **lymph-vascular system,** or lymphatic system, consists of lymph, lymph nodes, and lymphatics through which the lymph circulates.

These two systems are intimately linked with each other.

The Blood-Vascular System or Cardiovascular System

The blood-vascular system is a closed circuit system that consists of the heart, the arteries, capillaries, veins, and the blood. This system continuously circulates the blood throughout the body. Even though the blood-vascular system is considered to be a closed system, in which the blood normally does not leave the blood vessels, in the capillaries there is a constant and extensive interchange of fluids and the substances they contain.

The Heart

The **heart** is an efficient pump that keeps the blood circulating in a steady stream through a closed system of arteries, capillaries, and veins. The heart is a muscular, conical-shaped organ, about the size of a closed fist, located in the chest cavity between the lungs and behind the sternum. It is enclosed in a double-layered membrane, the **pericardium** (per-i-**KAR**-dee-um). The inner layer of the pericardium is a thin serous covering of the heart, while the outer layer is a protective fibrous connective tissue sac that is attached to the diaphragm, the vertebral column, the back of the sternum, and the large blood vessels that emerge from the heart. Between these two layers is a space, the **pericardial cavity,** that contains a serous fluid so that the heart is supported in position and at the same time allowed to move frictionlessly as it continually pulsates.

The walls of the heart consist of three distinct layers. The **epicardium** is the protective outer layer that includes the inner pericardium. This layer includes and supports the nerves, blood and lymph capillaries, and fat that surround the heart. The next thick layer is the cardiac muscle or the **myocardium** and is responsible for the muscular pumping action of the heart. The thin innermost layer is the **endocardium,** which provides a smooth protective covering that lines the inner chambers of the heart and heart valves and is continuous with the linings of the blood vessels (endothelium) (Fig. 5.47).

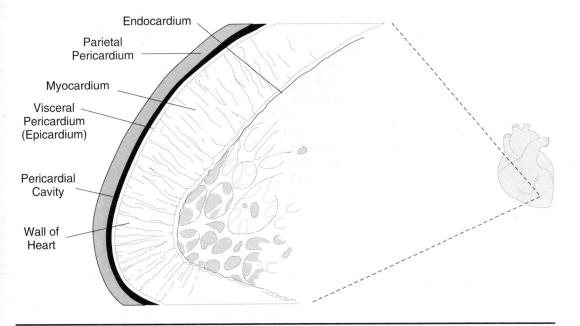

Endocardium
Parietal Pericardium
Myocardium
Visceral Pericardium (Epicardium)
Pericardial Cavity
Wall of Heart

Fig. 5.47 Wall of the heart, including pericardium.

The interior of the heart contains four chambers, two on each side of a muscular wall called the **septum** (SEP-tum). The upper thin-walled cavities, the right and left atrium (sometimes called the auricle), receive blood into the heart from the veins. The lower thick-walled chambers, the right and left ventricle, pump the blood out of the heart into the arteries. Four valves allow the blood to flow in only one direction. The **tricuspid valve,** located between the right atrium and right ventricle, allows blood to flow from the right atrium into the right ventricle and not the opposite direction. The **pulmonary semilunar valve,** positioned between the right ventricle and pulmonary artery, directs the blood from the right ventricle into the pulmonary arteries as it travels to the lungs. The **bicuspid (or mitral) valve,** located between the left atrium and ventricle, allows blood to flow only from the left atrium into the left ventricle. The **aortic semilunar valve,** situated in the orifice of the aorta, permits the blood to be pumped from the left ventricle into the aorta but not the reverse. With each contraction and relaxation of the heart, the blood flows in, travels from the atriums to the ventricles, and is then driven out to be distributed all over the body (Fig. 5.48).

The impulses that generate the rhythmical heartbeat originate within the heart muscle. A system of specilized cardiac tissue initiates rhythmic impulses that transmit throughout the cardiac muscle and stimulate it to contract. This occurs without stimulation by outside nerve fibers or other agents. Even though the rhythmic heart contractions are initiated within the heart muscle, there is a complicated neurological heart monitoring system that regulates

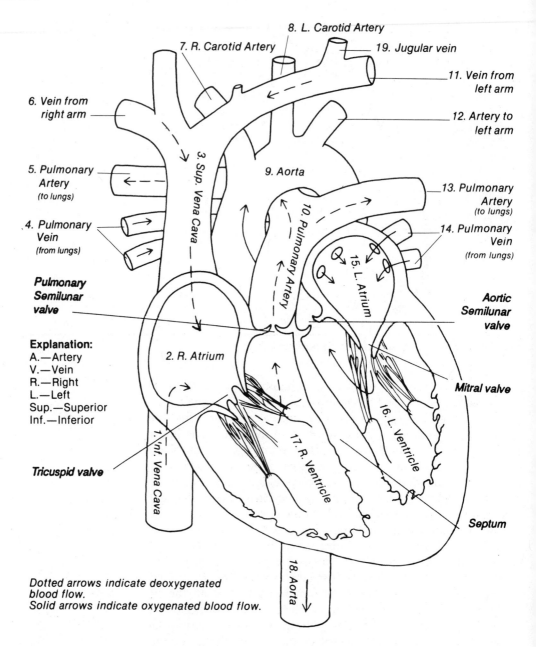

8. L. Carotid Artery

7. R. Carotid Artery

19. Jugular vein

11. Vein from left arm

6. Vein from right arm

12. Artery to left arm

5. Pulmonary Artery (to lungs)

3. Sup. Vena Cava

9. Aorta

13. Pulmonary Artery (to lungs)

4. Pulmonary Vein (from lungs)

10. Pulmonary Artery

14. Pulmonary Vein (from lungs)

15. L. Atrium

Pulmonary Semilunar valve

Aortic Semilunar valve

Explanation:
A.—Artery
V.—Vein
R.—Right
L.—Left
Sup.—Superior
Inf.—Inferior

2. R. Atrium

Mitral valve

1. Inf. Vena Cava

17. R. Ventricle

16. L. Ventricle

Tricuspid valve

Septum

18. Aorta

Dotted arrows indicate deoxygenated blood flow.
Solid arrows indicate oxygenated blood flow.

1. Veins of abdomen, pelvis and lower extremities empty into this vein. **2.** Receives impure blood from the vena cava. **3.** Veins of the head, neck, thorax and upper extremities empty into this vein. **4.** Conveys oxygenated blood from the lungs to the left atrium. **5.** Conveys venous blood from the right ventricle to the lungs. **7.** The principal large artery on the right side of the neck. **8.** The principal large artery on the left side of the neck. **9.** Main artery of the body; carries blood from the left ventricle to all arteries of the body. **10.** Divides into left and right branches and takes blood into the lungs. **15.** Receives purified blood through the pulmonary vein. **16.** From the left ventricle the aorta sends blood to all parts of the body except the lungs. **17.** Venous blood is carried through the pulmonary artery up to the lungs to be oxygenated and purified. **18.** A large vessel arising from the left ventricle which, by way of its branches, distributes arterial blood to all parts of the body. **19.** Any of several major veins of the neck.

Fig. 5.48 Anatomy of the heart.

the heart rate. Impulses from the **vagus** (**VAY**-gus) **nerve** and the **sympathetic nervous system,** help regulate the force of contraction and the heart rate. In a normal adult, the heart beats about seventy-two to eighty times a minute.

The Blood Vessels

The **arteries, arterioles, capillaries, venules, and veins** transport blood from the heart to the various tissues of the body and back again to the heart.

Arteries and Arterioles

Arteries are thick-walled muscular and elastic vessels that transport oxygenated blood (except for the pulmonary artery) under relatively high pressure from the heart. The main artery of the body is the **aorta** (ay-**OR**-tuh), which arches up from the left ventricle of the heart, extending over and down along the vertebral column. Arteries branch into smaller and smaller branches until eventually they become microscopic arterioles that control the rate of flow of blood into the capillaries. Arteries vary in size from the aorta, which is about an inch in diameter, to the microscopic capillaries, whose walls are just a single cell in thickness and are only large enough to pass one blood cell at a time.

The smooth muscle tissue in the walls of the arteries and arterioles is richly supplied with nerves from the sympathetic portion of the autonomic nervous system. Impulses from these **vasomotor nerves** cause the smooth muscles of the arterial walls to contract, reducing the diameter of the vessel. This action is called **vasoconstriction.** When the nerve impulses are inhibited, the muscles relax and the diameter of the vessel enlarges or undergoes **vasodilatation.** Changes in the diameter of the vessels affect the blood pressure and flow. The nerve response and control of the small arteries and arterioles regulate the flow of blood to the tissues in direct proportion to the tissue's specific needs.

Capillaries

Capillaries are the smallest microscopic, thin-walled blood vessels whose networks connect the small arterioles with the venules. The walls of the capillaries are extremely thin and permeable. The most important function of the capillaries is the two-way transport of substances between the flowing blood and the tissue fluids surrounding the cells. Substances move through the capillary walls either by the process of diffusion, filtration, or osmosis. of these, diffusion is the most prevalent.

In the process of **diffusion,** substances move from an area of higher concentration to an area of lower concentration. Blood entering the capillaries has a higher concentration of nutrients and oxygen than the fluid surrounding the cells, so the oxygen and nutrients diffuse into the tissue spaces. By the same account the concentrations of metabolic waste products and carbon dioxide are more highly concentrated in the tissue fluid and therefore tend to diffuse into the blood stream.

The pressure of the blood, especially at the junction of the arteriole and the capillary, tends to push fluids and substances through the capillary wall and into the tissue spaces through a process called **filtration.** Because of a high concentration of proteins and other substances retained in the plasma, there is an osmotic pressure created that tends to draw water into the capillaries from the tissue spaces at almost the same rate as the blood pressure forces fluid out. Through these processes substances can move back and forth between the blood stream and tissues to support the needs of the cells and at the same time maintain the volume of the blood at a normal level.

Veins and Venules

Venules (VEN-yools) are the microscopic vessels that continue from the capillaries and merge to form veins. Veins are thinner-walled blood vessels that carry deoxygenated and waste-laden blood from the various capillaries back to the heart. Many veins, especially those in the arms and legs, have a system of valves that prevent blood from flowing backward in the vein and act as a **venous pump** to move the blood toward the heart. These valves are flap-like structures that protrude from the inside walls of the vein in such a way that blood moving toward the heart pushes past the valve, but if the blood attempts to move in the reverse direction, pressure against the valve forces it closed and blood cannot pass. The venous pump is a phenomenon that results when muscles contract and exert external pressure on the veins, which tends to collapse them. As the vein is repeatedly collapsed, the blood is forced along through the system of valves toward the heart. Massage strokes are very effective at encouraging the blood to move through the veins and therefore should always be directed to follow the venous blood flow (Fig. 5.49).

The Circulation of the Blood

The blood is in constant circulation from the moment it leaves until it returns to the heart. There are two systems involved in circulation: pulmonary and systemic.

Pulmonary Circulation

Pulmonary circulation is the blood circulation from the heart to the lungs and back again to the heart. During the pulmonary circulation, the deoxygenated blood is pumped from the right ventricle of the heart, through the pulmonary arteries, to the capillaries of the lungs, where carbon dioxide is replaced by oxygen. The exchange is continuous. Freshly oxygenated blood returns to the left atrium of the heart through the pulmonary veins.

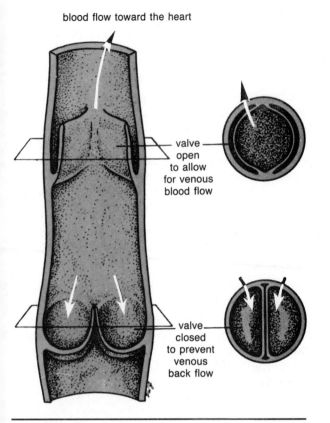

blood flow toward the heart

valve open to allow for venous blood flow

valve closed to prevent venous back flow

Fig. 5.49 Valves in the veins.

General or Systemic Circulation

General or **systemic circulation** is the blood circulation from the left side of the heart throughout the body and back again to the heart.

The course that blood travels is as follows:

1. The right atrium or auricle receives oxygen poor blood from the large superior and inferior vena cava.
2. From the right atrium, the venous blood passes through the tricuspid valve into the right ventricle.
3. From the right ventricle, the venous blood is pumped through the pulmonary semilunar valve and is carried through the pulmonary arteries to the lungs to be oxygenated.
4. The freshly oxygenated blood is collected from the capillaries into the pulmonary veins and returned to the heart.
5. The left atrium receives the oxygenated blood from the pulmonary veins.
6. From the left atrium or auricle, the oxygenated blood passes through the bicuspid or mitral valve into the left ventricle.
7. From the left ventricle the blood is pumped through the aortic semilunar valve and into the aorta.

8. From the aorta the blood is distributed to the major arteries throughout the body except for the lungs. The blood moves into ever-smaller branches of the arterial system until it flows into the arterioles.

9. From the arterioles the blood moves into the thin-walled capillaries where the oxygen, nutrients, and fluids move into the tissue spaces and the metabolic wastes and CO_2 are reabsorbed into the blood stream.

10. The blood is then collected from the capillary beds into the venules and then into larger and larger veins until the blood finally flows into the inferior or superior vena cava.

11. This cycle is repeated as the venous blood is brought back again to the right atrium or auricle of the heart (Fig. 5.50).

Disorders of the Blood Vessels

Atherosclerosis

Atherosclerosis is characterized by an accumulation of fatty deposits on the inner walls of the arteries. The development of the deposits, called plaque, seems to relate to the level of cholesterol in the blood. The deposits may interfere with blood flow or create a surface where blood clots may form. The walls of affected arteries tend to thicken, become fibrous, and lose their elasticity in a condition called **arteriosclerosis** (ar-**TEER**-ee-o-skler-**O**-sis).

Phlebitis

Phlebitis an inflammation of a vein which might result from injury, surgery, or infection. Symptoms include pain and inflammation along the course of the vein and swelling. A serious side effect is the development of clots that may block circulation (thrombophlebitis) (throm-bow-fle-**BYE**-tis) or break loose and float in the blood as an **embolus** (**EM**-bow-lus). If the floating embolus becomes lodged in an artery, the tissues supplied by that artery will stop functioning. If that happens in the lungs, heart, or brain, the consequences may be death.

Varicose veins

Varicose veins are characterized by protruding, bulbous, distended superficial veins particularly in the lower legs. Extensive back pressure in the veins due to prolonged standing or blockage causes the veins to enlarge and stretch to the point that the valves become incompetent. The weight of the blood further distends the veins and more valves become dysfunctional, perpetuating the condition. Increased pressure in the veins also increases pressure in the capillaries and often results in edema. Severe varicose veins are contraindicated for all but the lightest massage.

Edema

Edema is a condition of excess fluid in the interstitial spaces. Edema is characterized by swelling of the tissues due to the excess fluid.

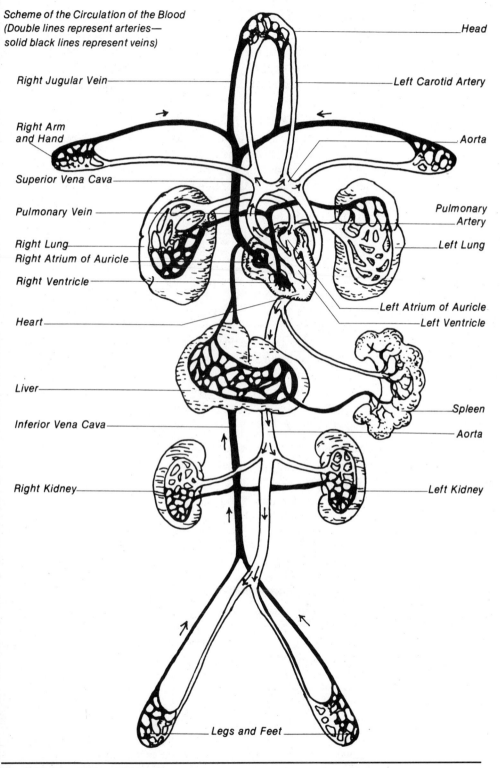

Scheme of the Circulation of the Blood (Double lines represent arteries— solid black lines represent veins)

Head

Right Jugular Vein

Left Carotid Artery

Right Arm and Hand

Aorta

Superior Vena Cava

Pulmonary Vein

Pulmonary Artery

Right Lung

Left Lung

Right Atrium of Auricle

Right Ventricle

Left Atrium of Auricle

Left Ventricle

Heart

Liver

Spleen

Inferior Vena Cava

Aorta

Right Kidney

Left Kidney

Legs and Feet

Fig. 5.50 Circulation of blood.

The cause of edema is an imbalance in fluid pressures within the capillaries. The pressure imbalance may be caused by obstructions in the veins or lymph vessels, high capillary pressure or porosity, or kidney malfunction that results in fluid retention.

The Blood

Blood is the nutritive fluid circulating throughout the blood-vascular system. It is salty and sticky, has an alkaline reaction, and maintains a normal temperature of 98.6° F (37° C). The amount of blood varies according to a person's size as well as some other factors. An average-sized male (about 160 pounds) will have approximately eleven pints of blood or about one sixteenth to one twentieth of the body's weight. The skin may hold as much as one half of all the blood in the body.

Chief Functions of Blood

1. The blood carries water, oxygen, food, and secretions to all areas of the body.
2. It carries away carbon dioxide and waste products to be eliminated through the excretory channels.
3. It helps to equalize the body temperature, thus protecting the body from extreme heat and cold.
4. It aids in protecting the body from harmful bacteria and infections through the action of the white blood cells.
5. It coagulates (clots), thereby closing injured blood vessels and preventing the loss of blood through hemorrhage.

Composition of Blood

The blood is a liquid tissue consisting of a fluid component (blood plasma) and a solid component which consists of red corpuscles, white corpuscles, and blood platelets. Plasma constitutes from 50 to 60 percent of the blood volume.

Blood Cells

Red corpuscles (red blood cells) or **erythrocytes** (e-**RITH**-row-sites) are double concave disc-shaped cells colored with a substance called **hemoglobin** (hee-mow-**GLOW**-bin). The function of the red corpuscles is to carry oxygen from the lungs to the body cells and transport carbon dioxide from the cells to the lungs. The red blood cells are confined to the blood vessels and do not circulate outside the blood vascular system. The red blood cells are formed in the red bone marrow. They are far more numerous than the white blood cells and account for as much as 98 percent of the blood cells.

The blood itself is bright red in the arteries (except in the pulmonary artery) and dark red in the veins (except in the pulmonary vein). This change in color is due to the color change of hemoglobin as the result of a gain or loss of oxygen as the blood passes through the lungs and other tissues of the body.

White corpuscles (white blood cells), also called **leukocytes,** differ from red blood cells in many respects. They are larger in size, colorless, and can change their shape and other properties according to their location and function. White corpuscles are produced in the spleen, lymph nodes, and the red marrow of the bones. Leukocytes can squeeze between the cells that comprise the capillary walls and move through the intercellular spaces with an ameba-like motion. The most important function of these cells is to protect the body against disease by combating different infectious and toxic agents that may invade the body. Most leukocytes actually engulf and digest harmful bacteria and other foreign elements in a process called **phagocytosis** (fag-o-sigh-**TOE**-sis). Our bodies also manufacture specialized leukocytes that produce antibodies that protect us from specific disease organisms and are an important part of our **immune system.**

Blood platelets or **thrombocytes** are colorless, irregular bodies, much smaller than the red corpuscles. They are formed in the red bone marrow. These bodies play an important role in the clotting of the blood over a wound (Fig. 5.51).

Blood Coagulation or Clotting

When a blood vessel is damaged, several things happen to prevent severe blood loss. The blood platelets adhere to the ragged edges of the injured vessel, especially to the collagen fibers surrounding the blood vessel. They immediately begin to change shape as protrusions form from their cell membrane and they stick together to create a platelet plug. Platelets also release **serotonin** (seer-o-**TOE**-nin) which is a vasoconstrictor that causes a vascular spasm that temporarily closes the blood vessel.

The tissue damage causes an enzyme to be released that acts on one of the components in the plasma (fibrogen) to activate and form threads of **fibrin.** The fibrin tends to stick to the damaged blood vessels, forming a meshwork that entraps other platelets and blood cells in a **blood clot.**

Plasma

Plasma is the fluid part of the blood, straw-like in color, in which the red corpuscles, white corpuscles, and blood platelets are suspended. About nine tenths of plasma is water. The remaining plasma is made up of about 7 percent proteins and 1.5 percent other substances. It functions to regulate fluid balance and pH and to transport nutrients and gases. Plasma is derived from the food and water taken into the body (Figs. 5.52 and 5.53).

Diseases of the Blood

Hemophilia

Hemophilia is characterized by extremely slow clotting of blood and excessive bleeding from even very slight cuts. This disease is

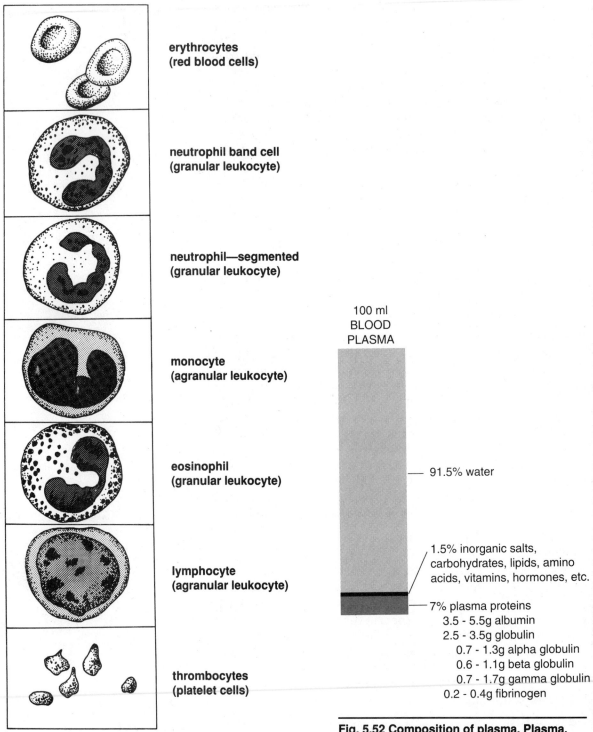

erythrocytes
(red blood cells)

neutrophil band cell
(granular leukocyte)

neutrophil—segmented
(granular leukocyte)

monocyte
(agranular leukocyte)

eosinophil
(granular leukocyte)

lymphocyte
(agranular leukocyte)

thrombocytes
(platelet cells)

100 ml
BLOOD
PLASMA

— 91.5% water

1.5% inorganic salts,
carbohydrates, lipids, amino
acids, vitamins, hormones, etc.

7% plasma proteins
  3.5 - 5.5g albumin
  2.5 - 3.5g globulin
    0.7 - 1.3g alpha globulin
    0.6 - 1.1g beta globulin
    0.7 - 1.7g gamma globulin
  0.2 - 0.4g fibrinogen

Fig. 5.51 Blood cells and platelets.

Fig. 5.52 Composition of plasma. Plasma, which is primarily water, contains about 7% protein and 1.5% other substances.

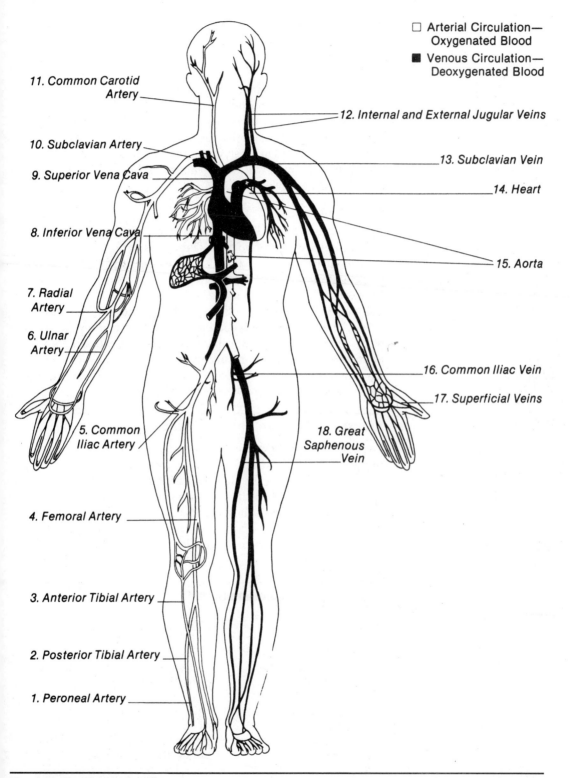

☐ Arterial Circulation—
   Oxygenated Blood
■ Venous Circulation—
   Deoxygenated Blood

11. Common Carotid
    Artery

12. Internal and External Jugular Veins

10. Subclavian Artery

13. Subclavian Vein

9. Superior Vena Cava

14. Heart

8. Inferior Vena Cava

15. Aorta

7. Radial
   Artery

6. Ulnar
   Artery

16. Common Iliac Vein

17. Superficial Veins

5. Common
   Iliac Artery

18. Great
    Saphenous
    Vein

4. Femoral Artery

3. Anterior Tibial Artery

2. Posterior Tibial Artery

1. Peroneal Artery

Fig. 5.53 Circulatory system.

hereditary, but men are the chief sufferers. Women may, however, transmit this blood condition to their sons.

Anemia

Anemia refers to a number of conditions in which there is a rapid loss or inadequate production of red blood cells. In this kind of condition the oxygen-carrying capacity is reduced, resulting in a lack of body strength and paleness of the complexion. A diet rich in iron, which is found in green vegetables, such as spinach, and organ meats, such as liver, will help to alleviate this condition. A physician should be consulted.

Leukemia

Leukemia is a form of cancer in which there is an uncontrolled production of white blood cells. These cells do not fully mature and remain virtually nonfunctional. As a result, the person's resistance to disease is reduced. There are two major types of leukemia: Myeloid leukemia begins in the bone marrow and lymphoid leukemia begins in the white-cell-producing portions of the lymphoid tissue. The leukemic cells soon metastasize into other areas of the body, producing leukemic cells and demanding excessive amounts of metabolic elements, resulting in severe tissue degeneration. Common effects are severe anemia, spontaneous bleeding, a tendency toward infections, and eventually death.

Arteries of the Head, Face, and Neck

The common carotid arteries are the main sources of blood supply to the head, face, and neck. They are located on either side of the neck, and each artery divides into an internal and external branch. The internal branch of the common carotid artery supplies the cranial cavity, whereas the external branch supplies the superficial parts of the head, face, and neck. The arteries, like the muscles and nerves, are named in accordance with the parts of the body that they serve (Fig. 5.54).

Important Arteries of the Body

NAME	FUNCTION
Head and Neck	
Facial Artery	Supplies blood to face and pharynx
Temporal Artery	Supplies blood to forehead, masseter muscle, and ear
Common Carotid Arteries:	
Internal branch	Supplies blood to cranial cavity
External branch	Supplies blood to surface of head, face, and neck

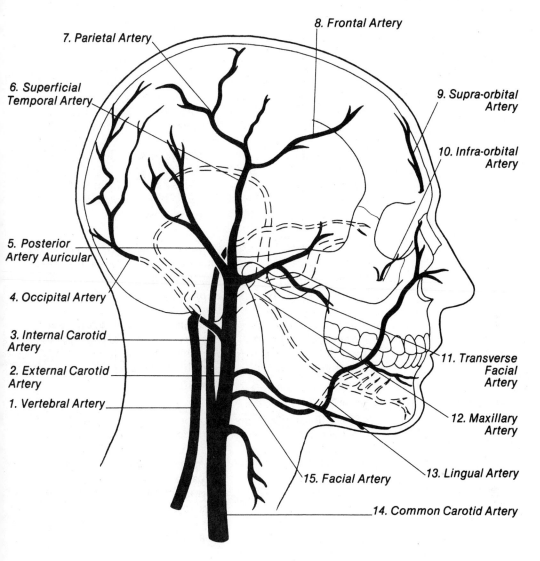

7. Parietal Artery

8. Frontal Artery

6. Superficial
Temporal Artery

9. Supra-orbital
Artery

10. Infra-orbital
Artery

5. Posterior
Artery Auricular

4. Occipital Artery

3. Internal Carotid
Artery

2. External Carotid
Artery

1. Vertebral Artery

11. Transverse
Facial
Artery

12. Maxillary
Artery

15. Facial Artery

13. Lingual Artery

14. Common Carotid Artery

1. Supplies muscles of neck, posterior fossa of skull. **2.** Supplies face, tonsils, root of tongue and submandibular gland. **3.** Supplies brain, sinuses, parts of the head. **4.** Supplies muscles of neck, ear area and scalp. **5.** Supplies area of ear, scalp and parotid gland. **6.** Supplies the masseter muscle. **7.** Located in the parietal bone of the skull. **8.** Supplies frontal bone, upper eyelid. **9.** Supplies root of orbit, frontal bone, upper eyelid. **10.** Supplies muscle of eye and upper lip. **11.** Supplies masseter muscle, parotid gland, skin of face. **12.** Supplies jaws, ear and deep structure of face.
13. Supplies membrane of tongue and mouth, gums, tonsils, soft palate, epiglottis. **14.** Right side supplies right side of head and face, left side supplies the left side of the head and face. **15.** Supplies face, root of tongue, submandibular gland.

Fig. 5.54 Arteries of the head, face, and neck.

Branches of External Carotid Artery

Ophthalmic artery	Supplies blood to the eyes
Supra-orbital artery	Supplies blood to the eye socket, forehead, and side of nose
Frontal artery	Supplies blood to the forehead
Parietal artery	Supplies blood to the crown and sides of head
Posterior auricular artery	Supplies blood to the scalp and back of ear
Submental artery	Supplies blood to chin and lower lip
Superior labial	Supplies blood to upper lip and center of nose

Trunk

Aorta	Forms main trunk of arterial system and subdivides to form large and small branches
Subclavian artery	Supplies blood to neck, chest, and upper part of back
Coronary artery	Supplies blood to heart muscles
Common iliac artery	Supplies blood to abdominal wall
External iliac artery	Supplies blood to lower limb
Internal iliac artery	Supplies blood to pelvic organs and inner thigh

Upper Extremities

(The following arteries are for one side of the body Fig. 5.55.)

Axillary artery	Supplies blood to shoulder, chest, and arm
Brachial artery	Supplies blood to the arm and forearm
Radial artery	Supplies blood to forearm, wrist, and thumb side of hand
Ulnar artery	Supplies blood to forearm, wrist, and small finger side of hand

Lower Extremities

(The following arteries are for one side of the body.)

Femoral artery	Supplies blood to lower part of abdominal wall, pelvic organs, and upper thigh
Popliteal artery	Supplies blood to knee and leg
Anterior tibial artery	Supplies blood to leg
Posterior tibial artery	Supplies blood to leg, heel, and foot
Dorsalis pedis artery	Supplies blood to foot

ARTERIES

VEINS

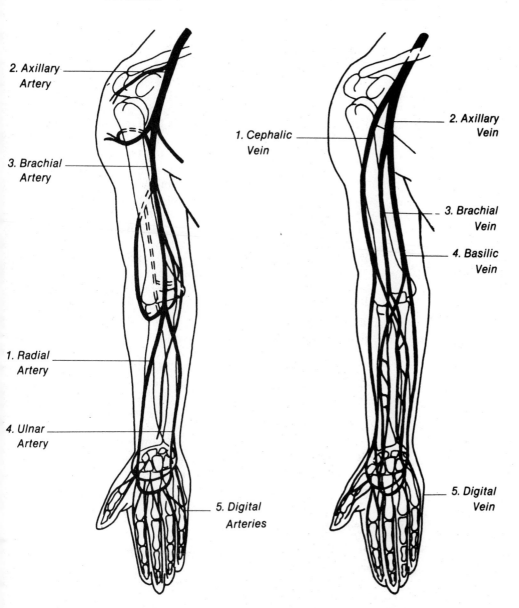

2. Axillary Artery

3. Brachial Artery

1. Cephalic Vein

2. Axillary Vein

3. Brachial Vein

4. Basilic Vein

1. Radial Artery

4. Ulnar Artery

5. Digital Arteries

5. Digital Vein

I. Arteries: Large thick-walled tubes comprising a system that carries blood directly from the heart to the main parts of the body. 1. Principal artery of thumb and deep palmar arch. 2. A continuation of the subclavian extending from the outer border of the first rib to the tendon of the teres major muscle where it becomes the brachial. 3. Distributes blood to various muscles of the arm, the humerus, elbow joint, forearm and hand. 4. Artery which supplies muscles of the forearm, shafts of radius and ulna, ulnal half of the hand and skin of these areas. 5. Arteries serving the dorsal areas of the fingers.

II. Veins: Blood vessels that carry blood from parts of the body back toward the heart. 1. The superficial vein rising from the radial side of the arm which supplies the biceps and deltoid muscles. 2. A continuation of the basilic ending in the outer border of the first rib in the subclavian vein. 3. Deep veins of the forearm and arm. 4. Veins beginning in the ulnar part of the dorsal network and extending to join the accessory cephalic vein. 5. Veins of the fingers.

Fig. 5.55 Blood supply of the arm and hand.

Important Veins of the Body

NAME	FUNCTION
Head and Neck	
Facial vein	Receives blood from face and empties into internal jugular vein
Internal jugular vein	Receives blood from cranial cavity and from surface of face and neck
External jugular vein	Receives blood from deep parts of face and from the surface of cranium
Temporal veins	Receives blood from the tempo-maxillary region of the head
Maxillary anterior vein	Receives blood from the anterior portion of the face
Ophthalmic vein	Receives blood from the eyes.
Supra-orbital vein	Receives blood from the forehead and eyebrow
Frontal vein	Receives blood from the anterior portion of the scalp.
Superior and inferior labial veins	Receives blood from the upper and lower lips (Fig. 5.56).
Trunk	
Innominate veins	Receives blood from internal jugular and subclavian veins
Coronary veins	Receives blood from heart muscles
Common iliac vein	Receives blood from external and internal iliac veins and empties into inferior vena cava
Inferior vena cava	Receives blood from abdomen, pelvis, and lower limbs
Superior vena cava	Receives blood from head, neck, thorax, and upper limbs.
Upper Extremities	
(The following veins are for one side of the body.)	
Cephalic vein	Receives blood from radial side (front) of arm
Basilic vein	Receives blood from ulnar side (outside) of arm
Axillary vein	Returns blood from arm to heart
Lower Extremities	
(The following veins are for one side of the body.)	
Great saphenous veins	Receives blood from the inner side of front leg
Small saphenous vein	Receives blood from back of leg
Popliteal vein	Receives blood from anterior and posterior tibial veins
Femoral vein	Receives blood from feet, legs, and thigh

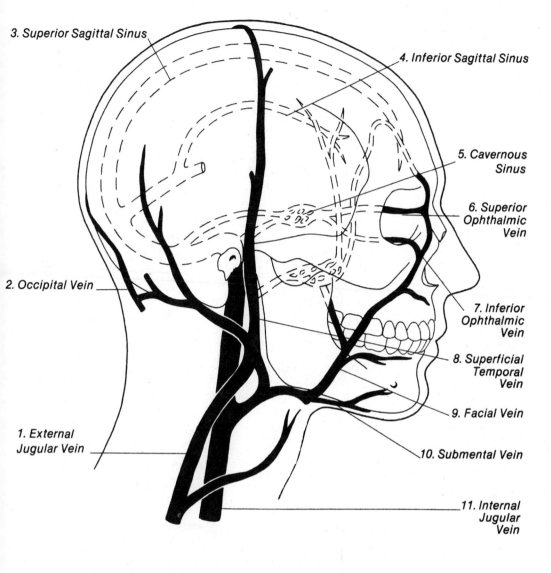

3. Superior Sagittal Sinus

4. Inferior Sagittal Sinus

5. Cavernous Sinus

6. Superior Ophthalmic Vein

2. Occipital Vein

7. Inferior Ophthalmic Vein

8. Superficial Temporal Vein

9. Facial Vein

1. External Jugular Vein

10. Submental Vein

11. Internal Jugular Vein

1. Vein located in side of the neck that drains the posterior part of the face area supplied by carotid arteries.
2. Drains into confluence of sinuses. **3.** A single long space located in midline above the brain. Ends in an enlargement called the confluence of sinuses. **4.** A small venous sinus of the dura mater, situated in the posterior half of the lower concave border of the cerebral falx. **5.** Situated behind the eyeball and drains the ophthalmic veins of the eye.
6. Drains veins of the eye. **7.** Veins supplying the eye area. **8.** Vein serving the temple region of the head on either side.
9. Vein supplying the anterior side of the face. **10.** A vein situated below the chin that follows the submental artery and opens into the facial vein. **11.** Vein located in side of the neck and drains the brain, face, neck and transverse sinus.

Fig. 5.56 Veins of the head, face and neck.

▼ THE LYMPH-VASCULAR SYSTEM

The lymphatic system acts as an aid to, and is interlinked with, the blood-vascular system. Lymph is derived from the blood and is gradually shifted back into the blood stream. The lymph-vascular system includes the lymph, lymphatics, lymph ducts, lymph nodes, and lacteals. Also considered a part of the lymph system are the tonsils, the spleen, and the thymus gland.

Function of the Lymph System

The lymphatics collect excess tissue fluid, invading micro-organisms, damaged cells, and protein molecules that are too large or too toxic to return directly to the blood system through the capillary walls. These materials are transported from the interstitial spaces through the lymph vessels, are filtered through the lymph nodes, and eventually rejoin the blood near the junction of the subclavian and jugular veins. The lymphoid tissue also produces lymphocytes, white blood cells that are an important element of the body's immune system (Fig. 5.57).

Lymph and Tissue Fluid

Lymph is a straw-colored fluid that is derived from and is very similar to the tissue fluid or interstitial fluid of the body part from which it flows. By bathing all cells, tissue fluid acts as a medium of

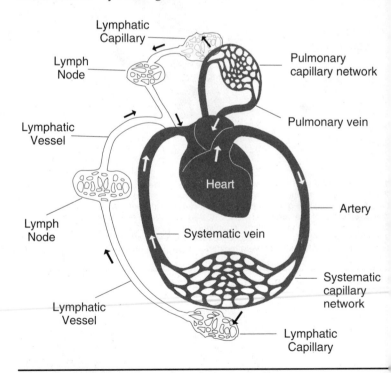

Fig. 5.57 Interaction of blood and lymph system.

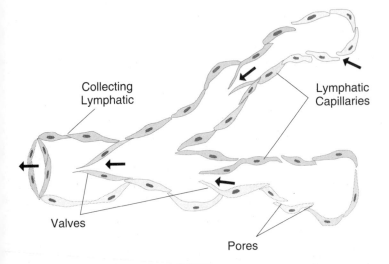

Fig. 5.58 Structure of lymphatic capillaries, showing the lymphatic valves.

exchange, trading to the cells its nutritive materials and receiving in return the waste products of metabolism. Most of the fluid that filters through the capillary walls to surround the cells is eventually reabsorbed into the capillaries. However, about 10 percent of the fluid enters the lymphatic capillaries and returns to the blood through the lymphatic system.

Lymph-Collecting Vessels

Lymph capillaries are located throughout the body with the exception of the epidermis of the skin, the central nervous system, the bones, and the endomyseum of most muscles. **Lacteals (LAK**-tee-als) are lymphatic capillaries located in the villa of the small intestine. The walls of the lymph capillaries are constructed of endothelial cells that overlap at the edges yet are not securely attached. This arrangement creates flap-like valve that allows fluid from the tissue spaces to enter the capillaries (Fig. 5.58).

Lymph Pathways

After being collected in the lymph capillaries, lymph flows into **lymphatics,** which merge into larger and larger lymphatics. The pathways of the lymphatics are closely associated with the veins of the body. The lymphatics continue to merge until the lymph flows into one of two large lymph ducts and finally back into the blood.

Lymph from the legs, abdomen, left arm, left side of the head, neck, and chest flows into the **thoracic duct (left lymphatic duct).** Lymph from the thoracic duct reenters the bloodstream through the left subclavian vein and from there flows into the superior vena cava and into the right atrium of the heart. Lymph from the right side of the head, neck, chest and the right arm flows into the right lymphatic duct. Lymph from the right lymphatic duct reenters the blood stream at the right subclavian vein.

Unlike the blood vascular system where the blood flows through a relatively closed circuit of arteries, capillaries, and veins, lymph moves through a closed end system from the body tissues to the heart (Fig. 5.59).

The Movement of Lymph

Lymph is collected from the interstitial spaces into the lymph capillaries. It travels through the lymphatics and lymph nodes, into the right or left lymphatic duct, and finally back into the blood stream. Unlike the blood vascular system where the heart pumps the blood, the lymph system has no internal pump. The structure and arrangement of lymphatics resemble those of the veins except that the lymphatic capillaries are closed, whereas the veins are a continuation from the arteries and capillary beds. Also resembling the veins, the lymph vessels contain a system of valves that allow fluid movement in only one direction. The action of external forces on this extensive system of valves creates a **lymphatic pump.**

Beginning in the smallest lymph capillaries, the endothelial cells that form the capillary walls overlap in such a way that they form microscopic valves that allow the movement of fluids into the capillary, but the slightest back pressure closes the openings so that once inside, the fluid does not escape. Within the lymph vessels, flap-like valves protrude from the inside of the vessel walls that prevent back flow.

When a segment of a lymph vessel is compressed, the pressure on the fluid in that segment forces the previous valve to close and the next one to open as the fluid moves through the valve and progresses toward the heart. The external pressure that activates the lymphatic pump is supplied primarily from the contraction of the skeletal muscles. Other factors that may contribute are movement of body parts, breathing, contractions of smooth muscles in the larger lymph vessels, arterial pulsation, and compression of tissues from outside the body (such as massage).

Lymph Nodes

Lymph nodes are made of **lymphoid tissue** and are located along the course of the lymphatics. They are oval or rounded masses from the size of a pin head to an inch in length and resemble the shape of a bean. Lymphoid tissue is a production site of **lymphocytes.** Lymph nodes contain a large concentration of lymphocytes and serve to filter and neutralize harmful bacteria and toxic substances collected in the lymph, thereby preventing the spread of infection to other parts of the body (Fig. 5.60).

Lymph nodes are found in the following regions of the body:
1. Back of the head, draining the scalp
2. Around the neck muscles, draining the back of the tongue, pharynx, nasal cavities, and the roof of the mouth

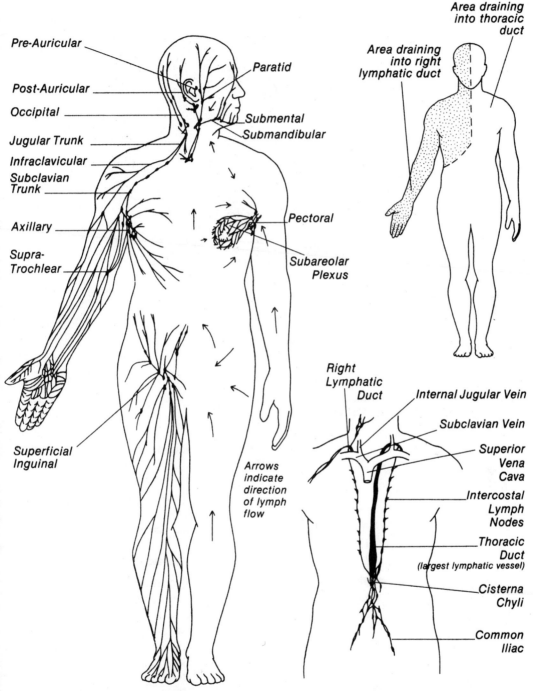

• Major locations of lymph nodes
• Lymphatic vessels are named according to their location

Fig. 5.59 The lymphatic system and lymphatic ducts.

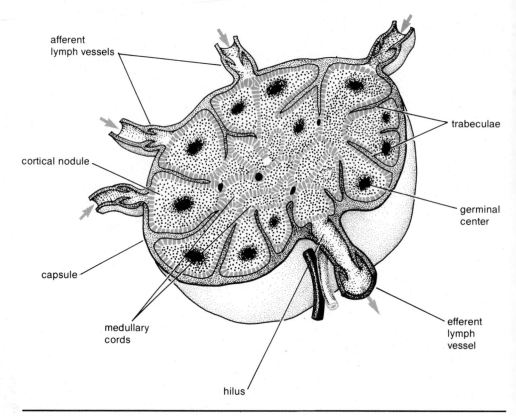

Fig. 5.60 Cross section of a lymph node.

3. Under the floor of the jaw, draining the floor of the mouth
4. Upper extremities, in the bend of the elbow, under the armpit, and under the pectoral muscle
5. Abdomen and pelvis, along the blood vessels in these regions
6. Lower extremities, in back of the knee and the groin.

Regional lymph nodes are named according to their location in the body:

Node	Location
Submandibular	Beneath the mandible
Occipital	Base of the skull
Axillary	Armpit
Inguinal	Groin
Supratrochlear	Elbow
Popliteal	Behind the knee
Mammary	Breast
Femoral	Thigh
Tibial	Leg
Cervical	Neck

Healthy tissue depends on good lymph circulation. Correct massage can increase lymphatic circulation and clear the lymph spaces as well as drain sluggish lymph nodes. The purpose of lymph drainage is to cleanse and regenerate the tissues and organs of the body. Massage stimulates the movement of lymph and the formation of lymphocytes that produce antibodies, increasing the body's resistance to infection.

REVIEW ▼

Important Veins of the Body

MATCHING TEST I

Insert the letter of the proper term in front of each definition.

_____ 1. Receives blood from eyes   a. Femoral vein

_____ 2. Receives blood from heart   b. Ophthalmic vein

_____ 3. Receives blood from face   c. Coronary veins

_____ 4. Receives blood from outer   d. Facial vein
       arm

_____ 5. Receives blood from legs   e. Basilic vein

TRUE OR FALSE TEST I

Carefully read each statement and decide if it is true or false; draw a circle around the letter T or F.

1. T F   Both the internal and external jugular veins return blood from the head, face, and neck to the heart.

2. T F   The inferior vena cava receives blood from the abdomen and upper limbs.

3. T F   The popliteal vein is located in the lower extremities.

4. T F   The innominate veins are found in the upper extremities.

5. T F   The superior vena cava receives blood from the head, neck, thorax, and upper limbs.

IMPORTANT ARTERIES OF THE BODY

MATCHING TEST II

Insert the letter of the proper term in front of each definition.

_____ 1. Supplies blood to heart   a. Ophthalmic artery

_____ 2. Supplies blood to eyes   b. Subclavian artery

_____ 3. Supplies blood to face   c. Frontal artery

_____ 4. Supplies blood to forehead   d. Coronary artery

_____ 5. Supplies blood to chest   e. Facial artery

TRUE OR FALSE TEST II

Carefully read each statement and decide if it is true or false; draw a circle around the letter T or F.

1. T F The posterior auricular artery supplies blood to the scalp.
2. T F The aorta does not form large and small branches.
3. T F The axillary artery supplies blood to the shoulder, chest, and arm.
4. T F The external branch of the common carotid artery supplies blood to the cranial cavity.
5. T F The external iliac artery supplies blood to the upper limb.

▼ SECTION QUESTIONS FOR DISCUSSION AND REVIEW

1. Name the important parts comprising the circulatory system.
2. What are the two divisions of the circulatory system?
3. What is the function of the heart?
4. Name the protective covering of the heart and describe its function.
5. Name the chambers of the heart in the order that blood would pass through them.
6. Which nerves regulate the heart beat?
7. What is the function of the arteries?
8. What is an arteriole?
9. Which nerves control the movements of the arterial walls?
10. What is the function of the capillaries?
11. What is the function of the veins?
12. What is a venule?
13. What is the purpose of the venous pump?
14. Name the main artery of the body.
15. Name two circulatory systems of the blood vascular system.
16. What vein carries freshly oxygenated blood?
17. Which constituents are found in the blood?
18. What is the primary function of the red blood cells?
19. What is the primary function of the white blood cells?
20. Which substances are carried by the blood to the body cells?
21. Which substances does the blood carry away from the body cells?
22. In what ways does the blood protect the body?
23. What is the normal temperature of the blood?
24. Name the parts of the lymph system.
25. What is the major function of the lymph-vascular system?
26. What is the major function of the lymph glands or nodes?
27. Which regions of the body contain lymph nodes?
28. From what is lymph derived?
29. Into which blood vessels does the lymph return?

30. What is meant by lymph drainage?

31. What are lacteals?

32. Of what value is massage to the health of the lymphatic system?

33. What determines names of lymphatics?

34. What is the lymphatic pump and how does it work?

35. Trace the flow of lymph from just before it enters the lymph system until it leaves.

▼ SYSTEM FIVE: THE NERVOUS SYSTEM

The nervous system controls and coordinates the functions of other systems of the body so they work harmoniously and efficiently. The nervous system is composed of the brain, spinal cord, and peripheral nerves. The primary function of the nervous system is to collect a multitude of sensory information, process, interpret, and integrate that information, and initiate appropriate responses throughout the body.

The functions of the nervous system are:
1. To rule the body by controlling all visible and invisible activities
2. To control human thought and conduct
3. To govern all internal and external movements of the body
4. To give the power to see, hear, move, talk, feel, think, and remember.

Neurons and Nerves

A **neuron** is the structural unit of the nervous system. A neuron is the **nerve cell** (cell body) including its outgrowth of long and short projections of cytoplasm, called **nerve fibers.** There are two types of nerve fibers. A neuron has numerous multibranched **dendrites** that connect with other neurons to receive information and a single **axon** that conducts impulses away from the cell body. The nerve cell stores energy and nutrients that are used by the cell processes to convey nerve impulses throughout the body. Neurons have the ability to react to certain stimuli (irritability) and to transmit an impulse generated by that stimulus over a distance or to another neuron (conductability). Impulses are passed from one neuron to another at a junction called a **synapse** (**SIN**-aps). When an impulse reaches the end of an axon, a chemical **neurotransmitter** is released at the synapse that acts on the membrane of the receptive neuron to pass the impulse along. Almost all the nerve cell bodies are contained in the brain and spinal cord, while their fibers extend outward to make up the nerves (Fig. 5.61).

Functionally, there are three types of neurons:

Sensory neurons (afferent neurons) originate in the periphery of the body and carry impulses or messages from sense organs to the brain where sensations of touch, cold, heat, sight, hearing, taste, or pain are interpreted and experienced.

Motor neurons (efferent neurons) carry nerve impulses from the brain to the **effectors** (the muscles or glands that they control).

Interneurons (internuncial neurons) are located in the brain and spinal cord and carry impulses from one neuron to another. They function to transmit and direct impulses from one place in the spinal cord or brain to another.

A nerve fiber is the extension from a neuron. A **nerve** is bundle nerve fibers held together by connective tissue that extends from

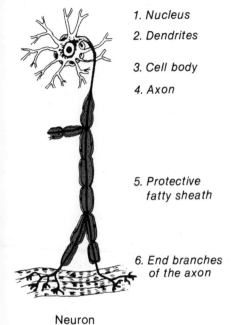

1. *Nucleus*

2. *Dendrites*

3. *Cell body*

4. *Axon*

5. *Protective fatty sheath*

6. *End branches of the axon*

Neuron

1. *Nucleus:* Nerve cells.

2. *Dendrites:* The branched part of a nerve cell that carries impulses toward the cell body.

3. *Cell body:* A nerve cell.

4. *Axon:* The central core that forms the essential conducting part of a nerve fiber.

5. *Protective fatty sheath:* A thin covering of fat.

6. The branched end of the axon.

Fig. 5.61 Common neuron.

the central nervous system to the tissue that the neurons enervate. Nerves have their origin in the brain and spinal cord and distribute branches to all parts of the body.

Sensory nerves, or **afferent nerves,** carry sensory impulses from a variety of sensory receptors toward the brain or spinal cord. **Motor nerves,** termed **efferent nerves,** carry impulses from the brain or spinal cord to the muscles or glands. Most nerves contain both sensory and motor fibers and are called **mixed nerves.**

Anatomically the nervous system is divided into two main divisions: the central nervous system and the peripheral nervous system.

Central Nervous System

The **central nervous system** (CNS) consists of the **brain** and **spinal cord.** The CNS is surrounded by bone and is covered by a special connective tissue membrane called the **meninges** (me-**NIN**-jeez). More specifically, the brain is housed in the cranium and the spinal cord is housed in the vertebral canal of the spine. The meninges has three layers. The outer layer, the **dura mater** (**DOO**-ruh **MAY**-ter), is a protective fibrous connective tissue sheath covering the brain and spinal cord. The **pia mater,** the innermost layer, is attached to the surface of the organs and is richly supplied with blood vessels to nourish the underlying tissues. Between the dura and pia mater is a thin net-like membrane called the **arachnoid mater,** sometimes referred to as the arachnoid space. The arachnoid mater provides a space for the blood vessels and the circulation of cerebrospinal fluid (Fig. 5.62).

Cerebrospinal fluid is a clear fluid derived from the blood and secreted into the inner cavities or ventricles of the brain. The fluid circulates through the ventricles and then down through the central canal of the spinal cord and into the arachnoid space. The brain and spinal cord are surrounded by cerebrospinal fluid and indeed seem to be suspended by the fluid. Cerebrospinal fluid carries some nutrients to the nerve tissue and carries wastes away, but its main function is to protect the CNS by acting as a shock absorber for the delicate tissue.

The Brain

The **brain,** the principal nerve center, is the body's largest and most complex nerve tissue containing in excess of ten billion neurons and innumerable nerve fibers. It is located in and protected by the cranium. It controls sensations, muscles, glandular activity, and the power to think and feel (emotions). The brain includes the following:

1. The **cerebrum,** the largest portion making up the front and top of the brain, presides over such mental activities as speech, sensation, communication, memory, reasoning, will, and emotions.

2. The **cerebellum,** the smaller part of the brain, located below the cerebrum and at the back of the cranium, helps maintain

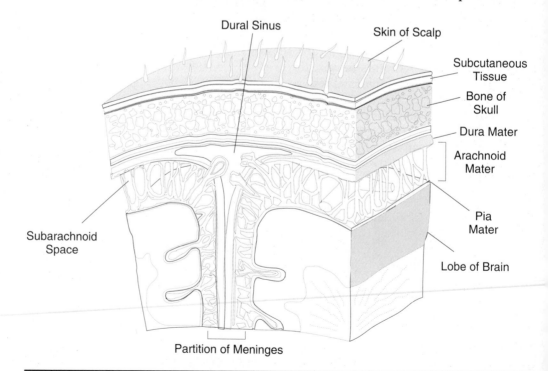

Fig. 5.62 Meninges of the central nervous system.

body balance, coordinates voluntary muscles, and makes muscular movement smooth and graceful.
3. The **brain stem** has three parts: the midbrain, the pons, and the medulla oblongata. These contain intricate masses of nerve fibers that relay and transmit impulses from one portion of the brain to another.

The midbrain contains the main nerve pathways connecting the cerebrum and the lower nervous system as well as certain visual and auditory reflexes that coordinate head and eye movements with things seen and heard.

The pons, located between the midbrain and the medulla oblongata, relays nerve impulses between the cerebrum and the medulla and from the cerebrum to the cerebellum.

The medulla oblongata is an enlarged continuation of the spinal cord that extends from the foramen magnum to the pons and connects the brain with the spinal cord. Control centers within the medulla oblongata regulate movements of the heart, and control vasoconstriction of the arteries and the rate and depth of respiration.

Spinal Cord

The **spinal cord** extends downward from the brain and is housed in and protected by the vertebral column. It extends down from the medulla oblongata to the level of the first lumbar vertebrae. The spinal cord consists of thirty-one segments, each segment being the site of attachment of a pair of spinal nerves. The spinal cord functions as a conduction pathway for nerve impulses traveling to and from the brain as well as a reflex center between incoming and outgoing peripheral nerve fibers (Fig. 5.63).

The Peripheral Nervous System

The **peripheral nervous system** consists of all of the nerves that connect the central nervous system to the rest of the body. It includes the spinal nerves, the cranial nerves, and all of their branches. Peripheral nerves send sensory impulses to the brain and spinal cord and transmit motor impulses from the brain to the muscles, glands, and visceral organs. The peripheral nervous system can also be divided into the **autonomic nervous system** and the **somatic nervous system.** Basically, the somatic system involves those nerves connecting the CNS, the voluntary muscles, and skin while the autonomic nervous system connects the CNS to the visceral organs such as the heart, blood vessels, glands, and intestines.

Cranial Nerves

There are twelve pairs of **cranial nerves** that connect directly to some part of the brain surface and pass through openings on the sides and base of the cranium. They are classified as **motor** or

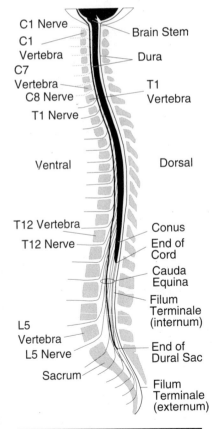

Fig. 5.63 Spinal cord and spinal nerves.

sensory nerves and **mixed** nerves, which contain both motor and sensory fibers.

The cranial nerves are named numerically according to the order in which they arise from the brain, and by names that describe their type, function, or location (Fig. 5.64).

Spinal Nerves

Thirty-one pairs of spinal nerves emerge from the spinal cord and are numbered according to the level of the vertebra where they exit the spine. All spinal nerves are mixed nerves that contain both sensory and motor nerve fibers to provide two-way communication between the CNS and the body.

Spinal nerves number:
- Eight pairs of cervical nerves
- Twelve pairs of thoracic nerves

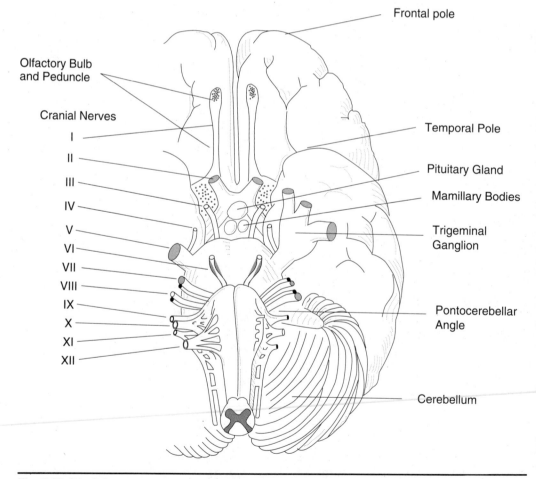

Fig. 5.64 Cranial nerves.

TABLE 5.3 CLASSIFICATION OF CRANIAL NERVES

CRANIAL NERVE	TYPE OF NERVE	LOCATION	FUNCTION
1. Olfactory nerve.	Sensory nerve.	Nose.	Sense of smell.
2. Optic nerve.	Sensory nerve.	Retina of eye.	Sense of sight.
3. Oculomotor nerve.	Motor nerve.	Muscles of eye.	Controls eye movements.
4. Trochlear nerve.	Motor nerve.	Obliquus superioris muscle of eye.	Rotates eyeball downward and outward.
5. Trigeminal or trifacial nerve.	Motor and sensory nerve.	Face, teeth, and tongue.	Controls sensations of the face and movements of the jaw and tongue.
6. Abducent nerve.	Motor nerve.	Recti muscles of eye.	Rotates eyeball outward.
7. Facial nerve.	Motor and sensory nerve.	Face and neck.	Controls facial muscles of expression and some muscles of the neck and ear.
8. Acoustic or auditory nerve.	Sensory nerve.	Ear.	Sense of hearing.
9. Glossopharyngeal nerve.	Motor and sensory nerve.	Tongue and pharynx.	Sense of taste.
10. Vagus or pneumogastric nerve.	Motor and sensory nerve.	Pharynx, larynx, heart, lungs, and digestive organs.	Controls sensations and muscular movements relating to talking, heart action, breathing, and digestion.
11. Spinal accessory nerve.	Motor nerve.	Shoulder.	Controls movement of neck muscles.
12. Hypoglossal nerve.	Motor nerve.	Tongue and neck.	Controls movement of the tongue.

- Five pairs of lumbar nerves
- Five pairs of sacral nerves
- One pair of coccygeal nerves.

The four upper cervical nerves form the **cervical plexus,** which supply the skin and control the movement of the head, neck, and shoulders.

The four lower cervical nerves and the first pair of thoracic nerves form the **brachial plexus,** which controls the movement of the arms by way of the musculo-cutaneous, radial, median, and ulnar nerves.

The next eleven thoracic nerves supply the muscles, skin, and organs in the thorax.

The first four lumbar nerves form the **lumbar plexus,** whose nerves supply the skin, the abdominal organs, hip, thigh, knee, and leg. The femoral and obturator nerves reach the upper parts of the leg.

Portions of the forth and fifth lumbar nerves, the first, second, third, and fourth sacral nerves form the **sacral plexus.** The spinal nerves that form the sacral plexus divide and merge to form several collateral nerves and one main branch, the **sciatic** (sigh-**AT**-ic) **nerve.** The sciatic nerve is the largest and longest nerve in the body. The sciatic nerve consists of two nerves in the same nerve sheath: the common peroneal nerve and the tibial nerve. The sciatic nerve serves the hamstrings and the lower leg and foot.

Another portion of the fourth sacral nerves, the fifth sacral nerve and the coccygeal nerve, forms the **coccygeal plexus** (kok-**SIJ**-ee-al **PLEK**-sus). The coccygeal nerves supply the skin and muscles around the coccyx (Figs. 5.65 to 5.67, pages 197 to 199).

The Autonomic Nervous System

Autonomic means self-governing. The **autonomic nervous system** regulates action of glands, smooth muscles, and the heart. The autonomic nervous system consists of motor neurons that originate in the central nervous system. The autonomic nervous system is further subdivided into the **sympathetic** and **parasympathetic** nervous systems.

The nerves of the **sympathetic nervous system** originate in the thoracolumbar (thoracic and lumbar portions of the spine) between T-1 and L-2 and enter a double chain of small **ganglia** (**GANG**-glee-uh) (masses of neurons) that extend along the spinal column from the base of the brain to the coccyx. Within these ganglia, neurons synapse with other neurons before continuing to their target organs. These ganglia are connected with each other and with the central nervous system by nerve fibers. The sympathetic nervous system supplies the glands, involuntary muscles of internal organs, and walls of blood vessels with nerves.

The activity of the sympathetic system is primarily to prepare the organism for energy expending, stressful, or emergency situations. Stimulation of the sympathetic nerves can bring about rapid responses, such as increased respiration, dilated pupils, and increased heart rate and cardiac output. Blood vessels dilate, and the liver increases conversion of glycogen to glucose for more energy. There is increased mental activity and production of adrenal hormones. All these activities prepare us to meet emergencies.

The **parasympathetic nervous system** balances the action of the sympathetic system. The general function of the parasympathetic division is to conserve energy and reverse the action of the

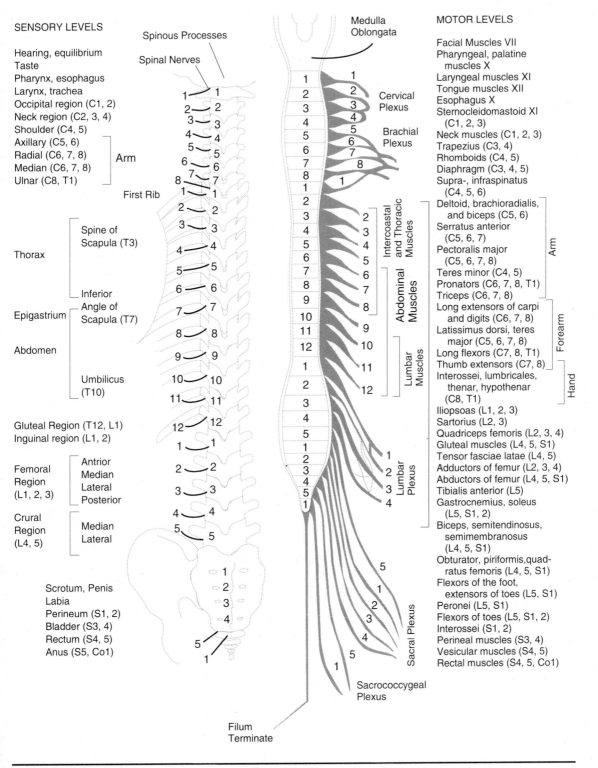

SENSORY LEVELS

Spinous Processes
Spinal Nerves

Hearing, equilibrium
Taste
Pharynx, esophagus
Larynx, trachea
Occipital region (C1, 2)
Neck region (C2, 3, 4)
Shoulder (C4, 5)
Axillary (C5, 6)
Radial (C6, 7, 8)   Arm
Median (C6, 7, 8)
Ulnar (C8, T1)

First Rib

Spine of
Scapula (T3)
Thorax

Inferior
Angle of
Epigastrium   Scapula (T7)

Abdomen

Umbilicus
(T10)

Gluteal Region (T12, L1)
Inguinal region (L1, 2)

Femoral   Antrior
Region   Median
(L1, 2, 3)   Lateral
              Posterior

Crural
Region   Median
(L4, 5)   Lateral

Scrotum, Penis
Labia
Perineum (S1, 2)
Bladder (S3, 4)
Rectum (S4, 5)
Anus (S5, Co1)

Medulla
Oblongata

Cervical
Plexus

Brachial
Plexus

Intercoastal
and Thoracic
Muscles

Abdominal
Muscles

Lumbar
Muscles

Lumbar
Plexus

Sacral Plexus

Sacrococcygeal
Plexus

Filum
Terminate

MOTOR LEVELS

Facial Muscles VII
Pharyngeal, palatine
  muscles X
Laryngeal muscles XI
Tongue muscles XII
Esophagus X
Sternocleidomastoid XI
  (C1, 2, 3)
Neck muscles (C1, 2, 3)
Trapezius (C3, 4)
Rhomboids (C4, 5)
Diaphragm (C3, 4, 5)
Supra-, infraspinatus
  (C4, 5, 6)
Deltoid, brachioradialis,
  and biceps (C5, 6)
Serratus anterior
  (C5, 6, 7)
Pectoralis major
  (C5, 6, 7, 8)
Teres minor (C4, 5)   Arm
Pronators (C6, 7, 8, T1)
Triceps (C6, 7, 8)
Long extensors of carpi
  and digits (C6, 7, 8)   Forearm
Latissimus dorsi, teres
  major (C5, 6, 7, 8)
Long flexors (C7, 8, T1)
Thumb extensors (C7, 8)
Interossei, lumbricales,
  thenar, hypothenar   Hand
  (C8, T1)
Iliopsoas (L1, 2, 3)
Sartorius (L2, 3)
Quadriceps femoris (L2, 3, 4)
Gluteal muscles (L4, 5, S1)
Tensor fasciae latae (L4, 5)
Adductors of femur (L2, 3, 4)
Abductors of femur (L4, 5, S1)
Tibialis anterior (L5)
Gastrocnemius, soleus
  (L5, S1, 2)
Biceps, semitendinosus,
  semimembranosus
  (L4, 5, S1)
Obturator, piriformis, quad-
  ratus femoris (L4, 5, S1)
Flexors of the foot,
  extensors of toes (L5, S1)
Peronei (L5, S1)
Flexors of toes (L5, S1, 2)
Interossei (S1, 2)
Perineal muscles (S3, 4)
Vesicular muscles (S4, 5)
Rectal muscles (S4, 5, Co1)

Fig. 5.65 Spinal nerves showing plexuses, motor and sensory functions.

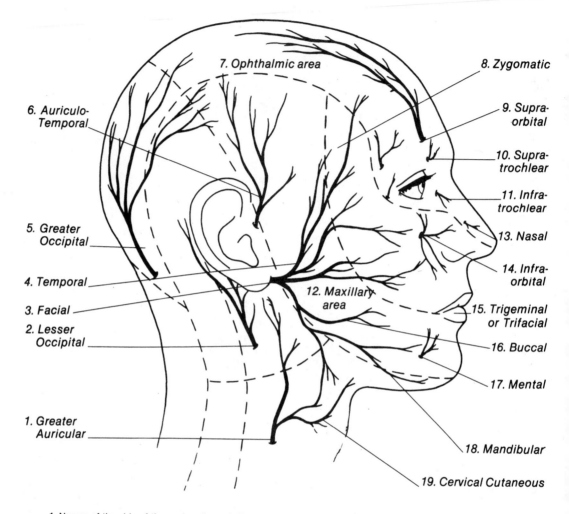

7. Ophthalmic area

8. Zygomatic

6. Auriculo-Temporal

9. Supra-orbital

10. Supra-trochlear

11. Infra-trochlear

5. Greater Occipital

13. Nasal

4. Temporal

14. Infra-orbital

3. Facial

12. Maxillary area

15. Trigeminal or Trifacial

2. Lesser Occipital

16. Buccal

17. Mental

1. Greater Auricular

18. Mandibular

19. Cervical Cutaneous

1. Nerves of the side of the neck and ear. **2.** Nerves of skin behind the ear and back of scalp. **3.** Nerves of muscles of expression. **4.** Nerves of the temporal muscle. **5.** Nerves of skin over back part of the head. **6.** Nerves of the side of the scalp. **7.** Nerves of tear glands, eye membrane, skin of forehead and nose. **8.** Zygomatic sensory nerve, a branch of the maxillary nerve which innervates the skin in the temple area, side of forehead and upper part of cheek. **9.** Nerves of the skin of the forehead. **10.** Nerves of the skin of upper eyelids and root of the nose. **11.** Nerves of skin of lower eyelids and sides of nose. **12.** Nerves of the nasal pharynx, teeth of the upper jaw and skin of the cheek. **13.** Nerves of skin and mucous membrane of the nose. **14.** Nerves of the skin of the cheek and lower eyelid. **15.** Nerves of skin of face, tongue, teeth and muscles of mastication. **16.** Nerves of buccinator and orbicularis oris. **17.** Nerves of lower lip and chin. **18.** Nerves of teeth and lower jaws and cheek area. **19.** Nerves which supply the skin of the jaw back of ear, lateral and anterior sides of neck and skin of upper anterior thorax.

Fig. 5.66 Nerves of head, face and neck.

sympathetic division. Parasympathetic nerve fibers that serve the organs and glands of the thorax and abdomen are part of the vagus nerve. Pelvic portions of the parasympathetic system arise from the second, third, and fourth sacral spinal nerves. Parasympathetic nerve fibers associated with parts of the head are included in the III, VII, and IX cranial nerves (Fig. 5.68, page 200).

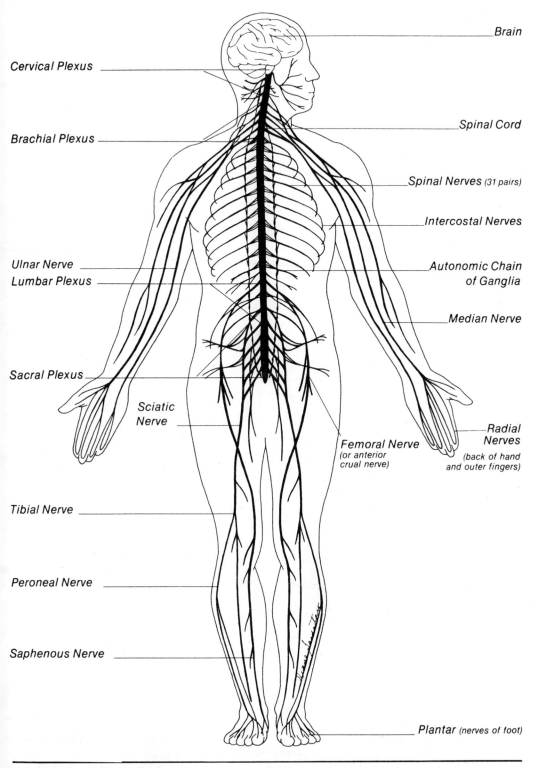

Cervical Plexus

Brachial Plexus

Ulnar Nerve
Lumbar Plexus

Sacral Plexus

Sciatic
Nerve

Tibial Nerve

Peroneal Nerve

Saphenous Nerve

Brain

Spinal Cord

Spinal Nerves (31 pairs)

Intercostal Nerves

Autonomic Chain
of Ganglia

Median Nerve

Radial
Nerves
(back of hand
and outer fingers)

Femoral Nerve
(or anterior
crual nerve)

Plantar (nerves of foot)

Fig. 5.67 The nervous system.

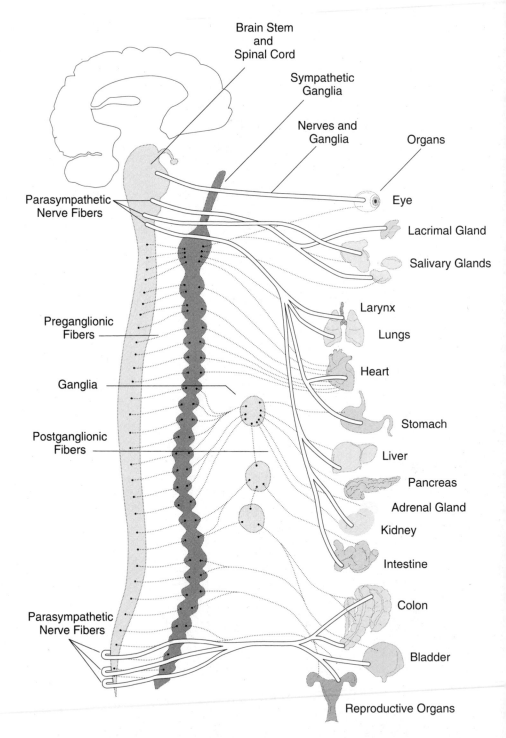

Fig. 5.68 The autonomic nervous system. Nerves of the sympathetic nervous system communicate through a chain of ganglia located along each side of the spine. Parasympathetic nerves arise from the Cranial nerves III, VII, IX, X and Sacral nerves 2, 3 and 4.

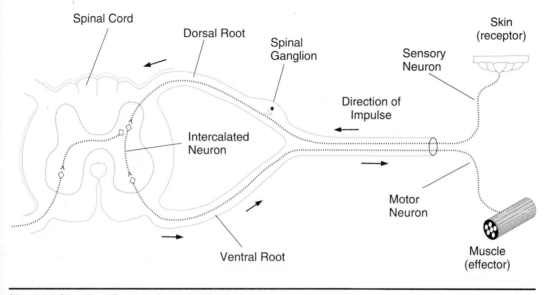

Fig. 5.69 Simple reflex arc; knee jerk reflex.

Reflexes and Reflex Arcs

A **neurological pathway** is the route that a nerve impulse travels through the nervous system. The usual nerve path consists of a stimulus that initiates an impulse along a sensory nerve fiber to the spinal cord to communicate with an indeterminable number of interneurons (depending on how complicated or intricate the response) and finally a response impulse along motor nerves to the associated effectors, producing the resultant action.

The simplest form of nervous activity which includes a sensory and motor nerve and few if any interneurons is called a **reflex.** The nerve pathway of a reflex is called a **reflex arc.** A simple reflex, such as a knee jerk, involves just two neurons (sensory and motor) that pass into and out of the spinal cord without influencing any other nerve centers. Another type of reflex called the withdrawal reflex (flexor reflex) occurs when a person touches something sharp or hot and immediately pulls away, thereby preventing excessive injury. Reflexes are automatic, unconscious, involuntary responses to a stimulus and are responsible for many of the body's activities, such as sneezing, coughing, and swallowing as well as many involuntary activities such as heart rate, breathing rate, and blood pressure. More complex reflexes affect parts of the body distant from the point of stimulation (Fig. 5.69).

The areas of the body that are particularly sensitive to reflex influences are:

1. The skin of the back between the shoulders
2. The side of the chest between the fourth and sixth ribs

3. The skin at the upper and inner portion of the thigh
4. The skin overlying the gluteal muscles
5. The sole of the foot.

Proprioception

Peripheral nerves are classified as either motor nerves or sensory nerves. Sensory nerves can be further classified as exteroceptors and proprioceptors according to their location and the sensations they record. **Exteroceptors** are located throughout the body and record conscious sensations such as heat, cold, pain, and pressure. **Proprioceptors** respond to the unconscious inner sense of position and movement of the body known as **kinesthesia** (kin-es-**THEE**-zee-uh). They sense where the body is and how it moves.

Proprioception is a system of sensory and motor nerve activity that provides information as to the position and rate of movement of different body parts to the central nervous system. Proprioception provides information as to the state of contraction and position of the muscles and in so doing helps to prevent injury to the joints and muscles from excessive stretches or contractions and makes possible the coordination of smooth and accurate motion.

Proprioceptors are specialized nerve endings located in the muscle, tendons, joints, or fascia. Two major categories of proprioceptors are the **muscle spindle cells** and the **golgi tendon organs.** Their sensory input goes no farther than the brain stem, so their activity is all unconscious.

Spindle cells are located largely in the belly of the muscle. They are made up of specialized contractile tissue called intrafusal muscle fibers. Coiled around the center of the intrafusal muscle fibers are the annulo-spiral or primary receptors. A secondary sensory nerve receptor, often referred to as a flower-type receptor, is located adjacent to the annulo-spiral receptor. These sensory nerve ends of proprioceptive neurons relay information directly to the spinal cord. These receptors continuously sense movement in the spindles and in the muscle fibers surrounding them, alerting the CNS as to the length and stretch of the muscle as well as how far and fast the muscle is moving.

The **golgi tendon organs** (GTO) are multibranched sensory nerve endings located in tendons in the area where muscle fibers attach to tendon tissue. The GTO measure the amount of tension produced in muscle cells as a result of the muscle stretching and contracting. They also monitor the amount of force pulling on the bone to which the tendon attaches.

The proprioceptive receptors located in and around the joints sense angulation and pressure. Other pressure-sensitive nerve endings are situated throughout all planes of connective tissue, and together these supply sensory information to the central nervous system to give a concise body image of soft tissue and of joint position and movement (Fig. 5.70).

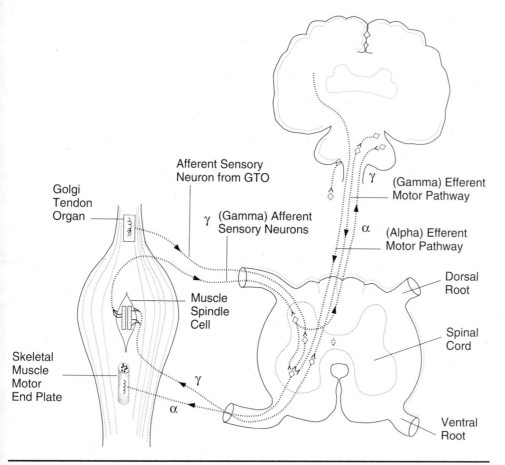

Fig. 5.70 Proprioceptors role in coordination of muscle movement.

How Proprioceptors Work

Proprioceptors sense tissue distortion. Each time the tissue is compressed, decompressed, twisted, or distorted in a specific way or there is a pressure on or movement in the body, these nerves record that change with the central nervous system. These messages feed the integrative areas of the brain with richer and more detailed information about every body part. The information is continually assembled into an overall body image that is the brain's way of knowing what the body is doing.

Neurological Disorders

Diseases of the nervous system have many causes. They may result from birth defects, trauma, or degenerative disease. They may be caused by infection, blood clots, tumors, or hemorrhage. Some diseases manifest as abnormal muscular activity, while others affect functional and mental activities. Only physiologically based diseases will be discussed here.

Degenerative nerve diseases such as **multiple sclerosis** (MS) and **Parkinson's disease** affect the ability to control the muscles. MS usually occurs in young adults between the ages of twenty and fourty and is the result of the breakdown of the myelin sheath, which inhibits nerve conduction. Symptoms include muscle weakness and loss of coordination and balance. Speaking becomes difficult and vision is affected. The progress of the disease varies with periods of remission and progression. There is no cure, but massage, physical therapy, and psychological counseling are useful in counteracting the effects of the disease.

Parkinson's disease occurs as the result of the degeneration of certain nerve tissues responsible for the regulation of certain body movements. It generally develops late in life and is characterized by tremors and shaking, especially in the hands. Muscles stiffen as movement slows and becomes more deliberate as many of the postural reflexes are lost. Massage is useful to relieve tension and relax muscles, especially in the shoulders, neck, and legs.

Trauma may result in a variety of dysfunctions depending on the severity and location of the injury. Head injuries may cause a loss of reasoning, speech, coordination, and often partial paralysis or mental retardation. A **spinal cord injury** usually results in paralysis of the parts of the body controlled by the spinal nerves that exit the spinal cord below the sight of the injury. If only the legs are affected, the condition is called **paraplegia.** If the arms and the legs are affected the condition is **quadriplegia.**

Stroke or cerebrovascular accident is the result of a blood clot or ruptured blood vessel in or around the brain and the subsequent destruction of nerve tissue. The effect of the stroke will depend on the location and extent of damaged tissue. Often a stroke will cause paralysis on one side of the body opposite the side of the brain in which the damage occurred. The extent of the paralysis is relative to the extent of the damage. The condition of unilateral paralysis caused by a stroke is called **hemiplegia.**

Epilepsy is a neurological condition in which there is abnormal electrical activity in the CNS without apparent tissue abnormalities. Epilepsy is characterized by seizures, some of which are so mild that they are barely noticeable while others may be so extreme that the person loses consciousness and is thrown into uncontrollable convulsions. People with epilepsy generally can live normal, productive lives with the use of appropriate medication.

Many diseases that affect the nervous system are the result of an invading virus or bacteria. Causes of such infections may vary from contaminated wounds and bites from animals or insects to infections elsewhere in the body. Viral infections include poliomyelitis, encephalitis, shingles, and rabies.

Poliomyelitis (po-lee-o-my-e-**LIE**-tis) or polio, is a crippling or even deadly disease that affects the motor neurons of the medulla oblongata and spinal cord, resulting in paralysis of the related muscle tissues. Symptoms of polio include fever, gastrointestinal discomfort, stiff neck, and headache. If detected early, its devastating effects can be minimized. The development of the Salk and Sabin vaccines has nearly eradicated this terrible disease.

Encephalitis (en-sef-a-LIE-tis) refers to several related viral diseases that cause an inflammation of the brain or the meninges. The infection is sometimes spread due to a carrier such as an animal or bird by way of a mosquito bite or may arise as a secondary infection from measles, mumps or chicken pox. Symptoms may include headache, fever, disoriented behavior, and often seizures. Serious cases may result in nerve or brain damage and cause paralysis, emotional disturbances, or even death.

Meningitis (men-in-JIGH-tis) is an acute inflammation of the pia and arachnoid mater around the brain and spinal cord. This is often a secondary infection due to bacteria traveling from the middle ear, upper respiratory tract, lungs, sinuses, or due to polio or mumps viruses. Symptoms include severe headache, stiff neck, high fever, chills, delirium, and often convulsions or even coma. Antibiotic treatment is usually effective. If untreated, permanent brain damage usually results with possible blindness, deafness, retardation, or paralysis.

Diagnosis of encephalitis and meningitis is made with a spinal tap or lumbar puncture, in which a hollow needle is inserted into the spinal canal in the lumbar area to determine the constituents and pressure of the cerebrospinal fluid.

Shingles is an acute inflammation of a nerve trunk by the herpes zoster virus. The symptoms include a band of pain around the torso and a rash with water blisters that erupt in a confined area on one side of the trunk. Seldom does the rash cross the midline of the body. Shingles may develop from an exposure to herpes or chicken pox, a reaction to a medication, or trauma. Massage is contraindicated due to the risk of infection and because it would be very painful. Immediate medical attention is recommended.

Neuritis literally means inflammation of a nerve. Neuritis affects the nerves of the peripheral nervous system. Since most peripheral nerves are both sensory and motor, neuritis may cause weakness or paralysis and be painful. The pain associated with neuritis is called **neuralgia.**

Generalized neuritis may be due to nutritional deficiency, alcoholism, chemical poisoning, allergies, and viral or bacterial infections. Usually the symptoms of neuritis will subside when the cause is removed. Rest, a diet rich in B vitamins, and therapy such as massage are helpful.

Sometimes neuritis will affect a specific nerve. Pain and/or partial paralysis along the course of the affected nerve could be the result of disease, pressure on, or injury to the nerve. A common form of neuralgia is the result of injury or pressure on the sciatic nerve called **sciatica.** The sciatic nerve is exposed to many sites of possible injury in the back, through the pelvis and along its course down the leg. Depending on the severity, sciatica results in pain down the back of the leg and into the foot that may be accompanied by muscle weakness or paralysis.

▼ TABLE 5.4 NERVES OF THE NECK

NAME	FUNCTION	DISTRIBUTION
Auricular, great	Sensation.	Skin of neck.
Colli, superficial	Sensation.	Skin of neck and throat.
Dental, inferior	Sensation-Motion.	Mylo-hyoid muscle.
Digastric	Motion.	Stylo-hyoid and posterior portion of digastric muscle.
Hypoglossal	Motion.	Genio-hyoid and omo-hyoid muscles.
Mylo-hyoid	Motion.	Mylo-hyoid and anterior part of degastric muscle.
Spinal accessory	Motion.	Neck muscles.
Stylo-hyoid	Motion.	Stylo-hyoid and posterior part of digastric muscle.
Suboccipital	Motion.	Muscles of back and neck.
Cervical, superficial	Sensation.	Skin of front of neck.
Occipital, greater	Sensation-Motion.	Muscles of back of neck.
Pneumogastric	Sensation-Motion.	Larynx or voice-box.

▼ TABLE 5.5 NERVES OF THE CHEST

NAME	FUNCTION	DISTRIBUTION
Pneumogastric	Sensation-Motion.	Heart and lungs.
Phrenic	Motion.	Diaphragm.
Suprasternal	Sensation.	Skin over top of breast bone.
Thoracic, external anterior	Motion.	Pectoralis major.
Thoracic, internal anterior	Motion.	Pectoralis major and minor.
Thoracic, external posterior	Motion.	Serratus anterior.
Thoracic, spinal	Sensation-Motion.	Muscles and skin of chest.
Cervical (8)	Sensation-Motion.	Trunk and upper extremities.
Dorsal (12)	Sensation-Motion.	Muscles and skin of chest and trunk.

TABLE 5.6 NERVES OF THE HEAD AND FACE

NAME	FUNCTION	DISTRIBUTION
Auriculo-temporal	Sensation.	Side of scalp.
Auditory	Sensory nerve of hearing.	Ear.
Abducent	Motion.	Obliquus externus muscle of eye.
Trochlear	Motion.	Obliquus superior muscle of eye.
Auricular, anterior	Sensation.	Skin of external ear.
Auricular, great	Sensation.	Side of neck and ear.
Auricular, posterior	Motion.	Epicranius and auricularis posterior muscle.
Buccal	Motion.	Buccinator and orbicularis oris muscles.
Dental, inferior	Sensation-Motion.	Teeth of lower jaw and skin of chin.
Facial	Sensation-Motion.	Muscles of expression.
Frontal	Sensation.	Skin of forehead.
Glossopharyngeal	Sensation-Motion.	Muscles and mucous membranes of pharynx and back of tongue.
Infra-orbital	Sensation.	Skin of cheek and lower eyelid.
Infra-trochlear	Sensation.	Skin of lower eyelid and side of nose.
Mandibular	Sensation-Motion.	Teeth and skin of lower jaw and cheeks.
Masseteric	Motion.	Masseter muscle.
Maxillary	Sensation.	Nasal pharynx, teeth of upper jaw and skin of cheek.
Mental	Sensation.	Skin and mucous membrane of nose.
Occipital, greater	Sensation-Motor.	Skin over back part of head.
Occipital, lesser	Sensation.	Skin behind ear and on back of scalp.
Oculomotor	Motion.	Levator palpebrae superioris, recti muscles and obliquus inferior muscle of eye.
Olfactory	Sensory nerve of smell.	Nose.
Ophthalmic	Sensation.	Tear glands, eye membrane, skin of forehead and nose.
Optic nerve	Sensory nerve of sight.	Retina of eye.
Orbital	Sensation.	Skin of temple.
Supra-orbital	Sensation.	Skin of forehead.
Pterygoid, external	Motion.	External pterygoid muscle.
Pterygoid, internal	Motion.	Internal pterygoid muscle.
Trigeminal or trifacial	Sensation-Motion.	Skin of face, tongue, teeth and muscles of mastication.
Supratrochlear	Sensation.	Skin of upper eyelid and root of nose.
Pneumogastric	Sensation-Motion.	Pharynx.
Temporal	Motion.	Temporal muscle.

▼ TABLE 5.7 NERVES OF THE ABDOMEN

NAME	FUNCTION	DISTRIBUTION
Hypogastric	Sensation-Motion.	Muscles and skin of abdominal wall.
Ilio-hypogastric	Sensation-Motion.	Muscles and skin of lower abdomen.
Ilio-inguinal	Sensation-Motion.	Obliquus internus abdominis muscle and skin of groin.
Intercostal	Sensation-Motion.	Muscles and skin of upper abdomen.
Lumar (5)	Sensation-Motion.	Front of lower abdomen.
Pneumogastric	Sensation-Motion.	Stomach.

▼ TABLE 5.8 NERVES OF THE BACK

NAME	FUNCTION	DISTRIBUTION
Coccygeal	Sensation-Motion	Coccygeus muscle and skin over coccyx of spine.
Gluteal, inferior	Motion.	Glutaeus maximus muscle.
Gluteal, superior	Motion.	Glutaeus medius muscle.
Intercostal	Sensation-Motion	Muscles and skin of back.
Subscapular	Motion.	Latissimus dorsi muscle.
Suprascapular	Motion.	Supra-spinatus and infra-spinatus muscles.
Spinal accessory	Motion.	Trapezius muscle.
Supraacromial	Sensation.	Skin over shoulder.
Iliac	Sensation.	Skin of gluteal region.
Sacral(5)	Sensation-Motion.	Multifidus muscles of spine and gluteal region.

TABLE 5.9 NERVES OF THE ARMS AND HANDS ▼

NAME	FUNCTION	DISTRIBUTION
Cervical (8)	Sensation-Motion.	Upper extremities.
Circumflex	Sensation-Motion.	Deltoid, teres minor, shoulder joint and overlying skin.
Cutaneous, internal	Sensation.	Skin of inner part of forearm.
Interosseous, anterior	Motion.	Deep flexor and pronator muscles of forearm.
Interosseous, posterior	Sensation-Motion.	Muscles and skin of back of forearm and wrist.
Median	Sensation-Motion.	Pronator and flexor muscles of forearm, external lumbricales, and skin of fingers.
Musculo-cutaneous	Sensation-Motion.	Flexors of upper arm and skin of external part of forearm.
Musclulo-spiral	Sensation-Motion.	Extensor muscles of entire arm and hand, and skin of back of forearm.
Radial	Sensation.	Back of hand and outer fingers.
Subscapular	Motion.	Teres major and subscapularis muscles.
Ulnar	Sensation-Motion.	Flexor carpi ulnaris and flexor digitorum profundus muscles, elbow and wrist joints and skin of fingers.

▼ TABLE 5.10 NERVES OF THE LEGS AND FEET

NAME	FUNCTION	DISTRIBUTION
Crural	Sensation.	Skin of upper thigh.
Musculo-cutaneous of leg	Sensation-Motion.	Peroneal muscles and skin of external part of lower leg and foot.
Obturator	Sensation-Motion.	Adductor muscles of thigh, hip and knee joints, and skin of inner portion of thigh.
Pectineal	Motion.	Pectineus muscle.
Popliteal, external Peroneal, common	Sensation-Motion.	Extensor muscles of lower leg and foot and overlying skin.
Popliteal, internal	Sensation-Motion.	Flexor muscles of lower leg and foot and overlying skin.
Sacral	Sensation-Motion.	Muscles and skin of lower extremities.
Saphenous, external	Sensation.	Skin of foot and toe.
Saphenous, internal	Sensation.	Skin of inner part of knee, leg, ankle, and dorsum of foot.
Sciatic, great	Sensation-Motion.	Flexor muscles of thigh, leg, foot, and skin of calf and sole.
Sciatic, small	Sensation.	Skin of back of thigh.
Tibial, anterior	Sensation-Motion.	Extensor muscles of foot and toes and skin of dorsum of foot.
Tibial, posterior	Sensation-Motion.	Flexor muscles of foot and toes, and skin of sole.
Cutaneous, dorsal	Sensation.	Top of foot.
Plantar	Sensation-Motion.	Sole of foot, deep muscles of foot and toes.

Nerves of the Head and Face

MATCHING TEST I

Insert the letter of the proper term in front of each definition.

_____ **1.** Sense of hearing   a. Facial nerve

_____ **2.** Sense of smell   b. Trifacial nerve

_____ **3.** Sense of sight   c. Auditory nerve

_____ **4.** Supplies skin of face   d. Olfactory nerve

_____ **5.** Supplies muscles   e. Optic nerve
of expression

TRUE OR FALSE TEST I

Carefully read each statement and indicate if it is true or false; draw a circle around the letter T or F.

1. T F The great auricular nerve supplies the epicranius muscle.

2. T F The frontal and supra-orbital nerves supply the skin of the forehead.

3. T F The abducent nerve supplies the obliquus superior muscle of the eye.

4. T F The trigeminal nerve supplies the muscles of mastication.

5. T F The auriculo-temporal nerve supplies the side of the scalp.

Nerves of the Neck and Chest

MATCHING TEST II

Insert the letter of the proper term in front of each definition.

_____ **1.** Supplies neck muscles a. Greater occipital nerve

_____ **2.** Supplies front of neck b. Phrenic nerve

_____ **3.** Supplies back of neck c. Pneumogastric nerve

_____ **4.** Supplies heart and d. Superficial cervical nerve
lungs

_____ **5.** Supplies diaphragm e. Spinal accessory nerve

TRUE OR FALSE TEST II

Carefully read each statement and decide if it is true or false; draw a circle around the letter T or F.

1. T F The cervical nerves supply the trunk and the lower extremities.

2. T F The suboccipital nerve supplies the back of the neck.

3. T F The dorsal and spinal thoracic nerves supply the muscles and skin of the chest.

4. T F The pneumogastric nerve supplies the heart and lungs but not the larynx.

5. T F Branches of the thoracic nerve supply the pectoralis major, pectoralis minor, and serratus anterior muscles.

Nerves of the Abdomen and Back

MATCHING TEST III

Insert the letter of the proper term in front of each definition.

_____ **1.** Supplies lower abdomen

_____ **2.** Supplies upper abdomen

_____ **3.** Supplies shoulders

_____ **4.** Supplies stomach

_____ **5.** Supplies trapezius muscle

a. Supra-acromial nerve

b. Ilio-hypogastric nerve

c. Pneumogastric nerve

d. Spinal accessory nerve

e. Intercostal nerve

TRUE OR FALSE TEST III

Carefully read each statement and decide if it is true or false; draw a circle around the letter T or F.

1. T F The sacral, coccygeal, and supra-scapular nerves supply various muscles of the spine.

2. T F The subscapular and supra-scapular nerves supply the same muscles of the back.

3. T F The lumbar nerves supply the upper part of the abdomen.

4. T F Superior gluteal nerve supplies the glutaeus medius muscle.

5. T F Subscapular nerve supplies latissimus dorsi muscle of the back.

Nerves of the Arms and Hands

MATCHING TEST IV

Insert the letter of the proper term in front of each definition.

_____ **1.** Supplies elbow joint

_____ **2.** Supplies shoulder joint

_____ **3.** Supplies skin of back of arm

_____ **4.** Supplies deltoid muscle

a. Median nerve

b. Ulnar nerve

c. Circumflex nerve

d. Radial nerve

_____ **5.** Supplies muscles   e. Subscapular nerve
              of forearm

TRUE OR FALSE TEST IV

Carefully read each statement and decide if it is true or false; draw a
circle around the letter T or F.

1. T F   The subscapular nerve supplies the teres minor muscle.

2. T F   The cervical nerves supply the upper extremities.

3. T F   The musculo-spiral nerve supplies the extensor muscles of
              the entire arm and hand.

4. T F   The musculo-cutaneous nerve supplies the pronator
              muscles of the upper arm.

5. T F   The ulnar nerve supplies the skin of the fingers.

Nerves of the Legs and Feet

MATCHING TEST V

Insert the letter of the proper term in front of each definition.

_____ **1.** Supplies soles of foot   a. Small sciatic nerve

_____ **2.** Supplies upper thigh   b. Obturator nerve

_____ **3.** Supplies inner portion   c. Crural nerve
              of thigh

_____ **4.** Supplies back of thigh   d. External saphenous nerve

_____ **5.** Supplies foot and toe   e. Plantar nerve

TRUE OR FALSE TEST V

Carefully read each statement and decide if it is true or false; draw a
circle around the letter T or F.

1. T F   The obturator nerve supplies the hip and knee joints.

2. T F   The internal popliteal nerve supplies the extensor muscles of
              the lower leg and foot.

3. T F   The sacral nerve supplies the muscles and skin of the lower
              extremities.

4. T F   The anterior tibial nerve supplies the flexor muscles of the
              foot and toes.

5. T F   The dorsal cutaneous nerve supplies the top of the foot.

SECTION QUESTIONS FOR DISCUSSION AND REVIEW

1. What is the primary function of the nervous system?
2. Name the main parts of the nervous system.
3. Name and describe the general structure of a nerve cell.
4. What abilities do neurons have that enable them to transmit nerve impulses?
5. What is a synapse?
6. Describe three types of neurons.
7. Describe the structure of a nerve.
8. What is an efferent nerve?
9. What is an afferent nerve?
10. What is a mixed nerve?
11. What are the two divisions of the nervous system?
12. What is the CNS and where is it located?
13. Define meninges and name its layers.
14. What is cerebrospinal fluid and what is its function?
15. What are the main parts of the brain?
16. Where is the peripheral system located?
17. What are the divisions of the peripheral nervous system?
18. How many pairs of cranial nerves branch out from the brain?
19. Identify the cranial nerves by name and number.
20. How many pairs of spinal nerves branch out from the spinal cord?
21. Describe how the spinal nerves are numbered.
22. What is a nerve plexus?
23. Name the important spinal nerve plexuses and the body areas they supply.
24. What is the function of the autonomic nervous system?
25. Name and contrast the two divisions of the autonomic nervous system.
26. Which organs are supplied by the sympathetic nervous system?
27. What is a reflex action?
28. What is proprioception?
29. Name two categories of proprioceptors including where they are located and the information they record.

SYSTEM SIX: THE ENDOCRINE SYSTEM

The endocrine system comprises a group of specialized glands that affect the growth, development, sexual activity, and health of the entire body, depending on the quality and quantity of their secretions.

The major function of the endocrine system is to assist the nervous system in regulating body processes.

Glands of the Body

Glands are specialized organs that vary in size and function. The circulatory and nervous systems closely interact with the glands. The glands act as chemical factories, with the ability to remove certain constituents from the blood to produce specialized secretions. There are two main classifications of glands. **Exocrine (EK-sow-krin)** or **duct glands** possess tubes or **ducts** leading from the gland to a particular part of the body. Various skin and intestinal glands belong to this group. The other group, known as **ductless** or **endocrine glands,** depend on the blood and lymph to carry their secretions to various affected tissues.

The chemical substances manufactured by the endocrine glands are known as **hormones.** Hormones, sometimes referred to as the body's chemical messengers, are specialized so that they act on specific tissues (target organs) or influence certain processes in the body. Some hormones stimulate other endocrine or exocrine glands. Some have a profound effect on physical or sexual development. Others regulate metabolism or body chemistry. (See Table 5.11 glands and their associated hormones.) The endocrine glands operate cooperatively with one another and the nervous system to maintain a state of homeostasis within the organism. Some of the endocrine glands exert a regulatory influence over the other glands. The effect of their hormones may either stimulate or restrain the activity of another gland. Under or over functioning of any ductless gland will upset the delicate balance of the entire chain of endocrine glands.

Among the important endocrine glands are the pituitary gland, thyroid gland, parathyroid glands, adrenal glands, sex glands (gonads), and pancreas. Other organs that have hormone-producing tissue include the pineal gland, the hypothalamus, the kidneys, the placenta, and intestinal mucosa.

Most diseases or dysfunctions of the endocrine system are the result of over activity or under activity of one or more glands. Over active or **hyperactive** glands oversecrete hormones due to lack of regulation or glandular tumors. Underactive or **hypoactive** glands secrete insufficient amounts of their hormones. Hypoactive glands may be diseased, underdeveloped, injured by trauma, surgery, or radiation, or they may not be receiving proper stimulation and

▼ TABLE 5.11 ENDOCRINE GLANDS AND THEIR HORMONES

GLAND	HORMONE	PRINCIPAL FUNCTIONS
Anterior pituitary	ACTH (adrenocorticotropin)	Stimulates adrenal cortex to produce cortical hormones; aids in protecting body in stress situations (injury, pain)
	TSH (thyroid-stimulating hormone)	Stimulates the thyroid to produce thyroxin
	FSH (follicle-stimulating hormone)	Stimulating growth and hormone activity of ovarian follicles; stimulates growth of testes; promotes development of sperm
	GH (human growth hormone)	Promotes growth of all body tissues
	LH (Luteinizing hormone)	Causes development of corpus luteum at site of ruptured ovarian follicle in female; stimulates secretion of testosterone in male
	Lactogenic hormone	Stimulates secretion of milk by mammary glands
Posterior pituitary	ADH (antidiuretic hormone; vasopressin)	Promotes reabsorption of water in kidney tubules; stimulates smooth muscle tissue of blood vessels
	Oxytocin	Causes contraction of muscle of pregnant uterus; causes ejection of milk from mammary glands
Adrenal cortex	Cortisol (95% of glucocorticoids)	Aids in metabolism of carbohydrates, proteins, and fats; active during stress
	Aldosterone (95% of mineralocorticoids)	Aids in regulating electrolytes
	Sex hormones	May influence secondary sexual characteristics in male
Adrenal medulla	Epinephrine and norepinephrine	Increases blood pressure and heart rate; activates cells influenced by the sympathetic nervous system plus many not affected by sympathetics
Pancreatic islets	Insulin	Aids transport of glucose into cells; required for cellular metabolism of foods, especially glucose; decreases blood sugar levels
	Glucagon	Stimulates the liver to release glucose, thereby increasing blood sugar levels
Parathyroids	Parathormone	Regulates exchange of calcium between blood and bones; increases calcium level in blood
Thyroid gland	Thyroid hormone (thyroxine and triiodothyronine)	Increases metabolic rate, influencing both physical and mental activities; required for normal growth
	Calcitonin	Decreases calcium level in blood

GLAND	HORMONE	PRINCIPAL FUNCTIONS
Ovarian follicle	Estrogens (e.g., estradiol)	Stimulate growth of primary sexual organs (uterus, tubes, etc.) and development of secondary sexual organs such as breasts, plus changes in pelvis to avoid broader shape
Corpus luteum (in ovaries)	Progesterone	Stimulates development of secretory parts of mammary glands; prepares uterine lining for implantation of fertilized ovum; aids in maintaining pregnancy
Testes	Testosterone	Stimulates growth and development of sexual organs (testes, penis, others) plus development of secondary sexual characteristics such as hair growth on body and face and deepening of voice; stimulates maturation of sperm cells

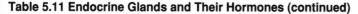

Table 5.11 Endocrine Glands and Their Hormones (continued)

regulation. Individual glands will be discussed as to their primary function and some effects of hyper- or hypoactivity (Fig. 5.71).

The Pituitary Gland

The pituitary gland is a small gland about the size of a cherry that produces a number of hormones that regulate many body processes. The pituitary gland is located in a depression just behind the point where the optic nerves cross on the floor of the cranium. The **pituitary gland** is often called the **master gland** because many of the hormones it secretes stimulate or regulate other endocrine glands. The pituitary gland is regulated by impulses and secretions from the hypothalamus. It has an anterior and posterior lobe, each of which secretes different hormones.

The anterior lobe of the pituitary produces and secretes the following:

Somatotropic or growth hormone. This hormone stimulates the growth of bones, muscles, and organs. A deficiency of this hormone will inhibit mental and physical growth.

Thyroid-stimulating hormone (TSH). This hormone regulates the thyroid gland.

Adrenocorticotropic hormone (ACTH) stimulates the adrenal cortex.

Gonadotropic hormones regulate the development and function of the reproductive systems in women and men.

Prolactin stimulates the production of milk in a woman's breast.

The posterior lobe of the pituitary stores and secretes the following:

Antidiuretic hormone stimulates the kidneys to reabsorb more water, thereby reducing urine output.

Oxytocin causes the uterus to contract (during and after childbirth) and causes the letdown of breast milk.

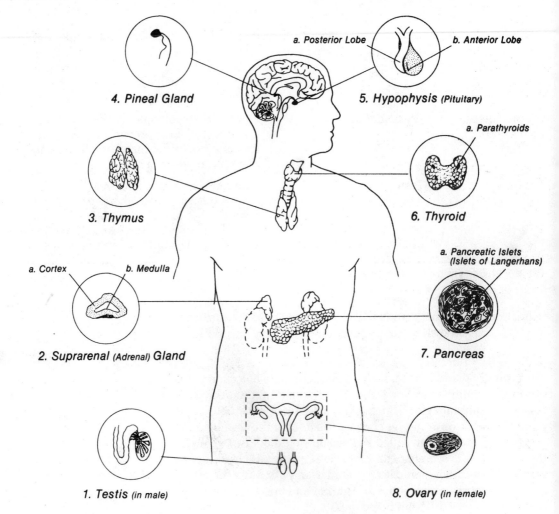

a. Posterior Lobe   b. Anterior Lobe

4. Pineal Gland

5. Hypophysis (Pituitary)

a. Parathyroids

3. Thymus

6. Thyroid

a. Pancreatic Islets
(Islets of Langerhans)

a. Cortex   b. Medulla

2. Suprarenal (Adrenal) Gland

7. Pancreas

1. Testis (in male)

8. Ovary (in female)

1. Two glandular male reproductive organs which produce testosterone, the hormone which controls sex characteristics in males. **2.** Two small glands located above the upper end of each kidney.
2a. External tissue. **2b.** Chromaphil tissue. **3.** The thymus is part of the lymphatic system located in the upper chest cavity along the trachea. Necessary in early life for development and maturation of immunological functions. **4.** A gland attached to the roof of the third ventricle of the brain. Function is stimulation of adrenal cortex.
5. Called the master or dominating gland. Controls skeletal growth, thyroid secretion and other metabolic processes. **5a.** Affects blood pressure, heartbeat, constriction and contraction of some muscles.
5b. Affects thyroid secretions. **6.** Gland that influences growth and development. Located in front of trachea below thyroid cartilage. **6a.** Four glands arranged in pairs that play a part in maintaining the normal calcium level of the blood, regulate phosphorus metabolism and play a part in the functioning of the nervous system and muscles. **7.** Located between the first and second lumbar vertebrae behind the stomach. Aids in the synthesis of sugar to glycogen, storage of glycogen, and conversion of glycogen to glucose in the liver.
7a. A special group of cells that secrete insulin, which is essential for normal glucose metabolism.
8. Two almond shaped bodies located on each side of the uterus that produce estrogen and progesterone and are essential in the development of female characteristics.

Fig. 5.71 The endocrine system.

Hyperpituitarism (high-per-pi-**TOO**-i-tar-izm) is most notably observed as the production of excessive amounts of growth hormone. If the hypersecretion occurs before puberty, the activity in the growth plates of the bones is accelerated and produces a giant, a condition known as **giantism.** If the hyperpituitarism occurs after puberty when a person has reached full height, the effects are different. The bones of the hands, feet, face, and spine enlarge in a condition called **acromegaly** (ak-row-**MEG**-a-lee). There is excessive growth in some soft tissues as the lips and nose enlarge and the lower jaw protrudes. Hyperactivity of the pituitary is usually due to a tumor.

Hypopituitarism can result from inadequate stimulation from the hypothalamus or from destruction of the pituitary gland. Since the secretions of the pituitary gland act to stimulate other endocrine glands, deficient pituitary secretions inhibit the actions of the target glands.

The Thyroid Gland

The thyroid gland, situated on either side of the trachea, produces three hormones. **Thyroxin and triiodothyronine** (trigh-ioh-o-do-**THIGH**-ro-neen) both act to stimulate the metabolic rate of the body. Thyroid hormones regulate the cellular consumption of oxygen and therefore the production of heat and energy in body tissues. The proper manufacture of these hormones requires adequate iodine in the blood. Proper diet assures adequate iodine, which helps to prevent goiter (enlarged thyroid).

Secretions from the pituitary gland control the rate of production of thyroxin. When the level of thyroxin in the blood is low, the pituitary releases **thyroid-stimulating hormone (TSH),** which stimulates the thyroid to produce more thyroxin to be secreted directly into the blood stream. When there is an adequate level of thyroxin in the blood, the pituitary stops releasing TSH into the blood and thyroxin production is inhibited.

The thyroid also produces **calcitonin** (kal-si-**TOE**-nin), a hormone that is antagonistic to the parathyroid hormone and helps control the calcium level of the blood.

Hyperthyroidism is the excessive functional activity of the thyroid gland. Often the thyroid gland enlarges to create a **goiter.** Symptoms of hyperthyroidism include heart palpitations, rapid pulse, profuse sweating, insomnia, nervousness, and excitability. **Graves' disease,** a form of hyperthyroidism, is characterized by strained, tense facial expression and bulging eyes.

Hyperthyroidism is generally treated by destroying some or all of the thyroid gland with radioactive iodine therapy or by surgically removing part or all of the thyroid gland.

Hypothyroidism is a condition of deficient thyroid activity. Symptoms are the opposite of hyperthyroidism with slow heart rate, sluggish mental and physical activity, bloated, edemic appearance, and muscle weakness. **Cretinism (KREE**-tin-izm) is congenital hypothyroidism due to an error in fetal development in which the thyroid fails to develop or is underactive. Thyroxin is essential to physical and mental health and development. Lack of it in young children results in a dwarfed stature and mental retardation. Hypothyroidism is easily treated with oral thyroxin supplementation.

Parathyroid Glands

Two pairs of parathyroid glands, situated on each lobe and behind the thyroid, produce **parathormone,** which regulates the blood level of calcium. When the blood calcium is low, the parathyroid secretes parathormone, which stimulates the activity of the osteoclasts in the bones. Thus calcium from the bones is absorbed into the blood. When blood calcium levels are high, calcitonin has an opposite effect as calcium is deposited in the bones. In this way parathormone and calcitonin have an antagonistic yet cooperative action in maintaining proper calcium levels in the blood.

Hyperparathyroidism causes loss of calcium from the bones and excessive excretion of calcium and phosphorus from the kidneys. The bones become brittle and prone to fracture and there is a tendency toward kidney stones and disease.

Hypoparathyroidism results in low blood calcium. The low blood calcium makes the nervous activity hypersensitive. The main characteristic of hypoparathyroidism is **tetany,** a sustained muscle contraction that usually affects the hands and feet.

The Thymus

The thymus is located behind the sternum and above the heart. It has endocrine and lymphatic functions and is active until puberty, at which time it begins to diminish. The thymus produces a number of related hormones that are essential in developing and maintaining our immune system. The main purpose of the thymus is to stimulate lymphoid tissue to produce lymphocytes.

The Pancreas

The pancreas is located behind the stomach and has both endocrine and exocrine functions. It produces digestive enzymes that are excreted into the small intestine through the pancreatic duct. This is the exocrine function. Scattered throughout the pancreas are small groups of specialized cells called **islets (islets of Langerhans)** that produce the hormones **insulin** and **glucagon,** which are secreted directly into the blood stream.

Insulin regulates the movement of glucose across the cell membrane so that when there is an increased level of glucose in the blood (such as after meals) secretion of insulin into the blood causes a rapid intake of glucose by most tissues in the body, especially the muscles, liver, and adipose tissue. Insulin also plays an important role in protein and fat transport and metabolism.

Diabetes mellitus is a condition caused by decreased output of insulin by the pancreatic islets. When insulin is deficient, blood glucose is elevated, and glucose is not transported across the cell membrane so there is not enough glucose in the cells for proper cell metabolism. Since the glucose is not used by the cells, blood glucose remains high and glucose is discharged by the kidneys into the urine. Glucose in the urine is the major sign of diabetes. Without being able to use glucose for metabolism, the body resorts to the abnormal breakdown of proteins and fats. Long-term fat and protein breakdown lead to serious complications of diabetes. Fat metabolism causes an increase in the lipids in the blood and a decrease in pH. The decrease in pH could cause the person to go into a coma. Increased blood lipids cause artherosclerosis. Circulation is generally poor. Occluded arteries in the heart can cause heart failure. Poor circulation to the retina of the eyes results in blindness. Vascular disorders in the legs result in poor healing and often gangrene, which sometimes leads to amputation.

Treatment of diabetes is in the form of controlled diet, exercise, and a controlled program of insulin injections.

Glucagon, also produced by specialized cells in the islets of Langerhans, has an effect antagonistic or the opposite of insulin. When the glucose level in the blood is low, glucagon acts to convert glycogen stored in the liver into glucose, thereby increasing the glucose level in the blood.

The Adrenal Glands

The **adrenal glands** are situated on top of each kidney. The adrenal glands each have two distinct parts, the **medulla** and the **adrenal cortex,** that produce different hormones.

The two principal hormones produced by the medulla are **epinephrine** (ep-i-**NEF**-rin) (also called adrenaline) and **norepinephrine.** Stimulation of the adrenal medulla comes from the sympathetic nervous system, and the actions of adrenaline and norepinephrine cause a similar effect throughout the body as direct stimulation to the organs by the sympathetic nervous system. Known as the "fight or flight" hormones, they cause the bronchioles to dilate, the heart rate to increase, the blood pressure to elevate, and glycogen to convert to glucose, flooding the blood stream and preparing the muscles to do an extraordinary amount of work to respond to any emergency situation.

The adrenal cortex produces a group of hormones called **corticosteroids** (kor-ti-ko-**STEER**-oyds). Over thirty steroids have been identified. One group, called **mineralocorticoids,** affects the extracellular electrolytes—especially sodium and potassium. The most important of these is **aldosterone** (al-**DOS**-ter-own) which regulates the sodium/potassium balance in the extracellular fluid and in the blood. In the absence of mineralocorticoid secretions, potassium levels would increase, sodium levels would fall, and the volume of blood would decrease. Without the administration of aldosterone or mineralocorticoid therapy, the patient would go into shock and die in a matter of days.

Another group, the **glucocorticoids,** affects carbohydrate, protein, and fat metabolism. Our bodies produce increased levels of these hormones in response to stress. The most important steroid of this group is **cortisol** (**KOR**-ti-sol), also known as **hydrocortisone.** These hormones have the ability to repress or resolve conditions of inflammation and enhance the rate of healing of damaged tissue.

The production of hormones by the adrenal cortex is stimulated by the adrenocorticotropic hormone (ACTH) from the pituitary gland.

Hyperadrenalism is the excessive release of adrenal hormones into the blood stream. The effects and symptoms of hyperadrenalism depend on which hormones are secreted in excess. **Cushing's syndrome** results from excess glucocorticoid production and is characterized by obesity (especially in the trunk), muscle weakness, elevated blood sugar, hypertension, and arteriosclerosis.

Hypoadrenalism, also called Addison's disease, is due to the failure of the adrenal cortex to produce aldosterone and cortisol.

The disease is characterized by weight loss, muscle fatigue or atrophy, low blood pressure, and darkened skin pigmentation.

The Sex Glands

The sex glands (gonads) are both duct and ductless glands. The male and female sex glands manufacture the reproductive cells and sex hormones that are required for fertility and reproduction. In the male, the **testes** produce **testosterone,** a potent androgen that is primarily responsible for the development of the reproductive structures. Another function involves the development of secondary sexual characteristics such as the voice, body hair, and body structure.

Estrogen and **progesterone** are the two essential hormones produced in the **ovaries** of the female reproductive system. In the female, estrogen nearly parallels the actions of testosterone regarding the development of secondary sexual characteristics. Estrogen also regulates the development of the reproductive organs, the mammary glands, and menstruation.

SECTION QUESTIONS FOR DISCUSSION AND REVIEW

1. What is the composition of the endocrine system?
2. What is the major function of the endocrine system?
3. What is an important difference between a duct and ductless gland?
4. Why are the glands dependent on an adequate nerve and blood supply?
5. Are sebaceous (oil) glands classified as duct or ductless glands?
6. What is the function of a ductless or endocrine gland?
7. Which glands function as both duct and ductless glands?

8. Which glands produce hormones?
9. Why are hormones important to the body?
10. Name the endocrine glands.
11. What is the nature of most endocrine dysfunctions?
12. Why is the pituitary gland called the master gland?
13. What are the two hormone-producing parts of the adrenal glands?
14. What is the endocrine function of the sex glands?

REVIEW ▼

MATCHING TEST I

Match the hormone in the left list with the gland that produces it by writing the appropriate letter in the space provided.

_____	1. Gonadotropic hormone	a.	Pituitary gland
_____	2. Adrenaline	b.	Thyroid gland
_____	3. Insulin	c.	Parathyroid
_____	4. Antiduretic hormone	d.	Thymus gland
_____	5. Thyroxin	e.	Adrenal cortex
_____	6. Testosterone	f.	Adrenal medulla
_____	7. ACTH	g.	Pancreas
_____	8. Cortisol	h.	Ovaries
_____	9. Progesterone	i.	Testes
_____	10. Aldosterone		
_____	11. Somatropic hormone		
_____	12. Glucagon		
_____	13. Epinephrine		
_____	14. Parathormone		
_____	15. TSH		

MATCHING TEST II

Match the hormone with the best description of its function by writing the appropriate letter in the space provided.

_____	1. Gonadotropic hormone	a.	Stimulates the thyroid
_____	2. TSH	b.	Affects growth
_____	3. Glucagon	c.	Regulates blood calcium
_____	4. Thyroxin	d.	Stimulates metabolic rate

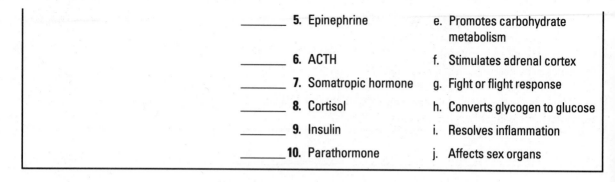

_____ **5.** Epinephrine	e. Promotes carbohydrate metabolism
_____ **6.** ACTH	f. Stimulates adrenal cortex
_____ **7.** Somatropic hormone	g. Fight or flight response
_____ **8.** Cortisol	h. Converts glycogen to glucose
_____ **9.** Insulin	i. Resolves inflammation
_____ **10.** Parathormone	j. Affects sex organs

SYSTEM SEVEN: THE RESPIRATORY SYSTEM

To carry on the vital functions of the organism, the cells of the body require a continual supply of oxygen and the removal of carbon dioxide. Without a constant supply of oxygen, a human being would die within a matter of minutes. The vital exchange of oxygen and carbon dioxide is accomplished by the respiratory system.

The respiratory system includes the nose, nasal cavity, pharynx, larynx, trachea, bronchial tubes, and the lungs. The lungs are composed of spongy tissue, blood vessels, connective tissue, and microscopic air sacs called **alveoli** (al-**VEE**-o-ligh). A network of very fine capillaries bring the blood in close contact with thin walls of alveoli (Fig. 5.72).

Respiration

Respiration is the exchange of carbon dioxide and oxygen that takes place at three levels in the body:
1. External respiration is the exchange between the external environment and the blood and takes place in the lungs.
2. Internal respiration is the gaseous exchange between the blood and the cells of the body.
3. Cellular respiration or oxidation occurs within the cell.

Respiration begins as air is inhaled through the nose and passes through the nasal cavity where it is warmed, moistened, and filtered. It passes through the pharynx and larynx and into the trachea. The trachea divides into two bronchi, which subdivide into the smaller and smaller branches of the **bronchial tree.** The air moves through the **bronchioles** until it reaches the ends of the air passages that terminate in clusters of air sacs called **alveoli.** The thin porous walls of the alveoli are surrounded by capillaries of the pulmonary circulatory system. The blood entering the lungs through the pulmonary arteries has a high concentration of CO_2 that has been picked up from the cells of the body and a low concentration of oxygen. The concentration of oxygen in the alveoli is greater than in the blood. Likewise, concentrations of carbon dioxide in the blood are higher than in the alveoli. Therefore, through the process of diffusion, CO_2 moves from the blood to the lungs and is exhaled while oxygen moves from the lungs into the blood stream and is carried by the red blood cells back to the heart and then circulated throughout the body.

Oxygenated blood moves into the capillaries of the general circulation. Differences in concentration of the gases between the blood and tissue fluid cause oxygen to diffuse into the tissue fluid while carbon dioxide diffuses out of the fluid and into the blood. A similar diffusion process takes place between the tissue fluid and the cells.

Once in the cells, the oxygen is used in cellular respiration to produce energy. Some of that energy is used by the cell to function.

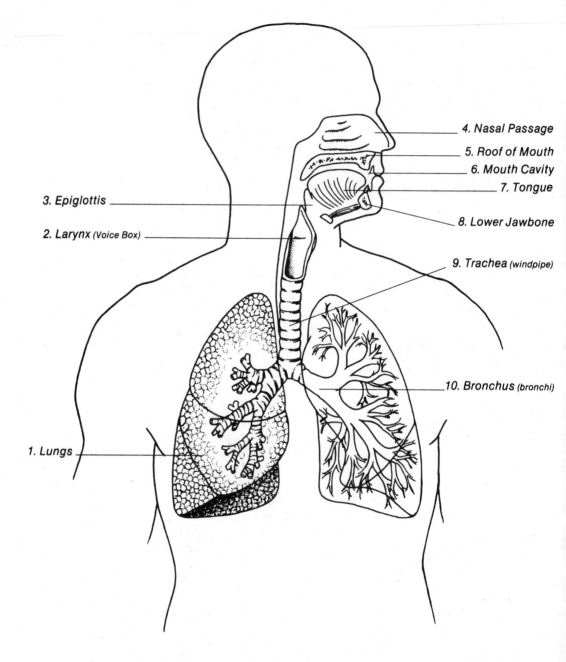

4. Nasal Passage

5. Roof of Mouth

6. Mouth Cavity

7. Tongue

3. Epiglottis

8. Lower Jawbone

2. Larynx (Voice Box)

9. Trachea (windpipe)

10. Bronchus (bronchi)

1. Lungs

1. Organs of external respiration located in lateral chambers of the thoracic cavity and consisting of three right and two left lobes. **2.** Situated between the tongue and trachea. Functions in production of vocal sounds. **3.** Forms part of larynx and assists in swallowing. **4.** Air passage extending from nostrils to pharynx. **9.** Located in front of esophagus. **10.** Air tubes entering the lungs.

Fig. 5.72 Respiratory organs and structures.

The rest is in the form of heat. The waste products of cellular respiration include carbon dioxide and water, which migrate back into the blood stream to be eliminated. The carbon dioxide is carried by the red blood cells and the plasma to the lungs, where it diffuses out of the blood into the alveoli to be expelled from the lungs with the next exhalation.

Breathing

External respiration, also called **ventilation** or **breathing,** involves the act of inhaling and exhaling air, resulting in an exchange of gases between the blood and air sacs. With each inhalation, the intercostal muscles contract, raising the ribs and expanding the thoracic cavity. At the same time the diaphragm contracts and is pulled down, causing the lungs to draw in air. Exhalation occurs as the intercostals and the diaphragm relax, returning to their neutral positions and pushing the air out of the lungs. Forced exhalation involves the contraction of the internal intercostal muscles, which collapse the rib cage, and the contraction of the abdominal muscles, which force the abdominal viscera against the diaphragm, further reducing the area of the thoracic cavity. The maximum intake of oxygen and expulsion of carbon dioxide is accomplished during deep breathing, which involves exaggerated movements of both the ribs and diaphragm.

Depending on the individual's lung capacity, the natural rate of breathing for an adult is between fourteen and twenty times a minute. The rate of breathing is increased by the demand for oxygen by such things as increased muscular activity.

A healthy respiratory system is maintained by avoiding air pollution, toxic chemicals, and smoking. Deep breathing, regular exercise, and a healthy diet all help to keep the respiratory system functioning normally. Should the massage practitioner notice that a client has trouble breathing normally, it is wise to suggest that the client see a physician. There is a great deal more to the respiratory system than has been covered in this brief overview. Study Fig. 5.72 to be sure you understand the location of the major parts of the respiratory system.

SECTION QUESTIONS FOR DISCUSSION AND REVIEW

1. What are the major organs of the respiratory system?
2. What is the function of the respiratory system?
3. What is the physical appearance of the lungs?
4. What are the three levels of respiration and where do they take place?
5. What is an alveoli and what is its function?
6. What is breathing?
7. What is the natural rate of breathing for an adult?
8. What is the diaphragm, and what function does it perform?

▼ SYSTEM EIGHT: THE DIGESTIVE SYSTEM

The human body is a living organism made up of millions of cells that perform a multitude of different tasks. Each cell must receive a continuous supply of nutrients to provide fuel for energy and nutritional elements for growth and regeneration. These nutrients come from the food we eat. Food that enters the mouth must undergo many changes before it can be used by the cells for nourishment. This process is carried on by the digestive system. The main functions of the digestive system are **digestion** and **absorption.** Digestion is the process of converting food into substances capable of being used by the cells for nourishment. Absorption is the process in which the digested nutrients are transferred from the intestines to the blood or lymph vessels so that they can be transported to the cells.

The digestive system is composed of the **alimentary canal** and **accessory digestive organs.** The alimentary canal, also known as the gastrointestinal or digestive tract, consists of the mouth (oral cavity), pharynx (throat), esophagus, stomach, small intestine, and large intestine. The accessory organs include the teeth, tongue, salivary glands, pancreas, liver, and gall bladder.

The alimentary canal is a muscular tube that is about five times as long as a person is tall and goes from the lips to the anus. The tube forms a continuous barrier so that material in the digestive tube can be acted on by the digestive juices although it is not yet part of the body or its cellular makeup.

The process of digestion changes the food into a nutritious fluid capable of being absorbed by the blood. Digestion is accomplished through physical and chemical means. The physical means involve the teeth, tongue, and involuntary muscles. The teeth tear and grind the food into small pieces while the tongue mixes and moves the food. Once the food is swallowed, the involuntary muscles mix the food with digestive juices and propel it through the alimentary canal. Food is acted on chemically by enzymes and a variety of digestive juices to break it down from complex food substances into simple nutritional molecules that can be absorbed into the blood stream and through the cell membranes.

The Path of Digestion

The mouth, called the **oral cavity,** prepares the food for entrance into the stomach. In the mouth the food is masticated (chewed) by the teeth and mixed by the tongue with secretions from the **salivary glands. Saliva** contains enzymes that begin to digest carbohydrates. The action of the teeth, tongue, and saliva prepares the food into a soft ball called a **bolus** that slides into the throat and is swallowed by voluntary and reflex actions of the muscles of the pharynx.

Structure of the Alimentary Canal

From the throat to the anus, the walls of the alimentary canal are similar in structure except for specialized modifications that perform particular functions. The wall of the alimentary canal consists of four distinct layers.

1. The **mucosa** (myoo-**KO**-suh) or mucous membrane is made up of epithelial cells, connective tissue, and a variety of digestive glands. This layer protects the underlying tissues and functions to carry on secretion and absorption.

2. The **submucosa** consists of connective tissue, nerves and blood and lymph vessels that serve to nourish the surrounding tissues and carry away the absorbed material.

3. The **muscular layer** has two layers of smooth muscle. The muscle fibers of the inner layer encircle the tube so that when they contract, the diameter of the tube decreases. The outer layer of muscle fibers is arranged longitudinally so that when they contract, the tube shortens.

4. The **serous layer** is the outer covering of the tube. On the stomach and intestines this layer is continuous with the peritoneum that lines the abdominal cavity (Fig. 5.73).

When food passes from the throat into the esophagus, the smooth muscles of the alimentary canal are stimulated and begin to produce a rhythmic, wave-like motion that will propel and churn the

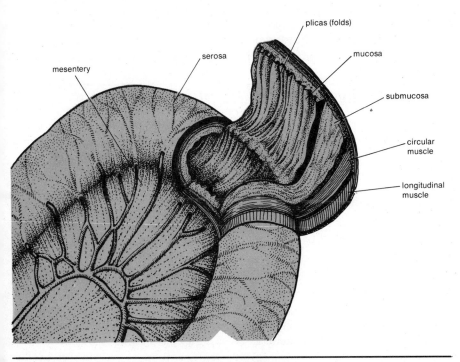

Fig. 5.73 Structure of the walls of the alimentary canal.

food throughout the length of the canal. The wave-like muscular action is called **peristalsis** (per-i-**STAL**-sis).

The Stomach

After food travels down the esophagus, it passes through the **cardiac sphincter** and enters the stomach, where it is churned with gastric juices secreted from glands in the wall of the stomach that contain **hydrochloric acid** and protein-digesting enzymes. The mixture of digestive juices, mucus, and food material is called **chyme.** From the stomach the chyme passes through the **pyloric sphincter** and into the duodenum of the small intestine. Sphincters are muscular valves that allow the passage of food substances in only one direction. The pyloric sphincter also plays an important role in determining how long food is held in the stomach.

The Small Intestine

The **small intestine** is the longest part of the alimentary canal. It consists of three parts: the **duodenum** (doo-o-**DEE**-num), **jejunum** (je-**JOO**-num), and **ileum** (**IL**-ee-um). Thousands of glands in the intestinal walls produce **intestinal digestive juices.** In addition to the intestinal juices, secretions of **bile** from the liver and **pancreatic fluids** from the pancreas are poured into the duodenum. Bile from the liver and gall bladder is carried through the **common bile duct** and is essential for the breakdown of fats. Pancreatic fluid enters the duodenum by way of the **pancreatic duct** and contains enzymes that act to digest proteins, carbohydrates, and fats.

The small intestine is lined with small, finger-like projections covering the intestinal walls called **villi** (**VIL**-eye) that greatly increase the surface area available for absorption. Each microscopic

▼ TABLE 5.12 GLANDS, DIGESTIVE JUICES AND ENZYMES

GLANDS AND JUICE	LOCATION	ENZYMES	CHANGES IN FOOD
Saliva (3) Salivary gland	Mouth	Salivary Amalase (ptyalin)	Begins digestion of starch into simple sugars
Gastric juice Stomach	Stomach wall	Pepsin	Begins digestion of protein into amino acids
Pancreatic juice Pancreas	Small intestine	Amalase Trypsin Lipase	Starches, proteins, fats
Juice from small intestine	Small intestine	Lactase Maltase Sucrase	Breaks down complex carbohydrates to simple sugars
Bile from liver	Small intestine	No enzymes	Breaks down fats into fatty acids

villus contains a network of blood capillaries and lymph capillaries (lacteals). The end products of digestion pass through the intestinal wall and are absorbed into the blood vessels and the lacteals. Nutrients absorbed into the blood stream are carried to the liver. Nutrients absorbed by the lymph flow through the cisterna chyli and the thoracic duct before entering the systemic circulation.

The Large Intestine

Once the digestive processes have been completed in the small intestine, the waste (unusable) materials (water and solids) moves through the **iliocecal valve** into a small, pouch-like part of the large intestine called the **cecum** (**SEE**-kum). The large intestine (colon) continues upward along the right side of the abdomen to form the **ascending colon.** Then it travels across the abdominal cavity and forms the **transverse colon.** It continues downward on the left side of the abdomen to become the **descending colon.** As the colon reaches the left iliac region, it forms an S-shaped bend known as the **sigmoid colon** that empties into the rectum. The **rectum** is a temporary storage area for waste. The distal part of the large intestine is the **anal canal,** which ends with the anus, from which fecal matter is expelled.

The functions of the colon include storing, forming, and excreting waste products of digestion and regulating the body's water balance. The colon aides in regulating the body's water balance by absorbing large amounts of water from the undigested material back into the body. Through a process of water absorption and bacterial action, the liquid state of the undigested and indigestible material in the colon is transformed into the semisolid **feces,** which is eliminated from the rectum. The bacterial action in the colon also synthesizes of some B-complex vitamins and vitamin K, which is reabsorbed into the blood stream (Fig. 5.74).

SECTION QUESTIONS FOR DISCUSSION AND REVIEW

1. Which structures compose the digestive system?
2. What is the function of digestion?
3. What is absorption?
4. What are the physical processes of digestion?
5. What chemical agents in the digestive juices aid digestion?
6. What digestive changes occur in the mouth?
7. Describe the general structure of the alimentary canal.
8. What is peristalsis or peristaltic action?
9. What digestive changes occur in the stomach?
10. Name the three parts of the small intestine.
11. Which glands supply digestive secretions to the small intestine?
12. What digestive changes occur in the small intestine?
13. Which structures absorb the end products of digestion?
14. From which organ is the undigested food eliminated from the body?

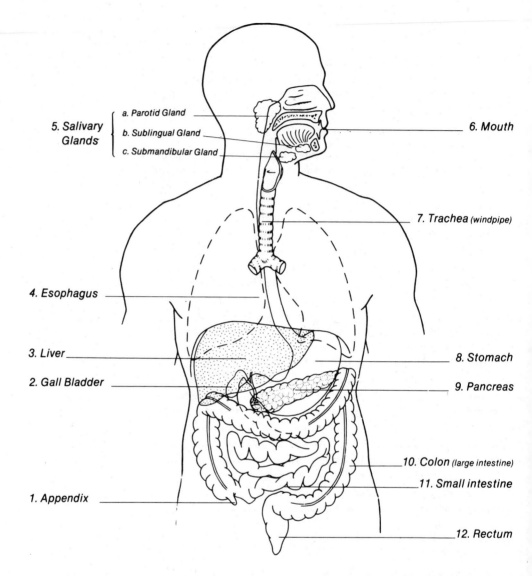

5. Salivary Glands
a. Parotid Gland
b. Sublingual Gland
c. Submandibular Gland

6. Mouth

7. Trachea (windpipe)

4. Esophagus

3. Liver

2. Gall Bladder

8. Stomach

9. Pancreas

10. Colon (large intestine)

11. Small intestine

1. Appendix

12. Rectum

1. A narrow tube attached to the cecum, a part of the colon. 2. The gall bladder is located on the underside of the liver. It receives bile from liver and expels the bile (as needed) into the duodenum. 3. Produces bile, which acts as fat solvent. The largest gland of the body, the liver functions to maintain and regulate homeostasis of body fluids and help to control body processes. 4. Moves food to the stomach.
5. Buccal glands. 5a. Located under and in front of ear. 5b. Located below the jaw and under the tongue. 5c. Located in floor of mouth beneath the tongue. 6. Principal functions of mouth and salivary glands are mastication and changing starch to sugar. 7. Windpipe (respiratory tract). 8. Serves as a receptacle for food; manufactures gastric juice during digestion. 9. Lies behind the stomach and produces enzymes which act on fat, proteins, starch and carbohydrates to complete the digestive process. Aids in regulation of glucose metabolism.
10. Responsible for absorption and elimination of foodstuffs. 11. Serves in the absorption and elimination of foodstuffs.
12. Serves to eliminate waste.

Fig. 5.74 The Digestive system.

SYSTEM NINE: THE EXCRETORY SYSTEM ▼

The Excretory Organs

The food we eat, water we drink, and air we breathe all play an important role in supplying the elements for the body's metabolic activity. As the cells metabolize these elements to produce their specialized substances and energy, waste products are formed that must be carried away and excreted from the body. If retained, these **metabolic wastes** would have a tendency to poison the body.

The function of the excretory system (including the urinary system) is to eliminate or excrete metabolic wastes and undigested food from the body. The organs of the excretory system are the kidneys, liver, skin, large intestines, and lungs.

1. The kidneys excrete uric acid, urea, electrolytes, water, and other wastes through the process of urination.
2. The liver produces urea, which is returned to the blood to be excreted by the kidneys. The liver also discharges bile through the gall bladder and into the intestines.
3. The skin eliminates water and heat through the process of perspiration.
4. The large intestine discharges food wastes through the process of defecation.
5. The lungs exhale carbon dioxide and water vapor through exhalation.

Urinary System

The urinary system includes two kidneys, two ureters, the bladder, and a urethra. The **kidneys** are bean-shaped glands located at the back of the abdominal cavity, between the tenth thoracic and third lumbar vertebrae, and kept in place by fibrous connective and fatty tissues. The kidneys are an efficient blood filtration system. The **nephron** (**NEF**-ron) is the functional unit of the kidney. There are two to three million nephrons in the kidneys. Each day the nephrons filter forty to fifty gallons of plasma from the blood. Ninety-nine percent of this fluid is reabsorbed into the blood stream. The kidneys excrete the remaining water and waste products through the **ureters.** As the kidneys filter the blood, they remove a certain amount of water and nitrogenous waste products of metabolism (such as urea, uric acid, as well as ammonia and some drugs). The **ureters** are tubes that carry urine from the kidneys to the **bladder,** where the urine is stored. The bladder is a hollow organ constructed of walls of elastic fibers and involuntary muscles that acts as a reservoir for the urine until it is excreted from the body. When the bladder accumulates about a pint of urine, sensors indicate that it is time to urinate. Voiding or emptying the bladder is accomplished by a voluntary relaxation of a sphincter muscle at the mouth of the urethra and the involuntary contraction of the muscles of the

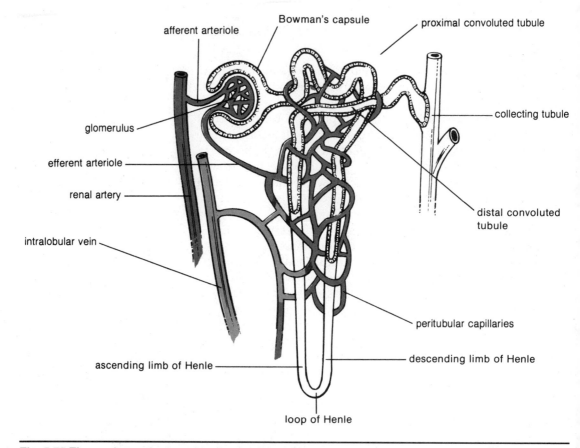

afferent arteriole

Bowman's capsule

proximal convoluted tubule

glomerulus

efferent arteriole

renal artery

intralobular vein

collecting tubule

distal convoluted tubule

peritubular capillaries

ascending limb of Henle

descending limb of Henle

loop of Henle

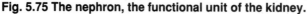

Fig. 5.75 The nephron, the functional unit of the kidney.

bladder. As the bladder contracts, urine is forced through the **urethra** and out of the body (Fig. 5.75).

A **urinalysis** is a chemical examination of the urine that is often part of the routine examination given by most physicians. The presence of white blood cells, blood, glucose, or other chemicals in the urine may be an indication of metabolic imbalance, infection, or numerous other conditions. Normal, healthy urine is a clear yellowish fluid. A change in the color of the urine, such as a reddish or brownish color, may indicate infection or other problems.

The kidneys also function to maintain the body's water balance and acid-base balance. Another function of the kidneys is the production of the hormone **renin**, which acts to regulate blood pressure. When the blood pressure is low, the kidneys are stimulated to release more renin into the blood stream, which causes blood vessels to contract, thereby raising the blood pressure (Fig. 5.76).

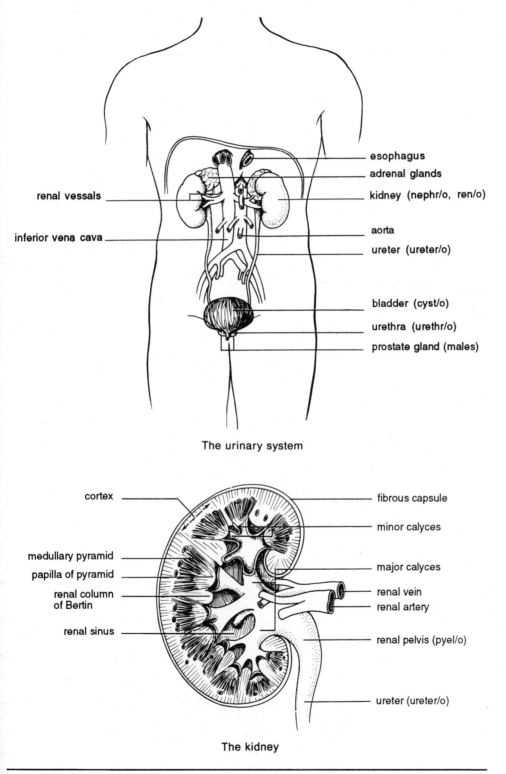

The urinary system

The kidney

Fig. 5.76 The urinary system.

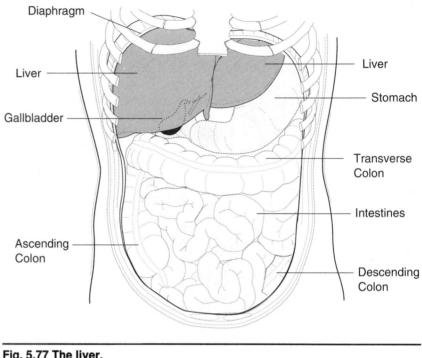

Fig. 5.77 The liver.

The Liver

The **liver** is the largest gland in the body and is situated on the upper right side of the abdomen, immediately below and in contact with the diaphragm. The liver performs many of the body's chemical functions. The liver neutralizes or detoxifies toxic substances that may have been absorbed from the intestines such as alcohol, food additives, and drugs. The liver functions in a great number of other metabolic processes that include converting glucose to glycogen, changing lactic acid to glucose, producing glucose from noncarbohydrates, changing carbohydrates and protein to fats for storage, producing cholesterol lipoproteins, and breaking down and reforming damaged red blood cells. The liver stores vitamins A, B, and B12 and glycogen. The main excretory function of the liver is the formation of urea, which is returned to the blood stream to be excreted by the kidneys. The liver also produces and excretes bile through the intestines. **Bile** is a bitter, alkaline, yellowish-brown fluid secreted from the liver into the duodenum and contains water, bile salts, mucin, cholesterol, lecithin, and fat pigments. Bile aids in the emulsification, digestion, and absorption of fats and the alkalization of the intestines (Fig. 5.77).

SECTION QUESTIONS FOR DISCUSSION AND REVIEW ▼

1. Name the five important organs of the excretory system.
2. What happens if waste products are retained within the body instead of being eliminated?
3. What is the function of the excretory system?
4. Name the parts of the urinary system.
5. What is the functional unit of the kidney?
6. Why do most physicians include urinalysis as a part of a routine physical checkup?
7. What colors of urine indicate a problem that needs checking by a physician?
8. Which organ of the body secretes bile?
9. What is the excretory function of the liver?

SYSTEM TEN: THE HUMAN REPRODUCTIVE SYSTEM

The reproductive system is the generative apparatus necessary for organisms to reproduce organisms of the same kind and ensure the continuation of their species.

Lower forms of life such as one-celled organisms do not need a partner to reproduce. They do so by nonsexual means, which is called **asexual reproduction.**

In humans (and most multicellular organisms), reproduction is sexual and requires a male and female, each having specialized sex cells. **Gamete** is the term used to describe a reproductive cell that can unite with another gamete to form the cell (zygote) that develops into a new individual. In the male these cells are **spermatozoa** (sper-ma-to-**ZOE**-uh) and in females, **ovum.** A **zygote** is the fertilized ovum, the cell formed by the union of a spermatozoon with an ovum. A **gonad** is a sex gland that produces the reproductive cell. In the female the gonad is the **ovary.** In the male it is the **testes** Fig. 5.78).

It is not within the scope of this book to describe in detail the entire process of human reproduction. The following is a brief summary.

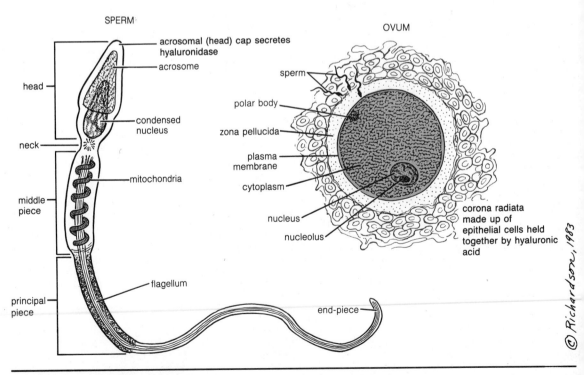

Fig. 5.78 Human sperm and ovum.

The Male Reproductive System

The functions of the male reproductive system are the production of sperm, the production of the male hormones, and the performance of the sex act. The reproductive system in males includes two testes, two vas deferens, two seminal vesicles, a prostate gland, the bulbourethral glands (Cowper's glands), and the penis.

The male gonads are located outside the body in a pouch situated at the base of and beneath the penis called the **scrotum.** The **testes** are two small, egg-shaped glands made up of minute convoluted tubules, lined with specialized cells that produce the spermatozoa. Other specialized cells in the testes form the male hormone **testosterone.**

Testosterone is essential to the development of the male sexual characteristics including body hair, masculine voice, sex organs, and sperm production. Spermatozoa are tiny detached cells, egg shaped and equipped with a tail that enables them to be motile or to swim. Of the millions of spermatozoa ejected during copulation, only one will fertilize the reproductive cell (egg) produced by the female. The others die within a short time.

The male reproductive system includes a duct system, tubes that transport the **spermatozoa** from the testes to the outside of the body.

The **epididymis** (ep-i-**DID**-i-mis), located in the scrotum, receives sperm from the testes and stores the sperm until it becomes fully mature. This tube extends upward to become the left or right **vas deferens (ductus deferens)** and continues through a small canal behind the abdominal wall and behind the urinary bladder. The sperm collects in the vas deferens until it is expelled from the body. The vas deferens join with the ducts of the seminal vesicles to form the **ejaculatory ducts.** These two ducts enter the prostate gland, where they empty into the urethra.

The Accessory Glands

The glands of the male reproductive system produce secretions that combine with the sperm to form **semen,** which is excreted from the body during ejaculation.

Seminal vesicles are two convoluted, glandular tubes located on each side of the prostrate that produce a nutritious fluid that is excreted into the ejaculatory ducts at the time of emission. The secretions of the seminal vesicles contain simple sugars, mucus, prostaglandin, and other substances to help nourish, protect, and aid the sperm as it travels into the female reproductive system. The **seminal fluid** forms the majority of the semen when ejaculated.

The **prostate gland** lies below the urinary bladder and surrounds the first part of the urethra. The prostrate secrets an alkaline fluid that enhances the sperm's motility (ability to swim). The fluid also neutralizes the acidic vaginal secretions, thereby protecting the

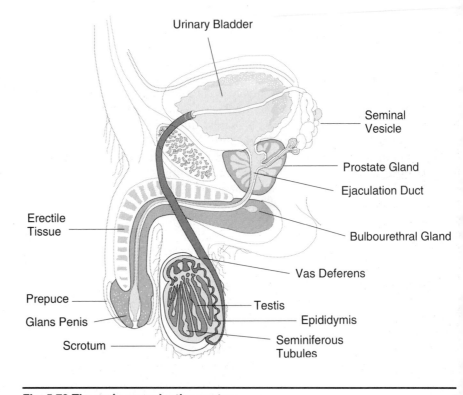

Fig. 5.79 The male reproductive system.

sperm and increasing its chances of reaching and fertilizing the ovum. Ducts from the prostate enter the ejaculatory ducts. The prostate gland is supplied with muscular tissue that reflexively contracts during the expulsion of the semen.

The Cowper's (bulbourethral) glands are two pea-sized glands located beneath the prostate gland. They are mucus-producing glands that serve to lubricate the urethra.

The **urethra** serves to convey urine from the bladder and to carry reproductive cells and secretions out of the body.

The **penis** is the male organ of copulation consisting of erectile tissue that may become engorged and erect in order to deposit the sperm-containing semen deep within the female's vagina (Fig. 5.79).

The Female Reproductive System

The functions of the female reproductive system are to produce the ovum and female hormones, to receive the sperm during the sex act, and to carry the growing fetus during pregnancy.

The reproductive system in females includes two ovaries, two fallopian tubes (oviducts), a uterus, a vagina, and the vulva or external genitalia.

The **vulva** forms the external part of the female reproductive system. It includes the outer lips called the **labia majora** and the inner, smaller lips called the **labia minora.** On a virgin, within the vulva a fold of connective tissue, the hymen, partially covers the external orifice of the vagina. The clitoris is a small sensitive body of erectile tissue located at the anterior junction of the labia. The mons pubis is a pad of fatty tissue over the pubic symphysis.

The Female Internal Organs

The **vagina** is a muscular tube or canal leading from the vulva opening to the cervix and is the lower part of the birth canal. The vagina is the organ that receives the penis and the ejaculated semen during sexual intercourse. Near the vestibule of the vagina are mucus-producing glands called **Bartholen's glands.**

The **uterus** is a pear-shaped, muscular organ consisting of an upper portion, the body, and the cervix or neck. The uterine cavity is small and narrow except during pregnancy, when it expands to accommodate the fetus and a large amount of fluid.

The **oviducts,** also called **fallopian tubes,** are the egg-carrying tubes of the female reproductive system. They extend from the uterus to the ovaries. The **ovaries** (female gonads) are a pair of glandular organs located within the pelvic area. The ovaries perform two functions. They produce the ovum and the female sex hormones, **estrogen** and **progesterone.** The **ovum** is the egg cell capable of being fertilized by a spermatozoon and developing into a new life (Fig. 5.80).

During each **menstrual cycle** (the periodically recurring series of changes that take place in the ovaries, uterus, and related structures in the female), a follicle develops in the ovary and produces estrogen (female hormone) as an ovum (egg) matures. Usually only one follicle matures each cycle (approximately every twenty-eight days). **Ovulation** is the discharge of a mature ovum from the follicle of the ovary. A hormone from the pituitary gland, called **luteinizing hormone,** transforms the follicle into the **corpus luteum.** This is a yellowish endocrine body formed in the ruptured follicle of the ovary that produces estrogen and progesterone. These hormones promote the lining of the uterus to thicken in preparation to receive the egg if it should be fertilized. Estrogen also controls the development of secondary female sexual characteristics (breast development, female body contours, etc.).

The ovum is carried into the fimbriated ends of the oviducts by the action of cilia, which produce a current in the peritoneal fluid. The ovum travels down the oviduct toward the uterus. If the ovum (egg) is fertilized by a sperm cell, pregnancy results. If the ovum is not fertilized, the built-up lining of the uterus sloughs off and is expelled along with the menstrual blood and secretions.

Menstruation is the cyclic, physiologic uterine bleeding that normally occurs at about four-week intervals (except during pregnancy) during the reproductive period of the human female. Menstruation begins at puberty and continues until **menopause,** which

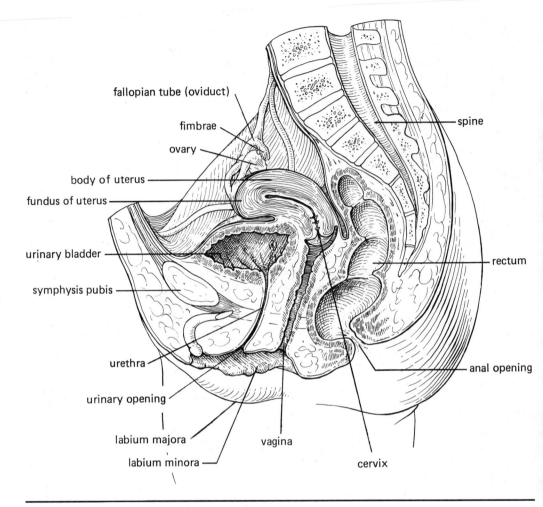

labels:
fallopian tube (oviduct)
fimbrae
ovary
body of uterus
fundus of uterus
urinary bladder
symphysis pubis
urethra
urinary opening
labium majora
labium minora
vagina
cervix
spine
rectum
anal opening

Fig. 5.80 The female reproductive system.

occurs at about ages 45 to 55. Menopause is the physiological cessation of the menstrual cycle and therefore the end of the child-bearing years.

Pregnancy

Pregnancy, or **gestation** (jes-**TAY**-shun), is the physiological condition that occurs from the time an ovum is fertilized until childbirth. During pregnancy the fertilized egg develops in the mother's uterus or womb from a single cell, through many stages to a full-term infant. The duration of pregnancy in women is approximately 280 days or forty weeks.

Embryonic life begins at conception, with the fertilization of the ovum by the sperm, which usually takes place within the first three days after ovulation and the first few hours after copulation. Of the millions of sperm deposited within the vagina, only several hundred reach the ovum. Of those that reach the ovum, only one will penetrate the covering to fertilize the egg. After fertilization the developing zygote travels down the fallopian tubes and becomes embedded in the uterine wall. The developing form first receives nourishment from the uterine fluids, and then the wall of the uterus until a placenta develops. From about the twelfth week, the developing fetus, enclosed in a protective fluid-filled amniotic sac with its own circulatory system, receives nourishment and disposes of its wastes by way of the placenta. The mother's blood and the blood of the fetus never interchange. From the beginning of the third month of pregnancy until birth, the developing child is called a **fetus.** During pregnancy the mother's metabolism changes due to the demands made on her body systems. Her lungs must provide more oxygen and her heart must pump more blood. The kidneys must excrete nitrogenous wastes from the fetus and the mother's body.

During pregnancy, the mother needs proper nutrition to provide for the growth of the fetus as well as to maintain the health of all organs as the body prepares for labor and birth.

Following the birth of the child, the mother should maintain her health and that of her child by attention to nutritional needs and by specific exercises to tone and strengthen her muscles.

SECTION QUESTIONS FOR DISCUSSION AND REVIEW ▼

1. What is the reproductive system?
2. What is the difference between asexual and sexual reproduction?
3. What is a gonad?
4. What is a zygote?
5. What are the parts of the male reproductive system?
6. What are the functions of the male reproductive system?
7. What are the parts of the female reproductive system?
8. What are the functions of the female reproductive system?
9. What is the difference between an embryo and a fetus?
10. What is ovulation?
11. What is the approximate duration of pregnancy in women?

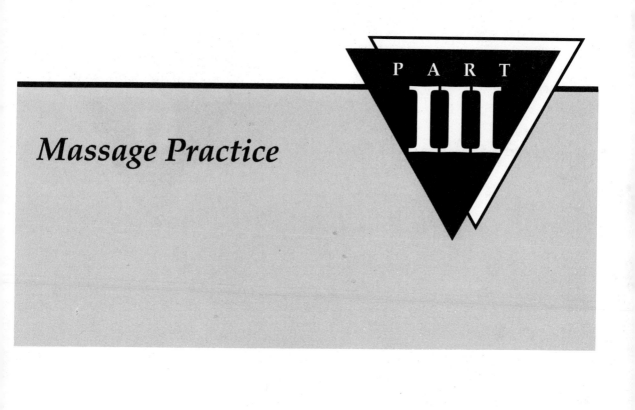

Massage Practice

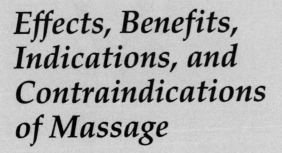

PART III

Effects, Benefits, Indications, and Contraindications of Massage

Learning Objectives

After you have mastered this chapter, you will be able to:

1. Explain the physiological effects and benefits of massage.
2. Explain the psychological effects and benefits of massage.
3. Describe the effects of massage on the circulatory, muscular, and nervous systems of the body.
4. Describe the effects of massage on the skin.
5. Explain the main contraindications for massage.

INTRODUCTION ▼

There is much historical evidence to indicate that massage was one of the earliest remedial practices for relief of pain and for the restoration of healthy body functions. Massage is a natural and instinctive method by which minor aches and pains can be soothed away while bringing relief from nervous tension and fatigue.

The term *massage* is applied to different practices, but in the following chapters the techniques of traditional western or what is commonly termed Swedish massage will be considered. The effects of massage differ from one client to another depending on the needs of the individual and the goals and intentions with which the massage is administered. This is why massage on two different people may render different results. In addition to physical effects from massage therapy, the client may experience mental and emotional reactions. Many healthy people believe that frequent massage helps them to remain physically, mentally, and emotionally fit. They enjoy the relaxed, refreshed, and invigorated feeling they get from a therapeutic massage.

Although massage is not a magic cure-all, it is a safe and beneficial health aid for everyone from infants to the elderly, except when there are certain contraindications. When there is doubt on the part of the practitioner whether to give massage or to recommend a particular exercise, the client should first have a physical checkup and obtain his or her physician's recommendations in writing.

EFFECTS AND BENEFITS OF MASSAGE ▼

Massage has direct psychological and physiological benefits. Physically, massage increases metabolism, hastens healing, relaxes and refreshes the muscles, and improves the detoxifying functions of the lymphatic system. Massage helps to prevent and relieve muscle cramps and spasms and improves circulation of blood and lymph, thereby improving the delivery of oxygen and nutrients to the cells as it enhances the removal of metabolic wastes. Since blood carries nutrients to the skin, massage is beneficial in keeping the skin functioning in a normal, healthy manner. Massage therapy is effective in pain management in conditions such as arthritis, neuritis, neuralgia, labor and delivery, whiplash, muscular lesions, sciatica, headache, muscle spasms, and many other conditions.

Psychologically, massage relieves fatigue, reduces tension and anxiety, calms the nervous system, and promotes a sense of relaxation and renewed energy.

There are indications that massage is beneficial in numerous conditions; however, in cases of injury or disease, the client's physician must be consulted before massage treatments are given. Massage has been credited with being of great benefit in helping patients recover from various illnesses or injuries. In some cases modalities that use heat, light, cold, water, and electricity may be recommended by the client's physician. A physician may recommend massage for both its physical and psychological benefits.

Physiological Effects of Massage

Skillfully applied massage is an effective means of influencing the structures and functions of the body. The specific effects of any massage will vary according to the intent with which it is given, the selection of techniques used, and the condition of the client. Depending on the type and manner of manipulation, a sense of mild relaxation, stimulation, or refreshment may follow massage. Under no circumstances should massage be applied so vigorously that it causes the client to feel exhausted or results in bruised or injured tissues.

There are two physical effects of massage, mechanical and reflex, which may occur separately or together. Mechanical effects are direct physical effects of the massage techniques on the tissues they contact. Reflex effects of massage are indirect responses to touch that affect body functions and tissues through the nervous or energy systems of the body. Gentle stimulation of the sensory nerve endings in the skin, as in superficial stroking, results in reflex effects, either locally or in distant parts of the body. When pressure is applied to the muscles, blood, and lymph vessels, or to any internal structure, both reflex and direct mechanical effects are experienced. Pressure on reflex points, active trigger points, and other pressure points reflexively affects functions or areas of the body away from the actual point of contact.

The immediate effects of massage are noticeable on the skin. Friction and stroking movements heighten blood circulation to the skin and increase activity of the sweat (sudoriferous) and oil (sebaceous) glands. Accompanying the increased flow of blood, there is a slight reddening and warming of the skin. Nutrition to the skin is improved. Massage treatments over a period of time impart a healthy radiance to the skin. The skin tends to become softer, more supple, and of finer texture.

The physiological effects of massage are not limited to the skin. The body as a whole benefits by the stimulation of muscular, glandular, and vascular activities. Most organs of the body are favorably influenced by scientific massage treatments.

Effects of Massage on the Muscular System

Massage encourages the nutrition and development of the muscular system by stimulating its circulation, nerve supply, and cell activity. Regular and systematic massage causes the muscles to become firmer and more elastic, while muscles too weak to be used voluntarily can be strengthened by active massage treatments. Massage is also an effective means of relaxing tense muscles and releasing muscle spasms.

The supply of blood to the muscles is proportionate to their activity. It is estimated that blood passes three times more rapidly through muscles being massaged than muscles at rest. Petrissage or kneading and compression movements create a pumping action that forces the venous blood and lymph onward and brings a fresh supply of blood to the muscles. Massage aids in the removal of metabolic waste products and helps nourish tissues.

Massage prevents and relieves stiffness and soreness of muscles. Muscles fatigued by work or exercise will be more quickly restored by massage than by passive rest of the same duration.

Muscle tissue that has suffered injury heals more quickly with less connective tissue build-up and scarring when therapeutic massage is applied regularly. Friction massage, when properly applied, prevents and reduces the development of adhesions and excessive scarring following trauma.

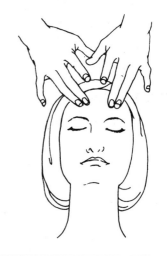

Massage can have positive effects on the range of motion of limbs that have a limited range due to tissue injury, inflammation, muscle tension, or strain. The client may have experienced discomfort or pain resulting in limited use of a limb or may have stopped using the limb. The limb will need to be taken through the range of motion passively and carefully and the range increased gradually.

Fig. 6.1 Active joint movements have beneficial effects similar to exercise.

Passive movement is the method by which joints are rotated through their range of motion with no resistance or assistance by muscular activity on the part of the client. Passive massage movements benefit circulation of the blood and lymph, nourish the skin, relax and lengthen the muscles, and soothe the nerves.

Active joint movement in massage refers to exercises in which the voluntary muscles are contracted by the client and either resisted or assisted by the therapist. Active joint movements have beneficial effects similar to exercise. They help to firm and strengthen muscles, improve circulation, and aid the function of related internal organs (Fig. 6.1).

Effects of Massage on the Nervous System

The effects of massage on the nervous system depend on the direct and reflex reaction of the nerves stimulated. The nervous system can be stimulated or soothed depending on the type of massage movement applied (Fig. 6.2).

Stimulation of the peripheral nerve receptors could have reflex reactions affecting the vaso-motor nerves, internal organs, pain perception, or the underlying joints and muscles of the areas being massaged.

1. **Stimulating massage techniques:**
   a. Friction (light rubbing, rolling, and wringing movement) stimulates nerves.
   b. Percussion (light tapping and slapping movements) increases nervous irritability. Strong percussion for a short

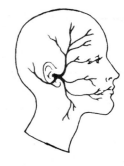

Fig. 6.2 Peripheral nerves.

period of time excites nerve centers directly. Prolonged percussion tends to anesthetize the local nerves.

c. Vibration (shaking and trembling movements) stimulates peripheral nerves and all nerve centers with which a nerve trunk is connected.

2. **Sedative effect of massage techniques:**

a. Gentle stroking, especially over reflex areas, produces calming and sedative results.

b. Light friction and petrissage (kneading movements) produce marked sedative effects.

Effects of Massage on the Circulatory System

Scientific body massage procedures effect the quality and quantity of blood coursing through the circulatory system. With the increased flow of blood to the massaged area, better cellular nutrition and elimination are favored. The work of the heart is lessened due to the improvement in surface circulation. Under the influence of massage, the blood-making process is improved, resulting in an increase in the number of red and white blood cells (Fig. 6.3).

An important principle to remember in Swedish massage is to always massage toward the heart. Massage movements should be directed upward along the limbs and lower parts of the body and downward from the head, thereby facilitating the flow of venous blood and lymph back toward the heart and other eliminatory organs.

Massage may influence the blood and lymph vessels either by direct mechanical action on the vessel walls or by reflex action through the vaso-motor nerves. Pressure against the vessels not only tones their muscular walls but also propels the movement of the blood. The vaso-motor nerves, by controlling the relaxing and constricting of the blood vessels, determine the amount of blood which will reach the area being massaged.

Massage movements affect blood and lymph channels in the following ways:

1. Light stroking produces an almost instantaneous though temporary dilation of the capillaries, while deep stroking brings about a more lasting dilation and flushing of the massaged area.

2. Light percussion causes a contraction of the blood vessels, which tend to relax as the movement is continued.

3. Friction hastens the flow of blood through the superficial veins, increases the permeability of the capillary beds, and produces an increased flow of interstitial fluid. This creates a healthier environment for the cells.

4. Petrissage or kneading stimulates the flow of blood through the deeper arteries and veins.

5. Friction, kneading, and stroking stimulate lymph circulation.

6. Compression produces a hyperemia (high-per-EE-mee-eh) or an increase in the amount of blood stored in the muscle tissue.

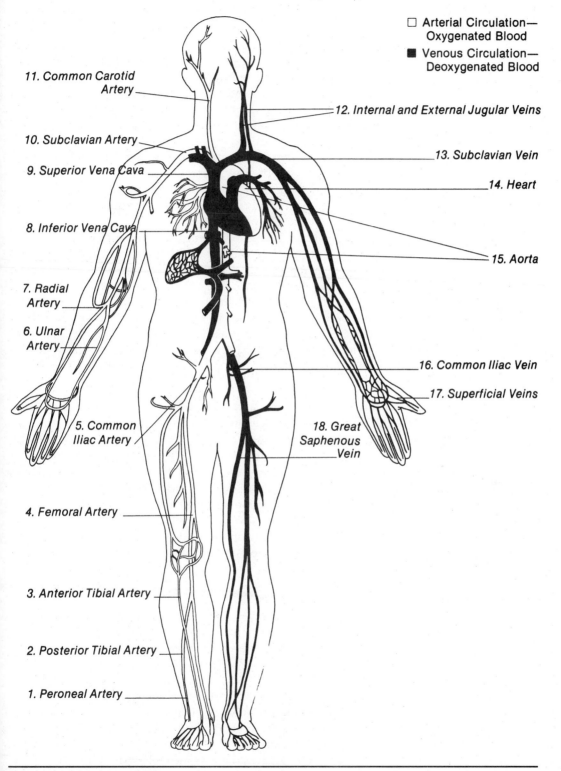

Arterial Circulation—
Oxygenated Blood

Venous Circulation—
Deoxygenated Blood

11. Common Carotid
Artery

12. Internal and External Jugular Veins

10. Subclavian Artery

13. Subclavian Vein

9. Superior Vena Cava

14. Heart

8. Inferior Vena Cava

15. Aorta

7. Radial
Artery

6. Ulnar
Artery

16. Common Iliac Vein

17. Superficial Veins

5. Common
Iliac Artery

18. Great
Saphenous
Vein

4. Femoral Artery

3. Anterior Tibial Artery

2. Posterior Tibial Artery

1. Peroneal Artery

Fig. 6.3 Circulatory system.

Psychological Effects of Massage

The psychological effects of massage should not be underestimated. If the client feels healthier, invigorated, and more energetic, the massage has been worth the effort. In treatment centers for addictions, massage has proven to be an effective therapeutic tool to rebuild a more positive self-image and sense of self-worth. People have regular massages as much for psychological as for physical benefit.

Many people suffer from stress and find that massage promotes relaxation as it soothes away minor aches and pains. For some clients, regular massage keeps them feeling more youthful and encourages them to pay more attention to proper nutrition, exercise, and good health practices.

Massage helps clients to become more aware of where they are holding tension, and where they have tight muscles or painful areas. The practitioner may discover areas the client may not have been aware of previously. By getting in touch with, or becoming aware of these conditions, the client can begin to focus on relaxing them both during the massage and on a daily basis. The client should be told that when muscles are tight there is constriction in the circulation to the affected area. Becoming aware of these trouble spots and responding to them is considered part of preventive maintenance.

▼ CONDITIONS GENERALLY RELIEVED BY MASSAGE

Almost all healthy people occasionally have some physical condition that can be improved by massage. When relief is obtained, there is also a renewed sense of well-being. No matter how well a client may be, a good massage will leave that person feeling even better.

The following conditions are most frequently relieved by regular massage treatment:

1. Stress and tensions are relieved. With the relief of tension and stress, the client feels better able to cope with day-to-day situations.
2. Mental and physical fatigue is relieved, leading to renewed energy and ambition.
3. Pain in the shoulders, neck, and back (usually caused by strained muscles or irritated nerves) is relieved.
4. Muscles and joints become more supple. Soreness and stiffness are relieved.
5. Muscle soreness from overexertion can be reduced or prevented.
6. Circulation is improved, thus improving skin tone.
7. Digestion, assimilation, and elimination are often improved.
8. Facial massage tones the skin, helps prevent blemished skin, and softens fine lines.
9. Headache and eyestrain are often relieved.
10. Deep relaxation is induced and insomnia relieved.

11. Muscular spasms are relieved.
12. Obesity (overweight) and flabby muscles can be improved when combined with proper exercise and diet programs.
13. Pain in joints, sprains, and poor circulation are relieved.
14. Increased circulation of nourishing blood to the skin and other parts of the body encourages healing.
15. Mental strain is reduced, resulting in better productivity.
16. Mildly high blood pressure is temporarily reduced.
17. Renewed sense of confidence and control is experienced.
18. Constrictions and adhesions can be reduced or prevented as traumatized muscle tissue heals.
19. Joint mobility can be increased.

CONTRAINDICATIONS FOR MASSAGE ▼

While there are many benefits from therapeutic body massage, there are also contraindications of which the professional practitioner must be aware.

Contraindication means that the expected treatment or process is inadvisable. In massage it means that conditions may exist in which it would not be beneficial to apply massage to a part or all of the body. The practitioner must know not only when massage is advised but, more importantly, when it should be avoided, or when certain strokes or movements should not be used.

When you define massage as a form of touch that is applied in a therapeutic manner, then it is true that massage of some form is beneficial to nearly everyone. However, there are situations where particular manipulations may not only be uncomfortable for the client but could be dangerous.

Many conditions are both indicated and contraindicated for massage. Many conditions respond favorably to massage, while others can be aggravated or worsened by specific massage techniques. Certain movements could do more harm than good. Such techniques are contraindicated. It is the responsibility of the practitioner to understand fully the indications and contra-indications for massage.

During the first interview or consultation with a client, it is important to obtain information about the state of his or her health and determine any reasons why massage treatments might be inadvisable. A client intake form that includes a medical history is helpful. Careful questioning about the client's conditions is essential in determining if contraindications exist. Often during the course of a massage, conditions that the client may not be aware of become apparent that are contraindicated and should be referred to the attention of a physician. When in doubt, caution is the best policy. The client can be asked (tactfully) to supply a physician's report and/or recommendations before beginning treatments, or the practitioner could ask the client's physician first if there are questionable circumstances.

Because massage requires a great deal of physical energy on the part of the practitioner, mechanical and electrical apparatus have been devised as aids to manual massage. The hand vibrator is an example. The same contraindications for manual massage also apply when any kind of helpful apparatus is used.

The major contraindications include the following:

Abnormal body temperature: 98.6° F (Fahrenheit), 37° C (Celsius) is considered normal body temperature, but it may vary depending on the time of day or other factors. The normal body temperature can vary from 96.4° to 99.1°F (35.8° to 37.3°C). Some doctors and therapists say that massage is not recommended when temperature exceeds 99.4°. If the client feels abnormally warm or feverish, his or her temperature should be taken to ascertain the advisability of massage treatment. Massage is contraindicated when the client has a fever. Generally a fever indicates that the body is trying to isolate and eliminate an invading pathogen. The body is stepping up its own action in order to confine, narrow down, and eliminate the problem. Therefore massage would tend to work against the defense mechanisms of the body.

Acute infectious disease: Typhoid, diphtheria, severe colds, influenza, and the like would preclude massage. Giving a massage to an individual who is coming down with an acute viral infection (cold or flu) will intensify the illness and expose the therapist to the virus. The client should seek his or her doctor's advice.

Inflammation: When there is acute inflammation in a particular area of the body, massage is not advisable because it could further irritate the area or intensify the inflammation. This is particularly true for spreading or penetrating types of massage manipulations. Inflamed joints do not indicate massage of the joint itself; however, there are some pressure point applications that are useful. Therapeutic touch, which is simply placing your hands on or near the inflamed area, may be helpful.

Although working directly on an area may be contraindicated, working on a reflex or related area or working in an area proximal to the affected area can be useful because it tends to stimulate circulation and the natural healing properties of the body. A **reflex** is a point that is distant to the affected area yet, when stimulated, has an effect on that area.

There are numerous types of inflammations. A word with the suffix -*tis* pertains to inflammation. For example, arthritis is an inflammation of the joints, neuritis is an inflammation of a nerve or nerves, dermatitis is inflammation of the skin, and so on. Caution must be used when a client has any kind of inflammation that could be aggravated by massage.

Inflammation due to tissue damage: When tissue is damaged, the body's natural response is inflammation. Inflammation is characterized by swelling, redness, heat, and pain.

If the tissue damage is of a traumatic nature and severe enough, blood vessels may be damaged, resulting in a hematoma (hee-muh-**TO**-muh). The area may become swollen and discolored. The bluish color is from blood escaping from the damaged blood vessels. Any reddening is a sign of inflammation. Inflammation is the body's natural defense mechanism to protect and speed healing to the tissues.

Inflammation from bacterial infestation: If there is pus or a pus pocket formed, massage is definitely contraindicated. Pus is a combination of dead white blood cells and bacteria. If it is disturbed, there is a chance of spreading infection. If the pus gets into the blood stream, there is a chance of a serious systemic infection.

Osteoporosis: This condition leads to deterioration of bone. In advanced stages bones become brittle, sometimes to the point that they are easily broken. Osteoporosis is prevalent in the elderly and in certain kinds of diseases. The symptoms of osteoporosis may include frailty and stooped shoulders. In women osteoporosis can be due to reduced estrogen levels. It is best to obtain the advice of the client's physician before giving massage when osteoporosis is indicated (Fig. 6.4).

Varicose veins: Varicose veins is a condition in which the valves in the veins break down because of back pressure in the circulatory

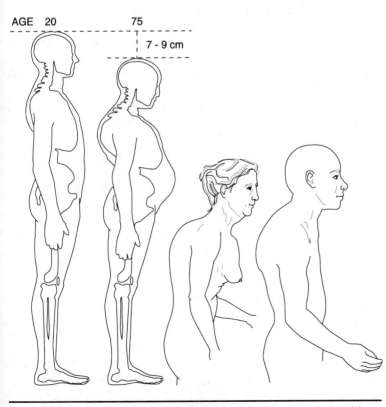

AGE   20   75

7 - 9 cm

Fig. 6.4 Symptoms of osteoporosis often include stooped shoulders.

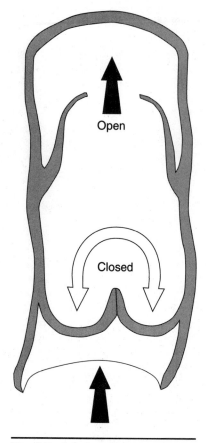

Fig. 6.5a A vein valve.

system. The veins bulge and rupture, usually in the legs. The development of varicose veins is often the result of gravity or obstructed venous flow, as the result of crossing the legs or other sitting postures that inhibit circulation to or from the legs. Varicose veins are often the result of standing for long hours. In women the pressure on the large veins in the pelvic area during pregnancy often contributes to this condition.

Blood is pumped through the veins by means of pressure originating in the heart and is helped along by contractions of muscle surrounding the veins. Veins are basically tubes consisting of a layer of endothelial lining and smooth muscle and are covered with connective tissue. Many veins, especially those in the arms and legs, have a system of valves that prevent blood from flowing backward in the vein and act as a **venous pump** to move the blood toward the heart. These valves are flap-like structures that protrude from the inside walls of the vein in such a way that blood moving toward the heart pushes past the valve, but if the blood attempts to move in the reverse direction, pressure against the valve forces it closed and blood cannot pass. The venous pump is a phenomenon that results when muscles contract and exert external pressure on the veins, which tends to collapse them. As the vein is repeatedly collapsed, the blood is forced along through the system of valves toward the heart (Fig. 6.5a).

Extensive back pressure in the veins due to prolonged standing or blockage causes the veins to enlarge and stretch to the point that the valves become incompetent. The weight of the blood further distends the veins and more valves become dysfunctional, perpetuating the condition. When veins become abnormally dilated due to excessive back pressure, they rupture and are called varicose veins. Blood then accumulates in enlarged portions of the vein. If the flow of blood becomes obstructed, clotting may occur. When this condition is accompanied by inflammation, it is painful and potentially dangerous. Increased pressure in the veins also increases pressure in the capillaries and often results in edema.

The practitioner will recognize varicose veins as bluish, protruding, thick, bulbous, distended superficial veins usually found in the lower legs. Also to be considered with caution are the small reddish groupings of broken blood vessels that often surround a small, protruding vein. Any deep massage on these areas may set a blood clot loose in the general circulation and cause a serious problem.

It is easy to see why massage would be contraindicated in cases of varicosities. However, massage proximal to the affected area might be very helpful, especially superficial (barely touching) techniques (Fig. 6.5b).

Phlebitis: Inflammation of a vein accompanied by pain and swelling is called **phlebitis** (fle-**BY**-tis). Phlebitis may be the result of surgery, or may be secondary to an infection or injury, or may have no apparent precursor. In many cases of phlebitis, a blood clot forms along the wall of the inflamed vein, causing the dangerous condition known as **thrombophlebitis.** If a piece of this clot loosens and floats in the blood, it is called an **embolus** (**EM**-bo-lus). If this embolus reaches the lungs, it can cause death by pulmonary embolism. If the embolus reaches the brain or the nourishing vessels of the heart, it can bring about stroke or myocardial infarction (heart attack).

Aneurosa: An aneurosa (an-yoo-**RO**-suh) or aneurysm (**AN**-yoo-rizm) is a localized dilation of a blood vessel or, more commonly, an artery. It can be caused by congenital defect, arteriosclerosis, hypertension, or trauma and is generally located in the aorta, thorax, and abdomen and sometimes in the cranium. Although this condition can appear, it is rarely encountered in the massage field, and if suspected, should be referred to medical attention.

Hematoma: A hematoma is a mass of blood trapped in some tissue or cavity of the body and is the result of internal bleeding. **Contusions** (kun-**TOO**-zhuns) or bruises are common types of hematomas that are generally not too serious. Contusions usually occur as a result of a blow that is severe enough to break a blood vessel. The escaping blood leaves the familiar black and blue spot. The blood quickly clots and, in a matter of time, the body naturally reabsorbs the cellular debris. The bruise changes color to greens and yellows and eventually disappears.

When the hematoma is in the acute phase, massage is contraindicated because of the risk of reinjuring the tissue. Once the bruise has changed colors, light massage will enhance circulation to the area and actually assist the healing.

A cranial hematoma is a serious condition that is usually the result of a blow to the head. A broken blood vessel inside the cranium forms a tumor-like mass that puts pressure on the brain. Depending on the location and severity of the hematoma, symptoms range from headache, confusion, and drowsiness to paralysis, loss of consciousness, and death. The only treatment for cranial hematoma is surgery to remove the pressure.

Edema: Edema (ed-**EE**-muh) is a circulatory abnormality that generally appears as puffiness in the extremities but is sometimes more widespread. Edema is an excess accumulation of fluid in tissue spaces; it has numerous causes. In some instances massage is indicated and in others, it is not. If edema is the result of back pressure in the veins due to immobility, massage and mild exercise may prove helpful. If, on the other hand, edema is the result of protein imbalance due to breakdown in the kidneys or liver, or is the result of increased permeability (allowing passage especially of fluids) of the capillaries due to inflammation, massage is contraindicated.

When edema is suspected, it can be easily detected by pressing a finger into the area. When the finger is removed and an indentation remains, edema is present. This indentation will take several seconds to return to the level of adjoining skin. This is called **pitting edema.**

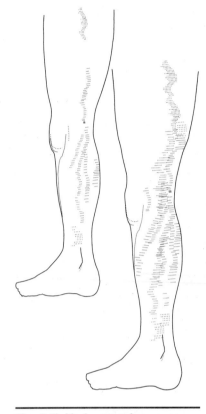

Fig. 6.5b Varicose veins appear as bluish, protruding, thick, bulbous, distended superficial veins usually found in the lower legs.

Edema can result from an imbalance of factors that regulate the interchange of fluids between the capillaries and tissue spaces. Other causes can be related to heart or kidney disease, poison in the system (affecting histamine levels that cause increased capillary permeability), or an obstruction of lymph channels. If edema is related to pregnancy and is caused by toxemia (poisons in the blood), massage is definitely contraindicated.

Obviously such conditions should be brought to the attention of a physician. It is essential that the reason for edema is known before massage is performed on the edemous tissue.

The practitioner should not try to reduce edema by direct massage on the area until channels leading out of the area have been flushed open. This means that if edema is in the feet, it is advisable to open channels in the abdomen, groin, and thigh before massaging the feet. Another consideration is to work on reflexes to increase lymph activity.

High blood pressure: High blood pressure refers to the pressure of the blood against the walls of the arteries. If the client has a history of high blood pressure, his or her physician should be consulted before treatment. The client may be taking medication to bring the condition under control. Unless it is severe, massage may be of assistance in relieving some of the hypertension that accompanies high blood pressure. Any massage that involves high blood pressure should be soothing and sedating. Low blood pressure is not a consideration in massage.

Cancer: Cancer is a disease that can be spread through the lymphatic system. Because massage affects the lymphatics, any massage that tends to increase lymph flow is contraindicated for cancer patients. However, there are exceptions where limited massage may be included in the daily regimen. For example, many physicians believe that an essential for those who are severely ill is caring, understanding, and human touch. A person who has been diagnosed as having cancer knows what to expect and knows which part of the body is affected. The practitioner can limit the massage to simple reflex and touch therapy to provide comfort to the client. The practitioner must remember that malignancies and cancers are contraindicated to circulatory types of massage.

Fatigue: In cases of chronic fatigue, the excretory system is already overburdened and there is little to nourish those overworked and exhausted tissues. When a client is suffering from chronic fatigue, massage should be extremely light and superficial to induce rest and relaxation. Over a period of time, massage helps to restore the client's energy.

Intoxication: Intoxication is a contraindication because it can spread toxins and overstress the liver.

Psychosis: Psychosis is another condition wherein it is advisable to work directly under the supervision of the patient's doctor.

Medication and drugs: There are times when a client will be taking specific medication or drugs and massage may or may not be recommended. If there is any question concerning the client's condition and possible harmful side effects a massage might cause, the client's physician should be consulted.

Skin problems: The following skin conditions are contraindications. Usually only the affected areas are of concern. For example, a minor laceration on the hand would not prevent massage of other healthy parts of the body. However, as has already been stated, when a condition is of a contagious nature, massage is not given.

Acne	Impetigo	Scratches
Boils	Inflammation	Skin cancer
Broken vessels	Lacerations	Skin tags
Bruises	Lumps	Sores
Burns and blisters	Moles	Stings and bites
Carbuncles	Pimples	Tumor
Eczema	Rashes	Warts
Hypersensitive skin	Scaly spots	Wounds

Hernia: Hernia is a protrusion of an organ or part of an organ, such as the intestine protruding through an opening in the abdominal wall surrounding it. This is also referred to as a rupture, and massage is not recommended over or near the afflicted area.

Frail elderly people: Frail elderly people may have fragile bones and very sensitive skin. However, gentle massage may be beneficial.

Scoliosis: When a client has scoliosis (sko-lee-O-sis), or crooked spine, massage must be recommended by the client's physician. Caution must be exercised (Fig. 6.6).

Specific conditions or diseases: It should be obvious to the practitioner that a client who is suffering from severe asthma (a chronic respiratory disorder), diabetes (deficient insulin secretion), or any type or heart or lung disease should be under the supervision of a physician. Massage would not be given without the physician's knowledge and advice. This is why it is important to take time during the first consultation (interview) to determine the client's state of health.

When making decisions whether to perform massage on a person who has a medical condition, be conservative. When in doubt, don't! Remember the first and foremost rule: "Do no harm!"

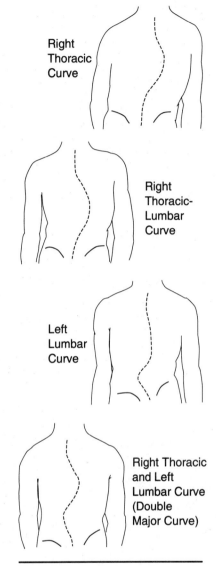

Right Thoracic Curve

Right Thoracic-Lumbar Curve

Left Lumbar Curve

Right Thoracic and Left Lumbar Curve (Double Major Curve)

Fig. 6.6 Scoliosis is an abnormal lateral curve of the spine.

MASSAGE DURING PREGNANCY

During a normal, healthy pregnancy, massage may be very beneficial in promoting relaxation, soothing nerves, and relieving strained back and leg muscles. Massage also tends to instill a feeling of well-being to both mother and unborn child. However, certain situations and conditions exist of which the practitioner must be aware.

Massage should always be soothing and relaxing. No heavy percussion or deep tissue massage should ever be done. Likewise, abdominal kneading or other deep abdominal massage should be avoided. Care should be taken to position the mother in such a way as to assure the comfort of both mother and unborn child.

When the client is supine (face up), pillows are used under the knees and head. In this position the weight of the fetus may press on the aorta in such a way to constrict the flow of blood to the lower body and the fetus. A half-sitting, or semireclining position might be preferred (Fig. 6.7a).

When the client is on her side, pillows are placed under her head and upper knee or between her legs (Fig. 6.7b).

During the second and third trimesters, lying prone (face down) places pressure on the abdominal area. This position is not only very uncomfortable, but it may be dangerous to the unborn child.

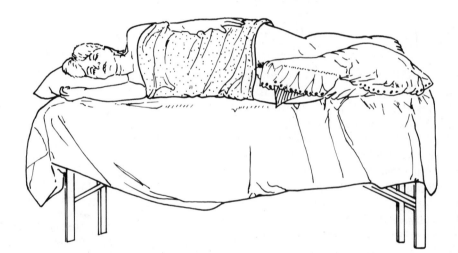

Fig. 6.7a In the supine, the pregnant client should be supported in a semireclining position to prevent pressure from the fetus on the major abdominal blood vessels.

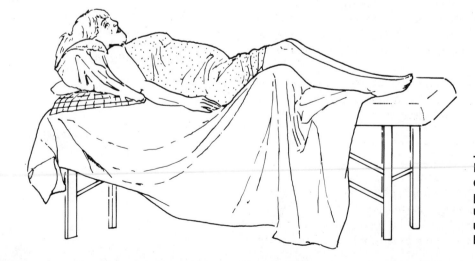

Fig. 6.7b When the client is on her side, pillows are placed under her head and upper knee or between her legs.

A prone position is not advisable unless proper and adequate support is provided. Special bolsters and massage tables are available that provide full and safe support so that even full-term soon-to-be mothers can lie face down and receive soothing massage to their back. If there is any question as to the state of health of either the mother or unborn child, the client's doctor must be consulted before massage is given.

MASSAGE FOR THE CRITICALLY ILL ▼

Massage is becoming a common part of preferred treatment with the critically ill. Many times conditions are present that are normally contraindicated for massage, however by making adjustments to the intent and delivery of the massage session, there is literally no contraindication for touch therapy. Depending on an individual's condition there are precautions and concerns as to how a massage will proceed.

Purpose

- The intent of massage for the critically ill is gentle and genuine caring touch therapy to bring comfort, pleasure, and relaxation to an individual at a difficult time of their life.

Benefits

- Helps control discomfort and pain
- Improves mobility
- Helps reduce disorientation and confusion by bringing person back to a more positive body awareness
- Reduces isolation and fear
- Helps to ease the emotional and physical discomforts of the individual
- Allows the individual to develop a more positive attitude about his or her situation or condition.

Considerations and Precautions

It is important for the practitioner to be conscious and aware of the individual's needs. Conditions dictate how much is done and what precautions are used. When in doubt about how or whether to proceed because of a person's condition, be sure to ask. Ask the client first. Generally they are very aware of any precautions concerning their condition. It is also important to communicate with their physician or the care giver in charge.

A critically ill person's physical and emotional condition is constantly changing. Continually assess the client visually, verbally and tactually and adjust the massage accordingly. The practitioner must be open to the needs of the individual at the moment.

Techniques

Many of the common massage techniques are designed for the relatively healthy person. When working with the critically ill, it is essential to be aware of each individual's needs and tolerances. Many massage techniques are made to stimulate circulation and stir up wastes and toxins. These may not be appropriate when massaging an individual with a critical illness. With the critically ill, the body may be having a hard time eliminating and not tolerate any more wastes being pushed into the system.

Techniques should soothe and add comfort. Touch, slow gentle stroking, and energy work are the most common choices for massaging the critically ill. Depending on the tolerance of the client, the length of a session may be abbreviated. Rather than a full massage that lasts an hour or more, the situation might call for a back and shoulders or just the feet that may last only fifteen minutes. This is a time to underdo rather than overdo. It is a time to be supportive and calming. The touch session may only involve holding the client's hand and being there for them.

Any and all contact that is made is an integral part of the session. Your mere presence is as important as the manipulations you use. Your actions, voice, breathing, and movements should all reflect the caring, nurturing and compassion of the session. In the words of Irene Smith of Service Through Touch:

> "We give massage primarily for relaxation and pleasure. The patient may be under a high level of stress due to fear, pain, and anxiety on the physical, emotional and spiritual levels. Slow, gentle, loving touch is used in order to offer the patient a time of peace and quiet. Peace and quiet and gentleness are three very valuable healing qualities."

▼ PRECAUTIONS FOR WORKING WITH HIV INFECTED INDIVIDUALS

The Human Immunodeficiency Virus (HIV) is the causative agent for Acquired Immune Deficiency Syndrome (AIDS).

Stages of HIV Infection

There is a continuum of stages of HIV infection. After being infected with the virus, there may be absolutely no symptoms for a long period of time. This period may be a matter of months or several years. When the immune system begins to weaken, mild symptoms appear. As the immune system continues to weaken symptoms become more severe. Symptoms continue to become more severe as the body loses its ability to fight off infections. When an HIV infected person has a T-cell count of 200 or less and/or is diagnosed with an **opportunistic infection** they have AIDS.

Opportunistic infections are caused by organisms that are commonly found in the environment and that many of us already have in our body. Normally our immune system protects us against these bacteria, protozoa, fungi and viruses. With the immune system weakened by HIV, the uncontrolled organisms become deadly. Common opportunistic infections associated with AIDS include:

- **Pneumocystis carinii pneumonia (PCP).** PCP is caused by a protozoan commonly found in our lungs. When the immune system is weakened as in AIDS, the organism multiplies and causes the disease. PCP is the most common opportunistic disease of persons with AIDS. Unless you have an immune deficiency there is no concern about catching PCP.
- **Cryptococcal meningitis.** Cryptococcal meningitis is caused by the fungus Cryptococcus neoformans. This fungus is found in the environment and grows in pigeon droppings. Dust containing the fungus is inhaled and it spreads to the meninges of the central nervous system creating the symptoms of the disease.
- **Toxoplasmosis.** Toxoplasmosis comes from a protozoan that is usually acquired through eating raw or undercooked meat. If the immune system is weak, the infection may spread to the heart, lungs, or brain. In AIDS patients, the infection often affects the brain resulting in lesions and neurological complications.
- **Candida.** The fungus Candida allicans is normally found in the intestines, mouth, and vagina. When a person's resistance is reduced due to illness, immunosuppressive drugs or broad spectrum antibiotics, Candida infections can occur. In people with AIDS Candida infection may appear in the mouth, where it is called thrush, or it may appear as a rash on the skin. Do not touch a Candida rash as it may be very sensitive and can spread from one part of the body to another.
- **Herpes.** There are three forms of the Herpes virus, all of which are very contagious.

  Herpes simplex I causes fever blisters and cold sores on the face and mouth.

  Herpes simplex II causes painful sores around the genitals and anus and is sexually transmitted.

  Herpes varicells-zoster is also called shingles and causes painful blisters that tend to follow specific nerve pathways.
- **Kaposi's Sarcoma (KS).** KS is a form of cancer of the cells that line certain blood vessels. KS produces lesions that may appear on the skin. The lesions may be bluish to reddish purple and may be smooth or raised. They may be closed in which case massaging over them is acceptable, or they may bo open in which case the same precautions as with blood products must be observed.
- **Other rashes.** The person with AIDS may have any number of rashes caused by fungi or reactions to medications. Most rashes are contraindicated to massage. Simply avoid the area where there is a rash and proceed to another area of the body.

Transmission of HIV

The virus that causes AIDS is transmitted from person to person only through the exchange of body fluid that contains the virus. The transmission of HIV requires three simultaneous conditions.

1. The virus requires a proper environment to survive. The virus is found in blood, semen, vaginal fluids and mother's milk in high enough concentrations to be virulent. HIV has also been found in sweat, tears and rarely in saliva.
2. The substance containing the virus must have a sufficiently large concentration of the virus in order to cause an HIV infection. There is no known case of HIV infection caused by contact with sweat, tears or saliva.
3. The virus must have a port of entry, that is there must be a way for the virus to enter the body. Some ways this may occur are: unprotected sexual activity, sharing needles used for injecting drugs or applying tattoos, receiving transfusions with infected blood, an infected mother to her unborn child or through nursing.

Precautions Against Infection

Understanding the stages of HIV infection and the factors necessary for transmission of HIV will help to guide the practitioner when determining what precautions to take.

Always be aware of standard infection precautions when working with any client. These precautions are designed to prevent blood or any other body secretions from entering the body through any opening of the body such as open sores or cuts.

The primary infection precaution is thorough hand washing. Thorough hand washing is accomplished by scrubbing the hands vigorously with a germicidal soap before and after each massage session. When deemed necessary, the hands may be washed during the session. The hands are washed before the session to protect the client who may be susceptible to infection. Thorough hand washing after the session protects the therapist and anyone the therapist comes in contact with after the session.

The Use of Gloves

The use of gloves is a secondary infection precaution and never replaces the need for thorough hand washing. Either vinyl or latex gloves may be used. When massaging with oil, latex gloves may break down or tear. Double gloving may be used when added protection is a concern. In situations where the client is susceptible to infection, sterile latex gloves may be used.

When a practitioner should use gloves:

• When handling blood, feces or any other body fluids or secretions or linens soiled with them.

- When the practitioner has an open sore, cut or broken cuticles on his or her hands.
- Whenever you as a practitioner do not feel comfortable without them. (Always explain to your client why you are wearing gloves and get their agreement before proceeding.)
- When the client request you wear gloves.

Caring for Equipment

Tables and other surfaces that have been contaminated with blood can be cleaned and sanitized with a solution of one part chlorine bleach to ten parts water. Alcohol can be used to disinfect surfaces contaminated by other body fluids and secretions.

Linens can be disinfected by washing them in hot water with detergent and a quarter cup of bleach and drying them in a hot dryer.

Following these general infection precautions does minimize the risk to you and your clientele however it does not eliminate the fact that some risk is involved. If any questions or concerns arise as a result of working with a person who has an HIV infection or any other infectious disease, contact your local infection control center. There is an infection control center located at your local hospital or medical center.

(For more information about Massage for HIV infected persons or Massage for the critically ill, contact Service Through Touch, 41 Carl St., San Francisco, CA 94117.)

ENDANGERMENT SITES ▼

Certain areas of the body warrant consideration when being massaged because of the underlying anatomical structures. Because of the possibility of injury to the structures by certain massage manipulations these areas are sites of potential endangerment. In most of these areas major nerves, blood vessels or vital organs are relatively exposed and vulnerable to deep manipulations or direct pressure. Following is a table of the endangerment sites, their location and the anatomical structures of concern.

TABLE 6.1 ENDANGERMENT SITES ▼

ENDANGERMENT SITES	LOCATION	STRUCTURES OF CONCERN
Inferior to the ear	Notch posterior to the ramus of the mandible	Facial nerve, external carotid artery, styloid process
Anterior triangle of the neck	Bordered by the mandible, sternocleidomastoid muscle and the trachea	Carotid artery, internal jugular vein, vagus nerve, lymph nodes.
Posterior triangle of the neck	Bordered by the sternocleidomastoid muscle, the trapezius muscle and the clavicle	Brachial plexus, subclavian artery, brachiocephelic vein, external jugular vein and lymph nodes.

(continued on next page)

▼ TABLE 6.1 ENDANGERMENT SITES (continued)

ENDANGERMENT SITES	LOCATION	STRUCTURES OF CONCERN
Axilla	Armpit	Axillary, median, musculocutaneous and ulnar nerves, axillary artery, axillary nerve and lymph nerves.
Medial Brachium	Upper inner arm between the biceps and triceps	Ulnar, musculocutaneous and median nerves, brachial artery, basilic vein and lymph nodes.
Cubital area of the elbow	Anterior bend of the elbow	Median nerve, radial and ulnar arteries, median cubital vein.
Ulnar notch of the elbow	The funny bone	Ulnar nerve
Femoral triangle	Bordered by the sartorius muscle, the adductor longus muscle and the inguinal ligament	Femoral nerve, femoral artery, femoral vein, great saphenous vein and lymph nodes.
Popliteal fossa	Posterior aspect of the knee	Bordered by the gastrocnemius (inferior) and the hamstrings (superior and to the sides). Tibial nerve, common peroneal nerve, popliteal artery, popliteal vein.
Abdomen	Upper area of the abdomen under the ribs.	Right side, liver and gall bladder: Left side, spleen; Deep center, aorta
Upper lumbar area	Just inferior to the ribs and lateral to the spine	Kidneys (avoid heavy percussion.)

▼ QUESTIONS FOR DISCUSSION AND REVIEW

1. What are the main physiological benefits of massage?
2. What are the main psychological benefits of massage?
3. What are the two physical ways massage affects the body?
4. Which body systems are said to benefit from regular therapeutic massage?
5. In what way does the muscular system benefit from massage?
6. What massage movements promote circulation in muscles?
7. How does massage relieve sore and stiff muscles?
8. What massage technique prevents the formation of adhesions and fibrosis in muscles?
9. What are the immediate effects of massage on the skin?
10. How does massage affect the nervous system?

11. What massage movements have a stimulating effect on the nervous system?
12. What massage techniques have a sedative effect on the nervous system?
13. What is the effect of massage on the circulatory system?
14. Why are all massage movements directed toward the heart?
15. Which massage movements increase the flow of blood and lymph?
16. In what way does improved circulation of the blood benefit the skin?
17. When should massage be avoided?
18. What is the meaning of contraindication as it relates to massage?
19. Why does the practitioner need to take the client's medical history?
20. Why should the therapist keep a fever thermometer on the premises?
21. What should the practitioner do when a client has a condition that appears to be a contraindication to massage?
22. What are the signs of inflammation?
23. How should massage be applied in the case of local inflammation?
24. How do you recognize varicose veins?
25. What is a hematoma and how is it massaged?
26. How does massage benefit a woman during a normal, healthy pregnancy?
27. How does massage benefit an individual who is critically ill?
28. How is the HIV/AIDS virus transmitted from person to person?
29. Why are certain areas of the body sites of potential endangerment?

Equipment and Products

Learning Objectives

After you have mastered this chapter, you will be able to:

1. *Prepare a checklist of supplies and equipment needed for therapeutic massage.*
2. *Describe various products and their use.*
3. *Select a massage table.*
4. *Check and adjust lighting for the massage room.*
5. *Check all equipment for safety and readiness.*

INTRODUCTION ▼

The practice of therapeutic massage is a part of the healthcare profession. It is important that a practitioner present himself or herself in a professional manner at all times. Professionalism is an attitude that is manifested in yourself and your business. Your clients will expect you to project a professional image by your speech, your appearance, your courtesy, and your good manners. Technical competence and the ability to express yourself are also professional ingredients. A massage practitioner should project an image of confidence and yet be relaxed. As a practitioner, your clothing must be appropriate for your work: neat, clean, and well fitted. You must be free of body and breath odors and have well-cared-for hands and nails.

The facilities in which you work should reflect a professional appearance yet at the same time be comfortable and relaxing.

YOUR PLACE OF BUSINESS ▼

The location of your massage business is an important consideration and will be discussed extensively in Chapter 19. The image of your place of business makes an impression on your massage clients and therefore must be considered when establishing a business.

A national survey of massage practitioners conducted by Knapp and Associates in 1990 indicates that approximately one third of massage therapists operate a private practice out of their home, one third from a private office or clinic, and the remaining third practice in another facility such as a health club, resort, health professional's office or salon, etc. Regardless of the location of the business, the internal environment of the facility reflects directly on the impression the client will have of the therapist and of the services the therapist offers.

Clients coming into your place of business will be influenced by the environment and the people with whom they come in contact. The decor should be professional yet comfortable, clean yet not sterile, relaxed and free of distractions and safety hazards. In a massage establishment, space should be allotted for the exclusive practice of massage. While this is necessary for a client's privacy and comfort, it also gives a more professional image. Some practitioners go to their clients' homes in addition to or rather than maintaining a studio and office space. The equipment used as well as the appearance and actions of the therapist when doing "outcalls" directly reflect on the perception of the client. Whether the massage facility is in the practitioner's home, the client's home, or a separate office, standards of cleanliness, safety, and professionalism must be observed.

Sanitation and Safety in Your Workplace

Whether working in a small salon or studio with little space or a large, luxurious spa, the space and equipment must be kept clean and neat. The massage facility and the equipment should be checked regularly to eliminate situations that may cause injury to the therapist or client. Passageways must be kept clear. Surfaces and linens must be sanitized and equipment checked against failure. The main concern is the protection of the client's health and comfort.

Equipment and Supplies

Equipment and supplies should be checked frequently to be sure they are in proper condition and that enough are on hand.

Each booth or room should have the appropriate furnishings and equipment for the treatments to be given. All equipment should be checked regularly for fitness and safety. All supplies must be kept in a clean, sanitized condition. Supplies such as oils, linens, and paper products should be selected and ready before the client enters the booth or room.

The following is a checklist of equipment and supplies generally needed. Add your own suggestions to this list.

MASSAGE ROOM EQUIPMENT

Supply and linen cabinets	Desk or table
Chair	Changing room equipment
Massage table	Hangers (clothing)
Stool	Chair or bench
Bolsters and pillows	Wraps or robes
Bolster and pillow covers	Small table
Sheets	Clock
Blankets	Covered waste basket
Indirect lighting	

THERAPY EQUIPMENT

Anatomical charts	Moist hot packs
Standard weight chart	Cold packs
Standard height chart	Electrical apparatus
Bathroom scales	Watch with second hand
Massage table	Cotton for facial cleansing
Heat lamp	Facial tissues
Massage vibrator	Cotton-tipped swabs
Shower room	Sterilizing agents
Shampoo slab	Table salt for salt glows
Bath cabinet	Record cards
Foot basin	Alcohol or other sterilizing agents
Bath tub	Analgesic oil for sore, stiff muscles

SUPPLY CABINET

Towels
Sheets
Pillows and cases
Bolsters and covers
Blankets or coverlets
Fever thermometer
Sphygmomanometer
Talcum powder
Massage creams, oils

EXERCISE EQUIPMENT

Weight lifts
Stationary bicycle
Stretching bars

 THE MASSAGE ROOM

Studio Space

A massage room needs to be approximately 10 feet wide and 12 feet long. This allows enough space for all needed equipment as well as enough room to move around the massage table. It also allows space for a desk, chair, and supply table or cabinet. A stool is also a handy item to have in the massage room, because there are times when the practitioner can sit down while working on the client's neck, face, feet, or hands. Sitting for a few minutes can give much needed rest when working long hours (Fig. 7.1).

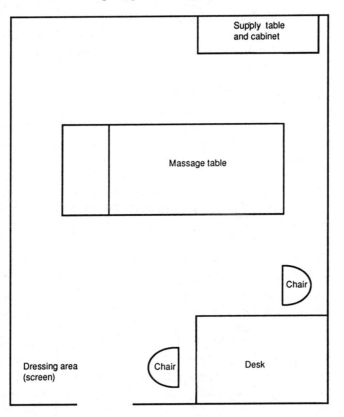

Fig. 7.1 The minimum size for a massage room is about 10 by 12 feet. This allows room for a table, desk, chairs, supply cabinet, and room to move around the table to perform the massage.

Temperature of the Massage Room

The temperature of the massage room should be comfortable. The room should be warm enough that the client does not chill. If the client becomes chilled, it is very hard for him or her to relax. About 75° Fahrenheit is warm enough for most clients and at the same time is cool enough to keep the practitioner from getting uncomfortably warm while working. The room should be warmed in advance because it is easy for the client to become chilled, especially after oil has been applied to the skin. In a room that is cooler, auxiliary blankets, electric mattress pads, or other heating devices must be used to ensure the client's warmth.

The massage room must be well ventilated. Performing a massage requires considerable exertion on the part of the practitioner. For proper relaxation, the client needs a good supply of fresh air. With poor ventilation, the room would become stuffy and the air may acquire an offensive odor. Proper ventilation assures an abundant supply of fresh air.

Lighting

It is difficult for either the practitioner or the client to be comfortable when the lighting in the room is harsh and glaring. In addition, colored lights such as red or blue can make the client feel uncomfortable. Reflective or soft, natural light is preferred. Dimmer switches enable you to change the light easily. Avoid direct overhead lighting or any light that could shine directly into the client's eyes (Fig. 7.2).

Use of Music

A stereo and supply of soothing taped music may provide another dimension to a relaxing massage. While you may like music playing while you work, you must remember that some people find it distracting and prefer absolute quiet. You may wish to have a selection of soothing music available and ask the client what he or she prefers. If there is outside noise that may be distracting, music will mask it. Obviously, you should not attempt to match the rhythm of massage movements to the tempo of the music.

The Massage Table

Your massage table is your main piece of equipment and, next to your hands, the most important regarding your comfort and that of your clients. One of your concerns should be that the table is stable, firm, and comfortable. If you will be working in an office or studio, a nonportable table may be your best choice. If your situation is temporary, or if you prefer the freedom of taking your equipment with you, choose a good portable table. If you travel to do massage,

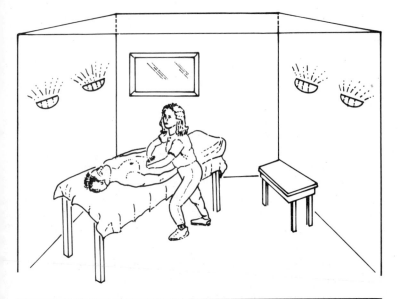

Fig. 7.2 Avoid direct overhead lighting in the massage room. Soft natural light from a shaded window or indirect light from wall or table lamps is preferred.

the table must be portable and light enough for you to carry. Regardless of your choice, check the construction carefully. The table should not shake, rock, or squeak. Seldom will new equipment display these problems, but you must consider what will happen after the table has been used for several hundred treatments.

A massage table allows you to move about or to change positions easily and when necessary, without breaking the rhythm of the massage movements.

The table must be the right height to give you the leverage needed and to prevent fatigue of your back, neck, arms, and shoulders. The height of the table is determined by your height so that you are not at a disadvantage when reaching and applying pressure. A good indicator for the proper height of a massage table is to stand in an erect yet relaxed manner and measure the distance from the floor to the styloid process on the ulnar (little finger) side of your forearm. This is approximately the optimum height for the table. Another way to test the height of a table is to place the palm of your hand flat on the table. While doing this, you should be able to hold your arm straight at your side.

Several studio and portable models have legs that can be adjusted up or down by removing and replacing wing nuts or thumb screws. These are advantageous if people of different heights use the same table, or if various techniques used require different table heights. Some studio tables have a height adjustment button and are operated by hydraulic force or electricity. Though costly, this type of table is very useful when dealing with the elderly or disabled, who might have difficulty getting on a table of normal height, or when several different practitioners use the same table.

The width of a massage table is approximately 28 inches with an additional inch allowed for padding, or approximately 29 inches wide. Tables narrower than 27 inches do not give enough arm support for large clients. Tables wider than 30 inches become awkward when the practitioner is required to reach to the opposite side of the client.

A good length for a massage table is about 76 inches. Most tables are about 68 to 72 inches long, which may be too short for tall clients. The padding on the massage table should be firm so that pressure applied by the practitioner to the client is absorbed by the client's body and not pushed into the table. About $1\frac{1}{2}$ to 2 inches of high-density foam is the best material to use. Padding should extend beyond the edge of the framework of the table by about half an inch all around to ensure the comfort of the client, who might place a hand or foot over the edge. A good quality vinyl is the best covering for the massage table because it is durable and easy to keep clean. Vinyl does not deteriorate when it comes in contact with oil and can be cleaned with a mild disinfectant after use.

Tables come in a variety of designs. Often the bed of a massage treatment table will fold up or down in a variety of configurations. This is to accommodate specific therapy situations and may be of no use to the general massage practitioner. An exception is the head piece that adjusts up or down to alleviate cervical strain. Accommodations for the face may be in the form of a hole in the end of the table or a padded extension to the end of the table. These additions allow the client to lie face down with the cervical spine straight, taking the strain off the neck and upper back.

Some massage tables include a number of accessories, like a face cradle. The face cradle is a valuable addition for the comfort of the client. Many tables have face cradles that adjust to a number of positions to ensure comfort. Some tables include side extensions to support the arms of larger clients.

The table is the massage therapist's main piece of equipment. A professionally designed massage table is recommended. Always buy equipment from a reputable company that stands behind its products. Be sure the items you purchase are guaranteed to hold up with reasonable use (Fig. 7.3).

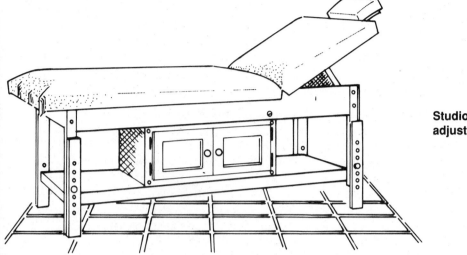

Studio table with adjustable head piece.

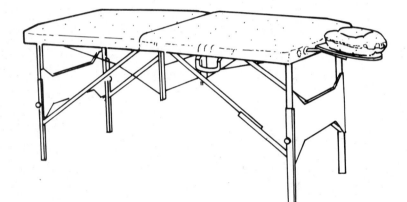

Portable table with detachable face rest.

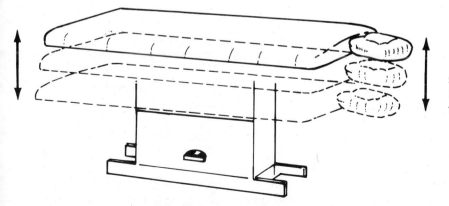

Studio model that hydraulically adjusts the height.

Fig. 7.3 Massage tables come in a variety of styles.

▼ SELECTING PRODUCTS

There is such a wide range of products on the market that it may be difficult to choose the powders, oils, creams, or lotions you will want to stock. Quality is important.

Oils and Powders

A good quality oil is the practitioner's most important product. Mineral oils are not recommended for massage because they are a petroleum-based product and tend to dry the skin and clog the pores. A combination of such oils as coconut, sweet almond, apricot, olive, peanut, sesame, grape seed, or sunflower oils are mild and easy to work with. A pleasant combination is coconut and almond oils. It is important to use fresh oil because rancid oil has a strong offensive odor. If oil gets on sheets and sets for a while, it will saturate the fibers and develop an offensive odor.

Oils, creams, and lotions have different qualities. Some glide better than others, while some absorb faster or become sticky. As a therapist, experiment with different products until you find the ones that you and your clients prefer. Once you have found your preference, it is more economical to buy in larger quantities. If you buy oil in bulk, some should be transferred to smaller bottles. These bottles should be kept filled to the top because it is the air space in the bottle that causes the oil to become rancid. When oil does not have a pleasant smell but is not rancid, a few drops of oil of lemon, clove, cinnamon, musk, or some other essential oil may be added. Usually a few drops of concentrate to a cup of oil will be enough to give a hint of scent. Oils and concentrated fragrances can be purchased from supply houses or are usually available at drug stores. Some practitioners like to mix their oils and then place them in attractive, easy-to-handle bottles with dispenser tops. This prevents spillage (Fig. 7.4).

Some clients may have very oily skin or may not tolerate oil. For these clients, talcum powder may be preferred. While talcum powder does not provide the lubrication you get with oil, the same massage movements can be done effectively with powder, and some clients prefer powder. You must avoid inhaling talc when using it for massage.

If you offer face massage, you will need cleansers for different skin types, toners or freshening lotions (astringent), moisturizers, and products suitable for any special face treatment you provide.

There are excellent creams and lotions on the markets. Always read the label to be sure you know the product's ingredients and that it is safe to use for massage. It is a good idea to have on hand a dictionary of cosmetic ingredients so you can look up unfamiliar words. When possible, consult a pharmacist or dermatologist. The FDA (federal Food and Drug Administration) endeavors to control

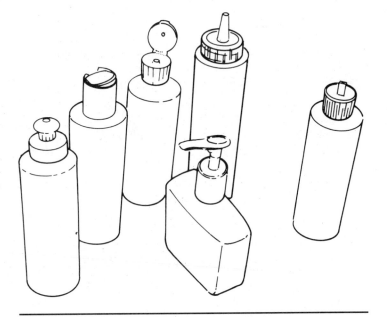

Fig. 7.4 Oil bottles with a variety of dispenser tops.

the distribution of products that contain harmful substances. How-ever, what may be harmless to the majority of people may cause an allergic reaction in someone with a sensitivity to a particular substance. During the consultation or before applying a substance to the face or body, it is best to determine if the client is allergic to any substance. When in doubt, give a patch test before proceeding with the application.

To give a patch test, first wash the area of the inner bend of the elbow with mild soap and warm water. Rinse the area, and then apply a small amount of the product to the skin. Allow fifteen to thirty minutes to see if there is a reaction, such as signs of itching, inflammation, and sensitivity, or a stinging sensation. If so, do not use the product. If there are no signs of inflammation or the afore-mentioned sensations, the product is considered mild enough to use.

Some people with allergies to fragrances and other cosmetic substances may need to have a patch test given twenty-four hours before a treatment. In such cases, the client will usually be under the care of a physician, who can give guidance on which products to use and which to avoid. Clients who are sensitive to some products may prefer to supply their own lubricants.

Most nonprescription products are considered safe for the gen-eral public. Most practitioners keep a variety of lubricants on hand to better serve the needs and wishes of their clients. Alcohol is kept available for sanitation purposes. It is also used to remove excess oil from the client's skin following massage, before he or she dresses.

QUESTIONS FOR DISCUSSION AND REVIEW

1. What kind of an image should a massage practitioner project to his or her clientele?
2. What are some important considerations when preparing a space to do massage?
3. Approximately how much space is optimal for a massage space?
4. Why should equipment and supplies be inspected periodically?
5. Why is it important to prepare a checklist of supplies and equipment?
6. What kinds of products are usually used for body massage?
7. What is the approximate temperature for the massage room?
8. Why is it important to be able to adjust the height of the massage table?
9. What type of lighting is preferred in the massage room?
10. Why should the client be asked if he or she would like background music?

Sanitary and Safety Practices

Learning Objectives

After you have mastered this chapter, you will be able to:

1. *Explain the need for laws that enforce the strict practice of sanitation.*

2. *Sanitize and sterilize implements and other items used in massage procedures.*

3. *Explain the difference between pathogenic and nonpathogenic bacteria.*

4. *Explain the importance of cleanliness of person and of surroundings as protection against the spread of disease.*

5. *Explain how various disinfectants, antiseptics, and other products are used most effectively.*

6. *Explain the role of safety in the massage therapy business.*

▼ INTRODUCTION

In recent years great progress has been made in the control and prevention of disease. In the medical profession sanitation and sterilization are required procedures that are taken for granted. Every state has laws that make the practice of sanitation and sterilization mandatory for the protection of public health. In the personal service professions, every precaution must be taken to protect the health of clients as well as the health of practitioners. The nature of the personal service business determines the procedures for the extent of sanitation and sterilization. For example, in the cosmetology profession, a comb or brush used on one client may not be used on another until it has been thoroughly cleansed and sterilized. The esthetician (skincare specialist) must apply products only with sterilized applicators. The massage practitioner may not use the same kinds of implements or have need for the same sanitation procedures; however, appropriate and recommended procedures must be followed diligently.

The massage practitioner need not be a biologist to have some understanding of bacteriology and to be aware of the importance of impeccable cleanliness at all times. Contagious diseases, skin infections, and other problems can be caused by the transfer of infectious material by unclean hands and nails and by unsanitary equipment and supplies. Therefore, the primary concern is that any item (for example, linens, apparatus) that comes in contact with the client is clean and sanitary. The practitioner's hands must be sanitized by washing with soap (preferably an anti-bacterial soap) and warm water before touching each client. The premises must also be clean at all times.

▼ PATHS OF DISEASE AND INFECTION

Bacteria are minute, unicellular microorganisms exhibiting both plant and animal characteristics. They are also called **germs** or **microbes** and are most numerous in dirt, refuse, unclean water, and diseased tissues. Bacteria exist on the skin, in the air, in body secretions, underneath the free edges of the nails, and elsewhere. There are hundreds of different kinds of bacteria that can only be seen under a microscope. Bacteria are classified as either **nonpathogenic** (harmless) or **pathogenic** (harmful). Nonpathogenic bacteria, the beneficial and harmless type, are the most numerous and perform useful functions, such as aiding the digestive process and other bodily functions. The saprophytes (**SAP**-ro-fights) are an example of nonpathogenic bacteria (Fig. 8.1).

Pathogenic bacteria, though not as numerous, are of greater concern to us because they produce disease. Parasites belong to this group because they require living matter for their growth and reproduction. We are primarily concerned with understanding

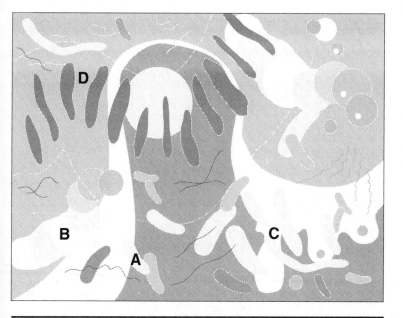

Fig. 8.1 A variety of nonpathogenic bacteria thrive in the large intestine: (A) bacteroides, (B) peptostreptococcus, (C) lactobacillus, (D) eubacterium.

and identifying pathogenic bacteria in order to deal with them more effectively. Figure 8.5 shows the three general forms of bacteria: **cocci** (**KOCK**-sigh), **bacilli** (ba-**SIL**-eye), and **spirilla** (spy-**RIL**-uh). To the right of the name and shape of the bacteria are listed the types of bacteria and the common diseases or conditions with which they are associated (Figs. 8.2 to 8.5).

Pathogenic bacteria become a menace to health when they are able to invade the body. Immunity is the body's natural ability to resist infection by harmful bacteria once they have entered the body. Healthy people are able to resist infection better than those with low resistance. Healthy skin is one of the body's most important defenses against invasion of harmful bacteria. Fine hairs in the nostrils, mucous membranes, and tears in the eyes also help to defend against bacteria. Inflammation (redness and swelling) is a sign that white blood cells, or corpuscles (**KOOR**-puhs-ls), are working to destroy harmful microorganisms that have invaded the body. The body also produces antibodies, which inhibit or destroy harmful bacteria. **Antibodies** are a class of proteins produced in the body in response to contact with antigens (toxin, enzymes, etc.) that serve to immunize the body against specific antigens.

A **virus** is defined as any of a class of submicroscopic pathogenic agents that are capable of transmitting disease. Viruses are parasitic in that they thrive only within the cells of a living host (plant, animal, or human). They invade living cells and control their activity to produce more viruses often along with toxic substances.

Cocci

Bacilli

Spirilla

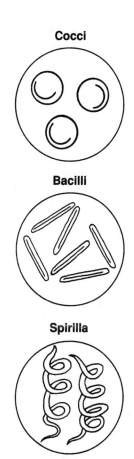

Fig. 8.2 Three general forms of bacteria.

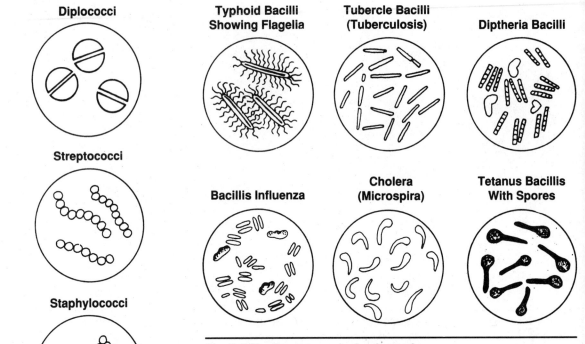

Diplococci

Streptococci

Staphylococci

Fig. 8.3 Groupings of bacteria.

Typhoid Bacilli Showing Flagelia

Tubercle Bacilli (Tuberculosis)

Diptheria Bacilli

Bacillis Influenza

Cholera (Microspira)

Tetanus Bacillis With Spores

Fig. 8.4 Six disease-producing bacteria.

The cell dies and releases the viruses to invade other cells. A virus may act as an antigen and cause the system to produce antibodies. The virus often has the ability to change its characteristics quickly, which makes viral infections hard to treat by chemical means. Viruses are the cause of many diseases such as the common cold, small pox, some forms of pneumonia, and childhood diseases like mumps and measles. A virus is also the causative agent for AIDS (Fig. 8.6).

The massage practitioner must take special precaution with a client who has a contagious disease or infection and suggest that the client see a physician. The practitioner also has a duty to protect his or her own health. For example, the practitioner's hands may pick up bacteria from the client's skin. If the hands are not cleaned, bacteria can be spread.

The best protection against the spread of disease is to keep yourself and your surroundings clean and sanitary. Maintaining high standards of cleanliness requires constant supervision. Board of health regulations should be observed in maintaining clean massage facilities at all times.

▼ MAINTAINING SANITARY CONDITIONS

The primary precaution in infection control is thorough hand washing. Thorough hand washing is accomplished by vigorously

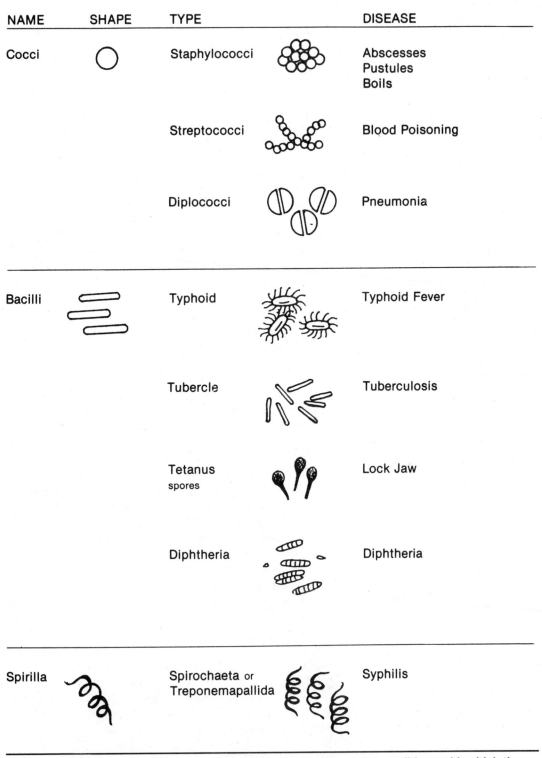

NAME	SHAPE	TYPE		DISEASE
Cocci	○	Staphylococci		Abscesses Pustules Boils
		Streptococci		Blood Poisoning
		Diplococci		Pneumonia
Bacilli		Typhoid		Typhoid Fever
		Tubercle		Tuberculosis
		Tetanus spores		Lock Jaw
		Diphtheria		Diphtheria
Spirilla		Spirochaeta or Treponemapallida		Syphilis

Fig. 8.5 Pathogenic (harmful) bacteria and the common diseases or conditions with which they are associated.

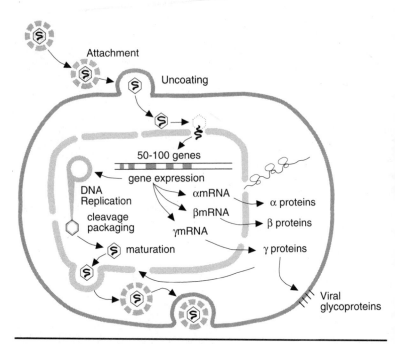

Fig. 8.6 Schematic of virus replication.

scrubbing the hands, preferably with an antibacterial soap and warm water. The hands are first moistened. The soap is applied and worked into a good lather. Special care is given to scrub between the fingers, between the finger and thumb, around the nails, and if appropriate up the arms. The hands are then rinsed thoroughly and dried with a clean towel.

The practitioner's hands should be washed before and after each session. Washing the hands before the massage protects the client. Thorough hand washing after the massage protects the practitioner and anyone the practitioner may come into contact with later.

It is important to keep the massage studio or work area, dispensary, implements, and equipment in a sanitary condition. Supplies such as towels, blankets, and sheets should be clean and fresh for each client. After each use, linens should be laundered in hot water and dried in a hot drier. If there is concern that the linens have been contaminated, one quarter to one half cup of chlorine bleach can be added to the wash water. Disposable products such as towels and sheets may be used and fresh ones supplied for each client.

Although the massage practitioner may not use a wide range of mechanical aids or electrical equipment, anything from body brushes to toenail clippers must be kept sanitized. There are disinfectants, antiseptics, and fumigants that kill or retard the growth of bacteria. Some are commercially prepared, economical to use, and quick acting. General antiseptics are alcohol, formalin, hydrogen peroxide, sodium hypochlorite, and boric acid. Disinfectants are stronger than antiseptics.

Sanitizers

A **wet sanitizer** is any receptacle large enough to hold a disinfectant solution in which the objects to be sanitized can be completely immersed. A cover is provided to prevent contamination of the solution. Wet sanitizers can be obtained in various sizes and shapes (Fig. 8.7).

Before immersing objects such as hand brushes in a wet sanitizer, be sure to: Wash them thoroughly with hot water and soap, and rinse them thoroughly with clear water. This procedure prevents contamination of the solution. In addition, soap and hot water remove most of the bacteria.

After items are removed from the disinfectant solution, they should be rinsed in clean water, wiped dry with a clean towel, and stored in a dry or cabinet sanitizer until needed.

Some implements can be washed with hot water and soap, immersed in alcohol, wiped dry, and then placed in a sterile container until needed.

A **dry** or **cabinet sanitizer** is an airtight cabinet containing an active fumigant. Objects are placed in a dry cabinet sanitizer, and a small tray at the bottom of the cabinet is used to place a fumigant such as borax formalin. Sanitized implements are kept clean in the cabinet until needed (Fig. 8.8).

Moist heat: This is the method of boiling objects in water at 212° Fahrenheit (100°C) for about twenty minutes. A vessel known as an **autoclave** is sometimes used in the medical field for sterilization purposes.

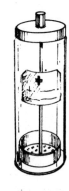

Fig. 8.7 Wet sanitizer.

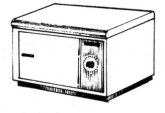

Fig. 8.8 Dry cabinet sanitizer.

Disinfectants

Some disinfectants in general use are:
• Quaternary ammonium compounds (quats)
• Ethyl or grain alcohol
• Formalin.

Quaternary ammonium compounds: These are available in tablet or liquid form under different trade names. The advantages claimed for these disinfectants are short disinfection time and that they are nontoxic, odorless and colorless, and stable. A 1:1000 solution is commonly used to sanitize implements. Immersion time ranges from one to five minutes, depending on the strength of the solution used. Implements such as manicuring and pedicuring tools, tweezers and spatulas can be immersed in this type of solution.

Ethyl or grain alcohol: This comes in liquid form. Electrodes and like implements can be sanitized in 70 percent solution. Alcohol can be used as a rinse to sanitize the hands.

Formalin: This is a sanitizing agent which can be used as either an antiseptic or disinfectant. It is composed of 37 to 40 percent formaldehyde gas in water. A 25 percent solution is generally used for brushes, which are immersed for about ten minutes. This preparation is two parts formalin, five parts water, and one part

▼ TABLE 8.1 APPROVED CHEMICALS

NAME	FORM	STRENGTH	HOW TO USE
Sodium Hypochlorite (household bleach)	Liquid	10% solution	Immerse implements in solution for 10 or more minutes.
Quaternary Ammonium Compounds	Liquid or tablet	1:1000 solution	Immerse implements in solution for 20 or more minutes.
Formalin	Liquid	25% solution	Immerse implements in solution for 10 or more minutes.
Formalin	Liquid	10% solution	Immerse implements in solution for 20 or more minutes.
Alcohol	Liquid	70% solution	Immerse implements or sanitize electrodes and sharp cutting edges for 10 or more minutes.

glycerine. The glycerine keeps metal from rusting. A 2 percent formalin solution can also be an effective sanitizing solution for the hands.

It is important to read directions on all containers when mixing any sanitizing agent.

Creosol or Lysol: (5 to 10 percent) can be used for the cleaning of floors, sinks, restrooms, etc. Commercially prepared solutions are available.

When in doubt about antiseptics and disinfectants approved for use in your studio or work area, consult your local health department or state board of health.

▼ SUMMARY OF PRECAUTIONS

1. Keep yourself and your clothing clean.
2. Wash and sanitize your hands with anti-bacterial soap and warm water before and after every client. A good hand brush should be used for scrubbing, particularly around the nails, and then the hands should be rinsed and wiped dry. If there is cause for suspicion of bacterial contamination, a mild alcohol solution can be used to rinse the hands.
3. Keep all products, implements, and areas used during massage in a sanitary condition. This includes surfaces where items are placed.
4. Keep supplies (oils, lotions, creams, etc.) organized with caps sealed.

5. Never remove a product from its container with your fingers. Use a spatula. Be sure all products have correct labels to prevent using the wrong product.

6. Linens and towels should be laundered in hot water and soap and dried in a hot drier. Chlorine bleach should be added for its germicidal benefits. Clean linens should be stored in closed cabinets. To prevent a rancid odor, sheets and towels should be laundered the day they are used. Generally, laundry products and fabric softeners will eliminate odor. However, once sheets and towels have become rancid, they should be discarded.

   Some oils (peanut, olive, mineral, almond) tend to be hard to remove from fabric. Oil will usually wash out if sheets and towels are laundered immediately. When it is not possible to launder as often as needed, practitioners should use disposable sheets. Commercial products are available to remove rancid oil and odors from linens.

7. Keep all areas of the workplace and furnishings clean. This includes restrooms, dressing rooms, and work space.

8. The place of business should be well ventilated and kept at a comfortable temperature. Floors, walls, windows, and the like should all reflect your concern for cleanliness and pride in your place of business. Practitioners should know and practice all the rules of sanitation issued by their state board and department of health.

SAFETY PRACTICES AND PROCEDURES FOR MASSAGE THERAPISTS ▼

Massage and massage therapy is a personalized health service that usually involves interaction between client and practitioner and does not involve the use of hazardous equipment or practices. However, there are safety issues that the massage student and practitioner must keep in mind. Safety is an attitude put into practice that is concerned with the prevention of situations and elimination of conditions that may lead to injury of the massage practitioner or client. To ensure the health and safety of everyone concerned, safety considerations must to focus on (1) the facility and equipment, (2) the massage practitioner, and (3) the client.

The Facilities

The facilities include the building that houses the massage facility, the facility itself, and the equipment and space within the facility. Safety precautions in the facility include housekeeping, sanitation, fire policy, and heating and ventilation.

Housekeeping/Sanitation

- Keep all halls and walkways clear.
- Keep all carpets vacuumed and cleaned.
- Keep all solid floors cleaned and sanitized.

- Sanitize all bathing facilities.
- Make sure all floors in wet areas are slip proof.
- Sanitize all equipment surfaces that come in contact with clients (table surfaces, linens, applicators and vibrators, etc.).
- Maintain hand-washing facilities (germicidal soap, sanitary towels, clean and sanitary area).

Equipment

- Check all equipment for stability (tables, stools, chairs, etc.)
- Each time a table is set up, check all hinges and locks for stability.
- Maintain all equipment (electrical cords, lubrication, etc.).
- Store equipment and linens properly.

Fire Safety

- Be familiar with the location and use of fire extinguishers.
- Clearly indicate fire exits.
- Be aware of evacuation procedures.
- Establish a policy regarding the use of open flames, candles, incense, etc.

First Aid

- Keep a maintained first aid kit on the premises.
- Make sure all personnel know the location of the first aid kit.
- As many staff members as possible should learn first aid and CPR techniques.
- Keep emergency information posted in plain view near all telephones including telephone numbers for the fire and police departments, ambulance, hospital, emergency room, doctors, and taxis.

Heat and Ventilation

The practice of massage generally requires that the massage room be somewhat warmer than normal. This necessitates either turning up the thermostat or using of auxiliary heating devices.
- Maintain and service heating and ventilation systems regularly.
- Use only UL-approved auxiliary heating devices.
- Regularly inspect auxiliary heating devices.
- Turn off auxiliary heating devices when not in use.

Practitioner Personal Safety

- When lifting equipment or clients, use proper body mechanics and lifting techniques to prevent muscle strain and injury (Fig. 8.9).
- Use proper body mechanics and techniques when practicing massage to prevent muscle strain and overuse syndromes resulting in back, shoulder, or arm injury.
- Use equipment and adjunctive modalities properly and according to manufacturers' instructions and recommendations.

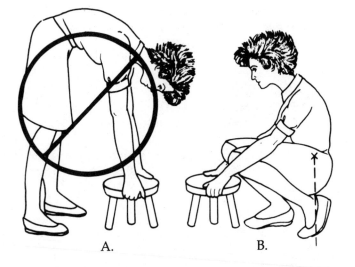

Fig. 8.9 Proper lifting. A. Lifting with poor body mechanics: using back muscles. B. Lifting with good body mechanics: using leg muscles with object close to body.

- All practitioners should maintain a current first aid and CPR certification.
- Know the location of the first aid kit.
- Wash hands before and after every treatment.
- Know contraindications for massage and perform only procedures that cause no injury and are within your scope of practice.
- When doing an outcall, inform an associate of the location, name of the client, the time of the appointment, and the time you plan to complete the appointment. When you have completed the appointment, contact your associate to indicate that you have finished.

Client Safety

- Understand the paths of infection and assure clients' protection with sanitary practices.
    a. Use clean linens with each client.
    b. Wash hands before and after each client.
    c. Provide sanitary bathing facilities and restrooms.
    d. Avoid open wounds and sores.
    e. Do not practice massage if you are ill and/or contagious.
- Provide safe, clear entryways and passages.
    a. Keep walkways clear and well lighted.
    b. Provide nonskid walkways and floors.
- Assist clients on and off of the massage table.
- Check to make sure clients are not sensitive or allergic to products used.

- Use proper procedures in dealing with illness and injury. Refer to proper medical authorities when conditions indicate.
- Do no harm!

▼ QUESTIONS FOR DISCUSSION AND REVIEW

1. Why do all states have laws pertaining to sanitation?
2. Why is it particularly important for a massage practitioner to practice rules of sanitation?
3. Why should the practitioner have some knowledge of bacteria?
4. What is the difference between pathogenic and nonpathogenic bacteria?
5. What is the main purpose of the body's production of antibodies?
6. Name three forms of pathogenic (harmful) bacteria.
7. What is the best prevention against the spread of harmful bacteria?
8. What should you do before using any disinfectant or antiseptic product?
9. Why are disinfectants used in the practice of massage?
10. What is the best method for keeping the hands and nails clean?
11. Which strengths of Creosol or Lysol are most suitable for cleaning floors, sinks, or restrooms?
12. What is sterilization?
13. What is safety?
14. What are the four areas of concern for safety in a massage practice?

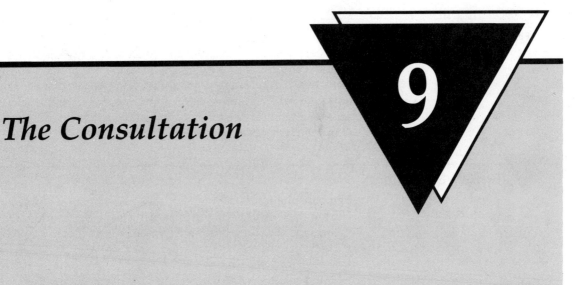

The Consultation

Learning Objectives

After you have mastered this chapter, you will be able to:

1. Explain the importance of the consultation before a massage.
2. Demonstrate how to screen clients while making appointments.
3. Demonstrate how to determine the needs and expectations of the client.
4. Explain why it is important to set policies during the first consultation.
5. Define a treatment plan.
6. Explain what records should be kept and why it is important to keep them updated.
7. Demonstrate how to take a person's pulse and temperature.

▼ INTRODUCTION

A consultation is a meeting in which views are discussed and valuable information is exchanged. During preliminary consultations between massage practitioners and prospective clients, clients give pertinent information about who they are and why they are seeking the services of the therapist. Practitioners inform clients about the services they provide.

▼ THE CONSULTATION

The consultation is a time to gather and exchange information. During the consultation the therapist has the opportunity to:
• Greet the client and introduce himself or herself.
• Determine the client's needs and expectations.
• Explain procedures.
• State policies.
• Perform preliminary assessment.
• Formulate a treatment plan.

An effective consultation depends on clear communication. The practitioner must not only be able to explain policies and procedures so the client can understand them, but must also listen to and understand clearly the needs and wants of the client. To communicate clearly, it is helpful for the practitioner to be aware of the client's level of intelligence and communicating style, as well as his or her emotional and mental condition. Communicate on a level with the client and in a manner he or she comprehends. Some people communicate better by seeing things or by reading or writing information. Others do better talking and listening or by being able to touch and feel things. Be aware of how the client best expresses himself or herself and respond in the same manner. Ask pertinent questions and listen closely to the responses. Above all, be honest and understanding of your client's point of view. It may be different from yours.

The consultation is an interview process that helps determine the course of treatment and sets the tone of the therapeutic relationship between therapist and client. Often the first consultation is the first time the therapist and client meet. First impressions are lasting impressions. The image the therapist exhibits will influence the client's respect and confidence. Be prepared by having everything needed for the interview and massage session organized and ready. Greet the client in a professional and friendly manner. Be courteous and sensitive. Keep the consultation relaxed yet directed toward pertinent information.

The preliminary consultation is the first opportunity for the client and therapist to meet one another and to clarify their intentions and expectations for the massage and to agree on some goals. The first consultation is the time for the client to learn about the kind of therapy the therapist uses and get some idea about the expected outcome. It is during this first consultation that the therapist learns about the client's conditions, needs, and expectations. The purpose of the consultation is to exchange information regarding the client's conditions and expectations and the services offered by the therapist and to determine if they are compatible.

The preliminary consultation is the most extensive; forms are filled out and policies set. However, each session should begin with a short question and answer session to determine any changes in conditions or course of treatment.

Making the First Appointment

Often the first time a client makes an appointment is the first time there is contact between the practitioner and the client. During this first contact, important information can be exchanged to determine if making the appointment for the massage is appropriate. The prospective client may be looking for services that the therapist does not provide, or it may be determined that massage is contra-indicated for the conditions of the would-be client. Screening prospective clients with a couple of questions can save valuable time for both the would-be client and the practitioner as well as eliminate difficult or inappropriate situations.

Three questions that will help screen prospective clients are:
• Have you had massages before?
• How did you find out about my services?
• What is your main reason for making this appointment?

Without going into detail, responses to these questions will clarify if an appointment is desired and appropriate. (We will discuss making appointments in Chapter 19.)

DETERMINING THE CLIENT'S NEEDS AND EXPECTATIONS ▼

To perform services that directly benefit clients, it is necessary to understand their reasons for seeking your services, their expectations, and any conditions they have that might benefit from your services. To get an understanding, you must ask questions and pay close attention to the responses. Two ways to ask questions are written and verbal. Written questions are in the form of intake and medical history questionnaires that the client fills out. When the forms are completed and you review them, a number of verbal questions may be appropriate to clarify the written answers or to gain more specific information about clients and their reason for coming. Important responses should be recorded in the client's file.

▼ EXPLAIN PROCEDURES AND STATE POLICIES

During the first consultation, practitioners clearly explain their operational and client interaction policies. When policies concerning such things as missed or late appointments, payment of fees, and sexual boundaries are clearly stated, misconceptions and awkward situations are avoided. Some practitioners include a disclaimer that their services are not a medical treatment. There is no specific manner to present these policies. They may be posted, printed on the intake forms, or verbalized. Regardless of how they are expressed, only set policies you are willing to uphold.

When the reasons for the client visit are clear and client expectations are stated, practitioners can explain the services they offer and how those services will be of benefit to the client. Practitioners can also explain any procedures they use during the treatment sessions or procedures clients will need to follow during their visits. It is important to keep clients informed about what is being done and why. This is especially important if it is the client's first visit to the place of business and/or first massage.

During the consultation, the client usually will want to know how the massage treatments will be beneficial. Being able to answer the client's questions adds to the practitioner's credibility as a professional and helps to build client confidence.

The following is a review of the benefits of massage that may be of interest to clients:

Circulatory system: Massage improves the circulation of the blood throughout the body, thus improving the supply of oxygen and nutrients to all cells, tissues, and organs. It helps to remove metabolic wastes from the body and can be beneficial in decreasing blood pressure.

Digestive system: Massage aids in relaxing the abdominal and intestinal muscles and improves functioning of the digestive system. Massage stimulates the liver and kidneys and helps to alleviate faulty elimination.

Lymph vascular system: Massage helps to increase lymph circulation, aids in the elimination of metabolic wastes, and stimulates the immune system.

Muscular system: Massage stimulates and tones muscles. It helps to relieve soreness and stiffness in muscles and joints and strengthens connective tissues. It aids in relaxation, relieves fatigue, and provides relief of muscle spasms.

Nervous system: Massage increases the blood supply to the nerves and brain. It stimulates motor nerve points, alleviates stress and tension, and promotes a sense of well-being.

Skin: Massage increases the supply of blood to the skin, thereby nourishing tissues. It improves skin tone, helps to firm facial muscles, and helps to keep the sebaceous (oil) glands functioning normally.

PRELIMINARY ASSESSMENT

To determine what massage procedures to perform on a prospective client or if it is advisable to refer the client to another health professional, the therapist must understand as much about the client and his or her condition as possible. An assessment that includes a client history, observation, and examination will help disclose problems and the physiological basis for the client's complaints.

The history includes information gained from the medical history form, answers to questions, and descriptions that clients offer. Observation includes noticing how clients hold their body and how they move. It includes noticing how they react to questions or manipulative tests. Examination uses various manipulative and verbal tests to help determine more precisely the tissues or conditions involved. (Assessment is discussed in Chapter 12.)

DEVELOP A TREATMENT PLAN

The treatment plan is an outline the practitioner can follow when giving massage treatments. The plan takes into consideration information from the intake and medical history forms, the interview, and preliminary assessment to formulate session goals and choose massage techniques. A general treatment strategy may cover several sessions, but every session should have a treatment plan.

The intake and medical history forms provide past information about the client. If this is not the first session, records from previous sessions provide valuable information. The interview provides additional information concerning the client's reasons for coming and preferences. A further assessment will indicate more about the client's current condition.

By combining and reviewing the information, a strategy or plan of action can begin to evolve. The client's needs, wants, and preferences become more apparent. Indications and contra-indications are determined. A discussion between the client and practitioner can prioritize what the client wants to work on. Options can be discussed.

Referral to other professional or health practitioners might be suggested. Goals for the session(s) are proposed. Modalities and techniques are chosen accordingly, and the plan is put into action.

CLIENT FILES

The client file is the vehicle that practitioners use to document the work they have done with the client. The information a practitioner keeps in the client files varies as much as the massage routines of different practitioners. Updated client files ensure the practitioner's access to current information regarding the client. Information that is often found in a client file includes intake information (name, address, phone, etc.), medical information and history, treatment plan and recorded notes, and financial and billing information. Keeping accurate records is a tedious but essential part of a professional operation.

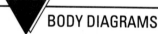

INTAKE AND MEDICAL HISTORY FORMS

Client intake forms and medical history forms provide vital information that the therapist uses to formulate a treatment strategy. The information requested on intake and medical history forms varies according to the kind of massage services offered or the needs of the therapist. Examples of intake and medical history forms have been included in this chapter to provide ideas.

By reviewing the forms, the therapist can reduce the time required to interview the client. After the prospective client has filled out the forms and the therapist has reviewed the information, the client is interviewed in order to elaborate on questions that may need more in-depth consideration. Information gained during the interview is recorded and becomes part of the client's permanent record.

When reviewing consultation forms with the client, it is important to be tactful. If a client questions why you are asking certain questions, explain your reasons. For example, on the form you ask: "What do you do with the majority of your time (hobbies, outside work)?" The client's answers give you clues about what area of the client's body may be carrying stress. The client's answer to the question, "Have you had any surgery?" gives you clues to health problems and contraindications. The question, "Have you received massages before?" allows you to determine what the client's expectation and preference may be. The question, "How did you find out about our massage services?" gives you information about the kind of advertising that is most effective (Fig. 9.1).

BODY DIAGRAMS

Body diagrams of the male or female figure are helpful when the client has some painful sore or stiff areas that may require attention. Give the client a few minutes to indicate these areas on the diagram, and then discuss the condition and allow the client to explain his or her symptoms. After clients have indicated the location of their discomforts on the diagram, ask them to touch or point to the area(s) on their own body. Add notes to the diagram to clarify and record clients' comments about their conditions.

The practitioner may direct more questions to assess the situation. Questions specifically relating to the client's condition will help to determine the course the massage sessions will take. Questions may also reveal other conditions that may or may not be related to the primary condition. Thorough assessment will also expose any contraindications for massage (Figs. 9.2 to 9.5, pages 298 to 301).

Massage Clinic
Client Information Form

Name_____ Birth Date_____

Address_____ Telephone_____

_____ Business Phone_____

    City   State   Zip   Social Security #_____

Occupation_____ Other Activities_____

General Health Condition_____ Blood Pressure_____

Have you had any serious or chronic illness, operations, chronic virus infections, or traumatic accidents? _____

Are you in recovery for addictions or abuse?_____

Are you under a doctor, chiropractor or other health practitioners care? _____

If so, for what condition/s? _____

Are you on any medication? _____ If so, what?_____

Do I have permission to contact your Doctor / Therapist?_____

Names of Doctors, Chiropractors or Health Practitioners:

Name_____ Name_____

Address_____ Address_____

Telephone_____ Telephone_____

Why did you come for our services? (relaxation, pain, therapy, etc.)_____

_____

What results would you like to achieve with our work?_____

Have you had any massage therapy before?_____ If so, by whom?_____

How did you find out about our services? _____

Were you referred to this office?_____ By whom?_____

In case of emergency notify: Name_____Phone _____

I have completed this information form to the best of my knowledge. I understand the massage services are designed to be a health aid and are in no way to take the place of a doctors care when it is indicated. Information exchanged during any massage session is educational in nature and is intended to help me become more familiar and conscious of my own health status and is to be used at my own discretion.

Our time together is precious and I agree to cancel 24 hours in advance. Unless there is an emergency, if I miss an appointment I agree to pay the full appointment fee.

Date_____ Signature_____

Fig. 9.1 Sample client intake information form.

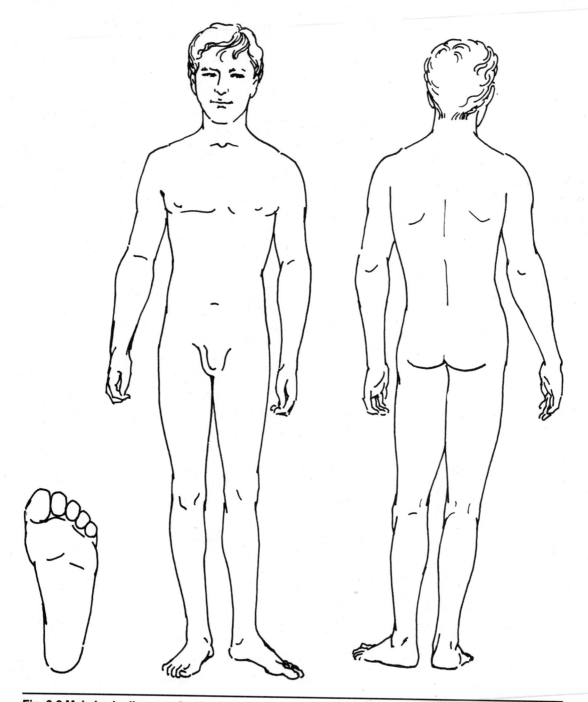

Fig. 9.2 Male body diagram. On the diagram, mark as follows: Put an X on any painful area. Shade in any stiff or sore areas. Circle areas of other concern and describe the condition.

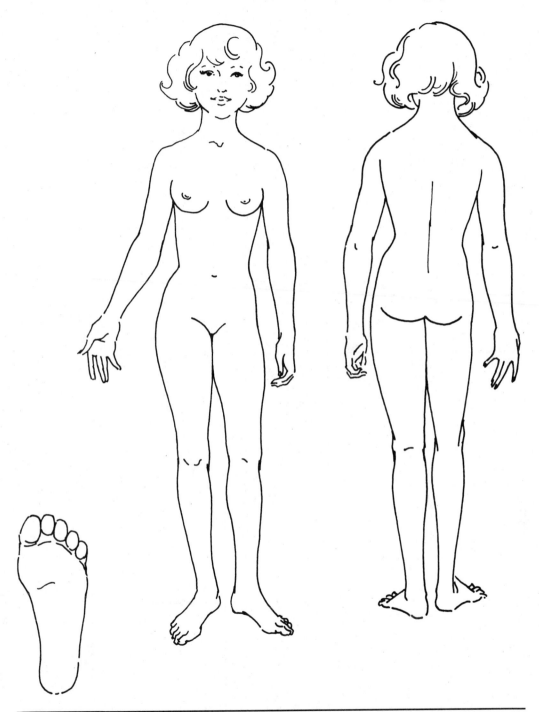

Fig. 9.3 Female body diagram. On the diagram, mark as follows: Put an X on any painful area. Shade in any stiff or sore areas. Circle areas of other concern and describe the condition.

Check Part of Body
Requiring Reducing Massage.

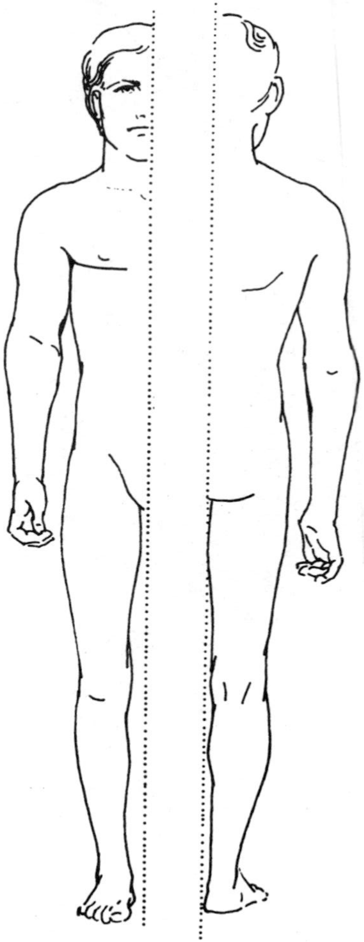

Measurements	1st	6th	10th							Remarks
Date										
Height										
Actual Weight										
Ideal Weight										
Weight Lost										
Weight Gained										
Wrist Pulse										
Body Temperature										
Exercise										
Cabinet Bath										
Body Massage										
Reducing Massage										

Final Results:

Additional Information:

Fig. 9.4 Information card (front side).

Name _____ Address _____ Tel. _____ Date _____

Month	1	2	3	4	5	6	7	8	9	10	11	12	13	14	15	16	17	18	19	20	21	22	23	24	25	26	27	28	29	30	31	Total
Jan.																																
Feb.																																
Mar.																																
Apr.																																
May																																
June																																
July																																
Aug.																																
Sept.																																
Oct.																																
Nov.																																
Dec.																																

Age _____
Occupation _____
No. of Visits _____
Source _____

Payment	Date	Amount

Medical Examination: Date _____

Doctor's Advice Regarding:

Body Massage: _____

Exercise: _____

Special Treatment (Baths) _____

Diet: _____

Additional Information _____

Doctor _____ Address _____

Fig. 9.5 Information card (back side).

▼ UPDATING RECORDS

It is necessary to keep records of all services. Records should be accurate and complete and should provide information concerning treatments given, products used, the state of the client's health, and accurate financial information. Any unique information regarding the client, reactions to treatment, or changes in the client's condition should be noted. All data should be recorded with each treatment, including any special information that may be needed as a reference.

Keeping accurate records of the client's condition, tolerance, and reactions permits you to render more effective treatments and to achieve better results.

Your concern for the client's well-being helps to establish mutual confidence. Reviewing updated records before a client comes in for a return visit refreshes your memory about the client's condition, treatments given, and the client's likes and dislikes. This not only allows you to plan the session, but it re-familiarizes you with the client, which impresses the client and increases his or her confidence in you. On the other hand, a practitioner who relies on memory and forgets important factors about a client from one session to the next may lose the trust which is so necessary in a therapeutic relationship.

The practitioner never discusses or gives out personal information about clients. All records should be kept in a secure place. A practitioner does not divulge information about a client's personal matters without the consent of the client, and then only when the exchange of such information is for the client's benefit. The practitioner often works closely with a client's physician when dealing with certain physical conditions; therefore the confidence of both client and physician must be respected.

When the practitioner feels that a client's physician should be consulted before beginning massage treatments, he or she should talk this over with the client.

▼ TAKING THE CLIENT'S PULSE AND TEMPERATURE

The client's temperature and pulse rate are taken and recorded, if necessary for the treatments being given. The client may not understand why pulse rate and/or temperature are taken and recorded. This can be explained by stating that an abnormally high temperature or pulse rate can be indications of health conditions wherein massage treatments may not be advisable. A marked elevation in body temperature tends to increase the pulse rate.

Under normal circumstances when the client is well, it is not necessary to take the pulse rate and temperature. However, if during the consultation the client appears flushed, unusually warm, and does not feel well, then it is best to take temperature and pulse rate.

To take the client's pulse:
1. Place three fingers (not the thumb) on the inside of the client's wrist and palpate the radial artery to feel the beat of the pulse.
2. Count the number of beats for a full minute on the second hand of your watch, or for 15 seconds × 4 (or 60 seconds).
3. Record the pulse rate (Fig. 9.6).

Normal temperature is about 98.6° Fahrenheit. The most convenient way to take temperature is by the mouth.
1. Wash your hands in warm soapy water and rinse them well.
2. Lower the mercury in the thermometer below the 98° mark by holding the thermometer firmly between your thumb and forefinger and giving your wrist a quick snap.
3. Clean the thermometer with an alcohol swipe, and rinse under cold running water.
4. Insert the bulb end of the thermometer into the client's mouth beneath the tongue. Have the client keep his or her lips closed for about three minutes.
5. Remove the thermometer from the client's mouth and wipe it from top to bottom with a tissue.
6. Locate the column of mercury on the triangular edge of the thermometer, and note the point where it has stopped. This should give you an accurate reading of the client's temperature.
7. Record the temperature on your chart, and explain the results to the client.
8. Wipe the thermometer from top to bottom with a piece of cotton moistened with soap and water, and then rinse it under cold water and immerse it in a sterilizing agent, such as 70 percent alcohol.

The client's height and weight may be recorded if relevant to the treatment. This step is essential if the client is having massage as part of a weight loss program.

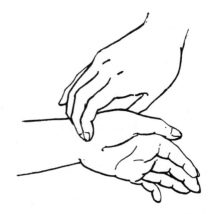

Fig. 9.6 The average resting pulse rate of an adult is between 60 and 80 beats per minute. The pulse is taken when the client is relaxed and after he or she has been resting for a short time. Position for palpating the radial pulse.

QUESTIONS FOR DISCUSSION AND REVIEW

1. Why is the consultation important to the success of the massage treatment?
2. What is included in a preliminary client assessment?
3. Why is a preliminary assessment advisable when doing therapeutic massage?
4. What is a treatment plan?
5. How is a treatment plan developed?
6. Why is it important to keep accurate records?
7. What information is included in a client's file?
8. Why is it important to inform the client of pre-massage procedures?
9. Why should the massage practitioner anticipate questions the client may ask and be able to answer them?
10. Why is it important to be prepared to take the client's pulse rate and temperature before giving the massage treatment?

Classification
of Massage Movements

Learning Objectives

After you have mastered this chapter, you will be able to:

1. *Describe the six major categories of massage movements.*
2. *Explain Swedish (classic) massage techniques.*
3. *Demonstrate mastery of basic massage movements.*
4. *Demonstrate passive and active joint movements.*
5. *Explain and demonstrate rhythm and pressure as applied to therapeutic body massage.*

INTRODUCTION

Massage movements are to therapeutic massage what words are to language or notes to music. To practice massage, some understanding of the movements is imperative. The more mastery therapists have of the movements, the better they are able to create a work of art each time they choose and combine movements according to each situation. There are any number of massage manipulations and possible combinations of strokes, so a massage can be tailored to the specific needs of each client. Regardless of whether a massage routine is standard or specialized to the specific needs of the client, there is much more to applying strokes than the movement of the hands. The continuous interaction of the client and therapist, the purpose for the session, and the intent with which each manipulation is delivered affect the delivery and outcome of the massage.

CLASSIFICATION OF MASSAGE MOVEMENTS

The following movements are the fundamental manipulations used in Swedish massage and are the foundation of most massage styles practiced today. The massage practitioner must understand the indications for and effects of the manipulations. Most massage treatments combine one or more of these movements, as divided into the six major categories:

1. Touch
   a. Superficial
   b. Deep
2. Gliding or effleurage movements
   a. Aura stroking
   b. Superficial
   c. Deep
3. Kneading movements
   a. Kneading or petrissage
   b. Fulling
   c. Skin rolling
4. Friction
   a. Circular friction
   b. Transverse or cross-fiber friction
   c. Compression
   d. Rolling
   e. Chucking
   f. Wringing
   g. Vibration
      • Manual
      • Mechanical
5. Percussion Movements
   a. Hacking
   b. Cupping

      c. Slapping

      d. Tapping

      e. Beating

  6. Joint movements

      a. Passive joint movements

      b. Active joint movements

        • Active assistive movements

        • Active resistive movements

The intention with which a massage is given or a technique is applied will greatly influence its effect. Each manipulation is applied in a specific way for a particular purpose. The practice of massage becomes scientific only when the practitioner recognizes the purpose and effects of each movement and adapts the treatment according to the client's condition and the desired results.

Control over the results of a massage treatment is possible only when the practitioner regulates the intensity of the pressure, direction of movement, and duration of each type of manipulation.

▼ UNDERSTANDING MASSAGE MOVEMENTS

The practitioner must understand the movement to be applied to a particular part of the body. For example,

- Light movements are applied over thin tissues or over bony parts.
- Heavy movements are indicated for thick tissues or fleshy parts.
- Gentle movements are applied with a slow rhythm and are soothing and relaxing.
- Vigorous movements are applied in a quick rhythm and are stimulating.

While applying the movements, the practitioner must pay close attention to the overall response of the client as well as the response of the tissue or body part to which the manipulation is being applied and adjust the application accordingly.

An important rule in Swedish massage is that most manipulations are directed toward the heart (centripetal). Many massage techniques are intended to enhance venous blood and lymph flow and therefore are directed towards the heart and other eliminative organs. Only strokes light enough that they don't affect fluid flow may be directed away from the heart. When a massage movement is directed away from the heart, it is said to be centrifugal.

The duration of a massage treatment should be regulated. Usually a therapeutic full-body massage takes about one hour, but some practitioners take more or less time. A prolonged massage can be fatiguing to some clients. When a student is learning massage, a full-body massage can take an hour and a half to two hours. This is not unusual because it takes practice for movements to become smooth and efficient. After a while, an hour will be plenty of time to accomplish the desired results. There are times when the practitioner will require more time, so the duration of massages varies. Knowledge and experience are prerequisites to judge the client's special need and adjust the massage session accordingly.

DESCRIPTION OF THE BASIC MASSAGE MOVEMENTS ▼

All hands-on therapies use physical contact as the primary modality. Indeed it is this caring human contact that makes massage therapy unique.

Touching: Touch, in the context of the classification of massage techniques, refers to the stationary contact of the practitioner's hand and the client's body. Touch is the placing of the practitioner's hand, finger, or body part (such as forearm) on the client without movement in any direction. The pressure exerted may vary from very light to very deep depending on the intention. Skillfully and purposefully applied touch achieves physiological and psychological (soothing) effects.

Gliding is the practice of gliding the hand over some portion of the client's body with varying amounts of pressure or contact according to desired results.

Kneading lifts, squeezes and presses the tissues.

Friction refers to a number of massage strokes designed to manipulate soft tissue in such a way that one layer of tissue is moved over or against another.

Vibration is a continuous trembling or shaking movement delivered by either the practitioner's hand or an electrical apparatus. Vibration may be classified as a type of friction.

Percussion is a rapid striking motion of the practitioner's hands against the surface of the client's body, using varying amounts of force and hand positions.

Joint movement is the manipulation of the joints or articulations of the client.

APPLICATION OF MASSAGE STROKES ▼

Touch

Touch is the first technique in developing a therapeutic relationship. Touch may be in the form of a hand shake or a pat on the shoulder. In the course of a massage, touch constitutes the first and last contact of the practitioner with the client. All massage techniques use physical contact, but the quality and sense of touch conveys the intent and the power of the movements. Touch is the primary communication tool used by the massage therapist. The sense of touch tells clients what is happening to their bodies and gives practitioners information about the condition and response of the tissues they are working on. The quality of touch continually transmits information from the therapist's hands to the client in

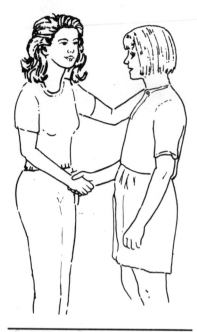

Fig. 10.1 A friendly greeting conveys a message of confidence and concern.

direct response to the information communicated by the client and his or her body (Fig. 10.1).

Light or superficial touch is purposeful contact in which the natural and evenly distributed weight of the practitioner's finger, fingers, or hand is applied on a given area of the client's body. The size of that area may be regulated as necessary by using one or more fingers, the entire hand, or both hands. Some therapeutic techniques employ touch almost exclusively (*jin shin do*, acupressure, polarity, therapeutic touch, *reiki*). Touch can be remarkably effective in the reduction of pain, lowering of blood pressure, control of nervous irritability, or reassurance for a nervous, tense client. If a person has signs of contraindications for a basic massage, or is in a fragile condition, a complete treatment using light touch exclusively is acceptable. The main objective of light touch is to soothe and to provide a comforting connection that is calming and allows the powerful healing mechanisms of the body to function (Figs. 10.2a and b).

Deep Touch Using Pressure

Deep touch is performed with one finger, thumb, several fingers, or the entire hand. The heel of the hand, knuckles, or elbow can be used according to desired results. The application of deep pressure is used when calming, anesthetizing, or stimulating effects are desired. Deep pressure may be used with other techniques such as cross-fiber friction, compression, or vibration. Deep pressure is useful in soothing muscle spasms and relieving pain at reflex areas, stress points in tendons, and trigger points in muscles. In addition to extensive use in trigger-point therapy, deep pressure is a tech-

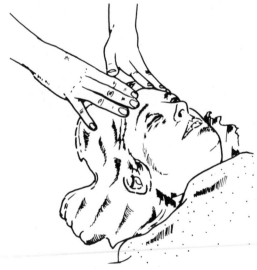

Fig. 10.2a Gentle contact allows the client to unwind.

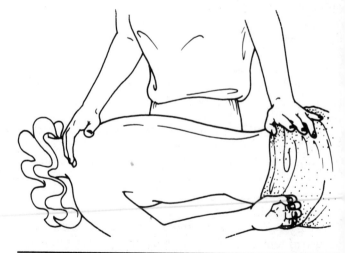

Fig. 10.2b A light touch at the base of the spine, the base of the neck, or the top of the head is a nice way to say hello or goodbye to the client's body

nique often applied in reflexology, sport massage, acupressure, and *shiatzu* (these methods will be discussed in Chapters 16 and 17). When using deep pressure, caution must be used to stay within the pain tolerance of the client (Figs. 10.3a to e).

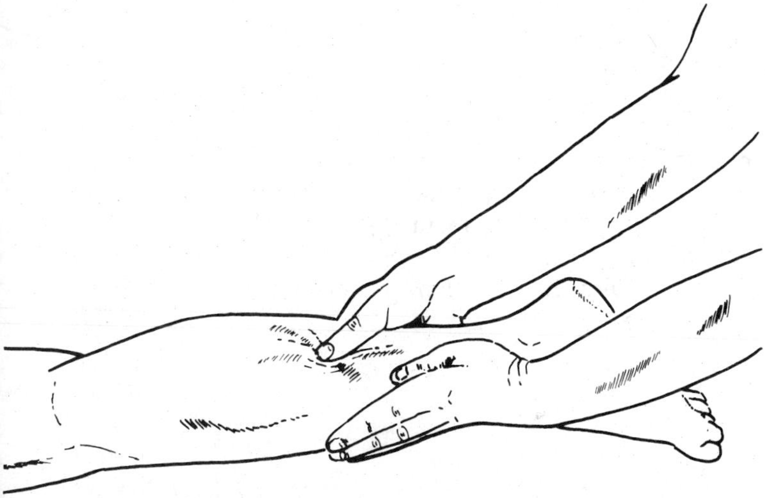

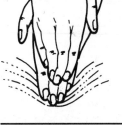

Fig. 10.3a Deep touch using thumb. Notice the alignment of therapist's thumb and arm to ensure that pressure is directed into client with minimal stress to therapist's joints.

Fig. 10.3b Deep pressure applied with braced fingers.

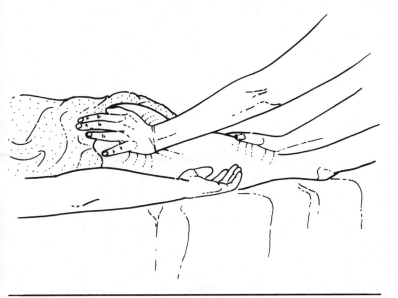

Fig. 10.3c Deep touch applied with heel of hand.

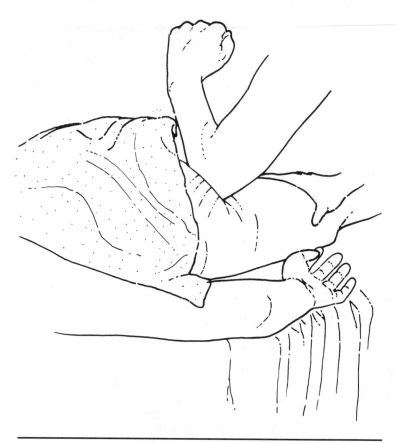

Fig. 10.3d Deep touch applied with elbow.

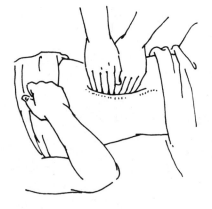

Fig. 10.3e Deep pressure to the abdominal area.

Gliding Movements

Gliding may be done using a varying amount of pressure and length of strokes. Gliding strokes glide over the client's entire body, body part (arm or leg), or a specific area (muscle or reflex).

Ethereal Body or Aura Stroking

This type of stroking is done with long, smooth strokes wherein the practitioner's hands glide the length of the client's entire body or body part, coming very close to but not actually touching the body surface. Generally the movement is in one direction only, with the return stroke being farther from the body. The intention is to affect the energy fields that, according to some philosophies, surround or permeate the body. The direction of the stroking may be along the surface of the body to enhance or impede the natural flow.

The application of this soothing stroke is done only when the surrounding circumstances are very quiet, relaxed, and the patient is receptive. It is sometimes used as the final stroke of a massage (Fig. 10.4).

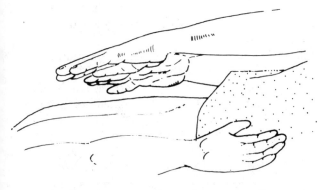

Fig. 10.4 Ethereal or aura strokes do not touch the surface of the client's body.

Feather stroking

Feather-stroking movements use very light pressure of the finger-tips or hands with long flowing strokes.

The application of feather stroking, sometimes called "nerve stroking," is usually done from the center outward and is used as a final stroke to individual areas of the body. Two or three such strokes will have a slightly stimulating effect on the nerves, while many repetitions will have a more sedating response (Fig. 10.5).

Gliding or Effleurage

Effleurage is a succession of strokes applied by gliding the hand over a somewhat extended portion of the body. There are two varieties of effleurage: superficial and deep. Superficial gliding strokes employ a very light touch. In gliding strokes, the pressure becomes firmer as the hand glides over the surface of the body. The technique of effleurage or gliding is accomplished either with the fingers, thumbs, the palm of the hand, the knuckles, or the forearm.

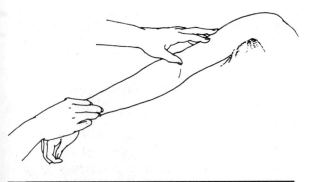

Fig. 10.5 Feather strokes (nerve strokes) use the lightest touch of the fingertips.

1. Over large surfaces, such as the limbs, back, chest, and abdomen, the gliding movement is performed with the palm of one or both hands.
2. Over small areas, such as the eyes or hands, the movement is performed with the fingers or thumbs.
3. For very deep gliding strokes, the palms of the hands, the fingertips, the thumbs, the knuckles or sometimes the forearms are used.

Superficial gliding strokes are generally applied prior to any other movement. The practitioner's hand is flexible yet firm and controlled so that as it glides over the body, it conforms to the body contours in such a way that there is equal pressure applied to the body from every part of the hand. Superficial gliding strokes accustoms the client to the practitioner's contact and allows the practitioner to assess the body area being massaged. Light strokes are used to distribute any lubricant that may be used and to prepare the area for other techniques. As the practitioner's hands glide over the tissues, they sense variations that indicate where specific techniques will be applied. Effleurage is interspersed between other techniques to clear the area and soothe the intensity of some deeper manipulations. Slow, gentle, and rhythmic movements produce soothing effects. Rhythmic strokes should be applied in the direction of the venous and lymphatic flow.

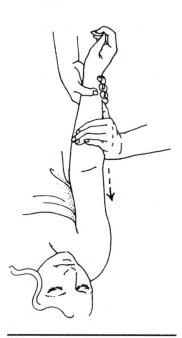

Fig. 10.6a Effleurage or gliding strokes are applied in the direction of venous blood and lymph flow.

Although superficial stroking appears to be simple, its technique is mastered only by long practice. The practitioner's hand should be relaxed in order to mold the surface of the body part being massaged. The pressure and speed of movement should remain constant. Upon completion of the stroke, the practitioner's hand may be elevated and directed to the starting point. In some cases, the hands stay in contact by exerting more pressure centripetally (toward the heart) and then reduce the pressure and lightly stroke (feather stroke) the body to return to the starting point of the stroke. In this way the practitioner always maintains contact with the client.

Superficial gliding strokes are a valuable application for overcoming a general tired feeling or restlessness. This movement is particularly soothing to nervous or irritated people. Nervous headaches and insomnia (sleeplessness) are often relieved by gentle gliding strokes of the forehead.

Deep Gliding

The term deep gliding indicates that the manipulation uses enough pressure to have a mechanical effect. The depth of the gliding movement depends on three factors: the pressure exerted, the part of the hand or arm used and the intention with which the manipulation is applied. Deep gliding strokes do not involve the use of excessive force. The pressure should never be so forceful as to cause bruising or injury to the tissues. Deep gliding strokes are especially valuable when applied to the muscles. It is most effective when the

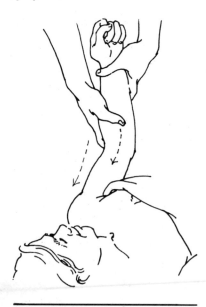

Fig. 10.6b A V-stroke can be used for superficial or deep gliding strokes.

part under treatment is in a state of relaxation. Then the slightest pressure of the surface will be transmitted to the deeper structures. Deep gliding strokes have a stretching and broadening effect on muscle tissue and fascia. It also enhances the venous blood and lymph flow. If the practitioner uses too much force, the client's body will respond with a protective reflex that will cause muscles to contract, thereby negating the desired effects of the treatment. Deep gliding strokes generally follow the direction of the muscle fibers. On the extremities the movements are always directed from the end of a limb toward the center of the body. Generally the movement is toward the heart or in the direction of venous and lymph flow, with the return stroke being much lighter and away from the center of the body. The exception to this rule is deep, short strokes applied to the muscle attachments and tendons. When directed from the tendon towards the muscle belly, these strokes tend to stretch the tendon and cause a reflexive relaxation of the muscle (Fig. 10.6a to g and 10.7a to g).

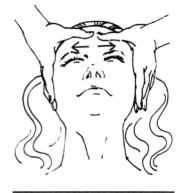

Fig. 10.6c Apply digital effleurage to the forehead.

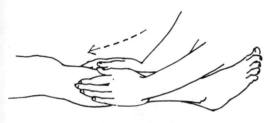

Fig. 10.6d Direction of effleurage on the lower leg. The same upward movements are applied when massaging the back of the lower leg.

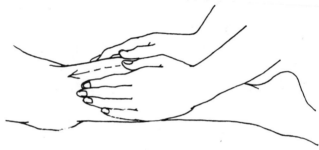

Fig. 10.6e Stroke the leg with two hands.

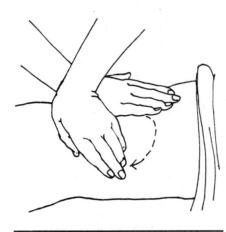

Fig. 10.6f Stroke the abdomen in a deep circular movement.

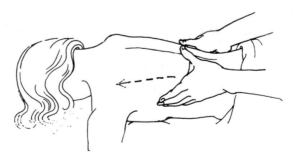

Fig. 10.6g Stroking the entire back.

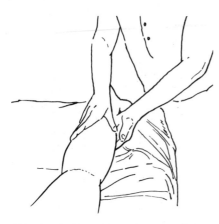

Fig. 10.7a V-stroke applied to the posterior leg.

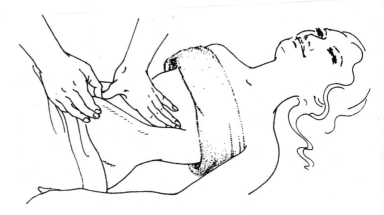

Fig. 10.7b Apply deep circular effleurage following the path of the colon.

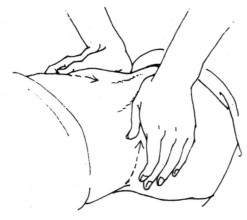

Fig. 10.7c Inward deep gliding strokes of muscles over the stomach area and the abdominal region.

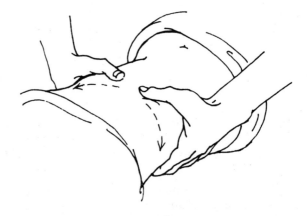

Fig. 10.7d Outward deep gliding strokes to the muscles of the stomach area and the abdominal region.

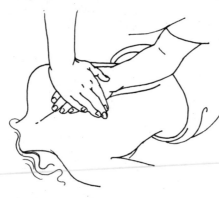

Fig. 10.7e Apply two-handed (deep) effleurage around the scapula. Note that one hand is on top of the other.

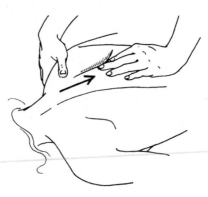

Fig. 10.7f Apply deep stroking under the scapula followed by rotation of the shoulder.

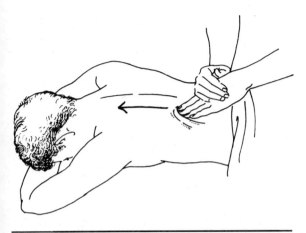

Fig. 10.7g Deep gliding strokes with braced fingers.

When using deep gliding strokes, the practitioner must use good body mechanics to prevent strain and overuse syndrome injuries. Hand and arm positions should direct the force of the manipulation into the client. The practitioner's shoulders remain down and relaxed, and hyperextension of the wrists, fingers, or thumbs must be avoided (Fig. 10.8).

Kneading Movements or Petrissage

In Swedish massage, kneading or petrissage is used on all fleshy areas of the body. Like deep gliding, kneading enhances the fluid

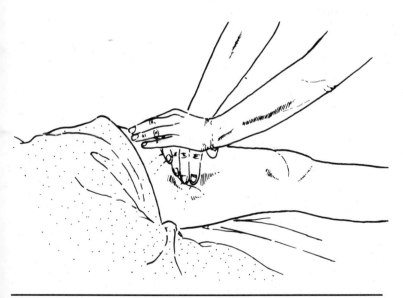

Fig. 10.8 When using deep techniques, the practitioner must use good body mechanics to direct the manipulation into the client and at the same time protect himself or herself from injury.

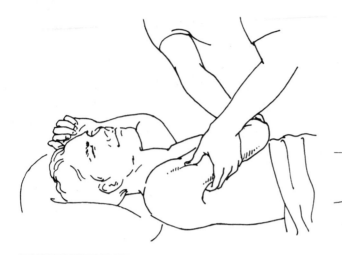

Fig. 10.9a Kneading the triceps.

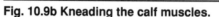

Fig. 10.9b Kneading the calf muscles.

movement in the deeper tissues. Skillfully applied, kneading helps reduce adhesions and stretch muscle tissue and fascia. In this movement, the skin and muscular tissues are raised from their ordinary position and then squeezed, rolled, or pinched with a firm pressure, usually in a circular direction.

On large areas of the body, two hands alternately press the flesh between the palmar surface of the fingers of one hand and the thumb and the nar portion of the opposite hand. Over smaller structures, such as the arms, the flesh is grasped between the fingers and heel of the hand or the thumb. In both cases the maximum amount of flesh is drawn up into the palm and gently and firmly pressed and squeezed as if milking the deep fluids. On an area such as the arm, one hand may be used to apply the manipulation while the other hand stabilizes the arm, or both

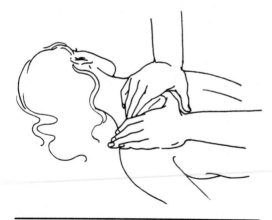

Fig. 10.9c Petrissage includes the trapezius muscles.

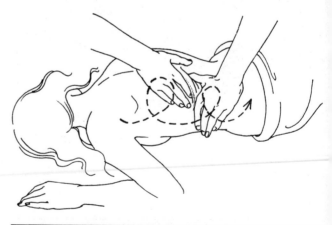

Fig. 10.9d Apply petrissage to the entire side that is opposite you. This takes several passes.

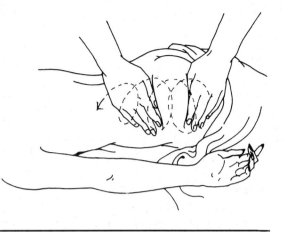

Fig. 10.9e Apply kneading over the gluteals.

hands may alternate grasping the tissue on each side of the arm. Over smaller structures, such as the hands or fingers, the flesh is held between the thumb and fingers.

Fulling is a kneading technique in which the practitioner attempts to grasp the tissue and gently lift and spread it out, as if to make more space between the layers of tissue or muscle fibers.

Skin rolling is a variation of kneading in which only the skin and subcutaneous tissue is picked up between the thumbs and fingers and rolled. As the fingers alternately and continuously pick up and pull the skin away from the deeper tissues, the thumb glides along in the direction of the movement stretching the underlying fascia (Figs. 10.9a to e, 10.10, and 10.11).

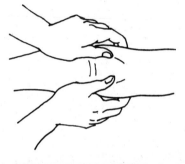

Fig. 10.10 For fulling movement, grasp the flesh between the fingers and palms of the hand.

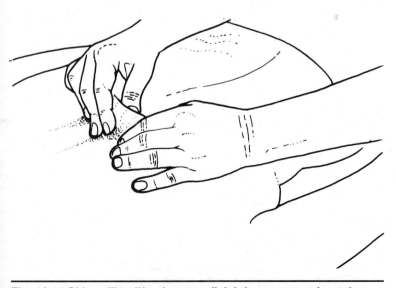

Fig. 10.11 Skin rolling lifts the superficial tissues away from the muscles and other deeper tissues.

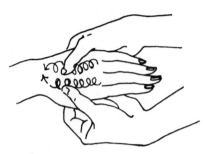

Fig. 10.12a Circular friction of the muscles of the hand.

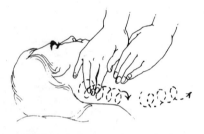

Fig. 10.12b Circular friction of the back of the neck.

Friction

Friction movements involve moving more superficial layers of flesh against the deeper tissues. Whereas kneading is done by lifting and pulling the flesh away from the skeletal structures and squeezing in such a way as to milk out the body fluids, friction presses one layer of tissue against another layer in order to flatten, broaden, or stretch the tissue. Friction is done in such a way that it also increases heat. As heat increases, the metabolic rate increases. Friction also increases the rate at which exchanges take place between the cells and the interstitial fluids (fluids situated between the cells and vessels in the tissues of an organ or body part). The added heat and energy also affect the connective tissue surrounding the muscles, making them more pliable so they function more efficiently.

Friction helps to separate the tissues and to break down adhesions and fibrosis, especially in muscle tissue and fascia. It softens the amorphous (massed) ground substance between layers of fascia. Friction also aids in absorption of the fluid around the joints. Friction has a marked influence on the circulation and glandular activity of the skin. With friction strokes the area usually becomes red. This indicates an increased flow of blood to the area and that more blood is being rushed to the surface of the skin.

Friction strokes involve moving a more superficial layer of tissue against deeper layers of tissue. This requires pressure on the skin while it is being moved over its underlying structures. The skin and the hand move as a unit against the deeper tissues. Over muscular parts or fleshy layers, friction is applied with the palms of the

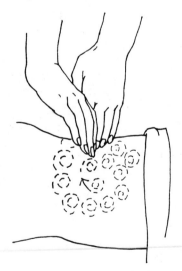

Fig. 10.12c Apply circular friction over the area of the intestines.

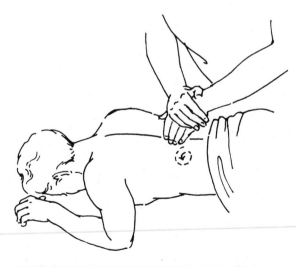

Fig. 10.12d Friction applied to the muscles along the spine.

hands, the flat of the fingers, or the thumbs. Over small surfaces, friction is applied with the fleshy parts of the fingertips or thumbs.

Friction movements may be circular or directional. In **circular friction** the fingers or the palm of the hand contact the skin to move it in a circular pattern over the deeper tissues. Circular friction is intended to produce heat and stretch and soften the fascia. Directional friction may be either cross-fiber or longitudinal friction.

Cross fiber friction, as the name implies, is applied in a transverse direction across the muscle, tendon, or ligament fibers. Cross-fiber friction is usually applied with the tips of the fingers or the thumb directly to the specific site of a lesion. The stroke is only long enough to cover the intended tissues. The fingers do not move over the skin but move the skin and superficial tissues across the target tissue.

Cross-fiber or transverse friction is a preferred technique for rehabilitation of fibrous tissue injuries. When the injury is healing, transverse friction, when properly applied, promotes the formation of elastic fibrous tissue. At the same time it reduces the formation of fibrosis and scar tissue so the healed injury retains its original strength and pliability. Applied to old injury sites, cross-fiber friction breaks down some of the adhesions and fibrosis, increasing pliability and reducing the chance of reinjury to the area.

In longitudinal friction, the practitioner's hand moves in the same direction as the tissue fibers. This tends to stretch the tissue and align the collagen fibrils within the fascia (Fig. 10.12a to f).

Another form of friction sometimes classified by itself is **compression.** As the name implies, compression is rhythmic pressing

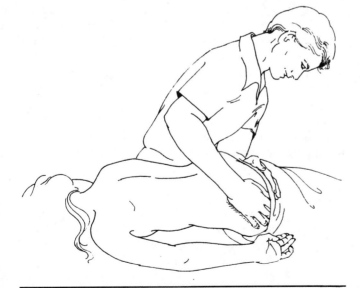

Fig. 10.12e Apply compression to the gluteal muscles.

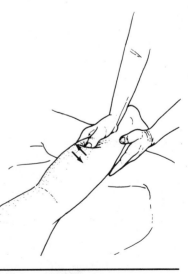

Fig. 10.12f Cross fiber to the musculo-tendinous junction of the posterior leg.

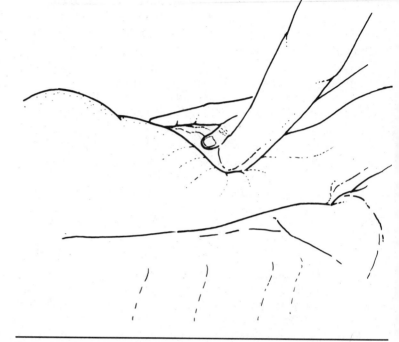

Fig. 10.13 Two-handed compression applied to the hamstrings.

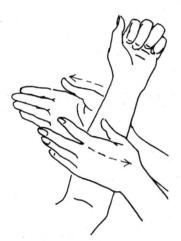

Fig. 10.14a Rolling the arm.

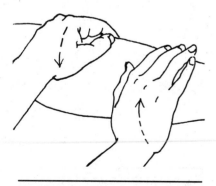

Fig. 10.14b Wringing the muscles of the leg.

movements directed into muscle tissue by either the hand or fingers. **Palmar compression** is done with the whole hand (palm side) or the heel of the hand over the large area of the body. Palmar compression is a rhythmical pumping action directed into the muscle perpendicular to the body part. Compression movements cause increased circulation and a lasting hyperemia in the tissue. Compression is a popular movement used in pre-event sports massage. The intention is to bring more blood and fluid into the tissues, preparing them to exert maximum energy sooner and for a longer period of time (Fig. 10.13).

Other manipulations that are considered friction include rolling, wringing, chucking, shaking, and vibration. Chucking, rolling, wringing, and shaking are variations of friction employed principally to massage the arms and legs.

Rolling

Rolling is a rapid back-and-forth movement with the hands, in which the flesh is shaken and rolled around the axis, or the imaginary centerline of the body part.

Chucking

The chucking movement is accomplished by grasping the flesh firmly in one or both hands and moving it up and down along the bone. It is a series of quick movements along the axis of the limb.

Wringing

Wringing is a back-and-forth movement in which both of the practitioner's hands are placed a short distance apart on either side of the limb. It resembles wringing out a wash cloth. The hands work in opposing directions, stretching and twisting the flesh against the bones in opposite directions.

Shaking

Shaking is a movement that allows the client to release tension and at the same time indicates to the practitioner where the client may be storing tension in a part of the body. The relaxed body part is gently yet forcefully shaken laterally or horizontally so that the relaxed flesh flops around the bone. The practitioner observes where the body moves freely and where it seems to be stiff. Rigidness indicates body areas that are tense and require more attention. The Trager method of bodywork uses shaking and rocking extensively to locate and release tension (Fig. 10.14a to h).

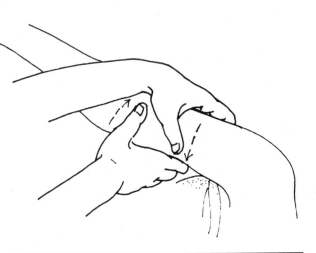

Fig. 10.14c Wringing the muscles of the arm.

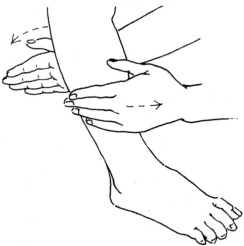

Fig. 10.14d Rolling the muscles of the leg.

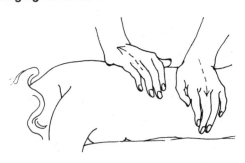

Fig. 10.14e Wringing the muscles of the lower back in a backward and forward movement.

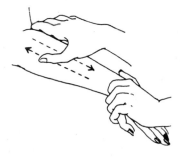

Fig. 10.14f Chucking the arm.

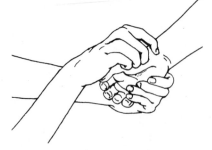

Fig. 10.14g Use the client's hand as a handle for shaking the hand during petrissage and applying friction to the hand.

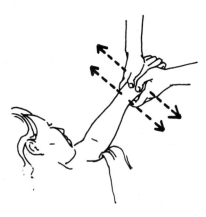

Fig. 10.14h Shaking applied to the arm.

Vibration

Vibration is a continuous shaking or trembling movement transmitted from the practitioner's hand and arm or from an electrical appliance to a fixed point, or along a selected area of the body. Nerve trunks and centers are sometimes chosen as sites for the application of vibratory movements.

The rate of vibration should be under the control of the massage practitioner. Manual vibrations usually range from five to ten times per second, while mechanical vibrations can be adjusted to give from 10 to 100 vibrations per second (Fig. 10.15).

There are a variety of mechanical vibrators on the market. They can be classified by size. A popular small model straps on the back of the practitioner's hand. Another popular size is held (usually with two hands) by the practitioner and moved over the client's body. A larger floor-standing model unit uses a flexible applicator arm to deliver its therapeutic affects (Fig. 10.16a to c).

Another way to classify mechanical vibrators is by the vibrating action they use. An oscillating vibrator has a back-and-forth movement. An orbital vibrator uses a circular motion. These vibrators produce a shaking movement when applied to the body. Another type of vibrator produces "thumping" action. This rapid percussion/compression is directed into the tissues rather than laterally, along the surface. Using vibrators may enhance the effects of the massage and at the same time reduce the physical exertion of the practitioner (Fig. 10.17a to c).

The effect of vibratory movements depends on the rate of vibration, the intensity of pressure, and the duration of the treatment. This form of massage is soothing and brings about relaxation and release of tension when applied lightly. It is stimulating when applied with pressure. A numbing effect is experienced when vibrations are applied for a prolonged period of time.

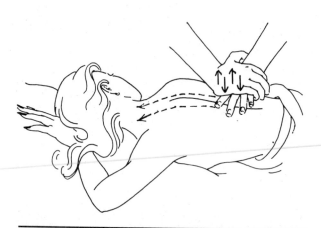

Fig. 10.15 Vibrating over each vertebra.

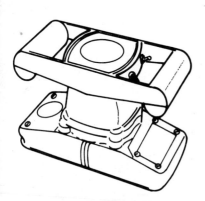

Fig. 10.16a Popular style of vibrator that uses an orbital movement.

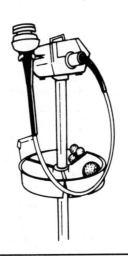

Fig. 10.16b The floor-standing model has a flexible shaft and a variety of applicator heads.

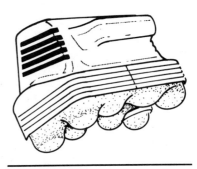

Fig. 10.16c Type of vibrator that uses a thumping action.

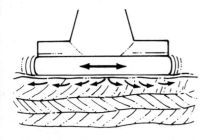

Fig. 10.17a Oscillating vibrators have a lineal back-and-forth action.

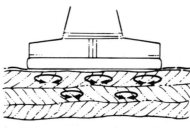

Fig. 10.17b Orbital vibrators have a circular action.

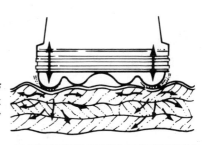

Fig. 10.17c "The Thumper™" uses a percussion/compression action.

PERCUSSION MOVEMENTS ▼

Percussion movements include quick, striking manipulations such as tapping, beating, and slapping, which are highly stimulating to the body. Percussion movements are executed with both hands simultaneously or alternately. The movements may be done in the following ways:

1. Tapping with tips of the fingers
2. Slapping with flattened palm and fingers of the hand
3. Cupping with the cupped palm of the hand
4. Hacking with the ulnar border of the hand
5. Beating with a softly clenched hand

Percussion movements do not use much force. Each blow to the body is a glancing contact wherein the practitioner's wrists remain very relaxed. Hacking is done with the hand and wrist relaxed and the fingers slightly apart. Each time the side of the hand comes in contact with the client, the fingers come together, creating a slight vibration. Beating likewise uses a soft fist and relaxed wrists. Slapping, cupping, and tapping use a relaxed wrist and a whip-like stroke of the hands and arms.

Tapping movements are employed on the face, chest, and back. Hacking and cupping movements are used when massaging the back, shoulders, arms, and legs. Beating and slapping are vigorous forms of percussion usually limited to the stimulation of heavy muscles and adipose (fatty) tissue found over the back, buttocks, and thighs. The beating and slapping movements should be used with discretion so the client is not overstimulated by the treatment. Cupping is used over the thorax when working with people who have a congestive lung condition.

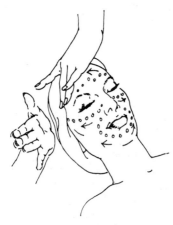

Fig. 10.18a Tapping with fingertips on the face.

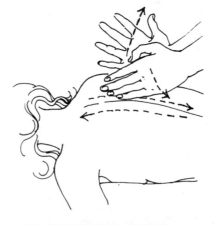

Fig. 10.18b Hacking movements on the back.

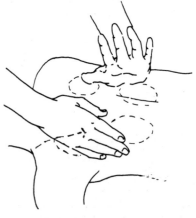

Fig. 10.18c Slapping movements on the back.

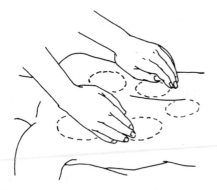

Fig. 10.18d Cupping movements on the thorax.

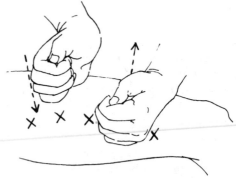

Fig. 10.18e Beating the muscles of the thigh.

The general effects of percussion movements are to tone the muscles and impart a healthy glow to the part being massaged. With each striking movement, the muscles first contract and then relax as the fingers are removed from the body. In this way, muscles are toned. Percussion movements should never be applied over muscles that are abnormally contracted or over any sensitive area (Fig. 10.18a to e).

JOINT MOVEMENTS ▼

There are a great variety of joint movements that can be used to manipulate any joint in the body, including joints of the toes, knees, hips, arms, the vertebrae, or even the less movable joints of the pelvis and cranium.

The basic classifications of joint movements are passive and active. **Passive joint movements** are done while the client remains quietly relaxed and allow the practitioner to stretch and move the part of the body to be exercised. In **active joint movements** the client actively participates in the exercise by contracting the muscles involved in the movement. For example, the practitioner straightens the client's arm while asking the client to hold against or resist the movement. Active joint movements may be subdivided into two categories: active resistive and active assistive.

Active assistive joint movements restore lost mobility when clients are having difficulty moving a limb. The client is instructed to perform a motion at the same time the practitioner assists the movement.

Active resistive joint movements help to strengthen muscles. The client is instructed to make a motion while the limb is held to resist movement. For example, the client is instructed to raise the left hand from the right hip to a position high above and to the left of the head. (The best form of instruction is to passively move the client's hand.) The therapist places one hand on the client's wrist and the other hand on the client's elbow and gives the command to lift. As the client lifts the arm, the therapist offers enough resistance through the entire range of movement so the client must apply some effort to make the movement.

Joint movements are used to help restore a client's mobility or increase flexibility in a joint. Often, passive and active joint movements will be combined. For example, to restore some mobility to a shoulder joint, the client is instructed to raise the arm to the point of discomfort (active unassisted movement). The therapist holds the arm in that position as the client is instructed to push against the therapist and attempt to continue the movement (active resistive joint movement). Then the client is instructed to relax as the therapist continues to move the client's arm (passive joint movement).

Joint movements may be applied with or without resistance, using either a forward, backward, or circular motion. To be most

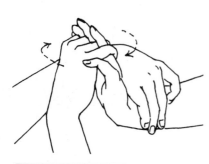

Fig. 10.19a Apply joint movements and rotation. Note the interlacing of the fingers.

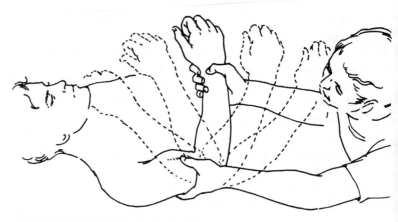

Fig. 10.19b Flexion and extension of the forearm.

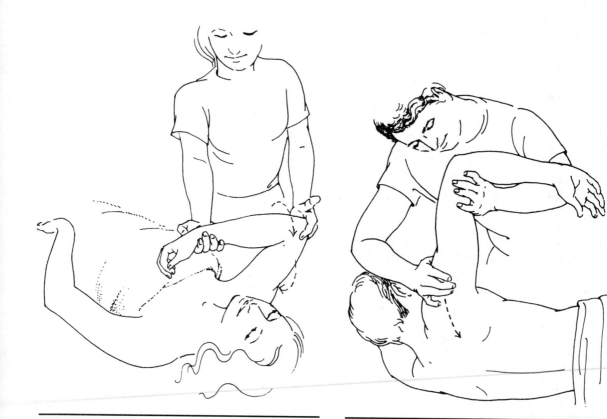

Fig. 10.19c Rotate the shoulder.

Fig. 10.19d Abduction of the arm. This is movement of a part away from the median line of the body.

effective, joint movements should be applied through the full **range of motion.** The range of motion is the movement of a joint from one extreme of the articulation to the other. All joints have normal restrictions that limit the range of motion. Those restrictions may be bone to bone, such as the extension of the elbow where the movement is stopped when the olecronon of the ulna contacts the humerus. Sometimes the restriction is due to pull on ligaments as in the hyperextension of the hip. Most often it is due to muscles. As the practitioner passively moves a joint to the end of its range, there is a sense that the limb is approaching the extent of its possible movement. The change in the quality of the feeling as the end of the movement is achieved is termed **end feel**. A hard end feel occurs when an abrupt clunk is felt at the end of the movement. This indicates that bone is making contact with another bone stopping the movement. A soft end feel occurs when, over the last few inches or degrees of the joint movement, there is a gradual and steady tightening until a soft barrier is reached. Soft tissue limits the range when there is a soft end feel.

Ideally every joint should move through its full range of motion freely, without discomfort. Often the range of motion is further restricted by tense muscles, injured or restricted tissues, inflammation, or other pathological conditions. The reaction of joint movements with these conditions is usually pain. The therapist must be aware of the end feel of the joints and the pain reactions of the client when doing joint movements. Joint movements have a great therapeutic benefit as an assessment tool and as a treatment to enhance function and mobility (Fig. 10.19a to j).

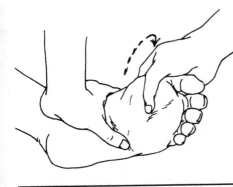

Fig. 10.19e Rotate and stretch the tarsals and metatarsals.

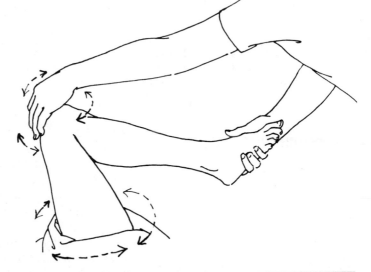

Fig. 10.19f Circumduction of the thigh.

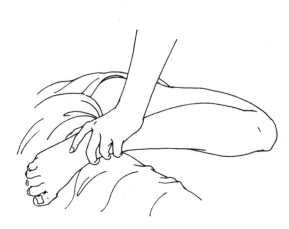

Fig. 10.19g Apply joint movements.

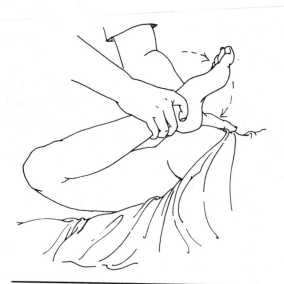

Fig. 10.19h Flexing the client's knee, pressing the heel against the gluteals.

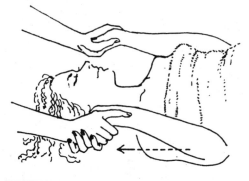

Fig. 10.19i Active movement: The client tries to move her hands above her head as the therapist either resists or assists.

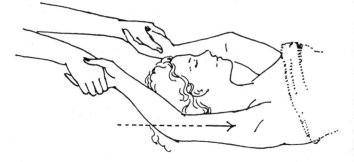

Fig. 10.19j Active movement: The client attempts to bring her arms back down to her side as the therapist resists the movement.

▼ RHYTHM AND PRESSURE IN MASSAGE

People have individual vibrations and their own sense of rhythm. The practitioner needs to remember that some people are high strung (tense), while others are very low key (relaxed). It is important to work with people according to their particular needs instead of following a personal agenda and possibly working against the client's natural rhythm. It is important to consider each individual situation when providing a therapeutic service. Usually someone coming for a massage is seeking a relaxing, rejuvenating experience. The rhythm must be steady and slightly slower than the client's pace in order to have a sedating effect. If the massage is part of an athletic training program, however, the rhythm may be more upbeat. Practitioners can develop skills to tune in to other people and work more effectively with them as individuals. Clients will return to the practitioner who is not only well trained, but sensitive and aware.

Breathing is a part of the body's natural rhythm and is important to the practitioner's stamina and ability to move easily while giving massage.

The practitioner must develop an awareness of the right amount of pressure to be used for various therapeutic situations and techniques. It is important to begin to massage in an area of the body cautiously, gently, and lightly and then apply more pressure as you become aware of underlying structures and the condition of tissues. This also helps you to note tension and stress build-up and determine how to proceed according to the client's body condition and sensitivity. The pressure varies with the technique used and according to the intended outcome. At no time should the pressure be so forceful as to cause injury to the tissues. The rule is to begin with a light and sensitive touch, and increase the pressure as you work into an area. As tension in the area begins to dissipate and the muscles relax, the client will let you in even deeper. When it is time to leave the area, back out gradually, smoothing the way as you go.

One of the primary indications of tension or dysfunction in the muscles and soft tissue is pain. Massage therapy is one of the best methods of locating and treating these conditions. Many massage techniques directly manipulate the painful areas and therefore are painful. People have different tolerances for pain. It is important not to work to a point that produces so much pain that the individual's pain threshold is crossed. Some deep tissue techniques advise that the most constructive therapy takes place at a depth and intensity that is barely tolerable to the client. When the pain threshold is violated, the client will tense up and the work will become less effective. Some bodywork does produce discomfort that is constructive; however, the pressure should never be so deep that it would hurt the client. Pain that hurts can not only damage the body, it can destroy the client's trust and ruin the therapeutic relationship. The first rule of massage and bodywork is: Do no harm!

QUESTIONS FOR DISCUSSION AND REVIEW

1. Name six basic classifications of movements used in massage.
2. What control should the practitioner have over the massage treatment?
3. Over which parts of the body are light movements applied?
4. Over which parts of the body are heavy movements applied?
5. In which direction is massage generally applied?
6. When are massage movements directed away from the heart?
7. What is the approximate duration of a full-body massage?

8. In terms of a massage technique, what is touch?
9. How is light touch administered, and what are its effects?
10. How is deep touch given, and when is it used?
11. How is aura stroking performed?
12. What is another name for feather stroking, and how is it used?
13. What is effleurage?
14. Which kind of effleurage requires the lightest possible touch?
15. Which kind of effleurage requires firm pressure?
16. What are the benefits of superficial gliding strokes?
17. What are the benefits of deep gliding strokes?
18. How is the kneading movement applied in massage?
19. What are the benefits of kneading?
20. What is the classical term that means the same as kneading?
21. For what part of the body is the fulling movement recommended?
22. What is the proper way to apply friction movements to the body?
23. What are the effects of friction on the connective tissue?
24. How is cross-fiber friction applied?
25. In what manner are compression movements applied to the body?
26. What are the benefits of compression movements?
27. What is the proper way to apply vibratory movements to the body?
28. What is a safe rate of vibration?
29. How can the practitioner control the effects produced by vibratory movements?
30. Why is excessive vibration harmful?
31. What is the proper way to apply percussion movements to the body?
32. Name the various forms of percussion movements.
33. What are the benefits of percussion movements?
34. To which parts of the body can joint movements be applied?
35. Name two types of joint movements.
36. Describe the difference between active assistive joint movements and active resistive joint movements.
37. What is range of motion?
38. Define *end feel*.
39. How is pressure regulated during a massage?
40. What is the significance of a pain threshold in the practice of massage?

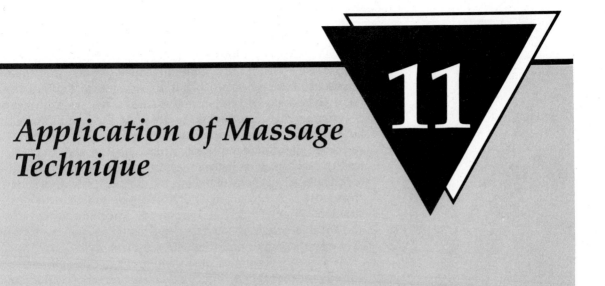

Application of Massage Technique

11

Learning Objectives

After you have mastered this chapter, you will be able to:

1. Demonstrate mastery of various hand exercises specifically for the benefit of massage practitioners.

2. Demonstrate correct standing posture and movements specifically for the benefit of massage practitioners.

3. Explain why it is necessary and desirable for the massage practitioner to develop coordination, balance, control, and stamina.

4. Explain why it is necessary and desirable for the massage practitioner to develop strong, flexible hands.

5. Describe the concepts of grounding and centering and how these practices benefit the massage practitioner.

▼ INTRODUCTION

In recent times the various movements used in body massage have been studied scientifically. Some movements are devised to induce relaxation while others are meant to invigorate and stimulate the body. The massage practitioner is primarily concerned with manual movements that have beneficial effects on the client's body and how to apply these movements correctly and effectively. The correct application of the massage movements described in Chapter 10 requires more than the use of the practitioner's hands against the client's skin. When done correctly, the therapists whole body is engaged in each movement. The feet are the foundation, the legs the strength, the pelvis and torso supply the power, the heart the love and compassion, and the arms and hands supply the intricate dexterity and communication with the client.

Massage is a strenuous practice and, when done correctly, requires a great deal of energy. By learning correct body mechanics and using good posture, the practitioner can reduce the effort and conserve energy when doing several massages a day.

▼ BUILDING STRENGTH AND FLEXIBILITY OF THE HANDS

The practitioner's hands are the most important tools used in massage. Hand mobility is important to maintain a regular rhythm and control when doing slow or fast movements. Flexible hands aid in working on the contours of the client's body and in controlling both speed and pressure. In addition to well-trained hands, the practitioner must have a good sense of balance and body control in order to move efficiently while applying various massage movements. While the hands are the main implements delivering the manipulations to the client, the positioning and the strength of the

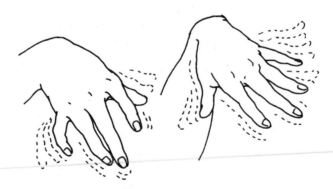

Fig. 11.1a Hold your hands at chest level and shake them vigorously for about ten counts. This exercise warms and limbers the hands.

entire body are essential to deliver effective massages over an extended period of time. The exercises shown will help develop strength, control, and flexibility of the hands (Fig. 11.1a–h and 11.2).

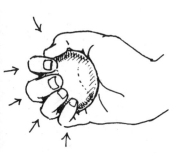

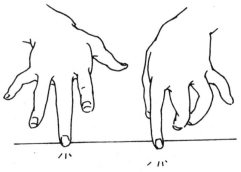

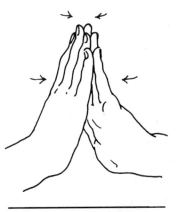

Fig. 11.1b Hold your hands at chest level. Use a small ball or clinch your hands into tight fists. Squeeze the ball or fists as hard as you can while counting to ten. Repeat this exercise several times. This exercise will strengthen your hands and wrists.

Fig. 11.1c Place both hands palm down on a flat surface. Begin with the thumbs and count each finger to the little finger and back to the thumbs. This exercise is similar to playing a piano or typing;. It is excellent for improving coordination and hand control.

Fig. 11.1d Place your palms together at chest level. Press one hand against the other back and forth. This will make your wrists supple and strong. Repeat the presses about ten times.

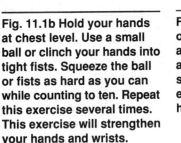

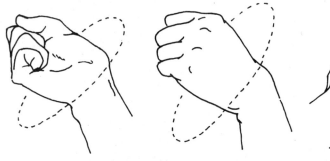

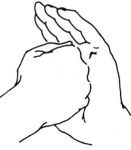

Fig. 11.1e Beginning with the thumb of the left hand, massage all the fingers of that hand by rubbing each finger from the knuckles of the hand to the tip of the finger. Repeat on the right hand. This exercise stimulates circulation and helps keep the hands supple.

Fig. 11.1f Hold your hands in fists at chest level. Rotate both hands in circles forward ten times, then reverse ten times. This exercise strengthens and limbers the wrists.

Fig. 11.1g Press the fist of one hand into the palm of the other, with each hand resisting the other. Do this ten times on each hand. This exercise will strengthen the entire arm and the hand.

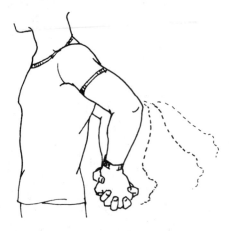

Fig. 11.1h Clasp your hands just below your waistline at the back of your body. Pull your arms upward while holding the tension for ten counts. Pull your arms downward for ten counts. This exercise strengthens the muscles of your arms, shoulders, and hands.

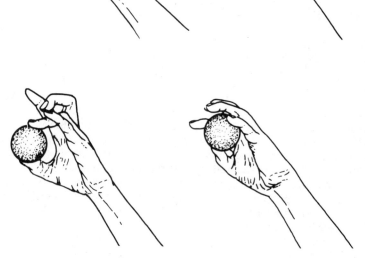

Fig. 11.2 Hold a semisoft foam rubber ball between the thumb and first finger. Squeeze the ball as hard as possible, ten times. Repeat, squeezing the ball with the second, third, and fourth fingers. Shake and massage that hand and repeat the exercise with the other hand.

▼ BODY MECHANICS

Even though the hands are the primary implement to touch the client, all of the practitioner's body is used to deliver massage manipulations. Proper positioning of the feet, the strength of the legs, the position of the back, shoulders, and head, and breathing all play an important role in the effective delivery of the massage, the level of fatigue, and the long-term health of the practitioner.

Body mechanics is the observation of body postures in relation to safe and efficient movement in daily living activities. Using good body mechanics increases the strength and power available in a movement while at the same time reducing the risk of potential injury to the practitioner.

Performing a full-body massage is a strenuous process. A professional massage therapist will perform six to ten massages a day. To do this, the practitioner must conserve his or her energy.

Even though the hands are the point of contact during a massage, if the practitioner depends solely on the hands and arms to do the massage, the hands and arms will fatigue quickly. When the arms are overextended to perform long strokes or reach a distant body part, control, force, and pressure are compromised. Overreaching usually requires bending at the waist, which puts the back in a strained position.

The practitioner can eliminate these problems by using good body mechanics and movement. By keeping the hands relatively close to the center of the body and the knees slightly flexed and feet apart, the practitioner uses the muscles in the legs and the movement of the whole body to deliver the strokes. When performing a manipulation that requires deep pressure or more force, the practitioner keeps the hand and arm in a stable position and leans the body into the movement. The practice of keeping the hands in good alignment and close to the practitioner's body and moving the whole body conserves energy and increases the power and strength when performing massage (Fig. 11.3).

The risk of injury is directly proportionate to the amount of stress and the amount of biomechanical deviation. This is easy to observe in acute injuries such as a sprained ankle or a strained back. If a force is applied when the body is not in proper alignment, the result

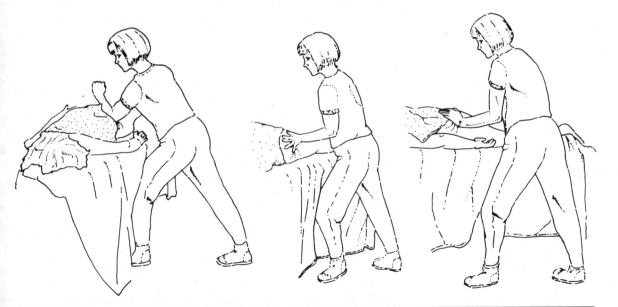

Fig. 11.3 Using good body mechanics and leaning into movements improves efficiency, power, and strength while reducing stress on the therapist.

could be a torn ligament, tendon, muscle, or even a broken bone. Poor body mechanics practiced over a period of time become bad postural habits that cause structural (biomechanical) deviations. When the stress of muscular activity or even gravity is added to the biomechanically weak structure, dysfunction, pain and injury will eventually result. This is precisely why many of your clients are seeking relief. It is important for the practitioner to avoid positions and practices that put undo stress on the back, neck, shoulders, arms, and hands.

As a massage therapist you must develop good body mechanics. Using proper body positioning and posture will enable you to deliver powerful strokes and manipulations with a minimum of effort. Proper position and alignment of the back, shoulders, arms, wrists, and hands, especially when delivering forceful movements, will reduce the chance of overuse syndrome and injury.

The quality, effectiveness, and efficiency of nearly any massage manipulation is enhanced by incorporating body mechanics and movement. Engaging the body when applying stroking, kneading, and friction produces deeper, smoother, and more penetrating results with less effort and fatigue.

▼ POSTURE AND STANCES

Correct posture and stances (foot positions) are important to the practitioner because they aid balance and allow the delivery of firmer, more powerful, more direct massage strokes. Proper stances allow the practitioner to lean into and out of the movements to deliver manipulations that penetrate with minimum effort and maximum effect. Correct posture is essential to conserve strength and prevent backache due to improper body mechanics that would put too much stress on the practitioner's arms and shoulders during the massage procedure. Good posture and body mechanics help sustain energy when it is necessary to work long hours, because they enable the practitioner to move around the table more freely and easily while maintaining the flow of movement and energy.

The most common stances are called the horse and the archer.

Horse Stance

In the horse stance, both feet are placed in line with the edge of the massage table. This is the most comfortable stance when doing petrissage on the legs or back. The knees are kept slightly flexed so the therapist can apply firmer pressure to the manipulations by shifting his or her weight and leaning into the client, thereby preserving the strength in the arms. The back remains erect and relaxed. The shoulders are comfortably dropped and back. The breathing is deep and full (Fig. 11.4).

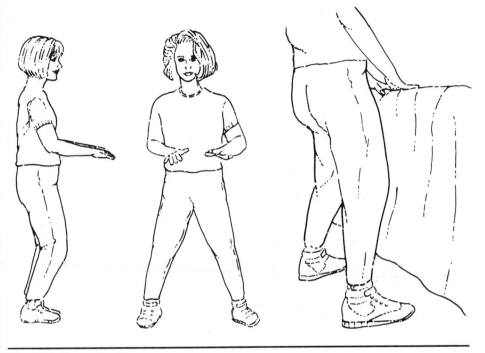

Fig. 11.4 Horse stance.

Archer Stance

The archer stance is the most commonly used position, especially when the practitioner's shoulders are at an angle (other than parallel) with the edge of the table or when the practitioner is stepping into a movement. For the archer stance, the feet are positioned so that an imaginary line drawn through the center of one foot at the arch passes through the other foot at midheel and the third toe. The feet may be close together or a full stride apart. This foot position provides a solid, stable foundation for the therapist to lean into or pull back on a manipulation. By shifting his or her weight from one foot to the other, the therapist can perform long rhythmic strokes without sacrificing good posture. This foot position also provides excellent mobility so the therapist can step into or away from a movement smoothly and at the same time maintain contact and pressure. This eliminates the need to bend at the waist. The mobility allows the therapist's hands to remain close to his or her body, where they retain more control and strength. Mobility uses the muscles of the legs to provide much of the movement and strength for many of the manipulations. This, along with the practice of leaning and stepping into or away from the movement, provides a large portion of the energy needed to deliver massage treatments.

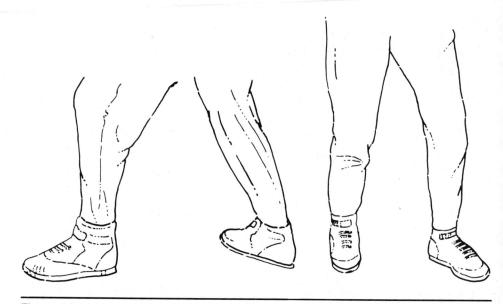

Fig. 11.5 In the archer stance, the forward foot is pointing in the direction of the movement.

In either stance the knees and ankles should be kept flexed slightly. Stiff, rigid knees contribute to fatigue, while locking the knees forces a posture that puts the back in danger of injury. The back remains relatively erect and stable. When it is necessary to lean over, the practitioner can step forward and bend from the hips, thereby maintaining the integrity of the spine.

Often the tendency when performing massage is to tighten and raise the shoulders. The shoulders should remain relaxed and dropped to ensure optimum nerve and blood supply to the hands and arms. It is also important that the breathing be deep and full to supply plenty of oxygen and eliminate carbon dioxide.

Correct stances make it easier to shift weight from foot to foot so movement is smooth, as in dancing. Correct stances give the practitioner more body power when leaning into the movements (Fig. 11.5).

▼ EXERCISES FOR STRENGTH, BALANCE, AND BODY CONTROL

Two techniques called centering and grounding are important to the practitioner because they provide a psychological, energetic, and physical base from which to work.

Centering: Centering is based on the concept that you have a geographical center in your body located about two inches below the navel in the pelvic area. The Chinese refer to this as the *tan tein* (don te-in). Many of the ancient writings about martial arts mention this concept. Having a sense of that center and moving from that center provides a quality of power, balance, and control.

Centering has both a physical and psycho-emotional context. Emotionally, being centered refers to a certain confident sense of balance and self-assurance. Being centered means you feel self-assured and emotionally stable. Being uncentered means you feel insecure and unstable. Feeling centered (in control) is of value because it is important to be able to handle problems that arise without becoming frustrated or emotionally overwhelmed. Centering is accomplished by concentrating on the geographical center (Tan Tein) and on being self-assured (Fig. 11.6).

Grounding: Grounding is based on the concept that you have a connection with the client and that you function as something of a grounding apparatus, helping the client to release unwanted tension and feelings of stress. Grounding is achieved by mentally visualizing yourself as having the ability to draw from a greater power or energy. By being grounded, you become a sort of conduit or conductor that allows the energies to pass through you. The negative energies can pass out of the client and the positive energies can be directed into the client through you. Grounding allows these energy transfers to take place without the practitioner being drained of your own energy or picking up any unwanted tension or stress from the client. Try thinking of yourself as a tree rooted to the ground. Controlled breathing is also helpful. The concepts of grounding and centering will become more clear as you master the following exercises (Fig. 11.7).

Exercise 1—Grinding Corn

This exercise helps you reach the full length of the part of the client's body that is being worked on by being able to shift your weight easily from one foot to the other while maintaining good posture and balance. The exercise is called grinding corn because the movement is similar to using an old-fashioned hand corn grinder. You may also think of it as a movement similar to polishing a car. Use your imagination.

Procedure: Place your feet apart (about the width of your shoulders) and tilt your pelvis forward and upward. Bend your knees, and sink down until you are in a semi-knee-bend. Do not go all the way down to a squatting position. Keep your back straight, and don't allow your head to jut forward. While maintaining this posture, hold your hands in front of your body (palms down) about the level of your waistline. Now begin to move both hands toward the right, forming a wide oval. This will look as if you are ready for a karate move.

After you get the feel of the standing position and hand movements, begin to move the right hand clockwise and the left hand counterclockwise. Shift your weight from foot to foot. Keep making the ovals (keeping your back straight) until you are comfortable with the movement. Lower your hands about six inches by bending your knees into a deeper knee bend. Continue practicing. As you

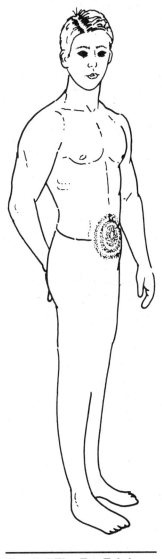

Fig. 11.6 The *Tan Tein* is the geographical and energetic center of the body.

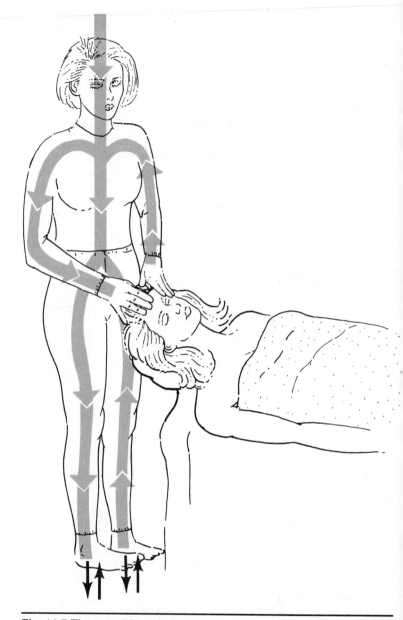

Fig. 11.7 The practitioner's body serves as a conduit for positive energy to be transmitted into the client and negative energy to be grounded out of the client.

continue the exercise, become aware of the centering concept previously described and allow your movements to be initiated from the pelvic area (about two inches below the navel), with the rest of your body following through. Remember, this is your geographical area or center which allows your entire body to move with balance and strength (Figs. 11.8a to c).

This exercise can be performed while standing next to a massage table. As you practice the movement, glide your hands lightly over the surface of the table. Gradually increase the area your hands cover until you are able to reach from one end of the table to the other and from one side to the other. To do this, shift your weight from one foot to the other. Be conscious of your balance, and do not compromise your back by extending or leaning too far.

As you master these techniques and continue to practice them, your arms, hands, and shoulders will become less fatigued because of the support supplied by the rest of your body.

Exercise 2—The Wheel

Procedure: First, take a deep breath and exhale slowly. Repeat this several times. This exercise helps you to relax. Take a comfortable stance with your feet about six inches apart. Turn the left foot out at a 45° angle. Shift most of your weight to the left foot while bending the left knee slightly. With the left heel remaining on the

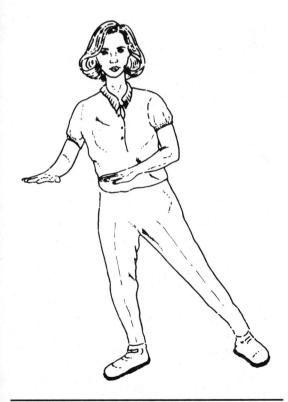 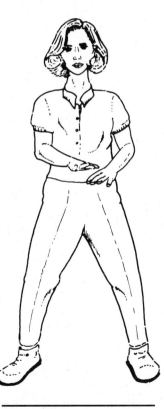

Fig. 11.8a Grinding corn: Move to the right, making large ovals with the hands and transferring the weight to the right foot.

Fig. 11.8b Grinding corn: front view.

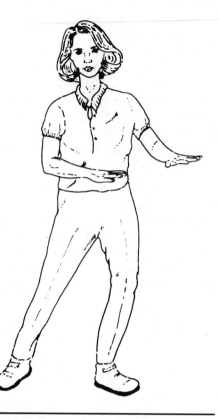

Fig. 11.8c Grinding corn builds strength in the legs as it teaches balance and coordination.

floor, step forward with the right foot. Remember to keep your hips and shoulders facing forward and your knees bent. The right foot should be forward about fifteen to twenty inches. Shift your weight forward to the right foot then back again to the left, in a smooth motion, so that 90 percent of your weight shifts from one foot to the other. Once you have the feel of the stance, take a deep breath and exhale slowly while placing your hands about six inches apart with palms facing one another. Begin making circles with your hands while imagining that you are rotating a large wheel that is suspended in front of you. The top of the wheel is about shoulder level, and the bottom is at the level of your pubic bone. As you shift your weight forward, reach out and rotate the wheel up. Shift your weight back as you rotate the wheel back and down. Continue the movement and breath deeply and slowly so that with each full revolution of the wheel, you take one full breath (inhale and exhale). Without breaking your rhythm, turn your right foot to a 45° angle and take one step forward. Repeat the exercise several times (Fig. 11.9a–c).

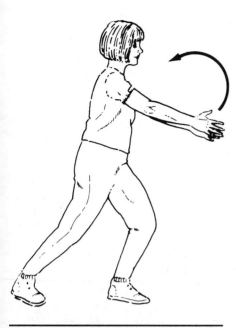

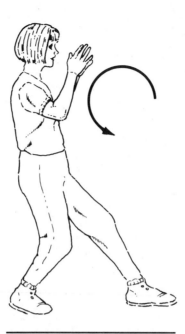

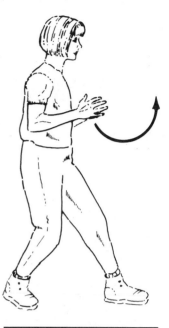

Fig. 11.9a The wheel is a good centering exercise that teaches deep breathing, balance, and moving from the center (Tan Tein).

Fig. 11.9b The wheel: The body weight shifts forward and back from one foot to the other.

Fig. 11.9c The wheel: The hands describe a large wheel. Each revolution of the wheel requires one full breath.

To complete the exercise, bring your feet together so that your weight is distributed evenly. Turn your palms facing downward and allow your hands to float down to your sides. Stay in this position for a few seconds to experience the feeling. As you master this movement, you will find that it is best accomplished by concentrating on originating the movement from the pelvic area (center or Tan Tein) and moving straight forward and backward while allowing the rest of your body to follow.

Exercise 3—Advance and Retreat

A variation of the wheel is a move that is valuable to the practice of massage. As the name implies, advance and retreat involves a powerful forward movement followed by a controlled withdrawal.

Procedure: The position of the feet is essentially the same as for the wheel or the archer stance. The back foot is turned approximately 45° while the front foot is pointing in the direction of the movement. The distance the feet are apart determines the length and the power of the movement. Optimally the feet should be between sixteen and thirty-two inches apart. The knees remain flexed as 80 percent of the body weight moves from one foot to the other. The hands are positioned at about belt level and close to the

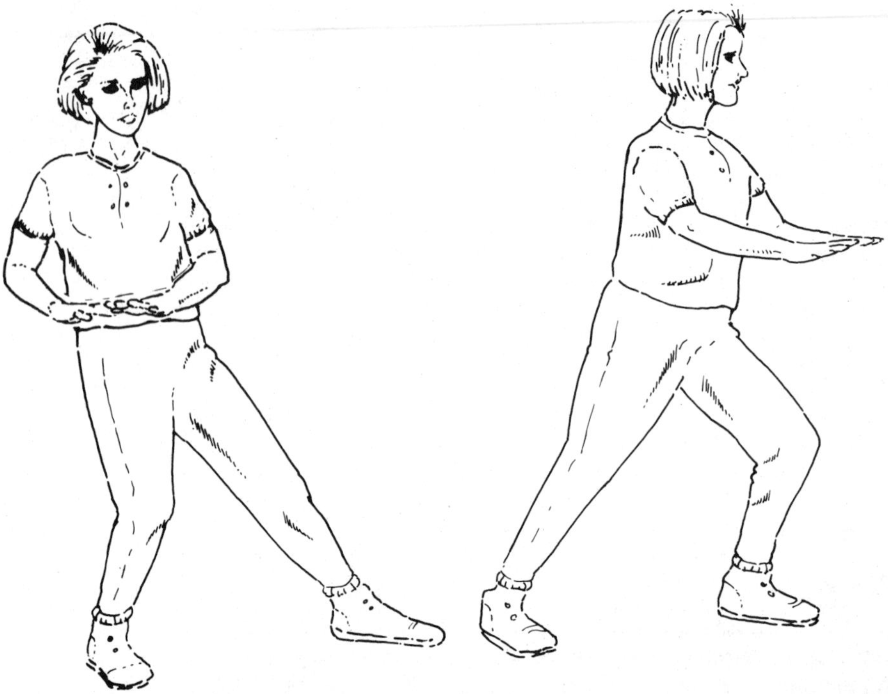

Fig. 11.10 Advance and retreat: The hands are held at the same height as the *Tan Tein*. The feet are in a wide archer stance. Retreat: Ninety percent of the weight is on the back foot. Hands are down to one side and upper body posture is erect. The body weight is shifted smoothly and powerfully forward. Advance: eighty percent of weight is shifted to the front leg. The arms are extended forward. The upper body maintains an erect posture.

side of the body. The primary movement is the hips and pelvis as they move straight forward and back. The hips do not move up or down, just straight forward and back. The torso remains perpendicular, and the hands accentuate the move only slightly. Change the position of the feet and the hands move to the other side of the body (Fig. 11.10).

Advance and retreat can be performed at the side of a massage table to illustrate the usefulness of the maneuver. Stand at the side of a massage table near one end, facing the other end. Turn the foot nearest the table 45°. Step forward with the outside foot. Bend both knees slightly. Rest both hands on the table beside and slightly in front of you. (Your hands should be close to your body and about the level or the Tan Tein.) Shift your weight from one foot to the other. Notice how much of the length of the table you cover while moving your arms very little (Fig. 11.11).

Exercise 4—The Tree

This exercise emphasizes the importance of posture and concentration and is combined with centering, grounding, and correct breathing.

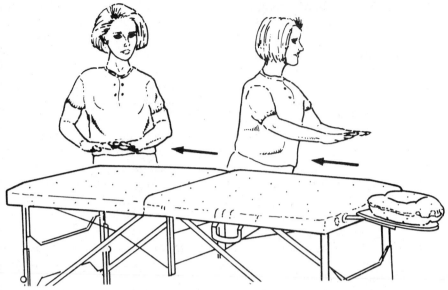

Fig. 11.11 Using advance and retreat at the massage table allows the practitioner to move the length of the table in one stroke while maintaining good body mechanics.

Procedure: Stand with your feet together, with your shoulders relaxed down and back. Pull your buttocks downward slightly. This will cause your pelvis to tilt upward. Take a deep breath and exhale slowly. Begin the exercise by turning the left foot out (bending the left knee) and shifting all your weight to the left foot. Keep your upper body erect. Move the right foot straight forward so that when the right leg is extended, the ball of the right foot rests lightly on the floor. Bring both arms up to about shoulder level to form a circle. This should look as if you are trying to reach around a large tree. Your fingers will be pointing toward each other, about two inches apart. Keep your head up, chin level, and gaze ahead. As you hold this pose, the leg bearing your weight may feel weak and begin to tremble. However, by maintaining the pose for about three minutes at a time and practicing your breathing exercises, you will soon experience a sense of renewed strength and power.

Change the pose to the left foot position (left foot forward) with your weight on the right foot, and continue to breathe deeply, exhaling slowly. Alternate the right and left feet, continuing to practice until you feel completely in control. To finish the exercise, bring your feet to a side-by-side position with your weight distributed evenly and your back straight. Allow your arms to float down to your sides. Take a moment to experience what is happening to your body (Fig. 11.12).

Although you may find these exercises tiring and sometimes boring, remember that there is no easy way to accomplish erect

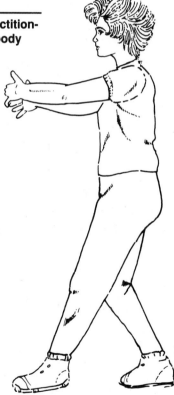

Fig. 11.12 The tree builds strength and endurance in the legs and shoulders as it encourages concentration and breathing.

posture, body strength, coordination, and proper breathing. Keep foremost in your mind that your goal is to be able to perform efficiently as a master of massage techniques. As you begin to do professional massage, you will see how these exercises increase your feeling of self-esteem.

▼ CONTACT WITH THE CLIENT AND QUALITY OF TOUCH

In administering a massage, there is much more to take into account than the application of strokes to various parts of the client's body. The practitioner must be aware of contact with the client and quality of touch, the constitution or composition for the massage itself, how the body is used in the application of the various movements, and the role breathing plays for both the practitioner and the client.

The way that touch is administered to the client determines the success of the massage and is often the reason a client will return and ask for a particular practitioner.

From the time a client enters a massage establishment, the confidence and ability of the practitioner are communicated. The confidence shown through the initial contact touch instills a certain trust in the recipient that encourages relaxation.

It is important for the practitioner to maintain contact with the client throughout the course of a full massage. If the client is in a state of wakeful conversation with eyes open and is following the moves of the practitioner, then there is verbal and visual contact. However, if the client is in a state of relaxation with eyes closed, the sense of touch is the only communication. If contact is broken, there is an immediate reaction of concern on the part of the client and relaxation may change to anxiety.

▼ THE MASSAGE SEQUENCE

Sequence refers to the pattern or design of a massage. Developing a good sequence is especially important because it coordinates and organizes the massage so there is smooth progression from one stroke to the next and from one body part to the next. Sequence provides a framework for a thought-out, logical progression and at the same time allows for flexibility and creativity.

The sequence of the overall massage is designed in a logical progression that leaves the client with a feeling of completedness. Although a sequence may vary according to the situation, a pattern should be used that ensures that every part of the body is massaged properly and thoroughly.

Massage movements for adjacent areas as well as bi-lateral body parts should follow in sequence. For example, when beginning with the hand, the massage should progress to the arm and then to the shoulder. Then massage the other hand, arm, and shoulder, followed by massage of both shoulders, the neck, and the head. Finally, massage the chest, abdomen, one leg and foot, followed by massage of the other leg and foot. This completes the massage for the front of the body.

There are many possibilities for putting it all together; therefore it is important to follow a plan that ensures completeness and balance.

Developing a sequence also insures a thorough massage that is balanced between one body part and another. The following is an example of an effective sequence to be used on each body area.

1. Make contact with, and undrape the body part to be massaged.
2. Apply massage oil with light effleurage.
3. Apply effleurage to accustom the body to your touch. Effleurage also flushes out the lymph and venous blood.
4. Apply petrissage, kneading the tissues to warm them. This also enables you to become aware of any areas of tension or congestion in the muscles.
5. Apply effleurage to flush the area.
6. Apply friction by using any of the recommended friction techniques.
7. Apply effleurage to the area again, because this flushes the area while linking and integrating the segmented parts back into the whole.
8. Do joint movements to restore mobility by reinforcing the possibility of movement. At the same time, joint movements stretch the muscles and connective tissues, and lubricate the joints.
9. Apply effleurage to flush out the loosened debris and to give a feeling of length to the body part.
10. Apply feather strokes. This stimulates the peripheral nervous system, smooths the energy field, and says good-bye to that part of the body.
11. Redrape the part of the body that has been massaged, undrape the next part, and continue until the client has been given a thorough massage.

PROFESSIONAL RULES TO REMEMBER ▼

Knowledge of the restrictions and limitations of massage is as important as knowledge of its proper use. A well-trained practitioner knows when a massage treatment is indicated, how it can be modified for the greatest benefit to the client, and under what circumstances it should not be applied.

Before beginning the massage routines discussed in the next chapter, review the basic rules for safe and effective massage procedures.

1. Everything used in massage treatments should be clean and sanitary.

2. Wash your hands thoroughly with soap and hot water and rinse and dry them before and after each treatment.
3. Keep your nails short and smooth to avoid scratching the client's skin.
4. Avoid chilling the client by contact with cold hands or by having the temperature of the room too low for comfort.
5. Avoid massage immediately after the client has eaten a meal.
6. Avoid heavy, rapid, or jarring movements that might convey fear of injury to the client.
7. Never use any form of heavy stroking against the venous blood supply.
8. When the client is obese, it may be necessary to apply massage with more strength but not to the point of discomfort for the client.
9. Never apply massage so vigorously that it causes fatigue in the client.
10. Allow the client to have a short rest period before and after the massage.

▼

QUESTIONS FOR DISCUSSION AND REVIEW

1. Why is it necessary for the massage practitioner to develop strong, flexible hands?
2. What is body mechanics?
3. Why is it important for the massage practitioner to practice good body mechanics?
4. How can the practitioner increase the power and strength in a movement and at the same time conserve energy?
5. Why are good posture and the use of proper stances important to the massage practitioner?

Procedures for Complete Body Massages

12

Learning Objectives

After you have mastered this chapter, you will be able to:

1. Demonstrate the steps in preparing a client for a massage session.

2. Demonstrate correct procedures for draping the client.

3. Explain the importance of assisting a client onto and off of a massage table.

4. Demonstrate a basic body massage (Massage 1).

5. Demonstrate massage variations (Massage 2).

6. Use correct anatomical terms when describing the part of the body being massaged.

7. Demonstrate correct posture and stances for the massage practitioner.

8. Demonstrate professional courtesies toward clients before, during, and after massage.

9. Understand when and where certain massage movements should and should not be applied.

10. Answer the client's questions concerning any aftereffects of massage.

11. Describe the four parts of the therapeutic procedure.

12. *Demonstrate assessment by passive, active, and resisted movement.*

13. *Explain how assessment findings are used to develop session strategies.*

14. *Explain the importance of evaluation.*

▼ INTRODUCTION

Massage procedure is the actual process of performing a massage therapy session. There are as many variations of doing a massage as there are therapists giving and clients receiving massages. Practitioners may adopt a routine and practice it on every client they see or the therapist may provide therapeutic services tailored to the specific needs of a client on the day of his or her appointment. Regardless of the style and content of the massage treatment, guidelines should be followed to ensure that the services received by the client meet high professional standards and the client's expectations. Clients who receive courteous professional services will regard the treatment with respect. They will repeat business and refer others to your service.

▼ PREPARING THE CLIENT FOR THE MASSAGE

When the preliminary interview is done and the client has completed any necessary forms, it is time to begin the actual massage. If this is the first time you have seen this client or if it is the client's first massage, an explanation of your services and clear instructions about what the client should do will eliminate false expectations and dispel much of the anxiety the client may have. At the end of the preliminary consultation when a strategy for the session has been formulated, briefly explain to the client what you will be doing and why. Show the client the facilities and explain the use of any equipment, such as steam baths or exercisers. Explain the dressing procedures and draping. Show the client the dressing room or area and explain the use of any wraps or drapes the client may use to get from the dressing area to the table.

Two commonly asked questions are "Do I have to take off my clothes?" And "How many of my clothes do I have to take off?" The most effective way to receive a massage is with all clothing removed. With proper draping, a client's modesty should never be compromised. However, many people (especially first timers) are not comfortable with all of their clothes removed. The client's comfort is of primary importance. Instruct the client that the best way to receive a massage is with all clothes removed and that draping will be used at all times. Also give clients the option to leave on whatever they feel comfortable with. Many people will choose to wear their underwear, but even if they choose to remain fully clothed, it is possible to perform a massage through clothing. As time goes on and clients receive more massages, they may become more accustomed to the procedure and comfortable with their own body.

ASSISTING THE CLIENT ON AND OFF THE TABLE ▼

For reasons of safety and liability, it is advisable that the practitioner assist the client onto the table at the beginning of a massage and into a sitting position and off the table at the end of the massage.

The table may be too high for some clients, or various disabilities may prevent easy access to the table. A foot stool is a useful item. It can be used as a step to assist some people onto the table and by the therapist to stand on for better leverage when performing some techniques.

The procedure you use may require the client to assume a specific position on the table. Careful instruction and physical guidance will assure that the client ends up in the proper place. By keeping a hand on clients and guiding them as they sit down on the table and then as they lie down, you greatly reduce the possibility of injury and clients are more likely to assume the position necessary to perform the massage. Maintaining contact as the client gets on and off of the table also provides a feeling of comfort and security.

Draping procedures must include techniques that allow these movements to be accomplished while keeping the client modestly covered (Fig. 12.1a and b).

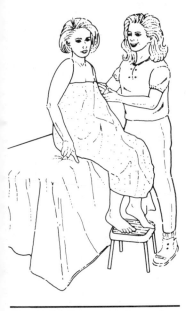

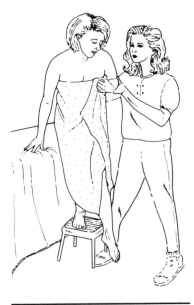

Fig. 12.1a A stepstool may be used to help the client get onto the table.

Fig. 12.1b It is helpful for the therapist to lend a hand as the client gets on and off the table.

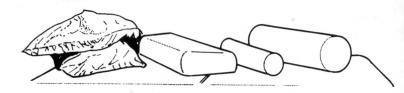

Fig. 12.2 A variety of bolsters can be used to position the client for comfort.

▼ POSITIONING THE CLIENT ON THE MASSAGE TABLE

The client should assume a position on the massage table that is comfortable and allows access to the body in order to perform the massage. Once the client is sitting on the table, instruct and assist him or her to lie down either face up or down, depending on the treatment to be given. When the client is lying down, he or she must be able to relax.

You might encounter a person who cannot comfortably lie on his or her back or face down without support. In such cases it is helpful to have foam cushions and bolsters in various shapes and sizes. These are made of fairly high-density foam and are covered with vinyl for easy cleaning.

Bolsters as wide as the table and four to eight inches in diameter can be used under the client's knees when clients are lying on their back. A bolster may be placed under the ankles when the client is lying face down. Positioning with bolsters provides more comfort for the client who has reduced flexibility in the ankles, knees, or lower back. Firm bed pillows may also be used (Fig. 12.2).

Another consideration for positioning the client face down is to have a support to place under the client's chest to take the pressure off the cervical spine while in the prone position. This support

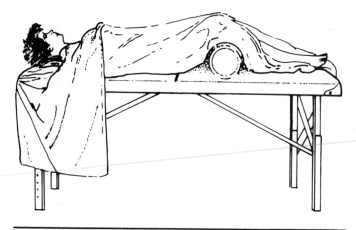

Fig. 12.3a In the supine position, a bolster behind the knees reduces tension in the back of the legs and the low back.

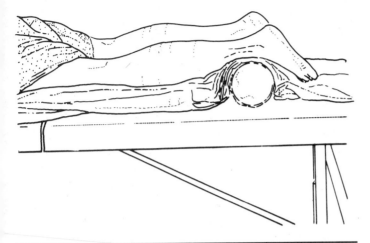

Fig. 12.3b In the prone position, a bolster under the ankles prevents hyperextension of the knee and ankle and relieves tension in the low back.

should hold the chest three to four inches off the table while allowing the head to rest forward comfortably.

Some people need support under the abdomen when they have severe low back discomfort. Elevating the midsection and abdomen six to eight inches in this manner helps you work on the back more effectively. A person who is unable to lie back with the head resting on the table will need support for head and neck as well as the small of the back and behind the legs (Fig. 12.3a to c).

You may have clients coming to you for massage who will have different problems. Some clients will be unable to lie face downward, and others will not be able to lie flat on their backs without

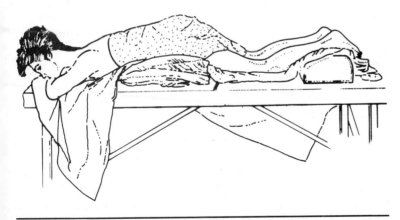

Fig. 12.3c Support under the abdomen relieves tension in the low back.

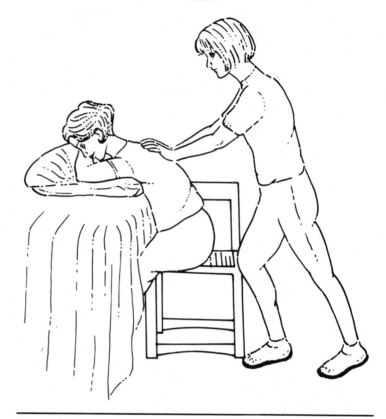

Fig. 12.4 If using a table is not practical, a supported seated massage is an alternative.

some kind of extra support. For this reason, extra supports should be a part of your professional equipment. For example, if a client is not able to get up on the massage table or lie down, you can use a chair and pillows to seat the person comfortably. You can then give a massage to the back quite easily (Fig. 12.4).

Having a variety of supporting pillows or bolsters as part of your equipment will enable you to position and support your client when necessary. All bolsters and pillows that come in direct contact with the client must have removable cloth slipcovers. Fresh clean covers are used for each client. Bolsters and pillows can also be placed under the bottom sheet next to the table to avoid contact with the client's skin.

▼ DRAPING PROCEDURES

The process of using linens to keep a client covered while performing a massage is called **draping.** This procedure allows for the client to be totally undressed and at the same time retain comfort, warmth, and modesty. It gives the practitioner the freedom to massage all parts of the body unencumbered by the client's clothing.

Proper draping ensures that the client stays warm, and feels safe and comfortable. Perspiration, oil, and being in a reclining position all increase the rate at which the body loses heat. The proper temperature for a massage room is between 75 and 80° F. If the area is cooler than this, extra precautions should be taken to make sure the client remains warm. It is much easier for a person to get chilled than to warm up. If a person is chilled, it is nearly impossible for him or her to relax.

Two items to keep on hand to deal with chilling are a twin-size electric mattress pad to put on the table under the sheet and a flannel blanket or sheet to put over the client after he or she is on the massage table and is properly draped.

By using proper draping (uncovering only the portion of the body that is being massaged) and by always concealing the client's personal parts, the practitioner maintains a professional and ethical practice while preventing embarrassment to either the practitioner or the client.

There are several methods of draping. All methods consist of techniques of maintaining personal privacy while getting the client from the dressing area to the hydrotherapy area and/or the massage table; using adequate draping while the client receives the massage; and keeping the client well covered while he or she gets up from the massage table and returns to the dressing area.

METHODS OF DRAPING ▼

There are several methods of draping that are easy and effective. In this chapter we will discuss three methods. Practice each of these until you are proficient. You may choose one style that works best for you, or you may combine portions of one method with another. While learning these various draping procedures, refer to the step-by-step directions and illustrations included in this chapter. The beginner should be careful to follow directions carefully and practice until he or she can drape a client smoothly and efficiently. It is also important to know how to instruct the client in how to change positions during the draping procedures.

Method 1—Diaper Draping

For this technique you will need a regular bath-size towel (two towels if the client is female) and a covering for the table. The table covering may be a small flat sheet, a cot-size fitted sheet, or a disposable paper sheet. The towel may also serve as the wrap the client uses to get from the dressing area to the table.

Diaper draping is suitable when the environment is very warm (80° F or warmer) so there is no chance of the client becoming chilled. This technique also ensures that the genital area is well concealed (Fig. 12.5a and b).

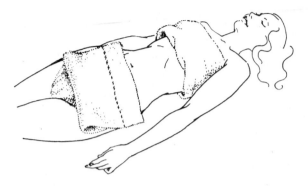

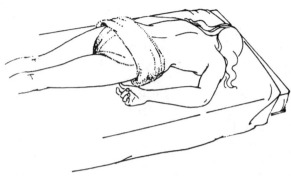

Fig. 12.5a The diaper draping method is used only when the massage area is sufficiently warm that the client will not chill.

Fig. 12.5b Fold the top of the towel neatly across the buttocks. Ask the client if the towel is comfortable and ask her to adjust it for comfort if necessary. This method makes it easy to work on the back of the body.

Method 2—Top Cover Method

This method uses a table covering as in method 1 along with a top covering that is large enough to cover the entire body. A large bath sheet towel or one half of a sheet will serve this purpose well. The minimum size for the top cover is seventy-two inches long and thirty-two inches wide.

The cover sheet may also serve as the wrap the client uses to get from the dressing area to the table.

The use of this type of draping ensures warmth and modesty while allowing easy access to each body part (Fig. 12.6).

Method 3—Full Sheet Draping

This method employs the use of a full-size double flat sheet (minimum width eighty inches) to cover the table and wrap the client. When working with a large client (200 pounds plus), it is necessary to use a queen-size sheet. When using this method it is necessary to supply an additional wrap for the client to get from the dressing area to the table. After the client is on the table the wrap is used to secure the sheet and to cover the client when he or she turns over and gets up after the massage (Fig. 12.7).

The following items may be used in the draping process.

Sheets

- Full double flat sheets (minimum width eighty inches)
- Cot-size fitted sheets
- One half of full double sheets, cut and hemmed to use as a table covering or a cover sheet
- Disposable sheets to use as table coverings when laundry is a problem

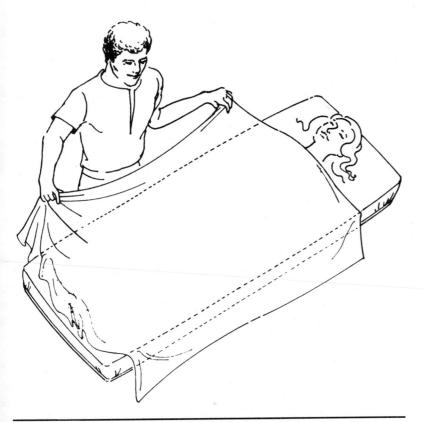

Fig. 12.6 As the client takes her place on the massage table, situate
the top cover lengthwise to cover all except her head. If the top cover
is also used as a wrap, it is rearranged from across the client's body to
a lengthwise position. If a terry wrap or towel is worn from the dressing
area, the top cover can be laid in place and the wrap discreetly slipped
from underneath.

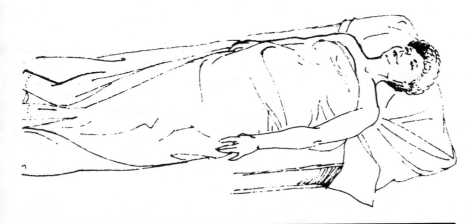

Fig. 12.7 Full sheet draping covers the client securely in a cocoon-like wrap,
and the client feels safe and warm.

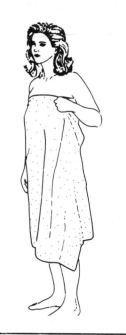

Fig. 12.8a The female wrap is long enough to cover the body and can be used as a top cover.

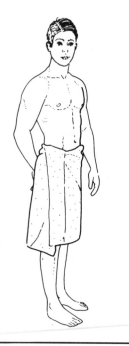

Fig. 12.8b The male wrap can be smaller but also must act as a modest covering.

Towels

- Bath-size towels for diaper draping and for personal use after hydrotherapy
- Bath sheets for body covers
- Terry cloth wraps to wear to and from the dressing area

Miscellaneous

- Pillow cases for covering pillows and bolsters
- Flannel sheets to use when extra warmth is needed
- Twin-size electric mattress pad for use on the table when warmth is a problem, such as working in a home where it is too cool

Remember that any materials coming in contact with the client's skin must be freshly laundered and sanitary. Clean linens must be used for each client.

Draping from the Dressing Area to the Massage Table

The first step in the draping process requires some form of wrap to be worn from the dressing area to either the hydrotherapy area or the massage table. The method of draping during the massage as well as the size and sex of the client will determine the type of wrap that is used. For diaper draping, a bath-size towel may be sufficient. In the cover sheet method, the cover sheet may be used. Terry cloth wraps can be provided instead of a towel for the client to wear in any method of draping. These wraps can be purchased in a department store or uniform department. The woman's wrap fastens above the breasts, while the man's wrap is a shorter version that wraps around and fastens at the waist. The length is usually just above the knees. These wraps are convenient because they secure and unfasten easily when the client is on the table, and they are easy to put back on after the massage. Wraps are available in small, large, and extra large sizes for men and women.

When using a wrap or a towel, the client arranges it so the open side is situated at the side of the body. As the client sits on the edge of the table, the wrap is lifted out of the way to avoid sitting on the wrap. The wrap is then unfastened as the client is instructed to lie down. As the client lies down, the wrap is smoothly slipped from under the body. In this way the client is lying down on the table with the wrap covering the body, not underneath (Fig. 12.8a and b).

An alternative to this procedure is to have the client lie on the table and then unfasten the wrap. Have the client lift his or her body slightly as you carefully slip the wrap from underneath.

Having gotten the client on the table, lying down, and covered by the wrap, you are ready to proceed with the draping of your choice and the massage.

When the massage has been completed and it is time for the client to get up and get dressed, a procedure must be followed that will maintain the client's privacy in a relaxed and efficient manner, while at the same time ensuring the client's safety. The illustrations shown (Fig. 12.9a to c) will be helpful.

It is important to be courteous and attentive toward your clients from the time they enter your place of business until they leave. You should show concern for their safety and comfort at all times. Some clients will want and expect help when getting on or off the massage table; others will indicate that they prefer helping themselves. When in doubt, ask. For example you might say "May I assist you?" or "Let me help you."

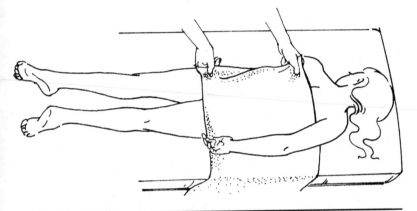

Fig. 12.9a The same wrap that the client wears from the dressing area to the massage table is used. The wrap is placed across the client's body, and other draping is removed. Instruct the client to lie on one side and arrange the wrap in such a way that it covers the back of the body with most of the wrap in front.

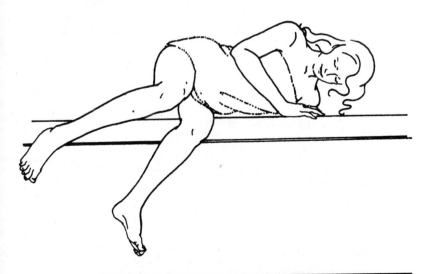

Fig. 12.9b From the prone position, the client draws her knees up so that her feet are just off the side of the table (women hold wrap over the breasts) and the practitioner assists her to a sitting position.

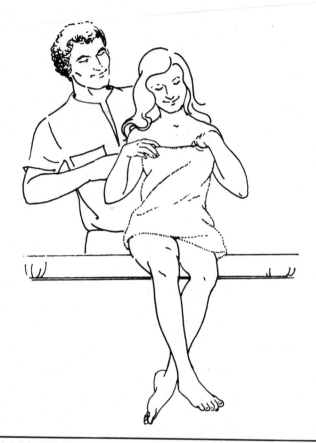

Fig. 12.9c At this point the wrap is refastened while the client is given a chance to regain composure. After a moment or two, the client is instructed to stand and return to the dressing area. As the client stands, it is advisable for the practitioner to keep one hand on the client's arm for balance and the other hand on the table to prevent it from tipping.

Alternate Method

An alternate and less desirable method is to leave the massage area while the client undresses, gets on the massage table, and uses the wrap (or towel) as a cover. At the end of the massage the practitioner leaves the room and allows the client to get off the table without assistance. This method is considered less professional because it increases the chances that the client could be injured when getting on or off the table.

Method 1—The Diaper Draping Method

Follow the illustrations for this method until you are able to remember how to do the entire procedure in a smooth and efficient manner (Fig. 12.10a to r).

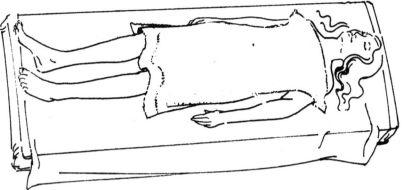

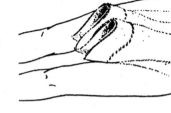

Fig. 12.10a A large terry towel is used for a covering. The towel must be long enough to cover the chest. It will come to just above the knees.

Fig. 12.10b Fold the lower end of the towel into smooth folds.

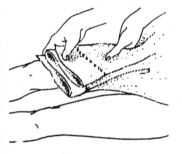

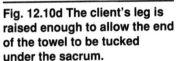

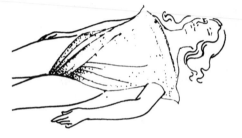

Fig. 12.10c The folds taper to fit the contours of the body.

Fig. 12.10d The client's leg is raised enough to allow the end of the towel to be tucked under the sacrum.

Fig. 12.10e The towel is in place.

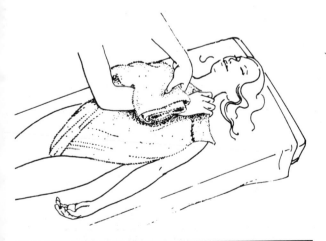

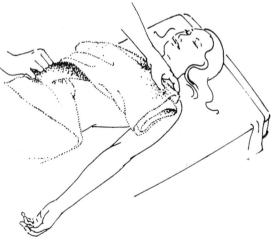

Fig. 12.10f To work on the abdomen, when the client is a woman, fold another towel to make a covering for the breasts, and place it over the first towel.

Fig. 12.10g Peel the first towel down while holding the folded towel in place over the breasts.

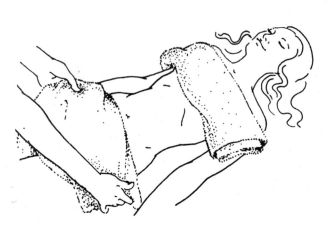

Fig. 12.10h Fold the top of the first towel neatly across the client's pelvic area.

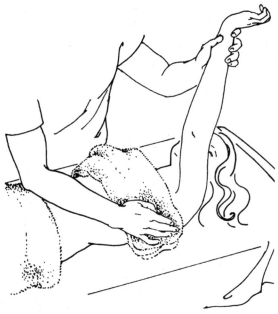

Fig. 12.10i Raise the client's arm and tuck the towel used for the breast cover neatly under the scapula to hold the ends of the towel securely in place.

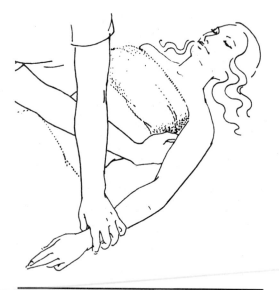

Fig. 12.10j Place the client's arm down and tuck the towel into place. Tuck the other side of the towel covering the breasts under the other scapula in the same manner.

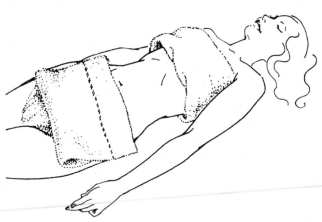

Fig. 12.10k This draping method allows you to work on the abdomen, chest, and sides of the body without exposing the breasts.

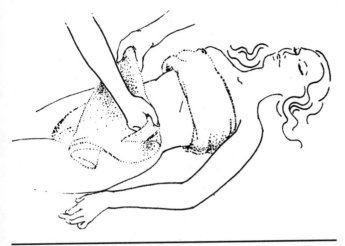

Fig. 12.10l To redrape the client, pull the towel up and over the folded towel that is covering the breasts.

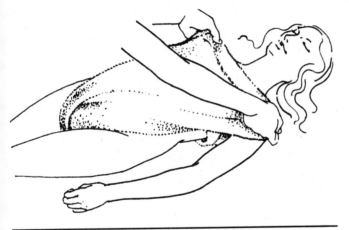

Fig. 12.10m Use the first towel as a covering while removing the towel that has been used as a breast covering.

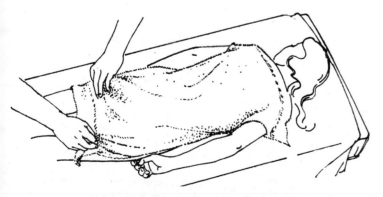

Fig. 12.10n Pull the other folded end of the towel from between the client's leg to enable her to roll into a prone (face down) position.

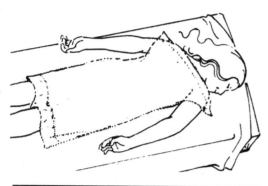

Fig. 12.10o The towel covers the client as she relaxes in the prone position.

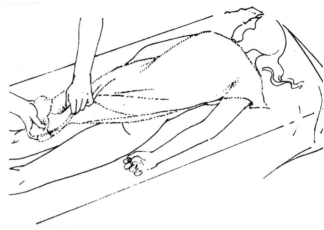

Fig. 12.10p Fold the lower portion of the towel into four folds again.

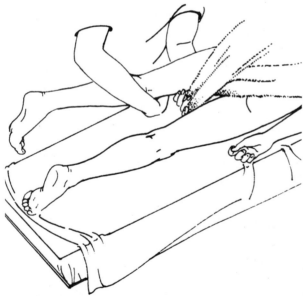

Fig. 12.10q Lift the client's leg and tuck the towel under the leg near the groin area so that it is held securely in place.

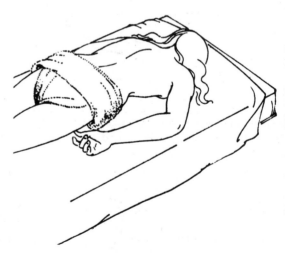

Fig. 12.10r Fold the top of the towel neatly across the buttocks. Ask the client if the towel is comfortable and ask her to adjust it for comfort if necessary. This method makes it easy to work on the back of the body. Following the massage, the procedure for getting the client off the table and properly draped is observed.

Method 2—The Top Cover Method

Follow the illustration for the method until you are able to remember how to do the entire procedure in a smooth and efficient manner (Fig. 12.11a to e).

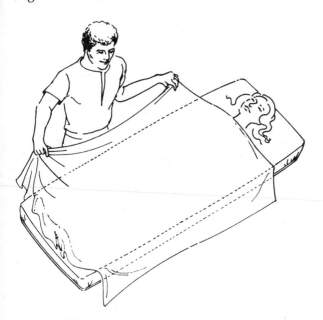

Fig. 12.11a As the client takes her place on the massage table, situate the top cover lengthwise to cover all except her head. If the top cover is also used as a wrap, it is rearranged from across the client's body to a lengthwise position. If a terry wrap or towel is worn from the dressing area, the top cover can be laid in place and the wrap discreetly slipped from underneath.

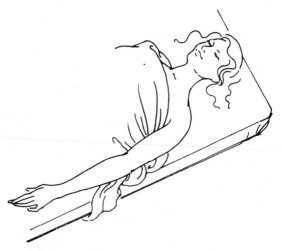

Fig. 12.11b As each arm is massaged, fold the top cover out of the way, exposing only the limb to be massaged.

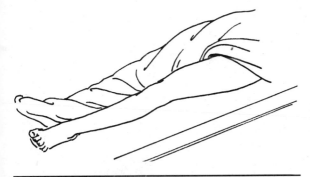

Fig. 12.11c To massage a leg, carefully tuck the cover under the opposite thigh with one hand while positioning the cover snugly along the inguinal crease, and then securing the wrap with your other hand.

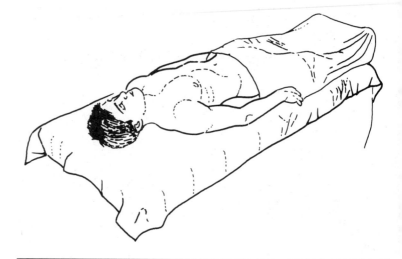

Fig. 12.11d To massage the chest and abdomen, neatly fold the top cover to the level of the hips. For a woman, the procedure described in Figures 12.10f through 12.10k may be used.

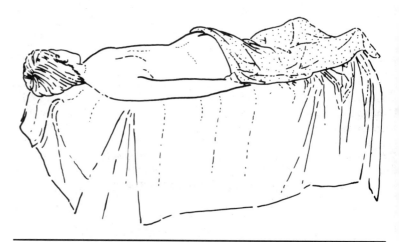

Fig. 12.11e To massage the back, neatly fold the top cover down to a level two inches below the beginning of the gluteal cleft.

When the massage is complete and it is time for the client to return to the dressing area, use the top cover for a wrap by turning the cover sideways before having the client come to a sitting position. If you choose to use a separate wrap, put the wrap in place, and while holding it with one hand, peel the top cover from underneath the wrap.

Method 3—Full Sheet Draping

The following is a step-by-step description of the full sheet draping method. It incorporates the use of a double-size flat sheet and a separate wrap or towel. First, prepare the massage table by unfolding the double-size sheet and placing it on the massage table (Fig. 12.12a to o).

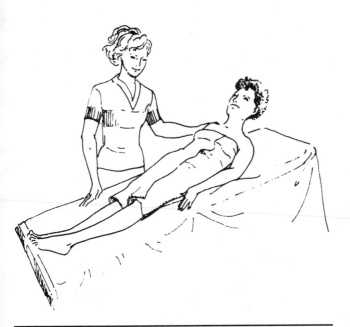

Fig. 12.12a Assist the client onto the table and into a supine (lying on her back) position. The wrap she wore to the table is used as a cover.

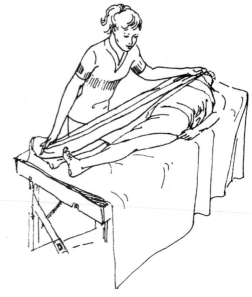

Fig. 12.12b Drape one side of the flat sheet over the client to cover her entire torso and one leg. The client may choose whether or not she wants her arms covered.

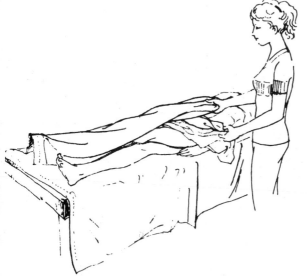

Fig. 12.12c Discreetly remove the wrap from underneath the draping.

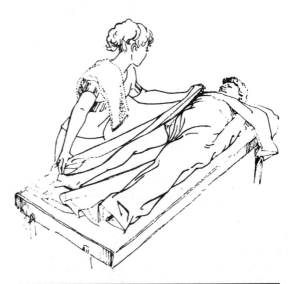

Fig. 12.12d Drape the other side of the flat sheet over the entire torso and the other leg.

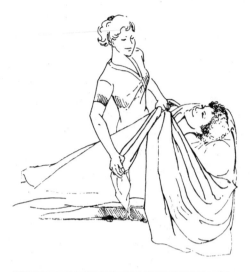

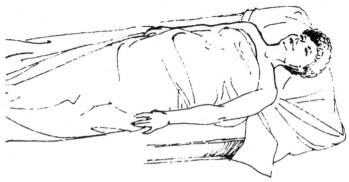

Fig. 12.12e The towel or wrap may be placed over the chest area to hold the drape in place. If it is not needed for this purpose, it may be placed aside for later use.

Fig. 12.12f If the client's arms are left outside the draping, there is no problem. (a) If the client prefers having her arms covered, then proceed with undraping them by holding the top of the draping, lifting it slightly, then reaching in with the other hand to grasp the client's wrist and lift her arm from beneath the drape. (b) After the arm has been massaged, the procedure is reversed, and the arm is placed back underneath the draping at the client's side.

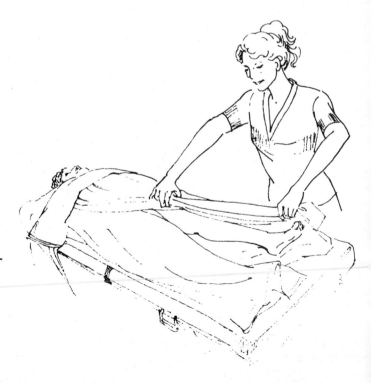

Fig. 12.12g Undraping the leg begins at the foot. Peel the sheet upward all the way to the iliac crest (hipbone). Remember that when initially draping the client, each leg was draped independently and was covered by only one layer of the draping sheet.

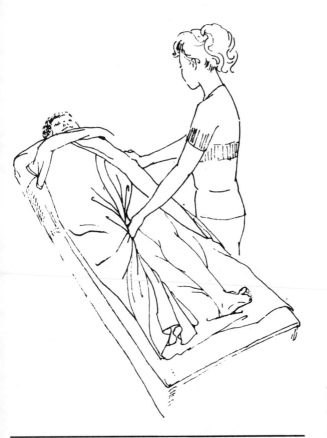

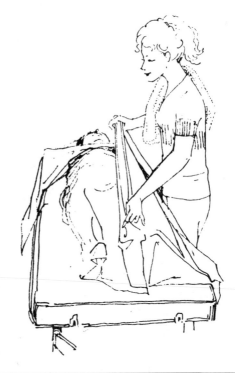

Fig. 12.12i Redrape the leg and the entire torso with the sheet on that side of the table, then proceed to the other leg in the same manner.

Fig. 12.12h Carefully tuck the drape covering the opposite leg under that thigh with one hand, while arranging the rest of the draping with the other hand across the torso and the genital area. This method assures that the client will be well covered when massaging upward to the hipbone and when performing leg stretches.

Fig. 12.12j Prepare to massage the upper part of the body by opening the draping to just above the pubic bone. When massaging a female client, fold the wrap (or towel) and use it as a breast covering. When massaging a male client, use the wrap to secure the draping at the level just above the pubic bone.

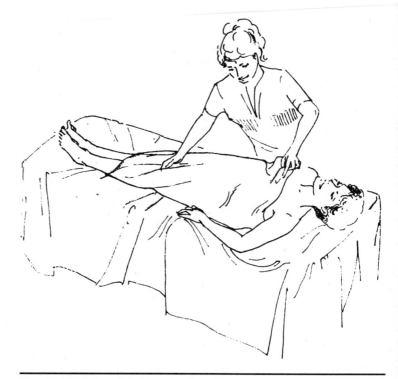

Fig. 12.12k When it is time for the client to turn over, use the wrap to cover the personal parts of the body.

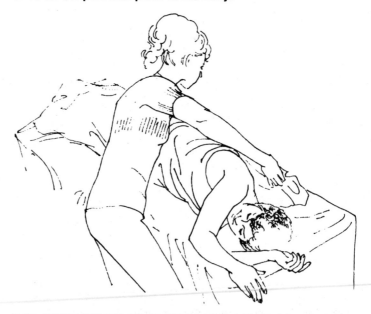

Fig. 12.12l Instruct the client to turn toward you by lifting her opposite shoulder first, then rolling onto her abdomen. Hold the wrap in place with your hands and the flat sheet in place by leaning against the table.

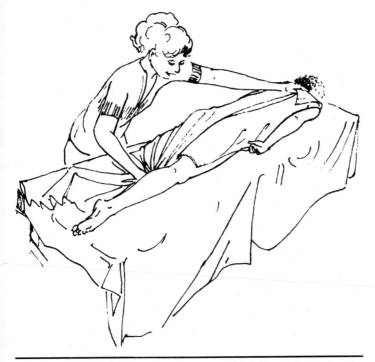

Fig. 12.12m With the client lying face down, place the wrap so that it covers the back down to the middle of the thighs. Drape the sheet over one leg and the back, then tuck it around under the same leg. Massage the other leg.

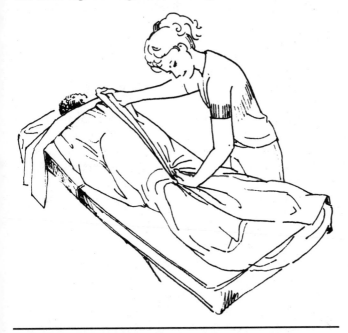

Fig. 12.12n Drape the leg after massaging it, and then undrape and massage the other leg in the same manner. Redrape the leg.

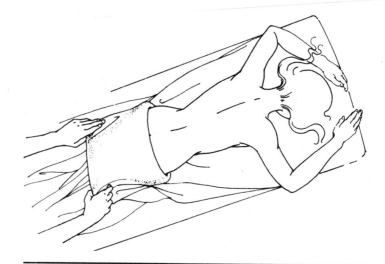

Fig. 12.12o Prepare to massage the back by peeling the wrap downward to expose the entire back. This method holds the leg draping in place and does not overly expose the gluteal area.

▼ MAINTAINING CONTACT WITH THE CLIENT

Before beginning a professional body massage, it is important to "tune in" to the client.

The massage begins when the client is positioned on the massage table and you, the practitioner, come in contact with his or her body. Once you undrape and apply oil to the part of the body to be massaged, you must remember to keep in contact with the client's body throughout the procedure. Try not to break the circuit of touch once it has been established between you and your client. Your goal is to maintain a constant flow without surges or breaks as long as contact is maintained. Once contact is lost, it can be somewhat startling to the client when you reestablish contact. Generally the person receiving the massage will have his or her eyes closed and will be in a relaxed, dream-like state as the massage progresses. As long as you maintain contact, the client will not be distracted from the relaxed state or psychic connection. It is important not to break contact until the massage is finished and the final strokes lightly feathered off.

If it is necessary to leave the client, this should be explained to the client. Explain that you must do something and will be right back. Recontact the client softly and inconspicuously. Another reason for continual contact with the client is that it allows him or her to become in touch mentally with that part of the body being massaged. For example, if a hand is being massaged and you move to an arm, as soon as contact is made, the client becomes aware of the arm and is anticipating the massage. This is why abrupt movements should be avoided at all times.

If you are massaging the client's arm and he or she is in a state of deep relaxation, and if the arm is dropped suddenly, contact is broken. This interrupts the pleasant state you have worked so hard to establish, and the client may not be able to relax again. There should be no element of surprise as the massage moves from one part of the body to another. To sum up, if you are to maintain trust on the part of the client, contact must be maintained throughout the massage procedure. The client usually comes to you for the purpose of relaxation and for the general sense of well-being that he or she receives from a good massage.

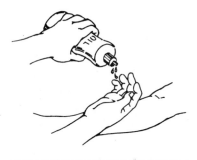

Fig. 12.13 Before beginning massage movements, undrape the body part and apply oil. With the back of your hands, maintain contact with the client's skin as you prepare to apply the massage oil.

Contact while Applying Oil

When you are ready to apply the massage oil to the client's skin, lay the back of your hand lightly against the part of the body to be massaged. Put enough oil in the palm of your hand to apply a thin film over the body part on which you are to work. Do not apply oil directly from the container to the body surface because it will feel cold to the client and will cause discomfort. Rub your hands together to warm the oil to body temperature. This also makes it easier to spread the oil over the client's skin (Fig. 12.13).

To apply oil efficiently, use long superficial strokes (effleurage) that cover the entire area to be massaged. As the oil is smoothed, strokes can become firmer. Effleurage is used to apply the oil and at the same time encourage the flow of body fluids toward the center of the body. Strokes should be continuous, pushing in the direction of the heart and then gliding back to the starting point. A good general rule is to keep the hand relaxed yet firm, so that even when passing over an obstacle such as the knee or shoulder, the hand is in complete contact with the client's skin.

PROCEDURE FOR A GENERAL BODY MASSAGE ▼

The Massage 1 routine is flexible in that some steps can be omitted and others included. The student should follow the instructor's directions. The main objective is to give a beneficial and relaxing massage that is suited to the client's desires and needs.

1. **Preliminary steps:**
   a. Obtain all necessary supplies and arrange as needed.
   b. See that the client has all items needed to prepare for the massage.
   c. Direct client to the dressing room and explain preparation procedures.
2. **Hydrotherapy** (optional):
   a. Select the bath most suitable for the client.
   b. Adjust the bath equipment and accessories.
   c. Take temperature of the bath.
   d. Assist the client as necessary during the bath. Give water to drink, and take pulse if necessary.

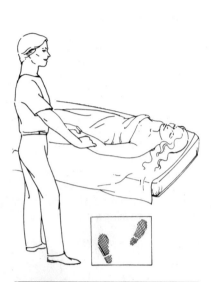

Fig. 12.14a Proper stance and posture is important. Proper posture reduces fatigue, and proper stance allows mobility and power.

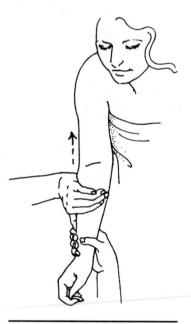

Fig. 12.14b Stroke the arm from the hand to the shoulder.

e. Assist the client as needed following the bath.

f. Allow the client to rest for a short period following the bath.

3. **Preparation for body massage:**

a. Wash and disinfect your hands.

b. Assist the client onto the massage table and into a supine (face-up) position.

c. Drape the client's body with sheet or towel, with the exception of the part to be massaged.

4. **Order of treatment (overview):**

The following procedure is suggested for a basic massage. However, it may be varied to suit the convenience of the practitioner and the needs of the client.

a. Begin with the hands and arms, right then left.

b. Proceed to front of the legs and feet, right then left.

c. Continue movements over chest, neck, and abdomen.

d. The client will turn over to assume a prone (face-down) position.

e. Begin with the back of the legs, right then left.

f. Finish the massage with the back of the body.

Following the massage the client should be allowed to rest for a short period and then be assisted from the table.

Step-by-Step Procedures for Massage 1

The following step-by-step procedure helps you to learn basic massage techniques quickly. Draping is performed and all preliminary steps are observed.

General Arm Massage

1. Raise the client's arm.
2. Stroke the arm three times.
3. Knead the arm from the shoulder to the elbow.
4. Stroke the arm from the elbow to the shoulder.
5. Bend the elbow and rest it on the table.
6. Knead the arm from the elbow to the wrist.
7. Stroke the arm from the wrist to the elbow.
8. Press the metacarpal bones back and forth.
9. Knead each finger and hand.
10. Rotate each finger.
11. Stroke the arm.
12. Roll the arm three times.
13. Apply joint movements to the arm.
14. Stroke the arm lightly three times.
15. Apply nerve strokes and redrape the arm.

Arm Movements for Body Massage Depending on the client's requirements, the following movements may be included or omitted (Fig. 12.14a to p).

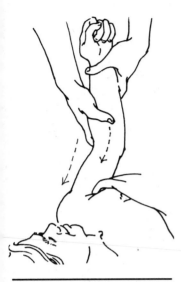

Fig. 12.14c Direction of effleurage and position of arm. The same upward movement is applied when massaging the back of the arm.

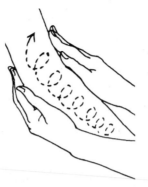

Fig. 12.14d Circular kneading of the arm.

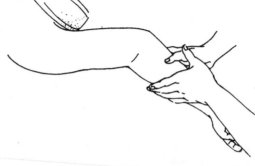

Fig. 12.14e Continue petrissage down the arm to the wrist.

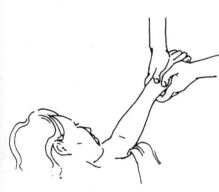

Fig. 12.14f Knead the carpals and metacarpals.

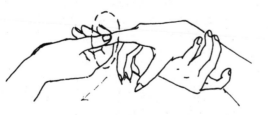

Fig. 12.14g Circular kneading of the fingers and hand.

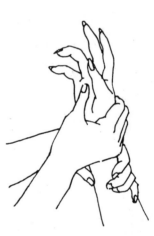

Fig. 12.14h While holding the client's hand, massage the palm, back of the hand, metacarpals, fingers, and upward over the wrist.

Fig. 12.14i Hold the forearm firmly. Rotate and circumduct the wrist. Knead and rotate each finger as you circumduct and apply traction.

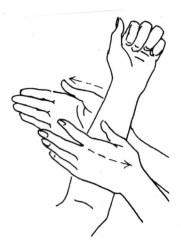

Fig. 12.14j Roll the arm.

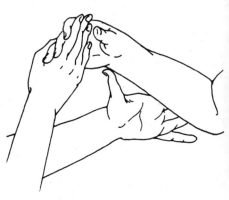

Fig. 12.14k Apply joint movements and rotation. Note the interlacing of the fingers.

Fig. 12.14l Rotate the forearm. Note how the fingers are used to steady the client's elbow.

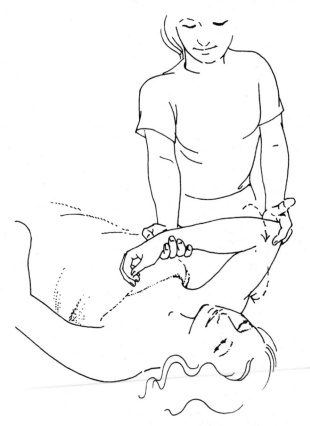

Fig. 12.14m Rotate the shoulder by moving the elbow. Note how the other hand supports the hand.

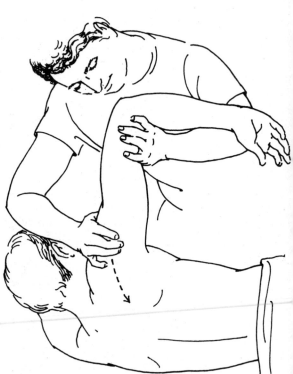

Fig. 12.14n Abduction of the arm. This is a movement of a part away from median line of the body.

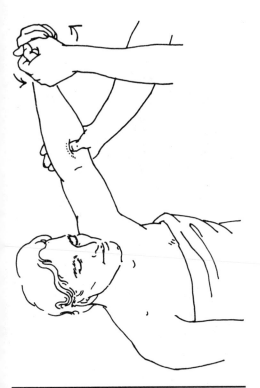

Fig. 12.14o Circumduction of the arm.

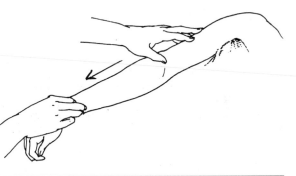

Fig. 12.14p Apply feather strokes (light effleurage) with your fingertips to complete the massage of the arm. The massage for the other arm is done in the same sequence of movements.

General Massage for the Foot and Leg

1. Stroke the leg three times.
2. Press metatarsal bones of the foot back and forth.
3. Knead each toe, around foot, ankle.
4. Rotate each toe three times.
5. Knead the leg three times.
6. Wring and roll the leg.
7. Stroke the leg three times.
8. Apply joint movements to the leg.
9. Stroke the leg lightly three times.
10. Apply nerve strokes and redrape the leg.

Massage for the Foot and Leg Depending on the client's requirements, the following movements may be included or omitted (Fig. 12.15a and b and 12.16a to r).

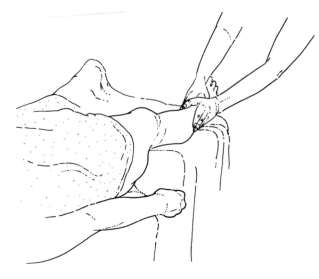

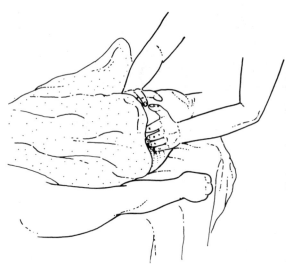

Fig. 12.15a Stroke the leg in long movements from the ankle to the hip. Apply more pressure on the stroke up the leg, and maintain light contact as your hands glide back to the starting point.

Fig. 12.15b A wide archer stance allows the therapist to stroke the entire leg using good body mechanics.

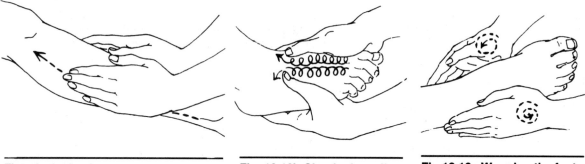

Fig. 12.16a Apply pressure on the stroke in the direction of venous blood and lymph flow.

Fig. 12.16b Circular kneading of the foot.

Fig.12.16c Warming the foot and ankles with circular rubbing movements.

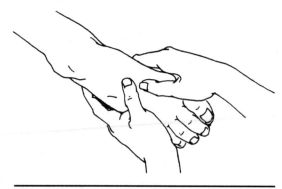

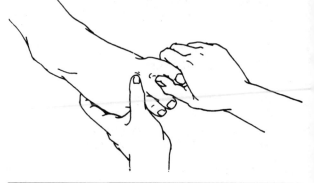

Fig. 12.16d Apply digital friction between the tendons and bones on all surfaces of the foot.

Fig. 12.16e Massage and rotate each digit.

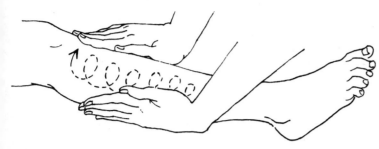

Fig. 12.16f Circular kneading of the leg and thigh.

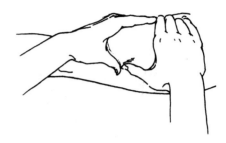

Fig. 12.16g Apply petrissage to the anterior leg.

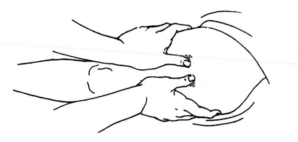

Fig. 12.16h Apply fulling (compression) movements.

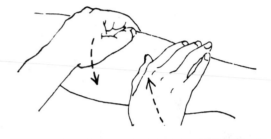

Fig. 12.16i Wringing the muscles of the thigh.

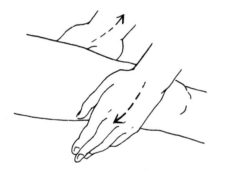

Fig. 12.16j Rolling the muscles of the thigh.

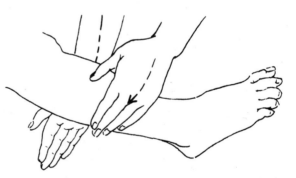

Fig. 12.16k Rolling the muscles of the leg.

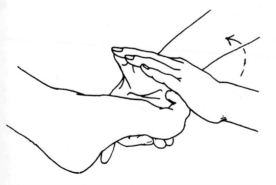

Fig. 12.16l Stretch the plantar surface of the foot and toes.

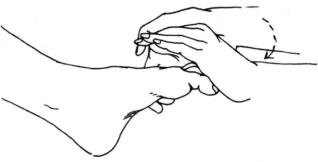

Fig. 12.16m Stretch the dorsal aspect of the foot and toes.

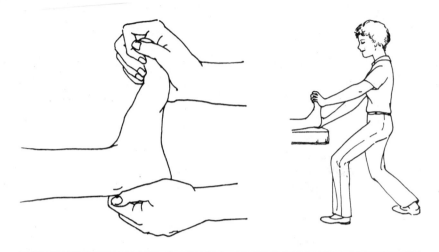

Fig. 12.16n Stretch the Achilles' tendon. Note the position of the hands.

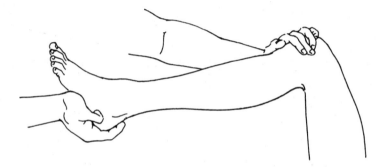

Fig. 12.16o Apply joint movements. The client's knee may be moved all the way to the chest, or this position may be used for joint rotations of the hip and knee in the range of motion. Note the position of the hands at the heel and knee.

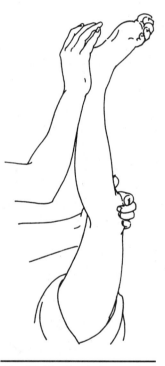

Fig. 12.16p Apply hamstring stretching movements.

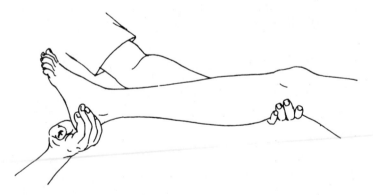

Fig. 12.16q Continue the stretching movements. Note how the hand is placed to support under the knee to avoid hyperextension of the leg.

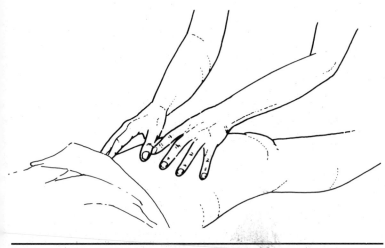

Fig. 12.16r Complete the massage of the front of the leg with a nerve stroke, then redrape and continue to the next part.

General Massage for the Chest and Neck

1. From the head of the table, stroke the back of the neck.
2. Knead back and sides of the neck and shoulders.
3. Stroke the chest three times. Stroke down between the breasts, around to the sides, coming up under each arm, and up and over the shoulders to the neck.
4. Apply deep gliding strokes along the ribs from the table toward the center of the chest.
5. Apply kneading to the pectoral muscles. (Avoid breast tissue on women.)
6. Repeat step #3.

Chest and Neck Movements Depending on the client's requirements, the practitioner may include or omit any of the following movements (Fig. 12.17a to h).

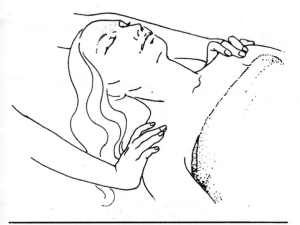

Fig. 12.17a Apply effleurage from the sternal notch, over the shoulders, and along the trapezius.

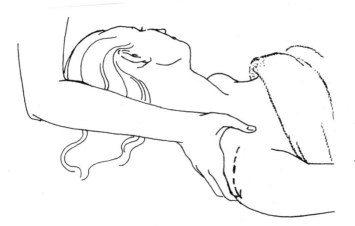

Fig. 12.17b Continue the movement across the shoulder and around the deltoid.

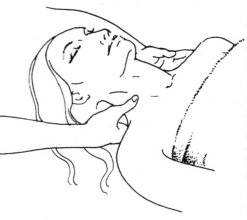

Fig. 12.17c Continue the movement up to the occipital ridge.

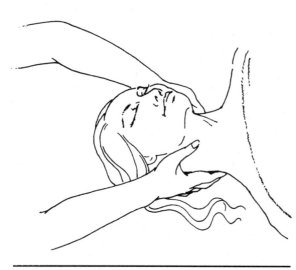

Fig. 12.17d Apply petrissage to the neck and shoulders.

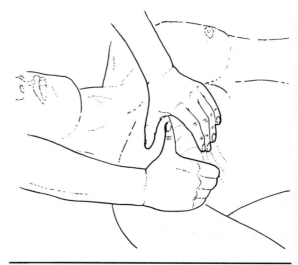

Fig. 12.17e Kneading and friction to the pectoral muscles.

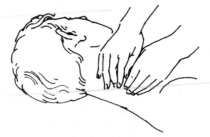

Fig. 12.17f Petrissage to back of neck and shoulder region.

General Massage Movements for the Abdomen

1. Stroke around the abdominal area in a clockwise direction three times.
2. Knead the abdominal muscles back and forth three times.
3. Vibrate the abdominal area with a circular motion over colon, intestines, stomach, and liver.
4. Stroke abdomen lightly three times.

Abdominal Movements for Body Massage Depending on the client's requirements, the practitioner may include or omit any of the following movements (Fig. 12.18a to d).

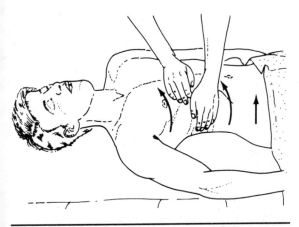

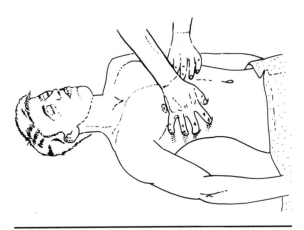

Fig. 12.17g Alternate hand stroking (shingles) is applied from the axillary area to the hips.

Fig. 12.17h Raking is done by flexing the tips of the fingers and stroking along the ribs from the table to the midline of the body.

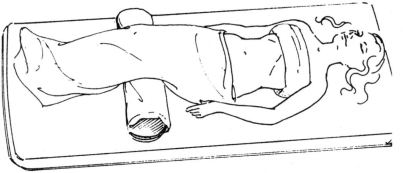

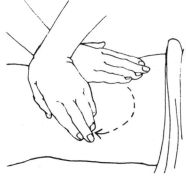

Fig. 12.18a This is the correct position and draping for massage of the abdomen. Oil is applied before beginning the massage. A folded towel is used to cover the female client's breasts. A bolster may be used to support the knees.

Fig. 12.18b Stroking the abdomen with deep circular movement.

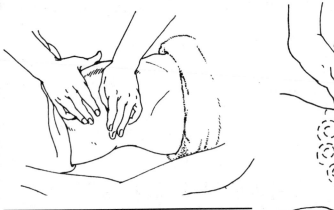

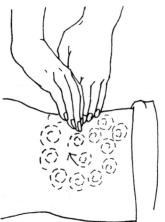

Fig. 12.18d Apply circular friction following the tract of the large intestine.

Fig. 12.18c Apply petrissage to the abdomen.

Changing Position

The client turns over to a prone, face downward position. Maintain proper draping to prevent exposure while turning client.

General Massage for the Back of the Legs

1. Undrape leg and apply oil.
2. Move legs apart and stroke leg three times.
3. Knead foot from toe to heel.
4. Knead leg from the heels to the hips.
5. Apply wringing and rolling.
6. Stroke each leg three times.
7. Apply nerve strokes and redrape.

Back of Leg Movements for Body Massage Depending on the client's requirements, the following movements may be included or omitted (Fig. 12.19a to g).

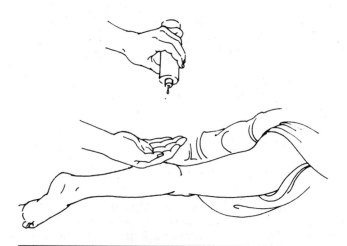

Fig. 12.19a Before beginning massage movements, prepare the posterior leg by draping and applying oil.

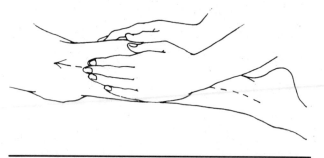

Fig. 12.19b Stroking the leg upward with both hands.

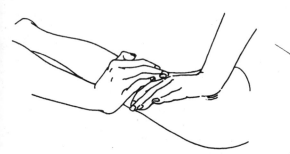

Fig. 12.19c Apply effleurage movements, leading with the little finger. Stroke toward the heart. Note: The leading hand is on the lateral aspect of the leg in order to travel up and over the gluteal muscles and the iliac crest and back down the lateral side of the leg. At the same time. the medial hand travels up to the gluteal crease and back down the medial side of the leg. Both hands return to the starting point to repeat the stroke three or more times.

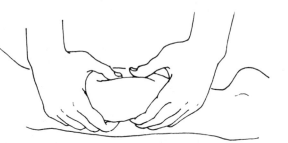

Fig. 12.19d Kneading the calf muscles.

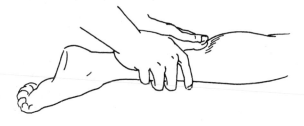

Fig. 12.19e Apply fulling or compression strokes to the entire leg.

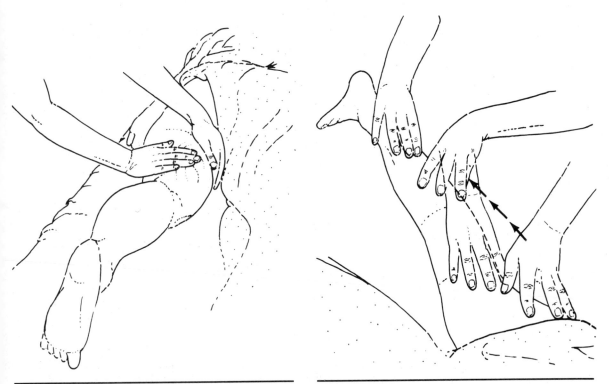

Fig. 12.19f Apply wringing to the back of the leg.

Fig. 12.19g Complete the massage of the posterior leg with several feather strokes (nerve stroke) from the hip to the foot.

General Massage for the Back of the Body

1. Undrape and apply oil to the back.
2. Stroke the back five times up the spine and down on each side of the body.
3. Place the hands flat on each side of the spine, and stretch them outward toward the shoulders.
4. Continue step 2 to cover the entire back.
5. Vibrate along each side of the vertebral column from the neck to the sacrum.
6. Knead the entire back and each side of the torso.
7. Apply deep gliding strokes from the table to the center of the back (shingles) from the hips to the shoulders.
8. From the head of the table, stroke the back three times. From the back of the neck, stroke down along the length of the spine, around to the side of the body, up the sides, around and over the shoulders, up to the neck, and repeat.
9. Apply light hacking movements along the spine, between the shoulders, over the gluteal muscles and the back of the legs. Avoid the kidney area.
10. Stroke the back lightly five times.
11. Apply nerve strokes to the entire back, redrape, and complete the massage.

Back Movements for Body Massage Depending on the client's requirements, the following movements may be included or omitted (Fig. 12.20a to l).

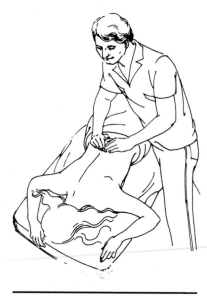
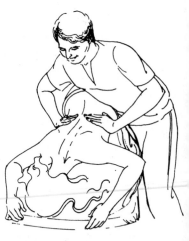

Fig. 12.20a Begin at the gluteal cleft and apply long strokes up along the muscles on each side of the spine.

Fig. 12.20b Continue with effleurage strokes up the back and over the shoulders.

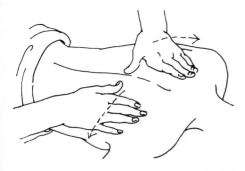

Fig. 12.20c Outward stretching of the muscles of the back.

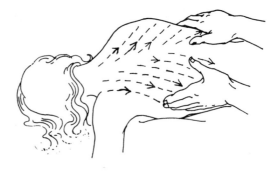

Fig. 12.20d Fan stroking of the back.

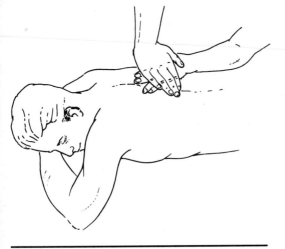

Fig. 12.20e Vibration movements are applied over each vertebra by placing the fingers of one hand on each side of the spinous process and the other hand on top. Vibrate back and forth as you move down along the spine.

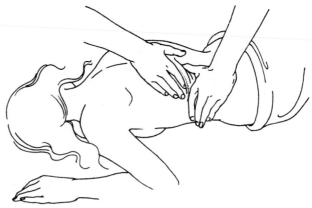

Fig. 12.20f Apply petrissage to the entire side that is opposite you. This takes several passes.

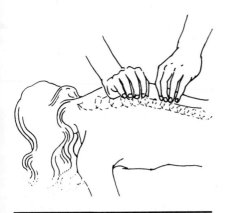

Fig. 12.20g Kneading around the spine.

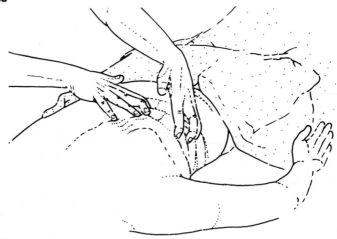

Fig. 12.20h Raking is applied in alternate strokes so the tips of the fingers glide between the ribs.

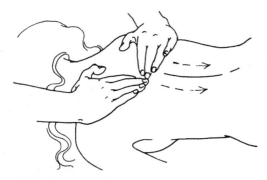

Fig. 12.20i Continue effleurage movements down the back, over and around the gluteal muscles, back up the sides, then over and around the shoulders to the nape of the neck.

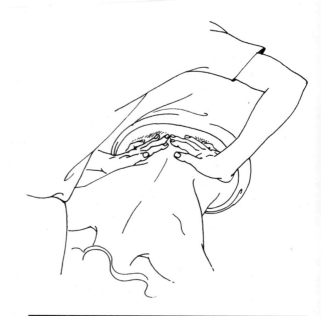

Fig. 12.20j The caring stroke continues down the back and over the gluteal muscles.

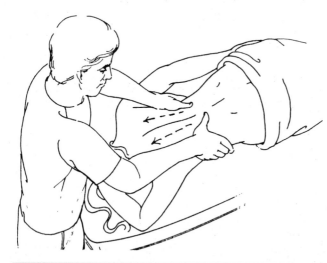

Fig. 12.20k The caring stroke is a continuous movement that proceeds up the side and around the shoulder to return to the starting point.

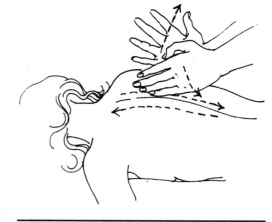

Fig. 12.20l Hacking movements on the back.

Completing the Treatment

1. After completing the final strokes, maintain light contact. Allow clients a few moments to savor the deep relaxation as they return to a more conscious state.

2. When they are ready, assist clients to a sitting position.
3. Suggest supplementary services and answer any questions clients may have.
4. When they are totally awake and reoriented assist clients off the table and direct them to the dressing area.
5. After clients are dressed, collect your fees and set up the next appointment (Fig. 12.21a and b).

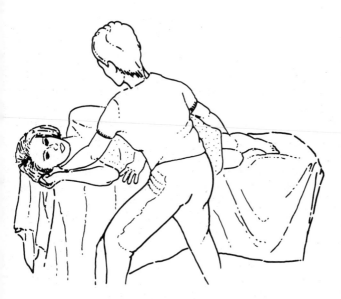

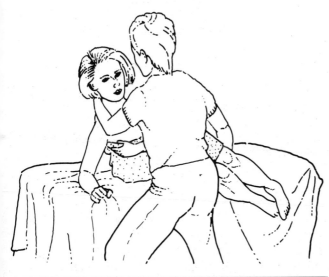

Fig. 12.21a and b If a client needs help sitting up, the client turns onto his or her side. The therapist places one hand under the neck and the other behind the knees and assists the client into a seated position.

Final Considerations

1. Complete the client's record card.
2. Place supplies in their proper place; discard used items.
3. See that all equipment and items, including massage table and bath, are properly prepared before the next client arrives.

▼ PROCEDURE FOR PROFESSIONAL BODY MASSAGE

Massage 2

Massage, like any other skill, requires practice and patience to learn the basics, build speed, and develop new techniques. Each time you give a massage you may find yourself becoming more innovative and more confident of your techniques. By the time you have learned Massage 1, you should be familiar with most of the terms for the various movements used in basic body massage. Massage 2 incorporates additional techniques to help you increase efficiency, remember sequence of movements, and readily identify movements and anatomy by proper names. While doing massage, pay attention to your hand positions and how you stand and move.

Massage 2 enables you to review what you have learned and allows for even more creativity in varying massage routines. Before beginning the massage, concentrate on projecting the manner, attitude, and appearance of the professional massage practitioner. Read directions carefully for each step. Once you have learned how to give a complete massage correctly and efficiently, you will not need to refer to your notes, illustration, or written guides. Your aim is to be able to give the complete massage in a knowledgeable and professional manner.

Preliminary Steps

1. Prepare all facilities and products.
2. If this is the client's first visit, be ready to greet her or him on time and introduce yourself. In many places of business the practitioner is addressed by his or her first name. For example, when introducing yourself to a new client you might say, "Good morning Mrs. Mason, I'm Carolyn. I'll be working with you today." You do not address the client by his or her first name unless it is customary to do so, or if the client has asked that you use his or her first name.
3. The first step with any client is the consultation or interview (see Chapter 9). Have the client fill out the information sheet first, and review it with the client to obtain more direct information. Discuss the client's needs and expectations and the kind of massage he or she prefers. This is the time to be observant of the client's physical condition and determine what benefits should be derived from the massage.

4. Put first-time clients at ease by showing the facilities and explaining the services.
5. When appropriate, take the client's temperature and blood pressure. Explain why these procedures are done.
6. Explain to the client how he or she is to prepare for the massage. Show the client to the shower or hydrotherapy area, depending on which services that client has decided on. Provide proper draping for the client from the dressing area to the massage table.
7. Assist the client (as necessary) to the massage table and explain the position, either supine or prone, he or she should assume. Drape the client appropriately and provide extra support (towels or bolster) under knees or head if necessary.

There are many possibilities for varying massage techniques for different clients. The following massage procedure will help you to become more proficient and creative.

Breathing for Relaxation

When the client is on the table, relaxed and comfortable, encourage him or her to breathe fully and deeply. Many people have never done this and may need some basic coaching. Help the client by using some of the following suggestions:

Tell the client to breathe through the nose deeply so that the abdominal area expands first, followed by the chest. Hold for a few counts, and then allow the breath to flow outward. Maintain the exhalation for a short time, and repeat the exercise a few times. Observe the client's breathing, and synchronize your own breathing. Have the client continue breathing freely for a few minutes to encourage relaxation and stress reduction.

Step-by-Step Procedure for Massage 2

Begin with the client lying supine on the massage table. Make initial contact (tune in) by first placing your hands on the frontal eminence of the client's forehead or the back of the neck, at the base of the head. If you prefer, you may begin by placing your hands on the client's shoulders. Hold the touch for a few seconds without moving (Fig. 12.22).

Massage the Face

1. Touch the frontal eminence and hold for about thirty seconds.
   a. Ask the client to inhale slowly, exhale, and continue breathing deeply.
2. Apply digital effleurage with your thumb from the centerline of the face to the hairline. Work gradually down the forehead to the eyebrow and across the eyes (the supra-orbital and suborbital ridges). The face is naturally oily and usually does not require the use of added lubricant. If a lubricant is needed, a cream or light lotion is generally preferred over massage oil.

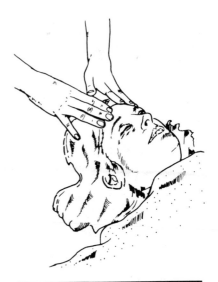

Fig. 12.22 A gentle contact to initiate the massage is a way for the therapist to say hello to the client's body and to center himself or herself.

3. Apply circular friction from the temples to the jaw. Massage along the hairline and in front of the ear, carefully massaging the temporomandibular joints.
4. Apply directional friction downward along the mandible, and circular friction under the mandible.
5. Apply light palmar friction on the cheeks.
6. Massage the ears.
7. Apply light effleurage from the centerline of the face to the hairline (Fig. 12.23a to g).

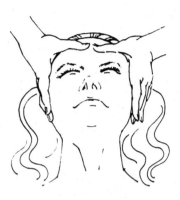

Fig. 12.23a Apply digital effleurage to the forehead, from midline to hairline.

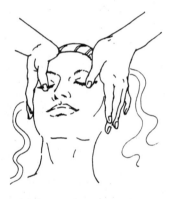

Fig. 12.23b Apply effleurage to the forehead and orbits.

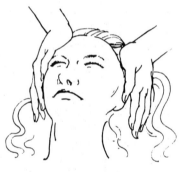

Fig. 12.23c Apply effleurage to the cheeks (zygomatics).

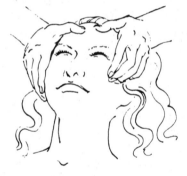

Fig. 12.23d Apply friction around the cheeks.

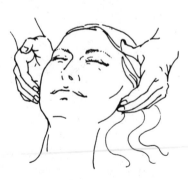

Fig. 12.23e Apply friction around the mouth (mandible) and jawline.

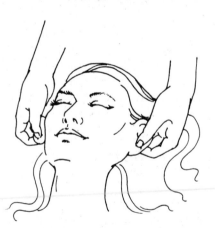

Fig. 12.23f Massage the ears with light friction movements applied with forefingers and thumbs.

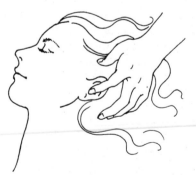

Fig. 12.23g Massage in and around the ears with light friction movement.

Massage the Scalp

1. Without using oil, apply gentle friction movements over the entire scalp. This is done in such a way as to move the scalp over the cranium and not the hair over the scalp.
2. Apply digital vibration using all five digits bilaterally.
3. Smooth the hair into its natural contour (Fig. 12.24).

Massage the Neck

1. Apply oil with a bilateral-lateral effleurage stroke beginning at the sternal notch and continuing over the shoulders, up the trapezius and the back of the neck, to the occipital ridge (Fig. 12.25a to c).

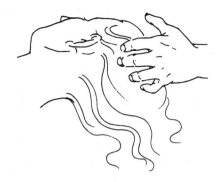

Fig. 12.24 Massage the scalp by making rotating movements with the fingertips.

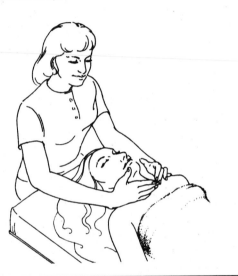

Fig. 12.25a Apply bilateral effleurage (beginning at the sternal notch). Use the hands simultaneously, leading with the little fingers.

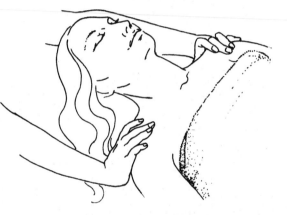

Fig. 12.25b Continue effleurage from the sternal notch, over the shoulders, and along the trapezius.

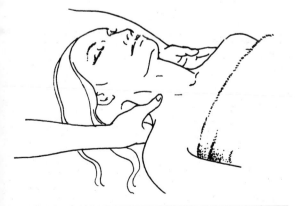

Fig. 12.25c Continue the movement up to the occipital ridge.

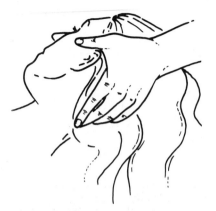

Fig. 12.26a Note placement of the hands in the "handle" position supporting the head.

2. Turn the client's head to one side, supporting it with your hand. Continue effleurage strokes, leading with your little finger and beginning just inferior (below) the mastoid process (bony bump below and behind the ear). Continue down the lateral aspect of the neck, over the shoulder and back up the trapezius to the occipital ridge. Repeat three to five times (Fig. 12.26a to d).

3. Thoroughly knead that side of the neck, paying attention to any tight areas.

4. Repeat effleurage stroke on neck and shoulders.

5. Apply circular friction to any congested or tight areas.

6. Apply V-stroke effleurage to side and back of neck (Fig. 12.27a to c).

7. Repeat effleurage.

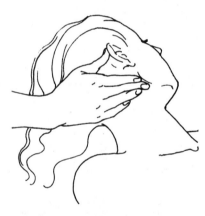

Fig. 12.26b Apply effleurage, leading with the little finger, just below the mastoid and continue down the neck.

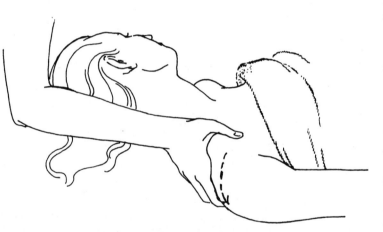

Fig. 12.26c Continue the movement across the shoulder and around the deltoid.

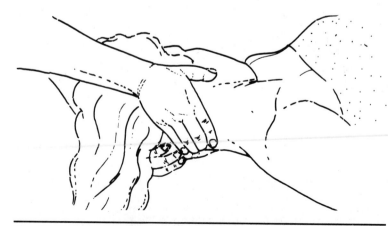

Fig. 12.26d Hand position at the completion of effleurage stroke.

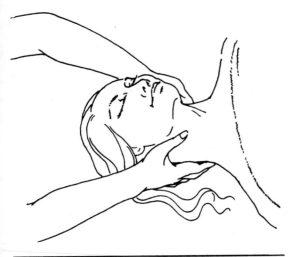

Fig. 12.27a Apply petrissage to the neck and shoulders.

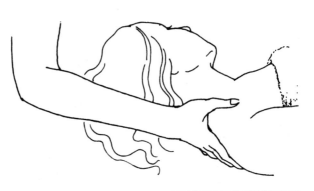

Fig. 12.27b Apply friction to the neck and shoulders.

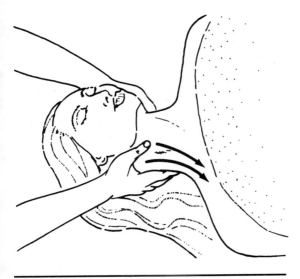

Fig. 12.27c Apply V-stroke to the neck and shoulders.

8. Turn the client's head to the opposite side and repeat the movements as you did in steps 2 through 6.
9. Return the client's head to the central position and apply bilateral-lateral petrissage and friction to the neck and shoulders.
10. Do the following joint movements: Tilt the head back with the chin up, then lower the chin down to the chest. Laterally flex the neck, moving the ear, first to the right shoulder, then to the left. Rotate the head to its full range of motion (lateral

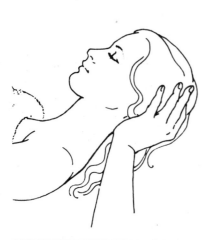

Fig. 12.28a Apply passive joint movements by rolling the head forward. Note placement of the hands on the client's head.

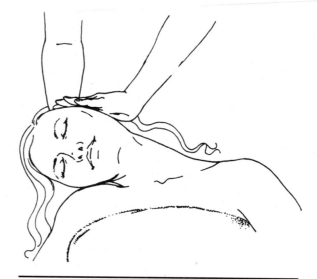

Fig. 12.28b Apply passive joint movements by moving the head from side to side.

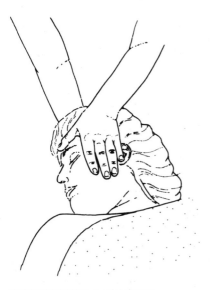

Fig. 12.28c Apply passive rotation to the neck, being careful to keep cervical spine straight.

rotation). The spine remains in a straight line. (*Note:* Joint movements of the neck are contraindicated in cases of osteoporosis.) (See Fig. 12.28a to c)

11. Hold the occiput in the palm of the hand or hook the fingers under the occiput and apply a slight traction to the neck.
12. Place one hand on each shoulder and gently alternately push them toward the feet, providing a gentle rocking motion (Figs. 12.29 and 12.30).
13. Repeat the stroking movement in step 1.

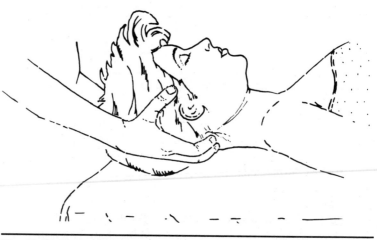

Fig. 12.29 Apply slight traction to the cervical spine by hooking the fingers under the occiput and pulling.

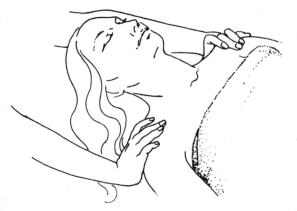

Fig. 12.30 Apply alternating pressure toward the feet to rock gently and stretch the shoulders.

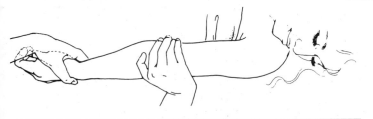

Fig. 12.31a Note the correct hand position and handle (the hand) to apply effleurage to the lateral aspect of the arm.

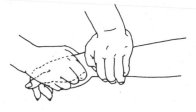

Fig. 12.31b Apply effleurage to the lateral aspect of the arm with your little finger leading. The stroke is continuous, up over the arm, over the shoulders, and back to the starting point. Use more pressure on the stroke up to the shoulder and a lighter, more superficial pressure on the return stroke. The client's arm is held in slight traction throughout the stroke. An alternative is to place the arm on the table for this stroke.

Massage the Arms

1. Undrape one arm to make contact and apply oil on the client's arm from shoulder to wrist, using light effleurage.
2. Locate the handle at the wrist, and put the client's arm in slight traction by holding it with the wrist handle. Apply effleurage. Apply more pressure from wrist to neck, then lightly stroke as you return to the wrist. Hold the thumb side handle (the client's wrist) with the arm that is closest to the client. Begin effleurage, leading with your little finger up from the wrist, up the arm, over the shoulder, and up to the back of the neck. Rotate your hand as it travels over the client's shoulder; at the same time apply slight traction to the handle. Proceed up the back of the neck and then down under the shoulder (trapezius area); then glide back to the starting point at the wrist. Repeat three to five times.
3. Change the handle to the ulnar side of the wrist. Lead with your little finger, apply effleurage up the medial aspect of the arm over the shoulder, around and down into the axillary portion of the arm, then return to the wrist. Do effleurage again three to five times (Fig. 12.31a to g).

Fig. 12.31c Note the hand position and handle to apply effleurage to the medial aspect of the arm.

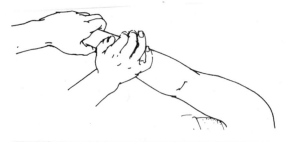

Fig. 12.31d Correct hand position for effleurage of the medial aspect of the arm.

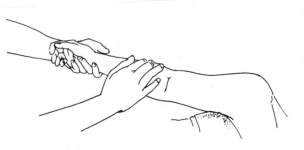

Fig. 12.31e Begin effleurage movements, leading with the little finger.

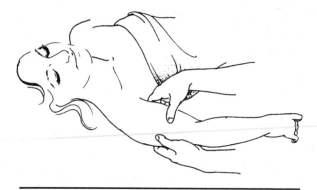

Fig. 12.31f Effleurage movements are continued up and over the shoulder, then back down the arm.

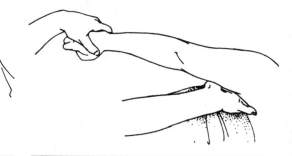

Fig. 12.31g Effleurage movements are continued up into the axillary area for a slight joint movement and stretch.

4. Using both hands, grasp the arm at shoulder level and apply petrissage, directing individual movements toward the shoulder while moving down the arm to the client's hand. On the upper arm, use both hands to alternately knead the biceps and triceps. On the lower arm, alternately knead the wrist flexors and extensors.

5. Wring and roll (using both hands) from the shoulder, moving down the arm and giving special attention to the muscles of the forearm (Fig. 12.32a to e).

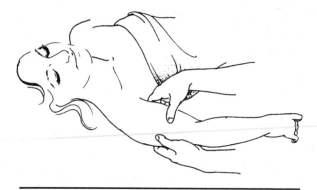

Fig. 12.32a Apply petrissage from the shoulder and continue down the arm.

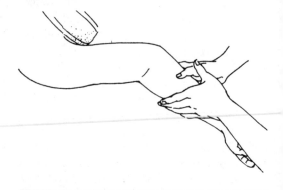

Fig. 12.32b Continue petrissage down the arm to the wrist.

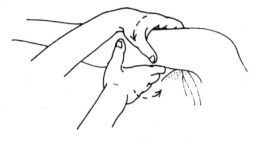

Fig. 12.32c Apply wringing movements from the shoulder to the wrist.

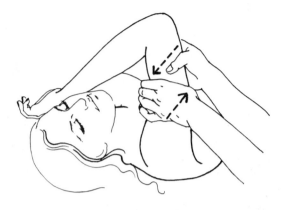

Fig. 12.32d An alternate position may be used for the wringing movements and kneading.

6. Apply V-stroke effleurage from wrist to elbow on the medial and lateral sides of the forearm.
7. Apply fulling to the forearm (Fig. 12.33a and b).
8. Repeat effleurage to the medial and lateral side of the arm.
9. Massage the hand and then do joint movements on the arm and hand.

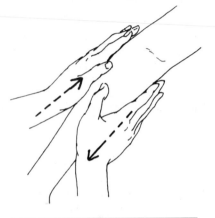

Fig. 12.32e Do rolling movements from the shoulder to the wrist.

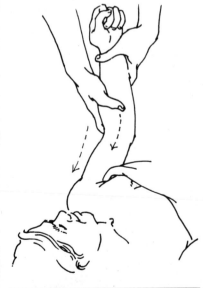

Fig. 12.33a Direction of V-stroke and position of arm. The same upward movement is applied when massaging the back of the arm.

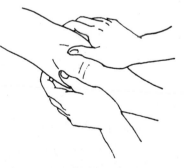

Fig. 12.33b Fulling the arm.

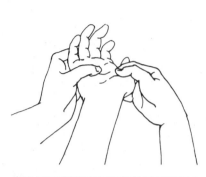

Fig. 12.34a Apply friction and petrissage to the palm of the hand, spreading the metacarpals.

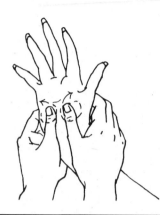

Fig. 12.34b With the client's elbow resting on the table, hold the hand upright and massage the palm of the hand with the cushions of your thumbs, using circular movements in alternate directions. This relaxes the hand.

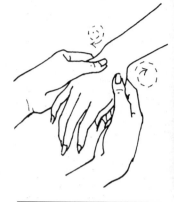

Fig. 12.34c Apply friction and petrissage to the wrist and muscles of the hand.

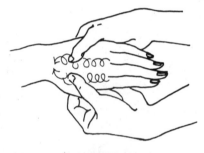

Fig. 12.34d Apply circular friction to the back of the hand.

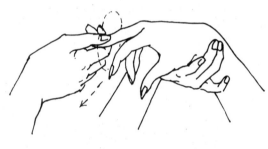

Fig. 12.34e Beginning at the base of each finger, apply friction and petrissage. Work downward to the tip of each finger.

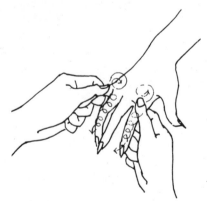

Fig. 12.34f Squeeze and gently twist each finger, beginning at the base and working toward the tip. Rotate each finger in large circles. Finish each finger with a gentle squeeze of the fingertip.

Massage the Hand

1. Apply petrissage to the palm of the client's hand.
2. Apply friction to the palm.
3. Apply petrissage to the back of the hand.
4. Apply friction to the back of the hand.
5. Do petrissage on each digit, including a joint movement (Fig. 12.34a to f).

6. Apply joint movement. Support the client's hand and rotate all fingers clockwise and counterclockwise.
7. Extend, flex, and rotate the fingers, wrist, and elbow.
8. Rotate the shoulder joint clockwise and counterclockwise.
9. Extend the arm straight above the client's head to stretch the entire arm.
10. Apply effleurage from elbow past axillary area (Fig. 12.35a to e).

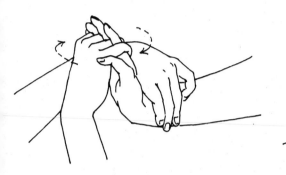

Fig. 12.35a Apply joint movements and rotation. Note the interlacing of the fingers.

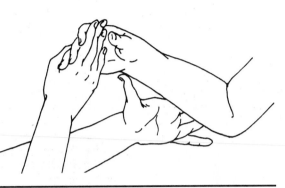

Fig. 12.35b Rotate the forearm. Note how the fingers are used to steady the client's elbow.

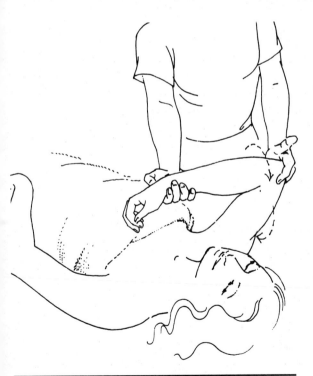

Fig. 12.35c Apply joint movements to the shoulder by moving the elbow in large circles. Note how the wrist is supported to prevent the client's hand from hitting him or her in the face.

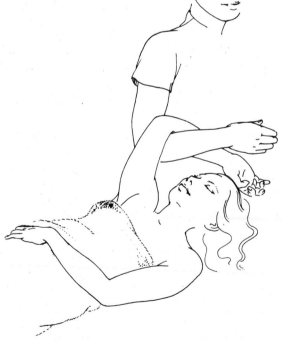

Fig. 12.35d Stretch the client's arm over your arm. A slight turn or stretch may be done with your hand holding the client's wrist.

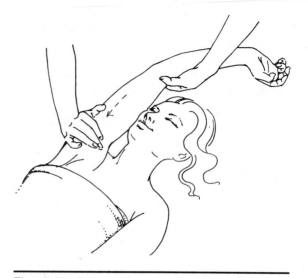

Fig. 12.35e Apply effleurage or compression to the axillary area.

11. Apply traction at the wrist while moving the arm from a position above the client's head and back down to the side.
12. Shake and vibrate the arm and hand.
13. Apply a final effleurage of the arm and hand, and rotate the shoulder.
14. Apply lateral effleurage; then feather downward with superficial strokes from the neck, down the arm, to the fingertips.
15. Redrape the client as necessary, and repeat the arm and hand massage for the other arm and hand (Fig. 12.36a and b).

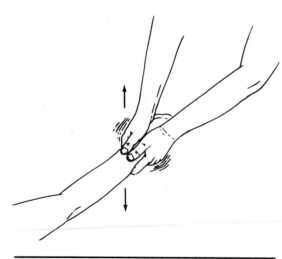

Fig. 12.36a Grasp the wrist securely, and vigorously shake the arm up and down.

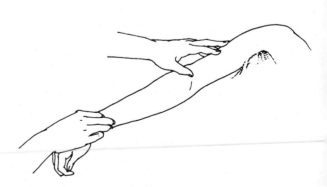

Fig. 12.36b Apply feather strokes (light effleurage) with your fingertips to complete the massage of the arm. The massage for the other arm is done in the same sequence of movements.

Massage the feet

1. Move to the feet, maintaining contact by using a light brushing stroke down the side of the body. Pause momentarily to allow the client to sense where you are before you begin massaging the feet. Undrape one foot and leg up to the hip.
2. Use just enough oil to allow your hands to work smoothly. (One or two drops are usually enough. Sometimes no oil is needed on the feet.)
3. Apply effleurage to each aspect of the foot to strip out the venous fluid. Stroke from the toes up to and past the ankle on the top, side, and bottom of the foot.
4. Apply petrissage and friction to the bottom of the feet from the ball of the foot to the heel. Use a closed fist or heel of the hand to do the pressing movements.
5. Apply kneading movements from the toes up to the ankles.
6. Apply small circular friction movements between each of the tendons on the top and sides of the foot.
7. Apply digital friction to each toe and between toes (Fig. 12.37a to f).

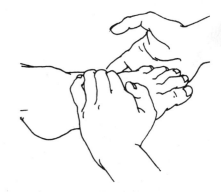

Fig. 12.37a Apply effleurage to both the top and bottom of the foot, working from the toes upward toward the heart.

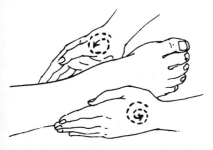

Fig. 12.37b Warming the foot and ankles with circular rubbing movements.

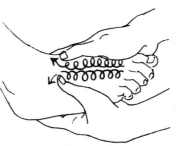

Fig. 12.37c Circular kneading of the foot.

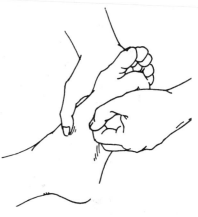

Fig. 12.37d Apply knuckles, stroking down the plantar surface of the foot.

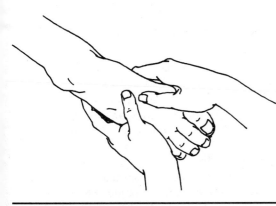

Fig. 12.37e Apply digital friction between the tendons and bones on all surfaces of the foot.

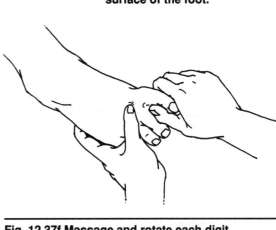

Fig. 12.37f Massage and rotate each digit.

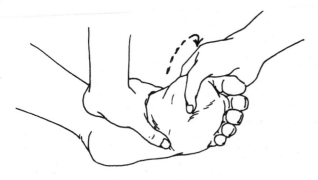

Fig. 12.38a Rotate and stretch the tarsus and metatarsus.

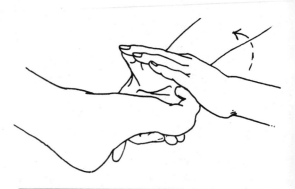

Fig. 12.38b Stretch the plantar surface of the foot and toes.

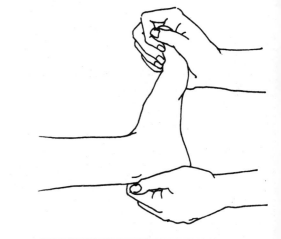

Fig. 12.38c Stretch the dorsal aspect of the foot and toes.

Fig. 12.38d Stretch the Achilles' tendon. Note the position of the hands.

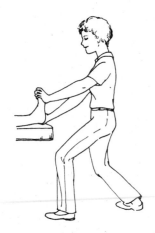

Fig. 12.38e Practitioner is always aware of using proper body mechanics.

8. Beginning with the toes, incorporate joint movements, first individually, then together. Apply plantar and dorsal flexion of the toes, then to the entire foot. Rotate the foot and ankle, then separate the toes (phalanges) and wring and roll the foot (Fig. 12.38a to e).
9. Repeat this entire procedure on the other foot and leg.

Note: You may choose to work on adjacent parts of the body in sequence (from one part to the adjoining part) rather than interrupting the flow of movement. After working on the foot, proceed directly to the front of the leg. Then continue to the other foot and leg.

Massage the Front of the Legs

1. Apply oil with light and continuous effleurage.
2. Apply effleurage with both hands, beginning at the ankle. Apply effleurage to the entire leg by leading with one hand on the lateral side of the leg and the other hand on the medial

aspect of the leg. Your hands should span the entire front of
the leg. Hand pressure may be increased with each effleurage
stroke and feathered back to the starting point. The medial
hand progresses to the groin and turns as it returns lightly
along the medial aspect of the leg to the beginning point at the
ankle. The lateral hand starts at the ankle, continues up the
lateral aspect of the anterior leg, all the way to the anterior
superior iliac spine (ASIS), along the iliac crest, and glides
back to the starting point. Repeat these movements three to
five times.

(Note: The leg is the longest part of the body. Be sure to use
proper body mechanics and movement when applying long
strokes to the leg (Fig. 12.39a to e)).

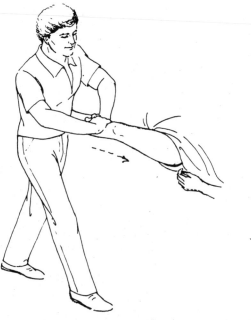

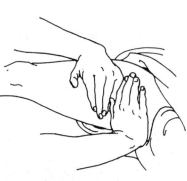

**Fig. 12.39a Apply effleurage to the leg.
Good posture and stance should be
maintained and the back kept straight,
with knees slightly flexed.**

**Fig. 12.39b The leading hand
should be on the lateral side of
the leg in order to travel up and
over the ilium and return back to
the starting point.**

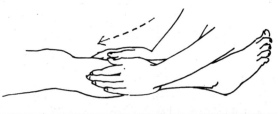

Fig. 12.39c Direction of effleurage on the lower leg.

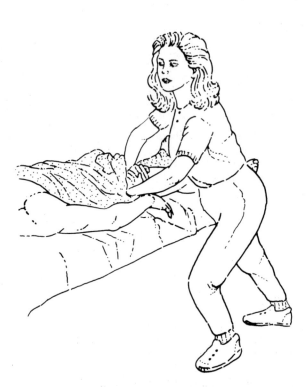

Fig. 12.39d Body position at the beginning of the gliding stroke on the anterior leg.

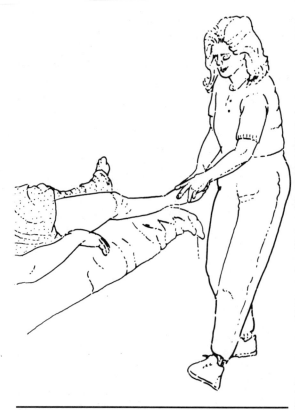

Fig. 12.39e Body position at the end of the gliding stroke on the anterior leg.

3. Apply petrissage, beginning at the ankle and proceeding up the leg along the fleshy parts along the side of the tibia to the knee.
4. Apply digital petrissage to the tendon areas around the patella. The thigh may require several passes up and down with this stroke because it is a large area.
5. Repeat effleurage (Fig. 12.40a to f).

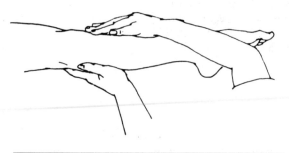

Fig. 12.40a Palmar friction of muscles of the leg and thigh.

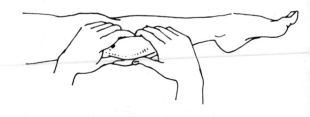

Fig. 12.40b Kneading of the calf muscles.

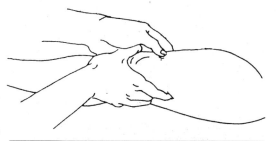

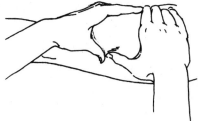

Fig. 12.40c Manipulate the kneecap by tracing circles with your thumb in opposite directions.

Fig. 12.40d Apply petrissage to the anterior leg.

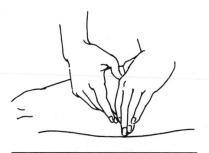

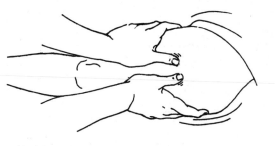

Fig. 12.40e Continue petrissage and wringing movements.

Fig. 12.40f Apply fulling (compression) movements.

Optional Position

(Bending the Knee) The following is an optional position for leg massage. In this position, the entire calf and thigh can be massaged easily. Position the client's foot flat on the table with the knee bent and the foot sixteen to eighteen inches from the buttocks. Wrap the foot with the drape and brace the leg either with your knee or by sitting on the table near the client's toes to keep the leg from sliding. Be sure the draping is intact to secure modesty of the pelvic area.

1. With the leg in the bent-knee position, apply effleurage from ankle to knee.
2. Apply petrissage from ankle to knee.
3. Repeat effleurage from ankle to knee.
4. While keeping the knee bent, apply a variety of friction techniques from ankle to knee. Pay special attention to areas that seem to be more congested or tight. Apply rolling, wringing, or cross-fiber friction in areas of tension.
5. Apply effleurage to the leg from ankle to knee.
6. Keeping the leg in the bent-knee position, apply effleurage from knee to hip, groin, and gluteal crease.
7. Apply petrissage to the entire thigh. Make several passes to cover the entire circumference of the leg.
8. Apply wringing, rolling, and chucking.
9. Follow with effleurage to the entire leg (Fig. 12.41a to e).

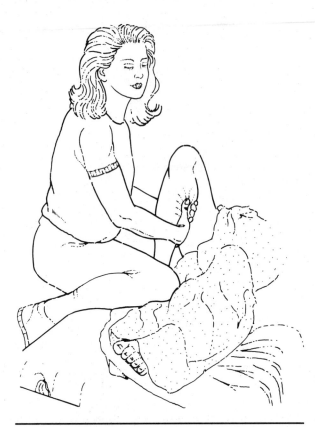

Fig. 12.41a Client's leg is supported in a bent position by therapist's knee (note draping so therapist's clothing does not touch client's skin).

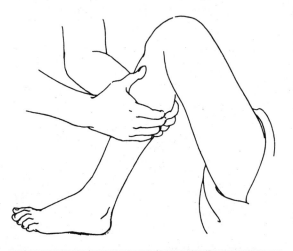

Fig. 12.41b In the bent-knee position, apply wringing and rolling movements to the calf.

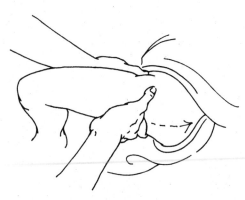

Fig. 12.41c With the client in the bent-knee position, apply effleurage to the thigh.

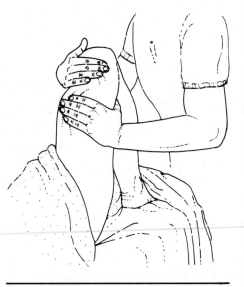

Fig. 12.41d Apply kneading and wringing to the thigh in the bent knee position.

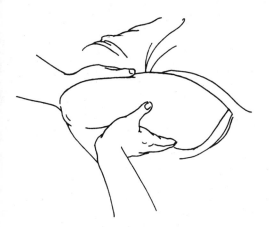

Fig. 12.41e Apply chucking to the thigh. With the client in the bent-knee position, manipulate soft tissue of the posterior aspect of the thigh and apply effleurage, petrissage, or rolling movements.

10. Apply joint movements. Grasp the ankle with one hand, and place the other hand just below the knee. Move the knee toward the chest while flexing it to the maximum. Pay attention to the degree of flexibility, and move the limbs firmly, but not forcefully, to their maximum range of movement. It is beneficial to have the client breathe deeply and then exhale as you apply downward pressure on the knee.

11. Move your hand around to grasp the ankle at the level of the Achilles' tendon; then elevate the foot toward the ceiling to extend the leg and flex the hip. Flex the hip to its maximum range of movement by moving the foot toward the client's head.

12. Flex the client's knee by bringing it toward the chest; then rotate the bent leg laterally, retaining slight pressure on the knee to maintain full range of motion as the leg rotates outward. Return the leg to the table by continuing the hip rotation and slowly straightening the leg. Your hand should support the back of the leg to prevent hyperextension as the leg is returned to the table. Repeat this procedure two times (Fig. 12.42a to e).

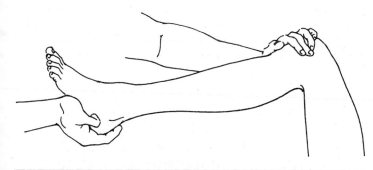

Fig. 12.42a Apply joint movements. The client's knee may be moved all the way to the chest, or this position may be used for joint rotations of the hip and knee in the range of motion. Note the position of the hands at the heel and knee.

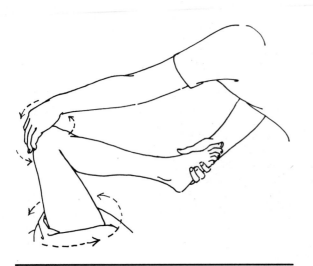

Fig. 12.42b Circumduction of the thigh.

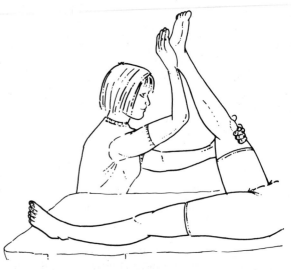

Fig. 12.42c Stretch the hamstrings by lifting the foot toward the ceiling and straightening the knee.

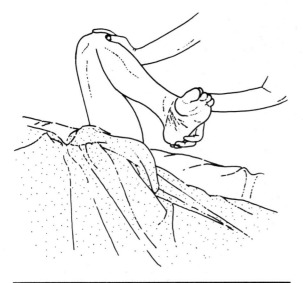

Fig. 12.42d Move the knee to the chest to stretch the hip and low back.

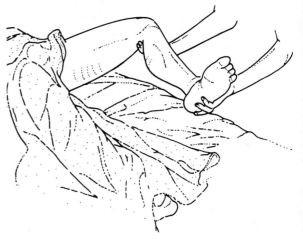

Fig. 12.42e Leg is rotated laterally. Note draping.

13. Move to the foot of the table and grasp the heel (handle) with the lateral hand (the one toward the outside of the leg you were working on). Rotate the foot and leg in the hip socket. This movement will be back and forth, and the foot movement will resemble a windshield wiper.
14. Dorsal flex and plantar flex the foot.
15. Place your other hand over the client's instep and apply slight traction. Shake the leg up and down. Keep the heel on the table to avoid hyperextension of the knee (Fig. 12.43a to d).

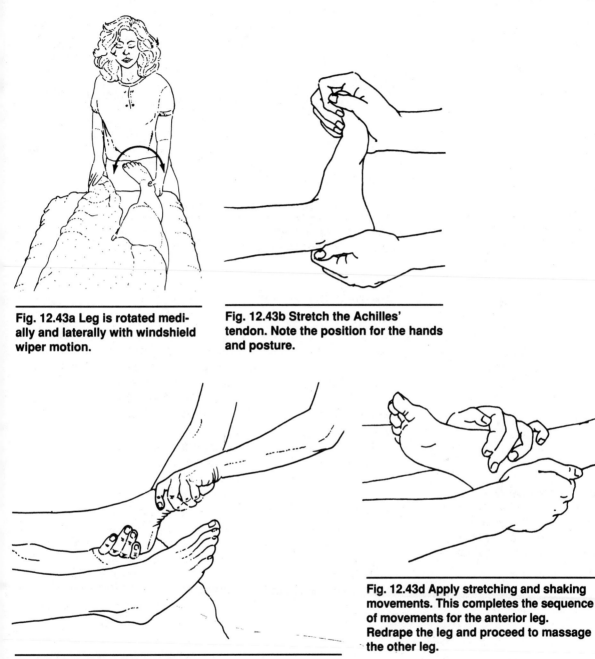

Fig. 12.43a Leg is rotated medially and laterally with windshield wiper motion.

Fig. 12.43b Stretch the Achilles' tendon. Note the position for the hands and posture.

Fig. 12.43c Plantar flex the foot.

Fig. 12.43d Apply stretching and shaking movements. This completes the sequence of movements for the anterior leg. Redrape the leg and proceed to massage the other leg.

16. Apply effleurage to the entire leg three to five times.
17. Apply feather (nerve) strokes from hip to toes, three to five times.
18. Redrape the leg and proceed to the other foot. Repeat the entire procedure on the other leg.

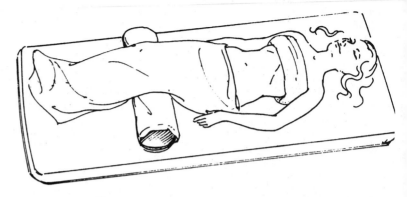

Fig. 12.44 This is the correct position and draping for massage of the abdomen. A folded towel is used to cover the female client's breasts. A bolster is used to support the knees.

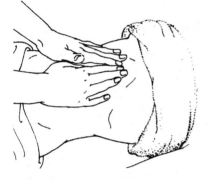

Fig. 12.45a Apply effleurage movements (leading with the little finger). The movement goes up, out, around, and down, then back to the center of the abdomen.

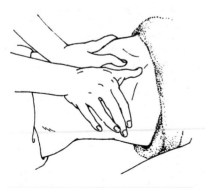

Fig. 12.45b The effleurage movements are repeated.

Massage the Abdomen and Chest

This part of the massage requires some special considerations. The need for draping usually varies when working with male and female clients. Women, for reasons of modesty may prefer having their breasts draped at all times. It is best to ask the female client what she prefers. Professional standards recommend that draping procedures (as directed earlier in this chapter) be followed. When asked, some clients will opt not to have the abdomen or chest massaged.

The following massage description refers to techniques used on the fully exposed torso, with added comments when using breast draping.

In preparation for massage of the abdominal region, use a bolster or pillow to elevate the client's knees and support them so that the abdominal muscles will remain relaxed. Draping should be open enough to allow massaging down to the top of the pubic bone, but secure enough to avoid exposure of the genital area (Fig. 12.44).

1. To begin, stand to the client's right to apply oil to the abdomen, chest, and sides of the body.
2. Do effleurage strokes on the abdomen and chest, over the shoulders, around and down the axillary areas, then down the sides of the crest of the ilium. Massage back to the center with a turn of your wrist and repeat the movements. When using breast draping, this stroke glides up as far as the drape will allow and then laterally over the ribs and down to the iliac crest. Massage should not be done directly over the sensitive area of the nipples on men or women (Fig. 12.45a to d).
3. Do circular effleurage on the abdomen in a clockwise direction following the path of the colon. On this stroke, one hand remains in constant contact doing circular massage. The other describes a semi-circle beginning at the lower right of the

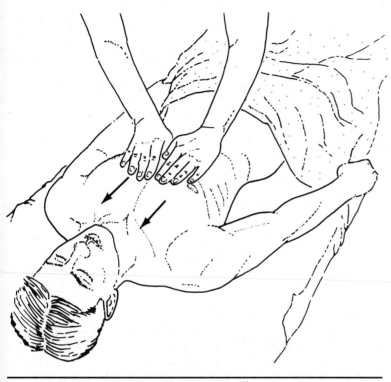

Fig. 12.45c When a breast drape is not used, the stroke continues up over the chest to the sternal notch.

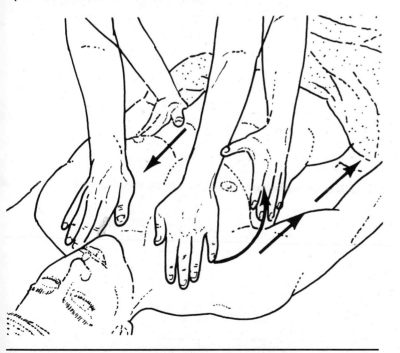

Fig. 12.45d The gliding stroke continues out over the shoulders, down the sides and back to the starting position.

client's abdomen, moving up the right side to the rib cage, across the abdomen just below the rib cage, then down the left side to an area just medial of the hip bone. Abdominal massage should always encourage the natural flow in the large intestines. Repeat the abdominal massage movements several times.

4. To massage the large intestine more thoroughly , apply circular friction to its entire length. Begin in the area of the lower left part of the abdomen. The circles should be on an oblique (deviation to the vertical or horizontal line) plane of the surface of the abdomen so that pressure is increased and decreased repeatedly over an area about two inches square, and at the rate of about 100 circles per minute. This movement encourages the contents of the colon toward the rectum. Proceed slowly back along the course of the colon all the way to the cecum, the first portion of the colon (Fig. 12.46a and b).

5. Knead the entire abdomen, massaging not only the abdominal muscles, but also stimulating the action of the abdominal organs.

6. Grasp as much of the abdominal tissue as possible and gently lift and shake it.

7. Do alternate hand strokes or shingles. Stand to one side of the client and reach over to the opposite side. Alternately pull your hands over the client's body toward you. As one hand nears completion of the stroke, the other begins a stroke. This movement begins just below the crest of the ilium (hipbone)

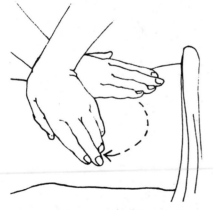

Fig. 12.46a Stroking the abdomen with deep circular movement.

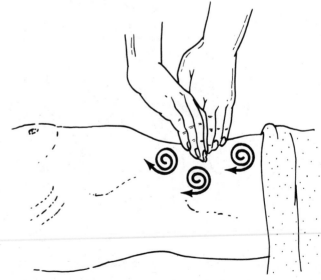

Fig. 12.46b Circular friction following the path of the large intestine.

and may continue all the way over the shoulder and up the neck. When working with breast draping, it is necessary to adjust the drape to continue this movement up to the axillary area and back down to the hip. When massaging the area of the ribs, flex your fingers slightly and rake gently between the ribs with your fingertips (Fig. 12.47a to g).

8. Move to the head of the table for the following stroke. This is referred to as the caring stroke and is a complete gliding stroke for the torso. This stroke can only be done when not using breast draping. Begin by placing your fingers (pointing toward each other) with palms flat on the client's skin at the

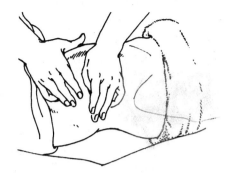
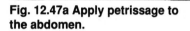

Fig. 12.47a Apply petrissage to the abdomen.

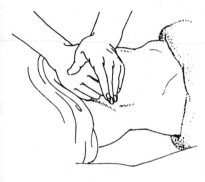

Fig. 12.47b Apply friction in small circles following the colon in reverse.

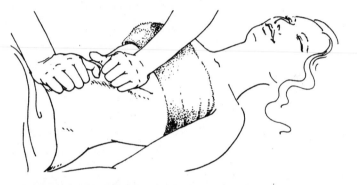

Fig. 12.47c Apply a shaking movement. Grasp the skin of the abdomen and shake it gently. This movement stimulates the action of the large and small intestines.

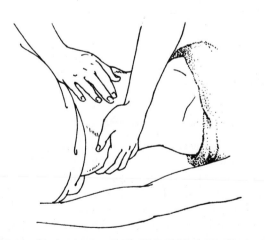

Fig. 12.47d Alternate-hand stroking movements (shingles) are applied from trochanter to axilla. Note: Shingles is the name often used to describe alternate hand effleurage in which one hand repeats the stroke as the previous hand is about to complete the stroke.

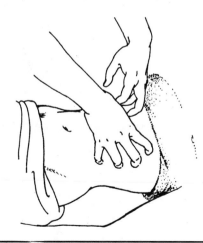

Fig. 12.47e Apply a raking movement several times with the tips of the fingers across the ribs and abdomen.

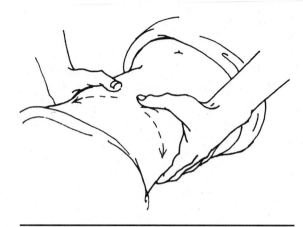

Fig. 12.47f Outward stretching of muscles of the stomach area and the abdominal region.

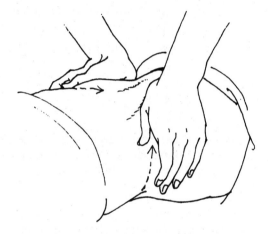

Fig. 12.47g Inward stretching of muscles over the stomach area and the abdominal region.

uppermost aspect of the chest. Stroke downward with the little fingers leading, over the chest and abdomen to the pubic bone. Rotate your hands over the client's hip bone, around the gluteus medius, around the sides, and back up to the axillary area. Rotate your hands as you continue upward, around the shoulders, up the trapezius muscles to the back of the neck, ending at the occiput. Rotate your hands as you move them back down to the starting point. Repeat the movement several times. Beware of any residual tension your hands might perceive, and spend a few extra moments to work on those areas. Then repeat the caring stroke (Fig. 12.48a to d).

This completes the massage of the front of the body.

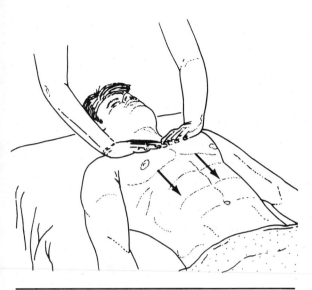

Fig. 12.48a Caring stroke covers the entire front of the body and the neck. It is not possible to do the full caring stroke on women when they are using breast draping.

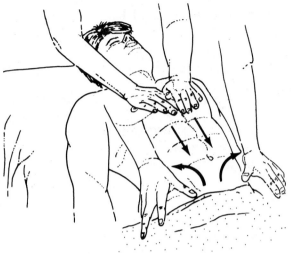

Fig. 12.48b The caring stroke begins at the collar bone with a stroke down the front of the body to the pubic bone.

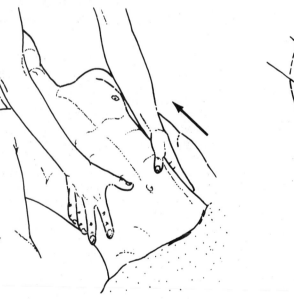

Fig. 12.48c Without losing contact, the hands rotate to the sides of the body and stroke up to the axillary area.

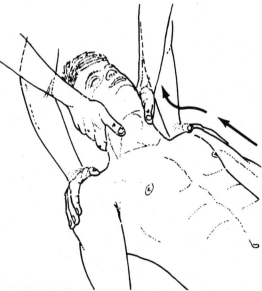

Fig. 12.48d The hands stroke up, over, and around the shoulders and up the neck. The stroke is repeated several times.

At this point, ask the client to turn over to a prone position. Be sure to follow proper draping procedures. Make the client comfortable by supplying a pillow or bolster to support the head, neck, back, chest, feet, or ankles as necessary.

Massage the Back of the Legs

1. Undrape one leg. This massage is similar to the procedures for the front of the legs.
2. Make contact with the client's skin and apply the oil with light effleurage strokes.
3. Apply effleurage, leading with your little finger of the lateral hand (medial hand following). Increase the pressure on the upward stroke with each pass. Repeat three to five times.
4. Apply petrissage to the calf and thigh upward to the crest of the ilium (Fig. 12.49a to g).

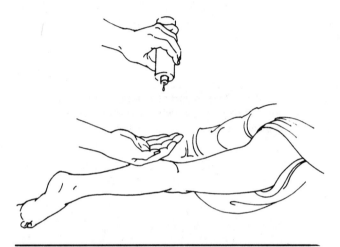

Fig. 12.49a Before beginning massage movements, prepare the posterior leg by undraping and applying oil. Keep the back of your hand against the client's skin while pouring the oil into your hand.

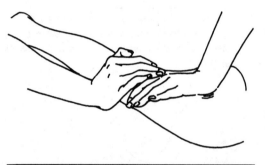

Fig. 12.49b Apply effleurage movements, leading with the little finger. Stroke toward the heart. Note: The leading hand is on the lateral aspect of the leg in order to travel up and over the gluteal muscles and the iliac crest and back down the lateral side of the leg. At the same time, the medial side of the leg. Both hands return to the starting point to repeat the stroke three or more times.

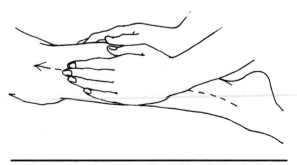

Fig. 12.49c Stroking the leg upward with both hands.

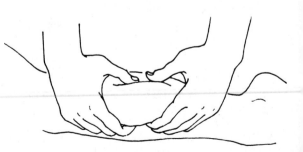

Fig. 12.49d Kneading the calf muscles.

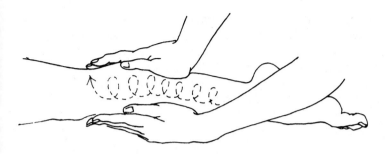

Fig. 12.49e Circular kneading muscles of leg and thigh.

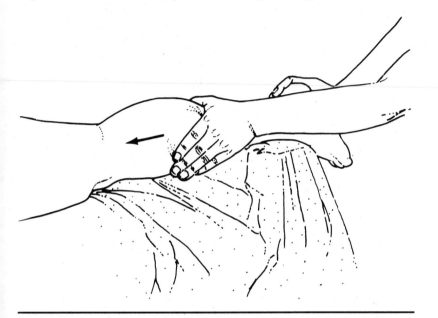

Fig. 12.49f Apply the V-stroke for deep stroking up the posterior leg.

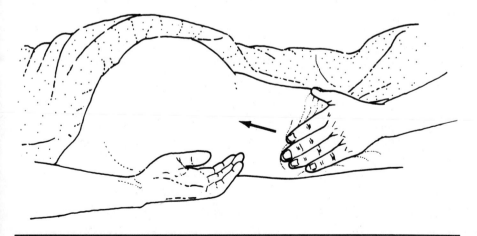

Fig. 12.49g V-stroke continues up the back of the thigh.

5. Repeat effleurage three to five times.
6. When there are particularly tight or tense areas, go over them with more specific friction movements such as compression, wringing, rolling, and deep friction. Using the heel of the hand can be quite effective over the gluteal muscles and the hamstrings (Fig. 12.50a to g).

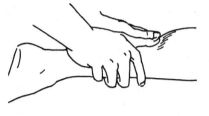

Fig. 12.50a Apply fulling strokes to the entire leg.

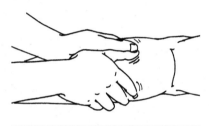

Fig. 12.50b Apply compression movements to the leg.

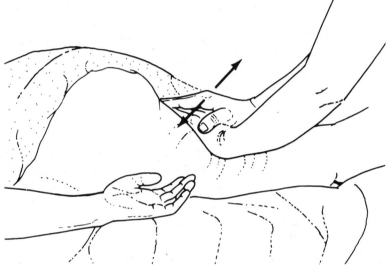

Fig. 12.50c Compression to the posterior thigh.

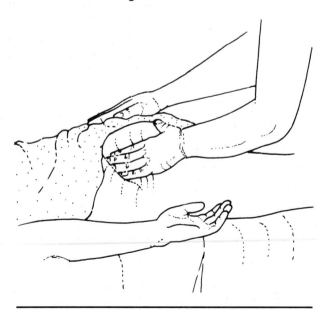

Fig. 12.50d Digital friction applied to the gluteal area.

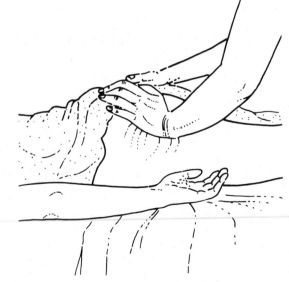

Fig. 12.50e Using heel of hand deep friction or deep pressure to the gluteal muscles.

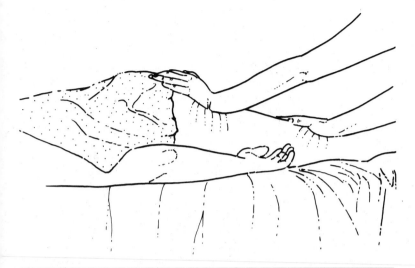

Fig. 12.50f When applying deep pressure always use proper body mechanics.

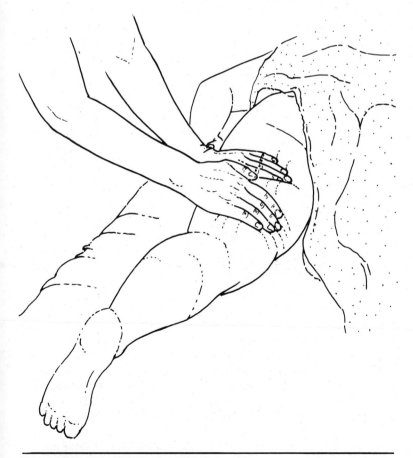

Fig. 12.50g Wringing back of thigh.

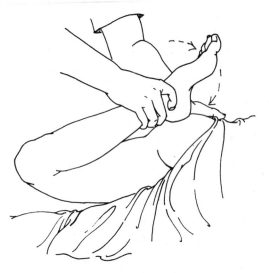

Fig. 12.51a Flex the client's knee, pressing the heel against the gluteal muscles.

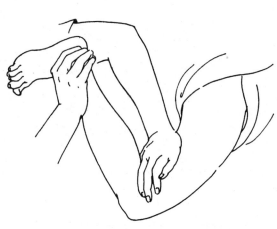

Fig. 12.51b Support the knee and circumduct the lower leg.

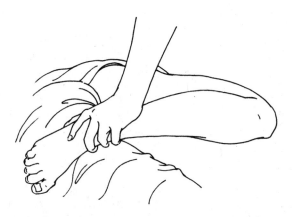

Fig. 12.51c Apply joint movements to flex knee and laterally rotate hip.

7. Repeat effleurage.
8. Apply joint movements. Grasp the client's ankle and move the foot toward the buttocks with gentle pressure to flex the knee and to stretch the muscles on the front of the thigh. Continue by making increasingly larger circles with the ankle to rotate the hip joint. Return the foot to the table (Fig. 12.51a to c).
9. Apply percussion (optional) over the leg (Fig. 12.52a and b).
10. Repeat effleurage as a finishing stroke, gently changing to feather (nerve) strokes.
11. Redrape the leg and repeat the entire procedure on the client's other leg.

Massage the Back

No massage is complete without a good back massage. It is important to give a good back massage because the client usually expects and looks forward to this part of the massage. There are hundreds of manipulations that may be done on the back. They range from extremely superficial stroking to deep tissue work using elbows and even knees when relieving tension around the spine, pelvis, and shoulders. The following is a basic soothing routine that is guaranteed to leave the recipient in a calm, relaxed state.

1. Follow proper draping procedures.
2. Stand to the side of the client. Apply oil with effleurage strokes.
3. Beginning at the top of the gluteal cleft, apply long effleurage strokes. Apply long gliding strokes up the spine to the nape of the neck.
4. Move your hands out and over the shoulders and down the sides to the hips. Rotate your hands and return to the starting point. Repeat the movement five to eight times. Use equal pressure on pulling and pushing strokes (Fig. 12.53a to d).
5. Apply petrissage. Begin with the gluteal region on the opposite side of the client from where you are standing. Knead the side of the body from below the hips up into the axillary area. Move hands to a position nearer to the spine (midway between the spine and extreme side of the body), then knead back down to the gluteal area. Work along the spine to include the trapezius muscles, the upper shoulders, and the neck.
6. Begin at the neck with alternate-hand strokes (shingles) from the side of the body to the spinal process. Move down to the top of the thigh and then back up to the top of the shoulder.

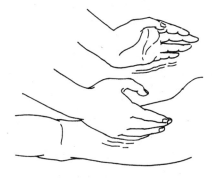

Fig. 12.52a Apply percussion to the posterior leg. The ulnar side of the hand aligns with the direction of the muscle fibers.

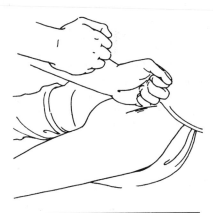

Fig. 12.52b Apply percussion (beating) to the gluteal area.

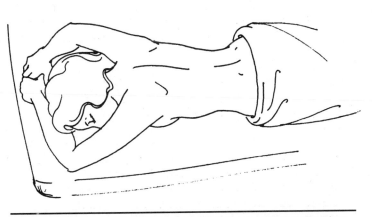

Fig. 12.53a Prepare for the massage of the back by adjusting the draping and applying oil with a light effleurage stroke.

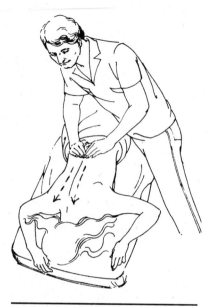

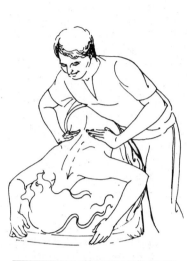

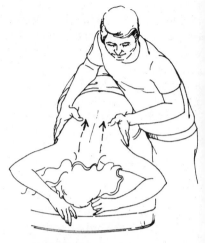

Fig. 12.53b Apply long strokes up the back beginning at the gluteal cleft. The ulnar side of the hand leads, with the fingers of one hand nearly touching the other at the midline of the back.

Fig. 12.53c Continue the long strokes up the back, to the neck, and over the shoulders.

Fig. 12.53d Continue with effleurage strokes back down the sides, returning to the starting point. Pressure is consistent throughout the entire stroke.

7. Change sides and repeat steps 2 through 6 (Fig. 12.54a to c).
8. Flex the client's elbow (closest to you), and place the client's hand on the table about six inches from the armpit. Some practitioners prefer to place the client's hand in the small of his or her back to abduct and elevate the scapula. In this position a number of kneading and friction movements can easily be performed on all sides of the scapula. Special

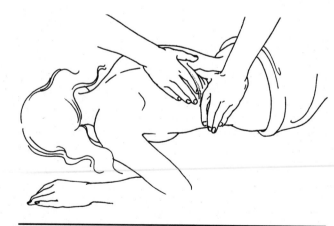

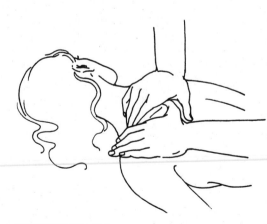

Fig. 12.54a Apply petrissage to the entire side that is opposite you. This takes several passes.

Fig. 12.54b Petrissage includes the trapezius muscles.

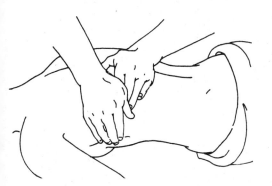

Fig. 12.54c Apply alternate-hand stroking movements, (shingles) up and down the entire side.

attention should be given the teres, trapezius, the rhomboids, and the infraspinatus muscles.

9. Apply joint movement. With the client's hand still in position at the side, grasp the top of the shoulder with one hand. Place your fingers neatly into a notch near the coracoid process, and use this hold as a handle. Place the other hand just inferior to the scapula so the inferior angle of the scapula fits neatly into the V formed between your thumb and index finger. Lift and rotate the scapula away from the rib cage. Although this may seem unnecessary, it is very effective in relieving a number of stress-related shoulder problems. Rotate the shoulder several times in both directions.

10. Abduct the elbow so the upper arm is at a square angle from the body and the forearm is relaxed at an angle from the upper arm. Support the arm with both of your hands just proximal to the elbow and gently swing the hand up and down, allowing the shoulder to rotate in a relaxed manner. Replace the hand and arm to the side of the body.

11. Repeat all the movements, eight through ten, on the other side of the back (Fig. 12.55a to e).

12. Apply deep kneading and friction to the gluteal area.

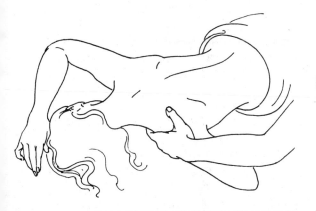

Fig. 12.55a Position the arm to elevate the scapula.

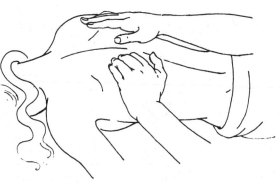

Fig. 12.55b Apply friction and compression movements to the muscles of the scapula.

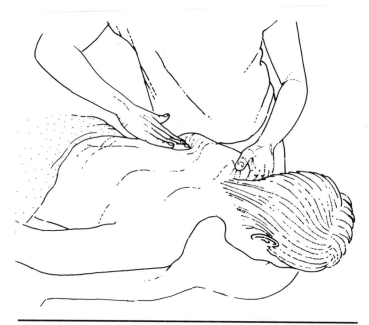

Fig. 12.55c Elevate the scapula and apply deep pressure and friction under the vertebral border.

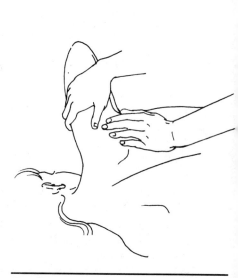

Fig. 12.55d Rotation of the shoulder is followed by stretching.

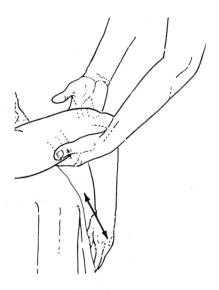

Fig. 12.55e Hold arm at elbow and rotate shoulder by swinging forearm back and forth.

13. Repeat effleurage on the entire back area.
14. Apply wringing friction to the back, moving back and forth across the back and working all the way up the neck and back down.
15. Apply circular friction on each side of the spine on the erector spine muscles.
16. Do "hand walking" bilaterally along the spine. Begin at the base of the spine just above the sacrum. Use the full palm side of your hand to apply deep effleurage from the spine to the side of the body. This is almost a compression stroke that slides. Use considerable weight on the strokes as you walk your hands up the client's back. Less weight is used in the area of the kidneys and the eleventh and twelfth ribs. Proceed with the walking movements up the back all the way to the area of the first thoracic vertebrae and then back down to the sacrum.
17. Do sacrospinalis vibration. Place the first two fingers of one hand to either side of the base of the client's spine, about two inches apart. Bend your fingers slightly, so they dig in on the medial edge of the sacrospinalis muscle and along each side of the spinus process. Place your other hand on the top of the hand resting on the client's back, and press down firmly while vibrating slowly (about 120 vibrations per minute) from side to side along the client's body. Slowly glide both hands up the spine, vibrating (jiggling) each spinal process back and

forth about three to ten times. Pay attention to any area along the spine that seems especially tense. These areas should be given extra attention. Work all the way up the spine to the seventh cervical vertebrae in this manner (Fig. 12.56a to h).

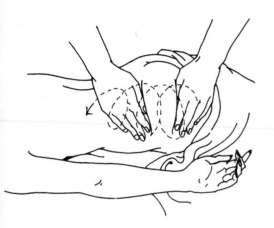

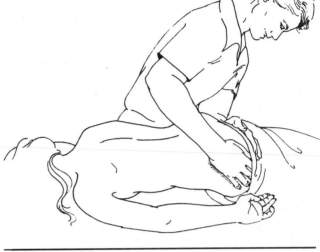

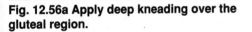

Fig. 12.56a Apply deep kneading over the gluteal region.

Fig. 12.56b Apply friction (compression) to the gluteal muscles.

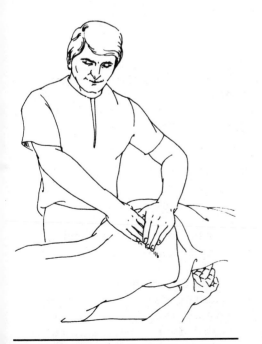

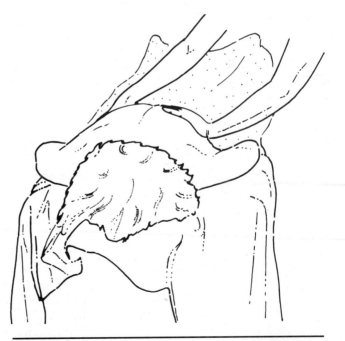

Fig. 12.56c Apply digital friction to the gluteal muscles.

Fig. 12.56d Apply wringing movements up and down the entire back.

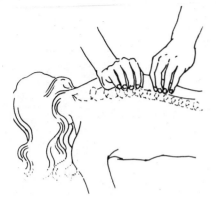

Fig. 12.56e Kneading around the spine.

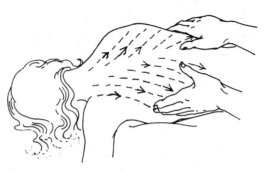

Fig. 12.56f Fan stroking of the back.

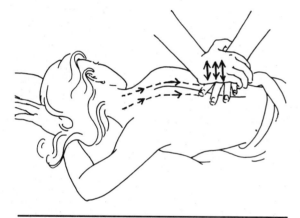

Fig. 12.56g Vibrating over each vertebra.

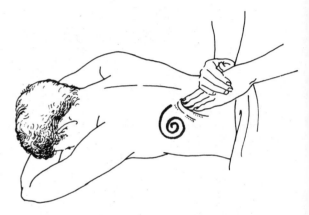

Fig. 12.56h Friction movements are applied to the muscles along the spine with the fingertips of one hand braced with the other hand. Movements are applied along both sides of the spine.

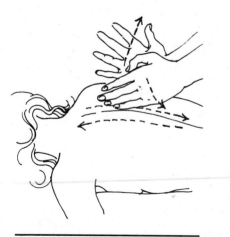

Fig. 12.57a Hacking movements on the back.

18. At this time a number of percussion movements are optional. Hacking may be done lightly over the entire back, including the gluteals and the back of the legs. (Avoid percussion over the area of the kidneys.) Beating movements may be applied over the thicker portions of the body. To end a stimulating massage, light slapping may be applied over the entire body (Fig. 12.57a to d).

19. A caring stroke completes the back massage. Remember that a caring stroke is an all-inclusive gliding stroke that is applied by standing at the head of the massage table. Place your hands on the upper back so that your fingers nearly touch in the area of the first and second thoracic vertebrae. Apply gliding strokes down the entire length of the spine. Your

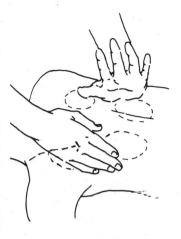

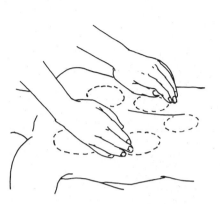

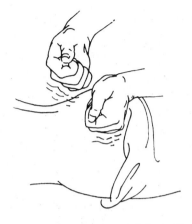

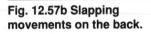

Fig. 12.57b Slapping movements on the back.

Fig. 12.57c Cupping along the back.

Fig. 12.57d Apply percussion with beating movements to the gluteal muscles.

hands glide over the gluteals and return up the lateral portion of the torso to the axillary area, slide smoothly over the deltoids up the trapezius to the occiput, and return to the starting point. Repeat the movements several times (Fig. 12.58a and b).

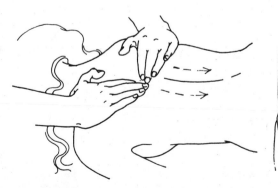

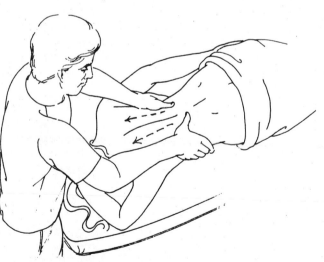

Fig. 12.58a Apply effleurage movements (caring stokes) from a position at the head of the client. The little finger leads the stroke, beginning at the nape of the neck.

Fig. 12.58b Continue effleurage movements down the back, over and around the gluteal muscles, back up the sides, then over and around the shoulders to the nape of the neck.

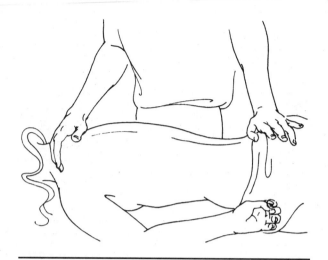

Fig. 12.59 A light touch to the base of the spine, the base of the neck, or the top of the head is a nice way to say hello or goodbye to the client's body.

A Finishing Touch

To complete the massage of the entire body, lightly place one hand on the sacrum and the other at the top of the spine and hold the position for several seconds. An option here is to apply a slight rocking motion (Fig. 12.59).

The state of relaxation brought on by massage makes the client mentally receptive, as in hypnosis. When fully relaxed, the client can be guided by the practitioner through some mental or physical exercise to enhance or relieve a particular condition. For example, the practitioner may place his or her hands on the client and make suggestions such as "You feel rested and relaxed," or "You will sleep better tonight because you are free of tension," or "You feel more relaxed than you have for some time." This type of positive suggestion should be made just before the client is fully awake.

Allow the client to relax quietly without being disturbed for several minutes. Assist the client to a sitting position. Be sure draping is properly placed and assist the client from the massage table as necessary. Show the client to the dressing area. After the client is dressed, take time to answer any questions or make recommendations.

Completion of the Massage

Following the massage, the client should be allowed to rest for a short while before going out to face the world again. This rest period is beneficial especially if you have done bodywork to the extent that some changes have taken place in the client's physical structure. A few moments of relaxation will help to integrate these changes into the client's psychological and neurological senses.

It is important to instruct the client in what to do and what to expect following the massage, especially clients who come to you for the first time. For example, when you ask the client to drink plenty of water to keep the system flushed out, explain that a massage, when done properly, can cause a lot of turmoil within the body tissues and that on the cellular level an increased rate of exchange of body fluids takes place. That increase means that some metabolic wastes have been expired from the cells and have been put into the general systemic circulation. This waste material has to be dealt with because it puts an extra burden on the excretory system. If this waste is not flushed out of the system, it will be reabsorbed into the tissues. An increase in the intake of water and other healthful fluids will assist in the process of elimination by supplying more fluids for the kidneys, the colon, the lungs and for perspiration.

You will need to give some guidelines as to the amount of water the client should drink. It is difficult to suggest a certain amount, but usually four quarts a day is about right. If the treatment was given in the afternoon, the client should drink about two quarts of water that day and four quarts the following day.

Aftereffects of Massage

Some clients experience certain aftereffects following massage and should be told that this is no cause for alarm. Usually the effects are felt following the first or second massage. Some people complain of a slight headache, upset stomach and nausea, or the feeling they get with the onset of a cold. Such reactions are due to an increase in metabolic waste material in the circulatory system. The particular symptom the client experiences depends on the organs that are being overtaxed. The intensity of the massage movements should be limited until the client has built up more tolerance. The client will seldom have a symptom that lasts for any length of time; however, he or she should be told to call you if there is a problem.

THERAPEUTIC PROCEDURE ▼

The previous procedure described a general full-body massage. This is only a recommended sequence that can be altered in many ways according to the preferences of the practitioner or needs of the recipient. This is a protocol for administering a relaxing and therefore therapeutic massage; however, giving massages according to a recipe or preset procedure may be less effective than following a therapeutic protocol to deliver a therapeutic massage. Often a person will seek the services of a massage therapist for relief of a specific condition. A relaxing full-body massage might be helpful, but it will probably not offer the relief of a more specific massage procedure. In these cases a therapeutic procedure specific to the client's complaint may be more appropriate.

Therapeutic procedure involves four basic steps:
1. Assessment
2. Planning
3. Performance
4. Evaluation.

Assessment involves reviewing any information available at the onset of the process to understand the present conditions.

During the planning stage, the information gained from the assessment is used to determine strategies and select therapeutic techniques to address specific conditions found during the assessment.

The performance is the actual application of the selected techniques.

The evaluation examines the outcome of the session in regard to the effectiveness of the selected procedure for the condition.

The therapeutic process can be implemented in many ways in the course of a massage therapy program. It is valuable for long-range goal setting, short-range planning, and during an actual massage session. In long-range goal setting, the assessment might be extensive and the planning encompass a number of sessions (six to ten). After the treatment strategy has been formulated and discussed and the treatments given, an evaluation is done to determine what progress has been made and what further therapy is needed.

Short-range planning might involve a single session. In this case, the assessment process may not be as extensive, but may focus more on a specific complaint. The client's needs are considered, indications and contraindications are determined, and a treatment strategy is decided on. The session is performed, and at the conclusion the outcome is evaluated as to the effectiveness of the session.

During a therapeutic massage session, the therapeutic procedure is constantly being applied. As the therapist proceeds through the massage, the hands are continuously assessing the condition of the tissues. The quality of the tissue, the constrictions in the tissue, or the movement of the limbs and the response from the client as different manipulations are being performed continuously provide information the therapist uses to plan the next manipulations. The evaluation process is also continuous as the therapist elicits feedback regarding the effectiveness throughout the treatment.

ASSESSMENT TECHNIQUES

To determine what massage procedures to perform on a prospective client or if it is advisable to refer the client to another health professional, it is necessary for the therapist to understand as much about the client and his or her condition as possible. An assessment that includes a client history, observation, and examination will help disclose problems and the physiological basis for the client's complaints.

History

A concise client history provides a wealth of background information about social, physiological, and psychological elements related to the complaints of the client. This information can be gathered by having the client fill out an information sheet and through a personal interview. Much of this takes place during the first consultation. A client information form may include questions about the client's age, occupation, hobbies, and reason for seeking your services. The form should contain questions about the client's medical history, including major illnesses, medications, surgeries, traumas, and allergies. If the client is under a doctor's care, find out who the doctor is and get permission to contact the doctor. Include questions about particular conditions the client has and the history of those conditions. Include a diagram of the body so the client can illustrate areas of concern (Fig. 12.60).

After reviewing the client information form, it may be helpful to augment the information with more questions so the client can describe the condition more elaborately. Take notes on the answers and include them in the client files for future evaluations. Find out when and how the condition started, what the client has done about it, what treatments the client has received and by whom, what has helped, what has made it worse, etc. Was there some incident that started the condition? Was the onset sudden or did it come on slowly? What has been the progression of the condition? Where in the body did the client first notice it? Is this the first time the condition has happened? If not how often, when was the last time, when was the first time?

If it is a painful condition, determine the location of the pain. Can the client put a finger or hand on it? Does it radiate or has it traveled from its original location? What affects it? What makes it worse or better? Does the time of day or activity affect it? What is the intensity, the duration, and the frequency of the pain? Does it come and go? How often and what instigates its return? Describe the pain.

Question the client about his or her tolerance of the condition and what he or she has done to cope with and correct the problem. Learn about the client and his or her willingness to do something about the condition.

Observation

The observation portion of a client assessment should begin when the client walks in the door and continue until he or she leaves. Watch for guarded movements the client uses to avoid or mask any pain.

Massage Clinic
Client Information Form

Name_____ Birth Date_____

Address_____ Telephone_____

_____ Business Phone_____

   City   State   Zip   Social Security #_____

Occupation_____ Other Activities_____

General Health Condition_____ Blood Pressure_____

Have you had any serious or chronic illness, operations, chronic virus infections, or traumatic accidents? _____

Are you in recovery for addictions or abuse?_____

Are you under a doctor, chiropractor or other health practitioners care? _____

If so, for what condition/s? _____

Are you on any medication? _____ If so, what?_____

Do I have permission to contact your Doctor / Therapist?_____

Names of Doctors, Chiropractors or Health Practitioners:

Name_____ Name_____

Address_____ Address_____

Telephone_____ Telephone_____

Why did you come for our services? (relaxation, pain, therapy, etc.)_____
_____

What results would you like to achieve with our work?_____

Have you had any massage therapy before?_____ If so, by whom?_____

How did you find out about our services? _____

Were you referred to this office?_____ By whom?_____

In case of emergency notify: Name_____Phone _____

I have completed this information form to the best of my knowledge. I understand the massage services are designed to be a health aid and are in no way to take the place of a doctors care when it is indicated. Information exchanged during any massage session is educational in nature and is intended to help me become more familiar and conscious of my own health status and is to be used at my own discretion.

Our time together is precious and I agree to cancel 24 hours in advance. Unless there is an emergency, if I miss an appointment I agree to pay the full appointment fee.

Date_____ Signature_____

Fig. 12.60 Client information form.

Look for bilateral symmetry both structurally and in the way the client moves. Throughout the assessment, it is helpful to compare one side of the body with the other. When doing many of the comparisons, look at the good side first to get an idea of personal norm for that individual, and then look at the affected side to assess the deviation from that norm. Note in the way a person moves if he or she holds one side of the body tighter or higher. Is the gait (walking) balanced and normal? Does the client stand erect, list to one side, or stoop?

Observing posture gives many indications of muscular imbalance and structural deviation. When observing a person, notice if one side of the body is held higher than the other. Notice the eyes, the ears, the shoulders, the hands, and the hips to see if they are level and even. Notice any rotation. Is either arm or leg rotated? Is the head rotated or tilted? Are the hips rotated or tilted? Posture is best observed when a person is standing erect and from all four sides. If a person has good posture, a plumb line will perfectly bisect the body when viewed from the front or back. From the side, the line would go through the ear, shoulder, elbow, acetabulum (as-e-**TAB**-yoo-lum), knee, and ankle. The farther out of balance the body is, the more strain is placed on the postural muscles. As a body ages, the pull of gravity tends to increase the deviations.

When the client lies down on the table in the supine position and is comfortable, again notice any deviations from bilateral symmetry. Observe the contour of the body as well as structural and skeletal symmetry. Is the client straight? Is the head tilted or turned? Is one leg rotated at a different angle? Are the hips level? Most minor postural deviations are caused by muscular imbalance. There is either muscle weakness (flaccidity), muscle tension, or both. Some forms of massage and soft tissue manipulation are very effective for relieving these imbalances.

Make note of abnormal marks, discoloration, varacosities, differences in skin texture, and scars. Check for skin conditions, redness, or swelling (signs of inflammation). Be aware of anything that might be a sign of former trauma or conditions that may indicate or contraindicate massage (Fig. 12.61).

Assess Range of Motion

Range of motion is the action of a joint through the entire extent of its movement. Assessing the extent and quality of that movement by testing the active, passive, and resisted (isometric) movement provides information about the tissues involved with the joint.

Dr. James Cyriax, an osteopath from England, has developed an extensive system of testing all the joints to isolate lesions in the hard and soft tissues. He has clarified and defined some terms and concepts that are invaluable when assessing range of motion. Those concepts include *contractile tissue, inert tissue, end feel,* and *capsular patterns*.

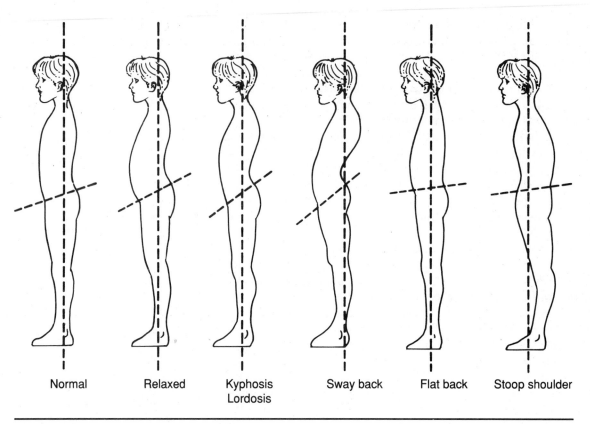

Normal   Relaxed   Kyphosis   Sway back   Flat back   Stoop shoulder
                     Lordosis

Fig. 12.61 Normal posture (with plumb line).

Contractile tissues are the fibrous tissues that have tensions placed on them during muscular contractions and include muscle tissue, tendons, and the muscle attachments.

Inert tissues are the tissues that are not contractile such as bone, ligament, bursae, blood vessels, nerves, nerve coverings, cartilage, etc.

End feel refers to the quality of the sensation the therapist feels as he or she passively moves a joint to the full extent of its possible range.

The **capsular pattern** refers to the proportional limitation of any joint that is controlled by muscular contractions.

When assessing range of motion, test the good side first to help determine an individual norm. First perform the active movements, then the passive, and finally the resisted movements. When testing, observe objective and subjective findings. Objective findings are things the therapist sees or feels such as muscle strength and degree of joint movement. Subjective findings include the amount of pain or discomfort the client feels and how he or she reacts to the pain. Objective findings generally can be measured where subjective findings are usually felt or perceived.

Assess Active Movements

Assessing active movement indicates the client's ability and willingness to move a limb through a range of motion. The client is instructed to move through a particular range of motion. The client makes the movement totally unassisted. If the entire movement can be made smoothly and painlessly, chances are there is no problem with that joint or the associated soft tissue. Both contractile and inert tissues are involved during active movement, so if there is an obvious limitation, pain, or hesitation during the movement, a closer assessment is needed.

If there was any pain during the movement, the therapist should note when in the movement the pain occurred, the intensity of the pain, the quality of the pain, and the client's reaction to the pain. If there is limitation to the movement, note where the limitation occurred and whether or not it was accompanied by pain.

Assess Passive Movement

When assessing passive movement, the practitioner moves the client's joint through the full range of motion while the client remains relaxed. During passive movement the practitioner determines the degree and quality of movement in a joint. The practitioner can sense if the joint is hyper- or hypomobile. The therapist also notes if there is any catches, crepitis, or pain involved. The reactions of the client must also be observed. Any apprehensiveness or unwillingness must be considered.

End feel plays a very important part in assessing passive movement. End feel is the feeling the therapist senses as he or she passively moves a limb to the limit of its range of motion. The quality of the end feel indicates the presence, type, and severity of lesions in the tissues associated with the joint.

There are three types of end feel considered normal: *hard, soft, and springy*.

Hard end feel is a bone-against-bone feeling. This is an abrupt, painless limitation to further movement that happens at the normal end of the range of motion such as knee or elbow extension.

Soft end feel is a cushioned limitation where soft tissue prevents further movement, such as knee or elbow flexion.

Springy end feel is the most common. Limitation is due to the stretch of fibrous tissue as the joint reaches the extent of its range of motion.

Normal end feel happens at the end of a normal range of motion and, unless carried to extremes, is painless. Pain or an observable limitation of movement indicates that some abnormal condition or lesion is present. If there is pain before reaching the end of the movement and there is no muscular resistance or spasm, bursitis or capsulitis might be involved. If the movement causes a sudden painful, muscle reaction or spasm, the body may be protecting an injury in the area. Cyriax calls this an empty end feel. The more acute and severe the injury, the more severe the pain and spasm. A medical referral and diagnosis should be recommended. Other abnormal patterns are similar to normal end feel, except that there is reduced movement or there is associated pain.

Passive movement assessment indicates the condition of the inert (noncontractile) tissues. Limitation of movement and pain are the indicators of malfunction. Full, painless range of motion indicates that the joint and associated structures are healthy. Range of motion that is limited with a painless, hard (bone-to-bone) end feel indicates osteoarthritis. Pain and limitation in all directions generally involve the whole joint and indicate capsulitis or arthritis. Pain or limitation in one direction and not another is usually due to stretching or compressing the involved tissue. More specific assessment must be done to isolate the involved tissue.

Assess Resisted Movement

Resisted or isometric movement is used to assess the condition of the contractile tissues (muscles, tendons, and attachments).

Indicators of lesions in the contractile tissue are weakness and pain. To perform resisted movement assessment or muscle testing, the therapist stabilizes a body part in a neutral position and commands the client to move that body part in a specific direction. As the client contracts the muscle, the therapist applies pressure to move the body part in the opposite direction so that the limb does not move. Eliminating any joint movement minimizes reactions of the inert tissues and indicates the relative strength and condition of the contractile tissues. Positioning the body part and instructing the client to make specific movements isolates specific muscles to be tested.

When contractile tissues are involved, active movement and resisted movement will both give positive results. Passive movement will show nothing except at the end of the movement where the contractile tissue is stretched and will react with pain or spasm.

Muscle testing provides information as to the condition of the muscles involved in a specific movement. As with the other physical assessment tools, it is important to compare one side of the body with the other. Test the good side first for comparison. A muscle test that is strong and pain free indicates healthy muscle tissue. A strong and painful muscle test indicates a lesion in the contractile tissue such as a minor (first-or-second degree) muscle strain. A weak and painless muscle test indicates interference with the nerve supply, circulation, or energy to the muscle. No strength in the muscle may be due to a severed muscle or tendon (third-degree strain) or a loss of enervation. A very weak and painful muscle test indicates a severe lesion, possibly a torn ligament or fracture.

In general, the more severe the condition, the more severe the pain.

Assess by Palpation

The sense of touch is one of a massage therapist's most powerful tools. It is what puts the therapist in touch with the client. It is the means of communication between the therapist and the client's body. Developing palpatory skills, sensing the difference in tissue quality and integrity, and responding with appropriate therapy techniques is the mark of a good massage therapist.

Although many massage therapists use palpation as the primary form of assessment, it is most accurate when used in conjunction with and after the afore mentioned assessment skills. Especially in pain conditions where there is radiating or referred pain, observation and examination isolate the cause of the pain and then palpation pinpoints the source.

The sensitive hands of the therapist can detect variations in temperature and skin texture. Elevated temperature can indicate fever or local inflammation. Palpation also detects abnormal sensations the client may be experiencing such as lack of sensation or increased or diminished sensation.

As with the other assessment techniques, it is important to make bilateral comparisons. Although many conditions affect both sides of the body, bilateral comparison helps establish what is normal for the individual and helps determine if the tissue in question is involved in the dysfunctional condition.

Assessment by palpation is both objective and subjective. As the therapist's hands palpate the body's tissues, the therapist must pay close attention to not only to the qualities of the tissue but also to the reactions of the client. The therapist begins lightly and proceeds to probe deeper into the tissues, noting any signs of tension or lesions.

Palpating bony landmarks helps when observing structural discrepancies such as a tilted or rotated pelvis. Palpating the bony tissue around joints may indicate abnormal development or calcification. The position and regularity of the skeletal structure is also noted.

Palpating the soft tissues helps the therapist determine the feel of the individual client's normal soft tissue, detect anatomical anomalies, and detect soft tissue lesions or pathology.

When palpating muscles the therapist observes tissue consistency and texture. A common palpable condition found in muscle that is usually associated with a lesion is a fibrous or taut band. Taut bands usually run the length of a muscle and feel like a hardened bundle that you can actually pluck. Taut bands are usually associated with a previous injury, a strained muscle, or a habitually overstressed area. Often a taut band will harbor one or more hypersensitive points (trigger points). Palpation effectively locates other hypersensitive points and areas. Finding and reducing taut bands and trigger points is one of the most effective ways of treating soft tissue pain and dysfunction.

Use Assessment Information to Plan Sessions

When the assessment has been completed, the therapist should have a clearer understanding of the client's condition. Using the assessment information, the therapist is better able to develop a strategy to best suit the needs of the client. Depending on the findings of the assessment, that strategy may include:

• Referral to another health professional for further assessment
• Referral to another health professional for treatment in lieu of or in conjunction with massage
• The initial number and frequency of sessions to be given
• The estimated length of the treatments and whether they are full body or specific to the condition
• The use of other modalities such as heat, ice, hydrotherapy, etc.
• What massage techniques will be used.
• What results are expected and by when.

Accurate assessment allows the therapist to design treatments with modalities and massage techniques and regimes that will best benefit the client.

The assessment findings and strategy can be discussed with the client so that he or she can be actively involved in the therapy process. Clients who actively participate in the therapy generally reap more benefits, respond to the therapy faster, and tend to follow through for a more lasting remedy. Discussing the assessment findings with clients teaches them about the functions of the body and the nature of the condition they have so they can make educated choices as to what changes they can make to help correct the condition. Discussing optional therapy strategies enables clients to be involved and make choices about what they want to do about their condition. Discussing therapy strategies with clients gives them a clear idea of what the therapy will consist of and what they might expect during the actual sessions.

When discussing assessment findings and treatment strategies with a client, use terminology the client can understand. Some clients will be more interested than others. Be clear in describing assessment findings. Use diagrams and charts to illustrate physical conditions when possible. Give enough information to inform clients without saturating them with unnecessary technicalities.

Performance

When the preliminary assessment has been done and a strategy has been developed, it is time to begin the actual therapy. Depending on the chosen strategy, a number of modalities may proceed or follow the actual massage. Hot packs, ice packs, ice massage, hot baths, or showers can be used previous to massage therapy to enhance the desired therapeutic effects. Used with other therapy modalities, various types of electrical stimulation, ultrasound, and exercise can be incorporated to produce excellent results.

The assessment and planning stages provide a blueprint for the procedures performed during treatment. Even though a proposed outline for the massage session is followed, there is still room to alter the treatment according the needs of the client's condition. Throughout the massage, the therapist continues the assessment as he or she works on each part of the body. In most therapeutic massages a routine is followed, but close attention is paid to the response of the client. Responses may be verbal, subtle movements or changes in the actual tissue that is being manipulated. The therapist continuously elicits feedback from the client and modifies the session to obtain the ultimate results.

Therapeutic massage is like an intense conversation. The therapist listens, observes, and examines the client to get an idea of the condition. Then the therapist's hands listen to the client's body and respond with manipulative touch. The body listens to the manipulations and responds. Hearing and feeling these responses, the therapist chooses the next delivery. And so goes the close interaction of a therapeutic massage.

Review Outcome in Relation to Intent of Session

Evaluation involves examining the outcome of the process in relation to the expected objectives. Evaluation is important in that the client and therapist can gauge the effectiveness of the selected course of therapy according to the success in attaining the goals. Examining the outcome is important when deciding ongoing therapy. It provides a rationale for applying similar therapies for similar conditions in the future. Evaluation is the grounds for altering portions or all of the process to better achieve desired results. Finally, evaluation helps determine if goals have been met and if a referral to another professional is warranted.

Evaluation is both subjective and objective. Much of the evaluation is based on how the client feels as a result of the therapy. Levels of posture, mobility, pain, and function can be reassessed to indicate the success of the treatment.

Evaluation is done at various times during the therapeutic process. After the assessment, an evaluation is done to decide how or if to proceed. If the decision is made to do several sessions, evaluations after each session help to determine the continued course of therapy. An evaluation at the end of the series helps to determine the course into the future.

QUESTIONS FOR DISCUSSION AND REVIEW ▼

1. How often should the practitioner wash his or her hands with soap and water?
2. Why is it advisable to assist a client on and off the table?
3. How can the practitioner prevent the chilling of the client's body?

4. Briefly describe three methods of draping.
5. Besides draping, how can the therapist ensure that the client stays warm?
6. How can the practitioner avoid scratching the client's body?
7. Which massage movements should be avoided because they convey fear of injury to the client?
8. Is it better to massage the body before or after a meal?
9. What is the average duration of a massage?
10. In which conditions should massage never be applied?
11. What preliminaries require attention before body massage?
12. Which position does the client usually assume first for body massage?
13. What is the usual order of massage movements?
14. What are the final considerations after completing body massage?
15. What are some undesirable aftereffects of massage and why do they occur?
16. Why should the client be advised to drink plenty of water?
17. What are the four steps of a therapeutic procedure?
18. What is the purpose of each of the steps of the therapeutic procedure?
19. How can the therapeutic procedure be implemented in therapeutic massage?
20. Name three important parts of the assessment process.
21. Name three types of movement tested when assessing range of motion.
22. According to Dr. James Cyriax, what is contractile tissue? inert tissue? end feel?
23. Name three classifications of end feel considered to be normal.
24. What are the characteristics of abnormal end feel?
25. How is a therapeutic massage like an intense conversation?
26. What are the important advantages of using the evaluation portion of the therapeutic process?

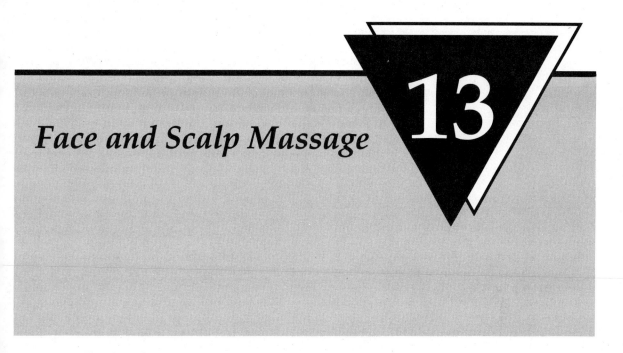

Face and Scalp Massage

13

Learning Objectives

After you have mastered this chapter, you will be able to:

1. Select and prepare the appropriate products and items needed to give a basic face or scalp massage.
2. Explain the benefits of face or scalp massage.
3. Explain contraindications for face and scalp massage.
4. Demonstrate corect procedures for cleansing the face.
5. Demonstrate corect procedures for giving a face massage.
6. Demonstrate corect procedures for giving a basic scalp massage.

▼ INTRODUCTION

Face massage benefits the skin by stimulating blood to the tissues, thereby nourishing the skin. Massage helps to tone the skin and keep underlying muscles firm. It also helps to keep sebaceous (oil) glands and the sudoriferous (sweat) glands functioning normally. The cleansing procedure removes surface as well as deeply embedded soil and helps to prevent problem blemishes such as blackheads, whiteheads, and pimples.

Practitioners may give a basic face and scalp massage as part of the complete massage service. Some clients may request one or both of these services, while others may not. Whether or not to include face or scalp massage can be determined during the consultation.

The face and scalp massages included in this chapter are basic cleansing and relaxing procedures.

▼ FACE MASSAGE

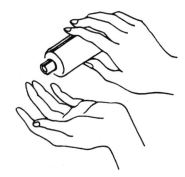

A face massage may consist of basic cleansing of the skin and gentle, relaxing massage movements, or it might include more extensive procedures using machines and various products. A complete face massage may be given as part of the therapeutic body massage, or it may be limited to a few rotary movements at the temples, around the forehead, and at the base of the skull. Generally, the massage practitioner gives only the basic, face massage.

An esthetician specializes in face massage and skin care. An esthetician may work with a dermatologist in the treatment of skin problems or in a salon where nonmedical, preventive skincare treatments are given. The esthetician does a variety of manual massage movements and may also use various machines and apparatus such as vaporizers, brushing and suction machines, as well as an assortment of products to achieve the desired results. Many estheticians are also qualified to give therapeutic body massage.

Whether the practitioner gives a partial or complete face massage, it is important to understand corect procedures. As with body massage, once the basic movements are mastered, the massage can be varied.

Fig. 13.1a Wash the hands with mild soap and warm water and rinse them thoroughly. Wipe the hands with alcohol and dry them carefully. Nails should be a reasonable length and smooth so they will not scratch the client's face during the facial procedure.

The Consultation

During the consultation it can be determined whether or not the client would like a face massage. Some women prefer not having their makeup disturbed. The client may have a skin condition such as an allergy which would be a contraindication for face massage.

Cleansing Procedures

If the client has a healthy skin and wishes a face massage, the following items to be used for the facial should be prepared in advance:
- Mild cleansing cream or lotion
- Mild astringent or skin freshening lotion

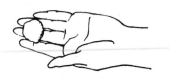

Fig. 13.1b Apply about one level teaspoon or less of the cleansing product to the fingers of either the right or left hand.

- A small towel or cape for the client's shoulders
- Cotton pads and pledgets to apply and remove cosmetics
- Cotton-tipped swabs and facial tissues to remove makeup from eye area and the lips
- A towel or headband to protect the client's hair.

Cotton pads should be prepared and moistened in cool water and then placed in a sterile container until needed (Fig. 13.1a to k).

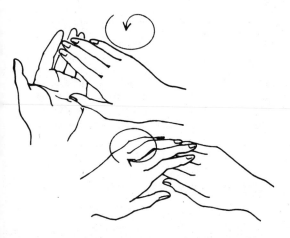

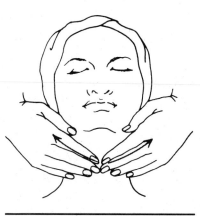

Fig. 13.1c With the other hand, distribute the product over both sides of the fingers. You are now ready to apply the product to the client's face.

Fig. 13.1d Place both hands palm down on the client's neck. Slide the hands back toward the client's ears until the finger pads rest at a point directly below the earlobes.

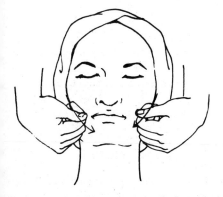

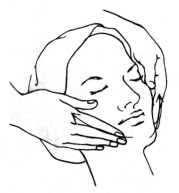

Fig. 13.1e Reverse the hands so the back of the fingers are resting on the skin. Slide the fingers along the jawline to the chin.

Fig. 13.1f Reverse the hands again, and slide the fingers back over the cheeks until the finger pads come to rest directly in front of the client's ears.

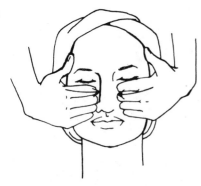

Fig. 13.1g Reverse the fingers again, and slide them forward over the cheekbones to the nose.

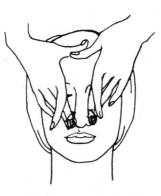

Fig. 13.1h With the pads of the middle fingers, make small circular motions on the flares of the nostrils.

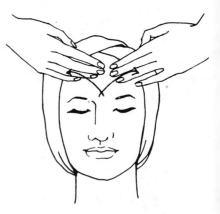

Fig. 13.1i Slide the fingers up to the forehead and outward toward the temples, and pause with a slight pressure on the temples.

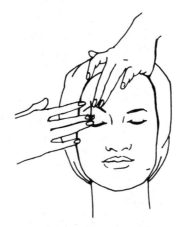

Fig. 13.1j Bring the left hand over and lift the right eyebrow with the middle and ring fingers. With the middle and ring fingers of the right hand, apply the cleansing product to the eyelid with downward strokes.

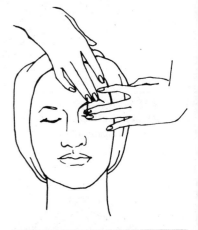

Fig. 13.1k Move the middle and ring fingers of the right hand over to the left side of the face, and lift the left eyebrow. With the middle fingers of the left hand, apply the cleansing product to the left lid with downward strokes.

Repeat the movements until the cleansing product has been applied thoroughly to the client's face and neck.

Removing Cleanser

Some professional practitioners prefer to use wet cotton pads when cleansing and working on the face. Others prefer to use facial sponges. Both methods are corect and equally professional. Many practitioners use both methods. In some areas, the facial sponges are not readily available, whereas cotton can be purchased at all drug and variety stores. Supply houses refer to cotton as "beautician's" cotton. Even when using sponges, some cotton is needed during the treatment for eyepads, and applying products such as astringent.

Procedure for Removing Cleanser with a Cotton Pad

It is important that the client be comfortable and relaxed throughout the face massage. Moistened cotton pads should be kept at a comfortable temperature, as very cold pads can be shocking and uncomfortable. Excess water should be squeezed from a prepared cotton pad so that no water drips on the client during the cleansing procedure (Fig. 13.2a to j).

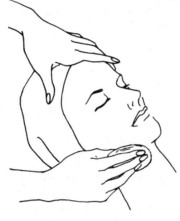

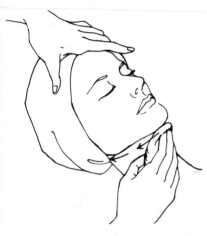

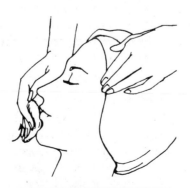

Fig. 13.2a Begin the cleansing procedure at the base of the neck, using upward strokes. If you are cleansing a man's face, do all the cleansing movements in the direction of the beard growth.

Fig. 13.2b Place the pad directly under the chin and slide it upward along the jawline. Stop directly under the ear.

Fig. 13.2c Repeat the movement on the other side of the face.

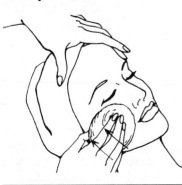

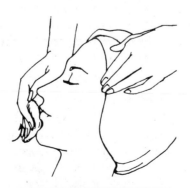

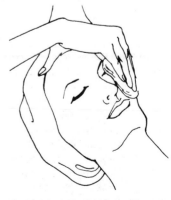

Fig. 13.2d Beginning at the jawline, use upward movements to cleanse the cheek.

Fig. 13.2e Continue the upward movement, crossing over the chin.

Fig. 13.2f Continue upward stroking movements to cleanse the cheeks.

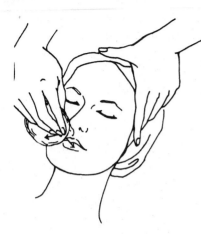

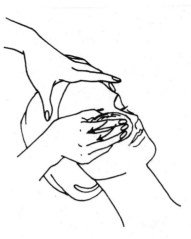

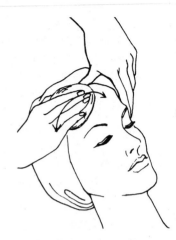

Fig. 13.2g Cleanse the area directly under the nose, Begin at the center, working outward toward the corners of the mouth. Alternate the movements back and forth three times on each side of the face.

Fig. 13.2h Begin on the bridge of the nose, and cleanse the right side and the area directly beside the nose. Repeat on the left side.

Fig. 13.2i Place the pad on the center of the forehead, and slide it to the right temple. Apply slight pressure to the temple. Repeat on the left side.

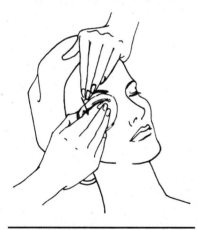

Fig. 13.2j With the middle and ring fingers of the left hand, lift the eyebrow. Use downward movements with the cleansing pad to cleanse the eyelids and lashes. Repeat the movements until both eyes are cleansed. Finally, take a clean pad and go over the entire face gently. Blot the face dry with a tissue if necessary. You are now ready to apply massage cream or lotion for the massage procedure. Use the same techniques as for applying cleansing lotion.

Manipulations for Face Massage

Effleurage

Effleurage is a light continuous movement applied to the skin with the fingers digital and palms (palmar) in a slow and rhythmic manner. Over large surfaces, the palm of the hand is used. Over small areas as on the face, the cushions of the fingertips are employed. Massage movements are generally directed toward the origin of the muscles in order to avoid damage to delicate muscular tissues.

For the correct position for stroking, the fingers should be slightly curved, with just the cushions of the fingertips (not the tips of the nails) touching the skin (Figs. 13.3 and 13.4).

The corect position for palmar stroking is to keep the wrist and fingers flexible, curving the fingers to conform to the shape of the area being massaged (Fig. 13.5).

Petrissage

Petrissage is a kneading movement whereby the skin and flesh are grasped gently between the thumb and the forefinger. As the tissues are lifted from their underlying structures, they are squeezed, rolled, or pinched with a gentle but firm pressure. When grasping and releasing the fleshy parts of the face, a smooth, rhythmic movement should be maintained. Kneading movements give deeper stimulation, improve circulation, and help to empty the oil ducts (Fig. 13.6).

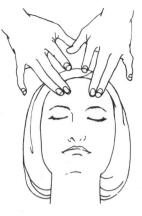

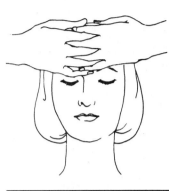

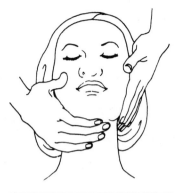

Fig. 13.3 Digital stroking of the face.

Fig. 13.4 Digital stroking of the forehead.

Fig. 13.5 Palmar stroking of the face.

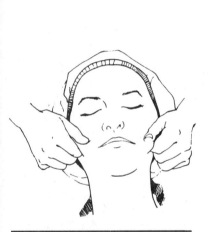

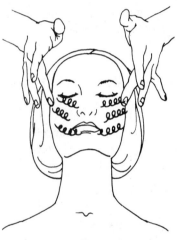

Fig. 13.6 Digital kneading of the cheeks.

Fig. 13.7 Circular friction of the face.

Friction

Friction is a movement that requires light pressure on the skin while it is moved over the underlying structures. The fingers and palms are employed in this movement. Friction has a marked influence on the circulation and glandular activity of the skin (Fig. 13.7).

Percussion or tapotement

Percussion or tapotement consists of tapping, slapping, and hacking movements. This is the most stimulating form of massage and should be performed with extreme care. In facial massage, only light digital tapping is used. In tapping, the fingertips are brought down against the skin in rapid succession. The fingers must be

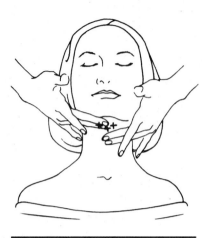

Fig. 13.8 Tapping under the chin.

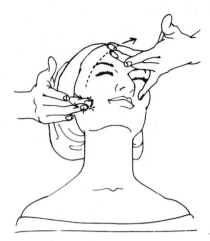

Fig. 13.9 Light slapping and lifting on the cheek.

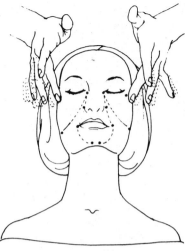

Fig. 13.10 Vibratory movement of the face.

flexible to create an even force over the area being treated (Fig. 13.8).

Slapping movements require flexible wrists to permit the palms to come in contact with the skin in very light, firm, and rapid movements. One hand follows the other in a rhythmic movement. When used in face massage, care must be taken to apply gentle movements only (Fig. 13.9).

Vibration (shaking movements)

Vibration is a movement accomplished by rapid muscular contractions in the arms while pressing the fingertips firmly on the point of application. It is a highly stimulating movement and should be used sparingly. It should never exceed a few seconds duration on any one spot (Fig. 13.10).

Muscular contractions can also be produced by use of apparatus such as mechanical vibrators. To obtain proper results from face massage, you should have a thorough knowledge of anatomy, especially of muscles, nerves, and blood vessels affected by massage. Almost every muscle and nerve has a motor point. The position of motor points will vary in location in individuals due to differences in body structure. A few manipulations on the right motor points will induce relaxation at the beginning of the massage treatment.

Massage Procedure

Apply the facial oil over the face and neck using the same movement as in applying cleansing lotion to the face and proceed with the massage (Fig. 13.11a to r).

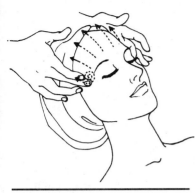

Fig. 13.11a Linear movement over the forehead. Slide the fingers to the temples, rotate with pressure on an upward stroke, slide to left eyebrow; then stroke the forehead across and back.

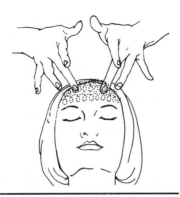

Fig. 13.11b Circular movement over the forehead. Begin at the eyebrow line, work across the middle of the forehead, and then toward the hairline.

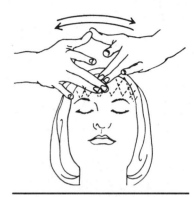

Fig. 13.11c Criss-cross movement. Begin at one side of the forehead, making cross movements and then working back.

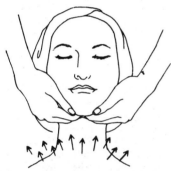

Fig. 13.11d Chin movement. Use light pressure with fingertips to lift chin.

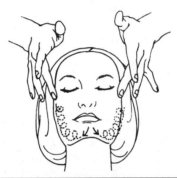

Fig. 13.11e Lower cheek. Use circular movement from chin to ear and rotate.

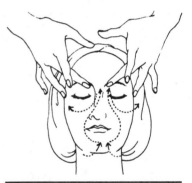

Fig. 13.11f Mouth, nose, and cheek movement. Make light circular movements from the chin.

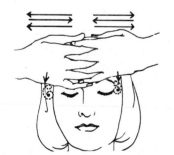

Fig. 13.11g Stroking movement. Slide the fingers to the center of the forehead and then, with slight pressure, draw the fingers toward the temples and rotate.

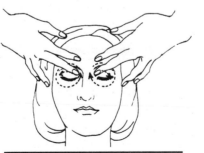

Fig. 13.11h Brow and eye movement. Place the middle finger at the inner corner of the eyes and the index finger over the brows. Slide the fingers to the outer corners of the eyes, under the eyes, and back.

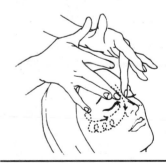

Fig. 13.11i Nose and upper cheek. Apply rotary movements across the cheeks to the temples, and rotate gently. Slide the fingers under the eyes and back to the bridge of the nose.

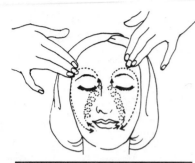

Fig. 13.11j Mouth and nose movement. Apply circular movement from the corners of the mouth up the side of the nose. Slide the fingers over the brows and down to the corners of the mouth.

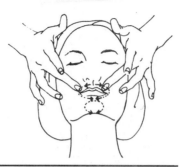

Fig. 13.11k Lip and chin movement. Draw the fingers from the center of the upper lip, around the mouth, and under the lower lip and chin.

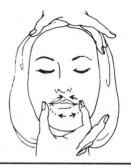

Fig. 13.11l Optional movement. Hold the client's head with the left hand, and draw the fingers of the right hand from under the lower lip and around the mouth.

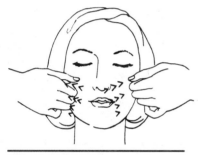

Fig. 13.11m Lifting movement of cheeks. Use knuckles to lift gently from mouth to ears, and then from nose to the top part of the ears.

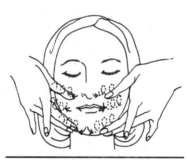

Fig. 13.11n Rotary movement of cheeks. Massage from chin to earlobes, and from the nose to the top if the ears.

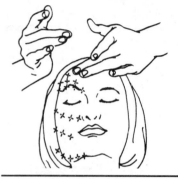

Fig. 13.11o Light tapping movement. Do light tapping movements from chin to earlobe, mouth to ear, and then across the forehead.

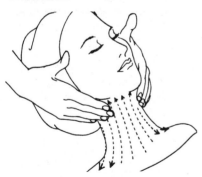

Fig. 13.11p Stroking movement of the neck. Apply light upward strokes over the front of the neck. Use heavier pressure in the sides of the neck in downward strokes.

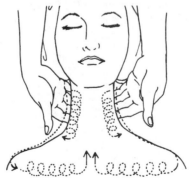

Fig. 13.11q Circular movements over the neck and chest. Beginning at the back of the ears, apply circular movement down the sides of the neck, over the shoulders, and across the neck.

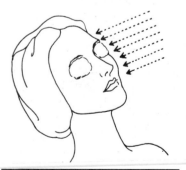

Fig. 13.11r Infrared lamp (optional). Protect eyes with eyepads. Adjust the lamp over the client's face, and leave it on for about five minutes.

CHEST AND BACK MASSAGE ▼

Chest, back, and neck manipulations are optional. Some practitioners prefer to treat these areas first before giving the face massage. A suggested procedure is as follows:

1. Apply and remove cleansing cream or lotion.
2. Apply massage cream or oil.
3. Give manipulations.
4. Remove cream or lotion with tissues or a warm, moist towel.
5. Dust the back lightly with talcum powder (Fig. 13.12a to c).

Following the complete face massage, cleanse the face with a fresh, moist pad, apply astringent (for oily skin) or skin freshening lotion (for normal and dry skin). Finish with a light application of moisturizing cream or lotion, or a protective cream or lotion.

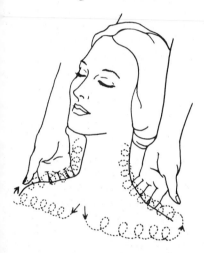 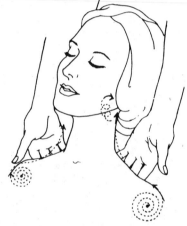 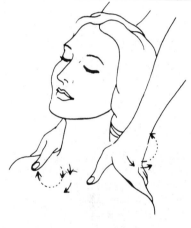

Fig. 13.12a Chest and back movements. Use rotary movements across the chest and shoulders and then the spine. Slide the fingers to the base of the neck and rotate three times.

Fig. 13.12b Shoulder and back movements. Rotate shoulders three times. Slide the fingers to the spine, then to the base of the neck. Apply circular movements up to the back of the ear, then slide the fingers to front of the earlobe and rotate three times.

Fig. 13.12c Back massage (optional). To relax the client, use thumbs and bend index fingers to grasp the tissue at the back of the neck. Rotate six times. Repeat over the shoulders and back to the spine.

SCALP MASSAGE ▼

In scalp massages, apply firm pressure on upward strokes. Firm rotary movements are given to loosen scalp tissues. These movements improve the health of hair and scalp by increasing the circulation of blood to the scalp and hair papillae. When giving a scalp massage, care should be taken to give the manipulations slowly, without pulling the hair in any way.

The massage practitioner does not confuse the basic relaxing scalp massage with full treatments of the scalp as given by a professional hair stylist or cosmetologist. The practitioner does not treat scalp disorders or massage the scalp if it is not in healthy condition. Basic manipulations are given by the massage practitioner as part of the massage treatment because they tend to promote relaxation. A good scalp massage can be beneficial in stimulating blood and lymph flow, in resting and soothing the nerves, and as an aid to keeping the scalp healthy and hair lustrous. This illustrated massage is designed for a client in a seated position. (Fig. 13.13a to f).

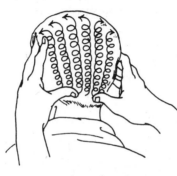

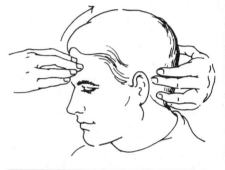

Fig. 13.13a Place the fingertips of each hand at the hairline on each side of the client's head, pointing the hands upward. Slide the fingers firmly upward, spreading the fingertips. Continue until the fingers meet at the center or top of the scalp. Repeat three or four times.

Fig. 13.13b Place the fingers of each hand on either side of the client's head behind the ears. Use the thumbs to massage from behind the ears toward the crown. Repeat four or five times. Move your fingers until both thumbs meet at the hairline at the back of the client's neck. Rotate your thumbs upward toward the crown.

Fig. 13.13c Step to the right side of the client. Place the left hand at the back of the head. Place the thumb and fingers of the right hand over the forehead, just above the eyebrows. With the cushion tips of the right hand, thumb and fingers, massage slowly and firmly in an upward direction toward the crown while keeping the left hand in a fixed position at the back of the head. Repeat four or five times.

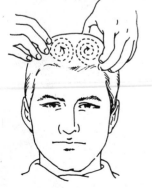

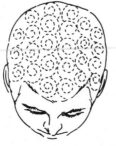

Fig. 13.13d Step to the back of the client. Place the hands on each side of the head, at the front hairline. Rotate the fingertips three times. On the fourth rotation, apply a quick, upward twist, firm enough to move the scalp. Continue this movement on the sides and tip of the scalp. Repeat three or four times.

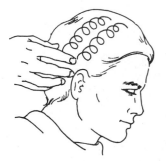

Fig. 13.13e Place the fingers (of each hand) below the back of each ear. Rotate the fingers upward from behind the ears to the crown. Repeat three or four times. Move the fingers toward the back of the head, and repeat the movement with both hands. Apply rotary movements in an upward direction toward the crown.

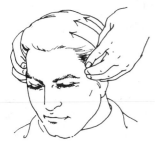

Fig. 13.13f Place both hands at the sides of the client's head. Keep the fingers close together, and hold the index fingers at the hairline above the ears. Firmly move both hands directly upward to the top of the head. Repeat four times. Move the hands to above the ears and repeat the movement. Move hands again to back of the ears and repeat the movement.

A Guide to Massage and Its Influence on the Scalp

MASSAGE MOVEMENTS	MUSCLES	NERVES	ARTERIES
Fig. 13.13a	Auricularis superior	Posterior auricular	Frontal Parietal
Fig. 13.13b	Auricularis posterior Occipitalis	Greater occipital	Occipital
Fig. 13.13c	Frontalis	Supra-orbital	Frontal
Fig. 13.13d	Frontalis	Supra-orbital	Frontal Parietal
Fig. 13.13e	Auricularis posterior	Occipitalis Greater occipital	Posterior auricular Parietal
Fig. 13.13f	Auricularis anterior and superior	Temporal auricular	Frontal Parietal

QUESTIONS FOR DISCUSSION AND REVIEW

1. When is a face massage not given?
2. What is the first important step in a face massage procedure?
3. How do movements in face massage differ from those used for body massage?
4. What are the main benefits of face massage?
5. Why is cleansing the face before massage so important?
6. What are the main benefits of scalp massage?
7. When does the practitioner avoid giving scalp massage?
8. What is the massage practitioner's main purpose in including face and scalp massages in his or her procedures?

Hydrotherapy

Learning Objectives

After you have mastered this chapter, you will be able to:

1. *Explain the use of heat and cold in body treatments.*
2. *Describe types of apparatus that may be approved for use by the massage practitioner.*
3. *Describe types of apparatus that may not be approved for use by the massage practitioner.*
4. *Explain precautions for suntanning.*
5. *Describe at least five ways of applying heat to the body.*
6. *Define cryotherapy and demonstrate at least three ways to apply it.*
7. *Explain hydrotherapy as a therapeutic aid.*
8. *Explain the effects of different water temperatures on the body.*
9. *Demonstrate a Swedish shampoo.*
10. *Demonstrate a salt rub.*
11. *Describe the effects of various water treatments on the body.*
12. *Explain contraindications, safety rules, and time limits for various bath treatments.*

Although body massage is generally done by hand, there is a wide range of treatments that combine manual massage and the use of various other modalities. These treatments are designed to encourage circulation, improve the body's efficiency in eliminating toxins, and promote relaxation.

THE USE OF ELECTRICAL MODALITIES ▼

A number of therapeutic methods that use electric stimulation have been found to be extremely beneficial in the treatment or rehabilitation of soft tissue or neurologic injuries. Examples include ultrasound, low- and medium-frequency electrical stimulation, electromagnetic stimulation, and others that use specific frequencies or pulses. Modalities requiring specific training should be performed only by qualified technicians under medical supervision. The use of most modalities using electricity is beyond the scope of therapeutic massage.

One popular electrical apparatus used for body massage is the vibratory massager. It is used to produce either a relaxing or stimulating effect depending on the method of application and the desired results. There are a variety of mechanical vibrators on the market. Using vibrators may enhance the effects of the massage and at the same time reduce the physical exertion of the practitioner.

The practitioner must have sound knowledge of procedures involving electrical equipment and its benefits as well as any contraindications of its use. While no machine can replace the well-trained hands of the practitioner, machines can offer advantages when used in conjunction with manual massage. The machine is mainly used as a means to conserve the practitioner's energy and to increase the benefits of various treatments. All electrical equipment must be inspected regularly to assure its safe operation.

SUNTANNING ▼

Overexposure to the sun can be harmful to the skin because the ultraviolet rays of the sun penetrate not only the epidermis but also the dermis, where the living cells are affected. One of the skin's main defenses against too much sun is its ability to tan. Tanning occurs as a result of the sun's ultraviolet rays reacting with melanin, a pigment in the epidermis, which darkens and acts as a shield to prevent damage to the underlying tissues. Excess exposure to the ultraviolet rays of the sun causes sunburn, which is considered to be the primary cause of skin cancer and premature aging of the skin. This is why it is so important to tan gradually and apply a good sunscreen before exposing the skin to the sun. Dark skin, due to its pigmentation, is not as affected by sun rays as light skin, which burns easily.

Sunburns, like all burns, are classified as first-, second-, and third-degree burns according to the depth and extent of tissue damage.

In first-degree burns there is pain and redness. The damage is done only to the epidermis or outermost layer of the skin. Normal healing occurs within a few days. Second-degree burns result in blistering and deeper damage to tissue. Healing may take one to three weeks. Third-degree burns are the most severe and can result in destruction of the epidermis and its appendages. Nerve fibers are destroyed and scarring usually occurs. Healing may take many months, and corrective surgery may be required.

The practitioner does not massage skin that is burned, peeling, or showing signs that it is too tender for the application of massage movements. However, the practitioner can do a valuable service by informing the client of the benefits and dangers of the sun and of suntanning equipment.

The client may not realize that when the skin is exposed to natural sunlight or to artificial ultraviolet radiation, the body's protective responses are generated so that the superficial layers of the skin begin to thicken and melanin (the coloring matter) begins to form in stages. People with very fair skin are more prone to spotting, freckling, and skin cancer. Premature aging of the skin is also accelerated, especially in thin, dry, sensitive skin. The client who insists on suntanning should be advised to use a good sunscreen product. Products are formulated for skins that tan easily and require minimum protection and for skins that require maximum protection.

The massage practitioner, though not so concerned with whether the client has a suntan, must be very concerned with any suntanning equipment (suntanning cabinets or beds) for which he or she may be responsible. Tanning cabinets or beds have escalated in popularity since their introduction to the United States in 1979. Before that, sun lamps and tanning booths were in use. These items emitted B rays (ultraviolet B), which caused sunburn; consequently this equipment had to be used with much care. Today's tanning beds, cabinets, and booths utilize ultraviolet A rays (UVA), which provide radiation that tans without burning.

A tanning bed is usually made of aluminum, with the upper and lower halves hinged so they can be moved up and down. The lamps are covered in acrylic, providing a cool surface for clients to lie on during the tanning session. The client must wear goggles (FDA mandatory) to avoid damage to the eyes. Most tanning beds also feature stereo headphones so the client can enjoy music while tanning. Suntanning cabinets or booths are similar, except that the client stands or sits. Some manufacturers declare suntanning beds and cabinets to have all the qualities of natural sunlight with none

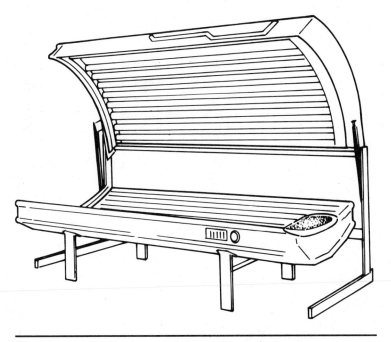

Fig. 14.1 Tanning beds use UVA rays to produce a tan.

of the hazards. There are others who warn against tanning by such artificial methods (Fig. 14.1).

We know that the sun has some healthful effects, such as acting on substances in the skin to manufacture vitamin D. Vitamin D is vitally important to healthy functioning of the nervous system and utilization of calcium for bone formation. UVA is also an accepted treatment for such skin conditions as psoriasis. However, the FDA advises that all forms of tanning be avoided by people who want to minimize the risk of skin cancer or premature aging of the skin. Those who insist on using a tanning bed for cosmetic purposes should take the following precautions:

• Always follow recommended instructions for use of the equipment.
• Wear protective goggles.
• Do not expect an instant tan. Begin with a shorter exposure time and build up to a longer (but safe) exposure.
• Be sure an attendant or someone familiar with the equipment is nearby in case of emergency.
• Report any injury from use of such equipment to the manufacturer and to the FDA.

The massage practitioner should be sure clients are advised about the use of any facilities or equipment in his or her place of business and should not allow the client to misuse equipment. Rules should be posted for the protection of both the client and owners.

THE USE AND EFFECTS OF HEAT AND COLD APPLICATIONS

The normal body temperature is 98.6°F. Physiologically the body strives to maintain this temperature. When heat or cold is applied to the body, certain physiological changes occur. The nature and extent of those changes depends on the temperature and duration of the application and the size of the body area and thermal conductivity of the body part involved. The greater the temperature differentiation, the more dramatic the effect. If the temperature of the treatment is the same as the body temperature, there is little or no physiological reaction. Treatments of short duration may have different effects than longer treatments. For example, a short application of cold (two to five seconds) has a stimulating effect whereas an extended application (ten to thirty minutes) will depress metabolic activity. Local applications have specific local effects, while general applications have systemic effects. Some thermal applications will have both direct local effects and reflex effects. The physiological effects from the application of heat and cold are predictable, which makes the use of heat and cold a powerful therapeutic agent.

Treatments using extreme temperatures or of long duration should be avoided or be used under very close supervision. Using thermal treatments below freezing or above 115°F may damage tissues. Prolonged general treatments below 70°F may cause hypothermia. Prolonged general treatments above 110°F may cause hyperthermia. Either condition is potentially dangerous.

The application of heat causes a vasodilatation and an increase of circulation in an attempt to dissipate the heat. A general application of heat will raise the body temperature, causing a fever-like reaction. There is profuse perspiration, the pulse rate increases, and the white blood cell count increases. A local application will cause local reddening (due to vasodilatation), increased metabolism and leukocyte migration to the area, relaxation of local musculature, and a slight analgesia.

The quick, short application of cold is stimulating, while prolonged application of cold depresses metabolic activity. General application of cold reduces the body temperature (hypothermia). While this has important therapeutic and medical advantages, it must only be done under strict medical supervision. Local applications of cold cause a reduction of nerve sensitivity, circulation, muscle spasms, and spasticity. They have a numbing, anesthetic, analgesic effect that makes them valuable in the relief of acute pain from bursitis, soft tissue injury, burns, and neuralgia.

APPLICATION OF HEAT

There are several sources for the application of heat. The choice of modality depends on the body part to be treated, its condition, and

the objectives of the application. Modalities for the application of heat include:
- Dry heat
    Heating pad
    Infrared radiation
- Moist heat
    Immersion baths
    Spray (pulsating spray)
    Moist heat pack
    Steam and sauna baths
- Diathermy
    Shortwave
    Microwave

Heating Pads

Heating pads are plastic-covered pads that contain electric heating elements similar to electric blankets. A heating pad supplies a local source of dry heat and is easy to apply. The heating pad is useful for local applications on one part of the body while the therapist works on another. There are usually three heat level settings. Some heating pads are manufactured for application of moist heat; however, manufacturers' instructions must be followed to prevent injury from burns or electrical shock.

Infrared Radiation

Infrared radiation may be produced from a bulb or an element. The warming effect of the sun is due to infrared radiation. As radiations are absorbed by the skin, heat is produced. The heat results in increased superficial circulation and sedation of sensory nerve endings. This results in the relaxation of tense or spasmed muscles, relief of pain, and increased availability of nutrients to the superficial tissues (Fig. 14.2).

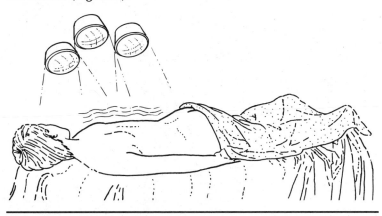

Fig. 14.2 As infrared radiation is absorbed into the skin, heat is produced.

Immersion Baths

Whenever a body part is submerged in water, it is considered an immersion bath. Depending on the objective of the treatment, various areas may be treated and various temperatures may be used. The use of water for therapeutic purposes is **hydrotherapy.** Water is an effective medium for the application of thermal procedures (hot or cold) because it surrounds the body part and is an excellent conductor of heat or cold. Hydrotherapy will be discussed more thoroughly later in this chapter.

Spray (Pulsating Shower)

There are a variety of pulsating shower heads on the market today. The pulsating shower is an effective means of combining moist heat and mild compression. This combination calms sensory nerves and increases peripheral circulation. Increased circulation restores nutrients as it clears away metabolic wastes. Sedated nerves mean reduction of pain, relaxation of tense or spasmed muscles, and reduced stress (Fig. 14.3).

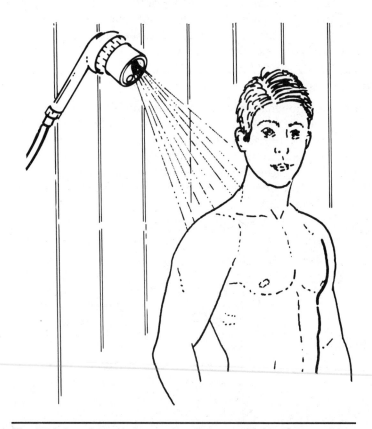

Fig. 14.3 A variety of shower heads are available that produce a pulsating spray of water.

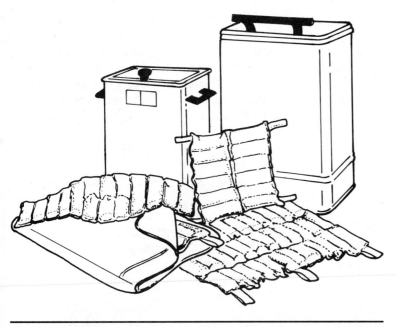

Fig. 14.4 Moist heat packs are heated in water in a hydrocollator before being applied to the body.

Moist Heat Packs

Moist heat packs are generally chemical gel packs that are heated in a water bath, wrapped in a terry cover, and placed on the body. A hydrocollator is used to heat and store the packs, which come in a variety of shapes, to conform to different areas of the body. The silica gel is formulated to retain heat and transfer it to the body part by means of conduction. Like heating pads, moist hot packs can be applied to one part of the body while the therapist works on another part (Fig. 14.4).

Steam and Sauna Baths

Heat in a steam bath is produced by a steam generator. Heat in a sauna is produced by a dry heat source. The temperature in a stream bath is 120 to 130°F while the temperature in a sauna may be 180 to 190°F. A steam bath may be a cabinet where the head remains outside of the heat or a steam room. Since the heat in a steam bath is supplied by steam, the air is supersaturated. This greatly reduces the body's ability to cool itself with perspiration. Saunas are always a room heated by dry heat. Evaporation of the body's perspiration has a cooling effect. This is why the sauna is so much hotter. Either one causes profuse sweating. Caution must be used to avoid overheating and to replace body fluids. Those with heart conditions, diabetes, and other conditions must first consult their physician.

Diathermy

Diathermy (**DIE**-uh-thur-mee) is the application of oscillating electromagnetic fields to the tissue. The oscillating fields cause a distortion in the molecules and an ionic vibration which produces heat. Diathermy requires the use of specialized equipment and training and is beyond the scope of practice of massage therapy.

▼ CRYOTHERAPY

The application of cold agents for therapeutic purposes is known as **cryotherapy** (**KRIE**-o-ther-uh-pee). The primary goal of cryotherapy is to reduce the tissue temperature. As cold is applied to the body, heat is drawn from the tissues, causing cooling. The local application of cold is beneficial on painful, inflamed, and swollen areas. It acts as an analgesic to reduce pain and causes vasoconstriction to limit swelling.

The application of extreme cold should be of short duration to prevent injury to the tissue from freezing. The application of ice will cause a series of sensations that can act as an indicator of the duration of the application. The first sensation of the application of ice will naturally be cold. Following the cold sensation will be pain, aching, and sometimes burning. Next will be the cessation of pain (the analgesic affect). When the third stage is reached, application should be temporarily suspended. Treatment may be repeated as necessary as often as once an hour.

Ice is first aid for traumatic soft tissue injuries. When a soft tissue injury such as a sprain or strain occurs, the standard first aid treatment is to apply RICE, an acrony in which R = rest, I = ice, C = compression, and E = elevation. This reduces swelling, pain, and the secondary tissue damage that results from excessive swelling. As soon as swelling has subsided, limited massage therapy can proceed on the healing tissue.

Ice therapy can be used by itself or in conjunction with other modalities. In the case of swelling due to local inflammation, ice offers tremendous relief from the swelling and accompanying pain. One of the best ways to increase circulation to an area to promote healing is alternate applications of heat and cold.

▼ APPLICATION OF COLD

Sources for the local application of cold include:
• Immersion baths
• Ice packs
    Commercial Ice bags
• Ice massage
• Compressor units with thermal packs and controls
• Vasocoolant sprays.

Immersion Baths

The entire body or a body part can be immersed in cool or cold water. Cool and cold baths will be discussed later in this chapter. When working with an extremity, such as a foot, ankle, hand, wrist, or elbow, an immersion icewater bath can be used. Prepare a basin or tub of 60 percent ice and water. Submerge the body part (foot, hand, forearm, or elbow) in the ice water until the feeling of cold or pain stops then remove the body part from the bath and proceed with therapy.

Ice Pack

Ice packs are used for the local application of ice on a specific body part. They are effective in relieving pain, preventing swelling, and decreasing inflammation. They are indicated for the early treatment of sprains, strains, and other soft tissue injuries. They are effective in the treatment of acute joint and nerve inflammation.

Reusable commercial ice packs are available in a variety of types and sizes. These are usually a sealed plastic pack containing a chemical gel. The pack is stored in the freezer until needed. The pack is wrapped in a terry cloth to prevent direct contact with the skin. Direct contact is unsanitary and may result in injury from freezing the tissue. The chemical gel in the pack stays pliable at freezing temperatures so the pack can conform to the area of the body to which it is applied (Fig. 14.5).

When commercial ice packs are not available, ice in a plastic bag is just as effective. A ZipLock® bag or a plastic freezer bag makes an excellent ice pack. Be sure there are no leaks in the plastic bag. Fill it one third of the way with broken ice cubes or crushed ice, seal it

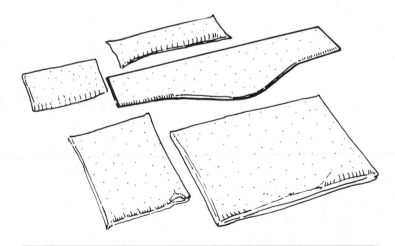

Fig. 14.5 Commercially manufactured cold packs are available in a variety of shapes and sizes. They are stored in a freezer until needed.

closed, and apply it directly to the affected area. The ice bag may be held in place by an Ace bandage or towel wrap.

A 2:1 mixture of crushed ice and isopropryl alcohol in a self-sealing plastic bag is an economic alternative to a commercial ice pack. The pack is stored in the freezer until needed. The mixture will not freeze solid and can be shaped to the contours of the body part to which it is applied (Fig. 14.6).

Another possibility for applying an ice pack is to fold or roll ice into a towel and apply the towel ice pack to the affected area (Fig. 14.7 a to e).

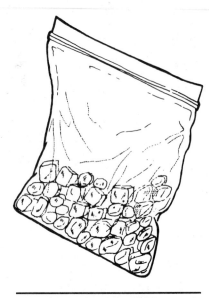

Fig. 14.6 An inexpensive ice pack uses ice chips or cubes in a sealed plastic bag.

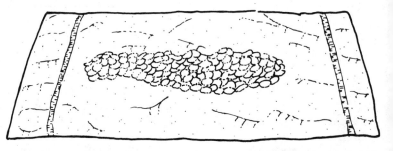

Fig. 14.7a Another alternative is to wrap ice in a towel and apply it to the affected area. Put crushed ice in the center of a towel.

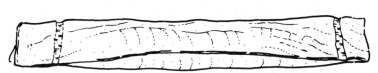

Fig. 14.7b Fold the sides of the towel over the ice. **Fig. 14.7c Fold the ends of the towel.**

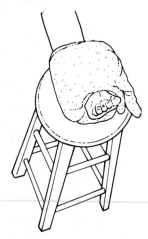

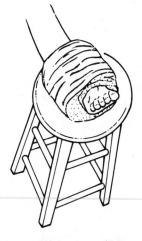

Fig. 14.7d Wrap the ice towel around the affected body part. **Fig. 14.7e Wrap the towel with an Ace bandage to secure it, and apply compression.**

Ice Massage

Another way cryotherapy can be applied is **ice massage.** Ice massage is a local application of cold achieved by massaging a cube of ice over a small area such as a bursa, tendon, or small muscle. Commercial ice cups are available that are filled with water and stored in the freezer until needed. They provide a mold for the ice cube that includes a handle frozen into the cube so the therapist can perform the ice massage without freezing his or her hand. Another way this can be achieved is to freeze water in an eight-ounce styrofoam cup. Remove the frozen cup from the freezer and cut the top half of the cup away. Use the base of the cup as a handle. An ice lollypop can be made by freezing a tongue depressor into a cup of water. The ice pop is removed from the cup and held by the stick for application. Ice massage is effective for reducing local pain, inflammation, and swelling and stopping muscle spasms (Figs.14.8a and b, 14.9a to c, and 14.10a and b).

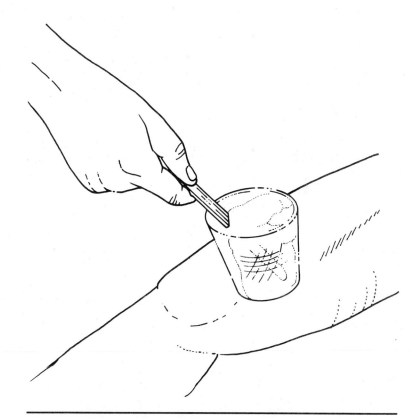

Fig. 14.8a A tongue depressor frozen into a paper into a paper cup of water makes an ice lollipop that can be used for ice massage.

Fig. 14.8b The tongue depressor acts as a handle when applying ice massage.

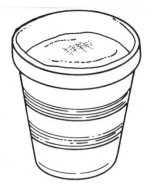

Fig. 14.9a Water frozen in a styrofoam cup works well for ice massage.

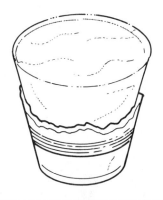

Fig. 14.9b When the water is frozen, peel the top half of the styrofoam cup away to make an ice cup with an insulated handle.

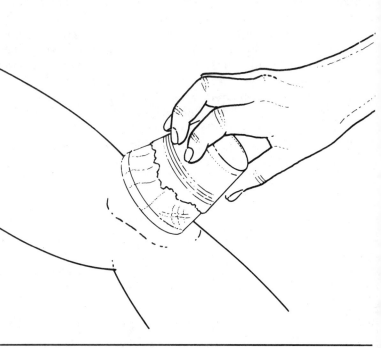

Fig. 14.9c Hold the bottom portion of the cup and apply ice massage.

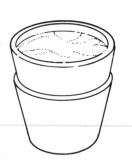

Fig. 14.10a Commercial ice cups are available.

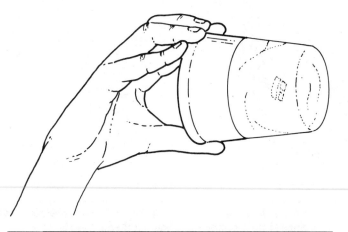

Fig. 14.10b When the ice is removed from the mold, a handle frozen into the ice protects the therapist's hand from the cold.

Controlled Compressor Units with Controls

Compressor units cool a fluid that is circulated through a pack that is applied to the body. The packs vary in size. A mat can be used for a general application. (These are employed for the control of high fever.) A smaller pack can be used for local application to an extremity. The temperature can be controlled by adjusting the controls on the unit. These units are relatively expensive and most commonly found in institutions that treat a large number of traumatic injuries.

Vapocoolant Sprays

Flori-methane is bottled under pressure and used as a vasocoolant spray. When sprayed on the skin, it evaporates very quickly, causing rapid cooling of the skin. It is an effective topical anesthetic used for trigger-point therapy and increasing the stretch in muscles. Caution must be used to avoid freezing the skin.

CONTRAST HEAT AND COLD ▼

The alternating application of heat and cold is one of the most effective methods of increasing local circulation. Contrasting hot and cold cause an alternating vasodilatation and vasoconstriction of the blood vessels in an area. Increased local circulation relieves stiffness and pain due to trauma and stimulates healing of injury and wounds.

Contrast baths require two tubs, one filled with hot water (105 to 110°F) and one with ice water. First immerse the body part in the hot water for three to five minutes or until the client becomes accustomed to the hot water (until the water no longer feels hot). Remove the limb from the hot water and place it in the ice water for thirty seconds to two minutes or until the client becomes accustomed to the cold water. While the client is in the cold bath, add hot water to the hot bath to bring it back up to temperature. Repeat the procedure three to six times, finishing with a cold application. Always complete the treatment with a soak in the cold tub.

HYDROTHERAPY ▼

Hydrotherapy (HIGH-dro-ther-uh-pee) is the application of water in any of its three forms (solid, liquid, vapor) to the body for therapeutic purposes. When properly used with body massage, hydrotherapy is an additional aid to the healthy functioning of the body.

Water has certain properties that make it a valuable therapeutic agent. It is readily available and relatively inexpensive to use. It has the ability to absorb and conduct heat. In its solid form as ice, it can be used as an effective cooling agent; in its vapor form it can be used for facials and steam baths; and in its liquid state it can be used for sprays and immersion baths.

The temperature of water affects the body; therefore it is important to understand how water temperature relates to body temperature. The normal temperature of the human body is 98.6°F or 37°C. The boiling point of water is 212°F or 100°C. The freezing point of water is 32°F or 0°C. Obviously we must not use water of too high or too low a temperature because it would be injurious to body tissues. Water temperatures above that of the body (98.6°F) are considered to be hot. Water that is slightly below normal body temperature is medium to warm (about 94 to 96°F). Water that is about 70 to 80°F is considered to be cool; and at 55°F and below, it is considered cold.

Changes in the body as a result of hydrotherapy are classified as thermal, mechanical, and chemical. Thermal effects of water are produced by the application of water at temperatures above or below that of the body. This is done by way of baths, wraps, and packs that raise or lower the temperature of the body. Mechanical effects are produced by the pressure exerted on the surface of the body by sprays, whirlpool baths, and friction. Chemical effects are produced by drinking water as an aid to digestion and elimination.

To use hydrotherapy effectively, the following supplies and equipment are needed:
• Bathtubs and showers
• Running hot and cold water
• Spray attachments
• Bath thermometer
• Towels, bath blankets, bath brushes, sponges, loofahs, bath mitts, etc.
• A slab usually of marble or simulated material
• A resting couch and blanket or other covering
• A robe and slippers for the client.

Bath Accessories

Soap, bath salts, oils, powders, and effervescent tablets are preparations that may be used during the bath. Soap is used for its cleansing action on the body. Bath salts increase the cleansing action of soap, especially in hard water. Bath oils also tend to increase the cleansing action of soap. Effervescent tablets produce bubbles of carbon dioxide gas that have a mild stimulating effect on the body. Dusting powders, body oils, and moisturizing lotions are used after the bath. Dusting powders impart fragrance and aid in drying the body. Body oils and moisturizing lotions help to lubricate the skin and replace natural oils lost during bathing. Following a hot bath or cabinet bath, a salt rub or Swedish shampoo may be given.

Water Treatments

The various procedures used in hydrotherapy may be classified as follows:

1. **Baths:** Practices whereby the body is surrounded by water, or vapor, such as in a whirlpool bath, tub bath, or steam bath
2. **Sprays:** The projection of one or more streams of water against the body, such as a shower or needle spray
3. **Sponging:** The application of a liquid to the body by means of a sponge, a cloth, or the hand
4. **Tonic friction:** The application of friction to the body with cold water so as to produce a stimulating or tonic effect
5. **Shampoos:** Cleansing measures accomplished with water and soap, such as a Swedish shampoo
6. **Whirlpool, Jacuzzi, hot tubs:** These are usually large tubs equipped with jets or agitators that causes the water to flow in different directions. The main benefit derived from this type of bath or water treatment is relaxation
7. **Special water treatments:** The use of compresses, packs, and fomentations.

Contraindications for Hydrotherapy

Water treatments that involve hot or cold applications should not be given when the client has cardiac impairment, diabetes, lung disease, kidney infection, extremely high or low blood pressure, or an infectious skin condition. The client's physician should be consulted when any questionable condition exists.

Body Reactions to Water Treatments

Water treatments are based on the simple physical property of water; namely, that heat, cold, or pressure can be conveyed to many blood vessels and nerves in the skin. The effects of water on the body vary according to the temperature and duration of the treatment and whether the application is general or local in character. The circulation of the blood and the sensations produced by the many nerve endings in the skin can be greatly influenced by skilfully applied water treatments.

The average temperature of the skin surface is about 92°F. Water approximating the temperature of the skin has no marked effect on the body. If water at a temperature different from that of the skin is applied, it will either transfer heat or absorb heat from the body. The difference in temperature has a stimulating effect on the vast network of blood vessels and nerves. The greater the difference between the temperature of water and that of the skin, the greater is the stimulating effect of the treatment.

Each water application initiates a series of predictable reactions that are the result of the body accommodating itself to the new environment. The body reaction may be either stimulating or sedating to the circulatory system, the nervous system, and the eliminatory process. The practitioner who uses hydrotherapy should be familiar with the specific effects of cold, hot, and warm applications on the body.

Effects of Cold Water

The specific effects of water applications on the body are an immediate and temporary effect or a secondary and more lasting effect. Cold applications are valuable in improving the circulation, stimulating the nerves, and awakening the functional activity of body cells. The prolonged use of cold applications has a depressing effect on the body and must be used cautiously under strict supervision.

The immediate effects of cold water applications are manifested in the following ways:

1. The skin is chilled.
2. Surface blood vessels contract and blood is driven to the interior of the body.
3. Nerve sensitivity is reduced.
4. The functional activity of body cells slows.

As soon as the cold application is discontinued, there is a secondary and more lasting effect on the body.

1. The skin becomes warmed and relaxed.
2. The surface blood vessels expand, bringing more blood to the skin.
3. Nerve sensitivity increases.
4. Adjacent body cells are stimulated in their functional activity.

Effects of Hot Water

The immediate effect of hot water applications is to draw the blood away from the interior and bring it to the surface temporarily. Local blood vessels dilate and circulation increases. A secondary and more lasting effect occurs after the hot application is discontinued. Then the blood goes back to the interior of the body. Long and continued hot applications increase all skin functions and cause profuse sweating. Moderately warm applications have a relaxing effect on the blood vessels, muscles, and nerves, and promote the functional activity of body cells.

Generally, the skin cannot tolerate hot water having a temperature in excess of 115°F. Above that temperature, water is injurious and may cause burns. However, the skin usually can tolerate steam vapor as high as 140°F. It is important to consider the client's sensitivity and tolerance to heat or cold.

A reliable bath thermometer is required to judge water temperature accurately. The temperature reading is obtained by moving the thermometer about in the water.

Kinds of Baths

The aim of all baths is the attainment of two objectives: external cleanliness and stimulation of bodily functions.

Depending on the temperature of water, the following kinds of baths are available for use.

1. Cold bath (40 to 65°F equal to 4.4 to 18.3°C)
2. Cool bath (67 to 75°F equal to 18.3 to 23.8°C)
3. Tepid bath (85 to 95°F equal to 29.4 to 35°C)
4. Saline (salt) bath (90 to 94°F equal to 32.2 to 35.5°C)
5. Warm bath (95 to 100°F equal to 35 to 37.7°C)
6. Hot bath (100 to 115°F equal to 37.7 to 43.3°C)
7. Sitz or hip bath (either hot or cold)

Cool Baths

Whether a cold bath is beneficial depends on its duration and the state of vitality and reserve strength of the client. If after a cold bath or shower the client comes out chilly, shivering, blue-lipped, or goose-fleshed, it indicates that his or her body reaction is not good. For the client who experiences a pleasant reaction and a feeling of warmth, the cold bath may be safely continued. A short cold bath or cold sponging of the body may be better tolerated if it is accompanied by friction and gentle rubbing with a rough towel.

The average time exposure for a cold bath or shower should be limited from three to five minutes.

A cool bath provides a satisfactory temperature for all-around bathing, particularly during warm weather. A tepid (slightly warm) bath exerts a soothing and relaxing effect on the body and is recommended for nervous and excitable people.

Saline (Salt) Bath

A saline (salt) bath, at a temperature of 90 to 94°F, produces a marked tonic effect by stimulating the circulation. The effect is similar to natural bathing in sea water. The amount of common salt to use is three to five pounds to a tub of water. The client is left in the saline bath for ten to twenty minutes.

Hot or Warm Baths

A warm or hot bath quiets tired nerves, soothes aching muscles, and helps to relieve insomnia. A cool shower should generally follow a warm bath because it forces some of the blood away from the skin, closes the pores, and leaves the body in a refreshed condition.

The warm or hot bath induces relaxation and relieves nervous tension. To accustom the body to the high temperature, first fill the tub with warm water. Have the client get in the warm tub, then gradually add hot water until the desired temperature is reached. The average time for hot baths or showers should range from five to twenty minutes. The following safety precautions should also be observed by the practitioner:

- Take the wrist pulse before and during the hot bath.
- Give the client water to drink during the hot bath.
- If the client complains of unpleasant reactions, place cold compresses over the forehead or on the back of the neck.

Very hot baths as well as very cold baths should be used only for clients who are in a healthy condition and who can withstand such treatments. For those clients whose health is not in the best condition, injurious effects may be produced. The hot bath or shower may give undue stimulation to the body and may overwork the heart. A cold bath or shower, on the other hand, is a tremendous shock to the nervous system.

Sitz Hip Bath

The sitz or hip bath is applied only to the hips and pelvic region of the body, which is kept immersed in either hot, tepid, or cold water; or alternately hot and cold water. For a hot sitz bath, five to ten minutes contact is usually sufficient. The time for a cold sitz bath varies from three to five minutes. The effects of a sitz bath depend primarily on the temperature of the water and its length of contact with the body. Generally, the sitz bath is given as a stimulant to the pelvic region. The temperature of the hot sitz is usually 105 to 115°F.

Besides being effective in overcoming chronic constipation, sitz baths are also beneficial for the kidneys, bladder, and sex organs.

A large basin or bathtub is suitable for a sitz bath. The bath is prepared by filling the basin or tub with water (of the correct temperature) to about a depth of four inches or enough to immerse the client's buttocks comfortably. When using a basin (the feet outside), a blanket should be placed around the feet for warmth and a towel can be placed under the knees for added comfort. The client sits in such a manner that the buttocks and upper thighs are immersed.

▼ SWEDISH SHAMPOO

A Swedish shampoo, or body shampoo, is really a cleansing bath applied over the entire body with the aid of a shampoo brush or bath mitt and soap and water. A good Swedish shampoo, when properly applied, does the following:

- Loosens dead surface cells of the skin
- Promotes the growth of new skin cells
- Imparts a healthy radiance to the skin.

Procedure for a Swedish Shampoo

Preparation

Apply warm water over a shower slab, and then have the client lie down on his or her back on the slab. The practitioner begins with the arms, then proceeds to the fronts of the legs, chest, abdomen, backs of the legs, and back of the body.

Shampooing the Arm

1. Apply sufficient soap to form a thick lather. Hold the client's left hand, and apply three long strokes over the entire surface of the arm.
2. Using a brush, apply circular and frictional movements over the entire left arm, and then use long strokes to brush the entire arm.
3. Repeat the movements over the right arm.

Shampooing the Legs

1. Apply sufficient soap on the brush to form a lather. Hold the client's leg just above the heel. Apply the brush in long strokes to the entire surface of the leg from foot to knee.
2. Continuing with the brush, apply friction three times over the leg from foot to knee.
3. Lift the knee (by placing hand under the bend of knee), and apply three strokes followed by friction over the entire surface from hip to knee.
4. Repeat the entire procedure on the other leg.

Shampooing the Chest and Abdomen

1. Apply soap by hand over the chest and abdomen (between and around the breasts).
2. With a brush, apply gentle friction over the upper chest, between the breasts, and up the sides. Brush under the arm, down the side, and across the abdomen to the other side. Brush up the side, under the arm, and down the side again.
3. Apply the brush in three long strokes over the center of the chest, down each side, and across the abdomen.
4. Have the client change to a prone (face-down) position.

Shampooing the Backs of the Legs

1. Apply sufficient soap to the brush to form a thick lather.
2. Lift the left foot at the ankle, and brush the sole of the foot, using three strokes over the entire surface.
3. Using the brush, apply friction over the same area.
4. Lift the knee by placing a hand underneath the kneecap. Apply the brush in three long strokes over the entire surface from heel to hip. Apply the brush with friction over the same area.

5. Apply three long strokes over the same area from heel to hip.
6. Repeat the same procedures over the back of the right leg.

Shampooing the Back of the Body

1. Apply soap with hands over the entire back.
2. Apply the brush over the spine and down, and then up the sides (three times) using long strokes.
3. Using the brush, apply friction three times over the same area of the back and sides of the body, and then apply three long strokes over the lower part of the back.

Finishing the Body Shampoo

Apply warm or cool shower or spray to remove all traces of shampoo from the client's body. Dry the body thoroughly and then apply dusting powder or body oil. Allow the client to rest on a comfortable surface (massage table) for about thirty minutes before leaving.

▼ SALT RUB

A salt rub is a frictional application of wet salt over the client's body. It may be given as a separate treatment or after any hot bath or cabinet bath. The benefits of a salt rub are derived chiefly from its stimulation of the circulation and its tonic value to the body. This treatment should be recommended only to clients who can withstand a high degree of stimulation. The salt rub should not be given if there is any indication of skin disease or open wounds.

Procedure for a Salt Rub

Have two to three pounds of salt and all other supplies and equipment ready before the client arrives. Adjust the room to a comfortable temperature, and apply warm water over the slab just before having the client lie on it in a supine position.

The treatment begins with the arms and then proceeds to the legs, chest, abdomen, and finally to the back of the body.

Application to the Arm

1. Moisten the salt slightly, and apply it over the client's arm from the hand to the shoulder.
2. Using both hands, rub salt quickly into the skin, going three times up and down over the entire surface of the arm.
3. Apply three long strokes up and down over the same area.
4. Rinse the salt thoroughly from the area with warm water.
5. Repeat the entire procedure over the other arm.

Application to Legs

1. Moisten the salt slightly and then apply it from ankle to hip. Using both hands, rub the salt quickly into the skin, going three times up and down, covering the entire front surface of the leg.

2. Apply three long strokes over the same area.
3. Rinse the salt thoroughly from the area with warm water.
4. Repeat the procedure over the other leg.

Application to Chest and Abdomen

1. Moisten the salt slightly, and then apply it over the chest and abdomen.
2. Using both hands, rub salt quickly into the skin, covering the entire surface of the chest (except the breasts) and then the entire surface of the abdomen.
3. Apply three long strokes from chest to abdomen.
4. Rinse the salt thoroughly from the area with warm water.

Application to Back

1. Have the client change to a prone position.
2. Moisten the salt slightly and then apply it over the entire back, from top of shoulders to buttocks.
3. Using both hands, rub salt quickly into the skin over the entire surface.
4. Apply three long strokes over the same area.
5. Rinse the salt thoroughly from the area with warm water.

Final Steps

1. Apply a warm and then cool shower or spray to remove all traces of salt from the client's body, and then dry the body thoroughly.
2. Apply dusting powder or body oil.
3. Allow the client to rest on a comfortable surface (massage table) for about thirty minutes before leaving.

CABINET BATH

Bath cabinets are also known as vapor or steam cabinets, electric bath cabinets, and electric light cabinets. As used in body massage treatments, they are constructed in an upright or reclining position to accommodate the client's body while leaving the head exposed. When in operation, heat is generated and warm, moist air surrounds the client's body. The heat, besides having a relaxing effect on the client, induces profuse perspiration. The intensity and duration of the heat can be controlled by a switch for low, medium, or high heat, and by an automatic time clock. At the discretion of the practitioner, heat (dry, moist, or both) and therapeutic lights (ultraviolet or infrared rays) can be used separately or in conjunction. The manufacturer's instructions are the most reliable guide for the proper use and care of the bath cabinet.

Not all clients react the same way to the cabinet bath. Knowing the condition and tolerance of the client is of assistance in controlling the temperature and duration of this treatment. A client in a weakened or nervous condition should be given gentle treatments of short duration until improvement is shown. Always consult a physician before administering cabinet baths for a client with a systemic disorder such as heart trouble, high blood pressure, or any severe illness.

Length of Treatment

The exposure time in a cabinet bath ranges from ten to fifteen minutes. During this time, the practitioner should attend to the comfort and safety of the client and not to his or her reactions to the heat treatment. The client's heat tolerance will be greater if there is a gradual rise in the temperature of the bath cabinet. Postpone treatment if the client is ill, has an abnormal pulse or body temperature, and reacts unfavorably to the treatment.

The heat treatment induces profuse perspiration. To replace the fluids lost and to prevent body weakness, the practitioner should give the client water to drink at periodic intervals. If the client complains of a headache or a throbbing in the head during the treatment, cold compresses can be applied.

Following the cabinet bath, a mild tonic such as a tepid shower, a Swedish shampoo, or salt rub followed by a tepid shower may be given. After this treatment, keep the client warmly wrapped to prevent chilling of the body (Fig. 14.11).

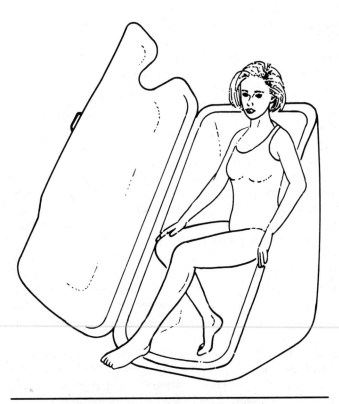

Fig. 14.11 Client sitting in a vapor cabinet bath.

WHIRLPOOL BATH ▼

A whirlpool bath is a partial immersion bath in which the water is agitated to produce a slight pressure on the body. A whirlpool bath is beneficial to circulation, soothing to the muscles, and relaxing to the nerves. Whirlpool baths are often used by physicians as part of physical therapy for conditions such as arthritis, sprains, strained muscles, and relief of pain. The following supplies and equipment are needed:

1. Whirlpool tub
2. Bath mats and towels
3. Robe and sandals (disposable paper sandals)
4. Lotion or oil
5. Bath thermometer
6. Ice bag (optional)
7. Material for cold compress, if needed
8. Tank suits for women and trunks for men.

Procedure

1. Fill the whirlpool tub to the recommended depth and test the temperature. Generally, the most desirable temperature is about 105 to 110°F, but the bath may be cooler.
2. Add the recommended antiseptic agents to the water.
3. Instruct the client in how to enter the tub safely.
4. The treatment time is usually about fifteen to thirty minutes.
5. Instruct the client about rest period, showers, and drying off.
6. Complete the client's records noting benefits, reactions, effects, etc.
7. Be sure the tub is sanitized thoroughly before it is used again.

FRICTION BATH ▼

The friction bath is given with terry towels, friction, or loofah mitts and applications of cold water. This treatment is beneficial in that it stimulates circulation and metabolism. The following supplies and equipment are needed:

1. Bath towels
2. Bath blankets
3. Loofah or friction mitts
4. Cold water and appropriate basin (temperature between 40 and 75°F).

Procedure

1. Be sure the room is at a comfortable temperature.
2. Explain the procedure to the client. Have client lie face down on a bath blanket.

3. Keep the client's body covered except for the area being treated.
4. Apply friction movements first to the arms. Wring the towel or mitts out in the water and then briskly rub the part for five to ten seconds. Be aware of sensitivity of the client's skin, and do not apply excessive pressure that may cause pain.
5. Dry the part with a towel while applying light friction movements.
6. Cover the finished part and proceed to the next. Generally, you will do the arms and legs and then the back and chest areas.
7. Following the treatment, be sure the client is warm and dry. Allow a short rest period following the friction bath.
8. Keep a complete record of the friction treatments, and note benefits or any adverse reactions.

▼ RELAXING NEUTRAL TUB BATH

The neutral tub bath is basically for relaxation and has a sedative effect. The body is immersed in a tub of water at a neutral temperature (about 94 to 98°F) for about fifteen to twenty-five minutes. The following supplies and equipment are needed:

1. Bathtub and bath thermometer
2. Bath towels and mat
3. Shower cap, robe, and slippers for client
4. Bath oil and lotion
5. Bath sheets
6. Compress cloth and basin of cool water
7. Air pillow and towel.

Procedure

1. Check the room temperature to be sure it is comfortable for the client.
2. Instruct the client regarding bathing and dressing procedures.
3. Fill the tub to the appropriate level.
4. Test the temperature of the water to be sure it's comfortable. A recommended range is 94 to 98°F.
5. Assist the client into the tub, and place an air pillow or towel underneath his or her head.
6. Cover the client's body with a large towel or bath sheet.
7. Allow the client to relax for fifteen to twenty-five minutes. Warm water may be added if desired.
8. Assist the client out of the tub, and dry his or her body with a towel while applying light friction.
9. Supply the client with robe and slippers.
10. Allow the client time to rest. Complete the client's records, noting benefits of the bath or any adverse reactions. Be sure the tub is sanitized thoroughly before the next bath.

RUSSIAN BATH

The Russian bath is a full-body steam bath for the purpose of causing perspiration. The primary benefits are cleansing, relaxation, and improved metabolism. The following supplies and equipment are needed:

1. Steam room with a slab or table for reclining
2. Padding and bath sheet for slab
3. Towels for neck and protection
4. Air pillow with a towel to cover
5. Shower cap to protect hair
6. Robe and slippers
7. Compress cloth and basin of cool water
8. Pitcher and glass of drinking water
9. Appropriate product to add to the bath.

Procedure

1. Prepare the steam room for the desired temperature. Usually this is 110 to 140°F.
2. Take and record the client's pulse and temperature.
3. Have the client lie on the slab. Adjust the pillow underneath the client's head.
4. Cover the client with a large towel or bath sheet.
5. Apply a cool compress to the head if desired.
6. Check pulse as necessary.
7. Give client instructions about drinking water during treatment.
8. Allow the client to relax for five to fifteen minutes.
9. Instruct the client to shower in a warm to cool shower following the steam bath.
10. Assist the client in drying off following the steam bath.
11. Allow the client to rest following the treatment.

QUESTIONS FOR DISCUSSION AND REVIEW

1. What precautions should be observed when using any electrical apparatus?
2. What are the concerns of the practitioner when advising a client about suntanning?
3. What are the effects of the application of heat?
4. Define *cryotherapy*.
5. What are the effects of the local application of ice?
6. What does the acronym RICE stand for and how is it used?
7. What is a contrast bath?
8. What is the main effect of a contrast bath?
9. Define *hydrotherapy*.
10. How are the effects of water treatments controlled?

11. What are the qualities of water that make it a valuable therapeutic tool?
12. Describe the three classifications of effects hydrotherapy has on the body.
13. What are the contraindications for performing hydrotherapy?
14. In which three ways are cold applications beneficial?
15. When are cold applications undesirable?
16. What are the benefits of hot water applications?
17. How high a temperature can the skin safely tolerate?
18. What are the two objectives of baths?
19. What is the temperature of a warm bath? A hot bath?
20. What is the average duration of a cold bath, cold shower, or cold sitz bath?
21. What is the average duration of a hot saline or sitz bath?
22. What is a Swedish shampoo?
23. When is a salt rub usually given?
24. What is the purpose of the cabinet bath?
25. What safety precautions should be observed during the operation of a bath cabinet?
26. What are the main benefits of a whirlpool bath?
27. What is a Russian bath and what are its benefits?

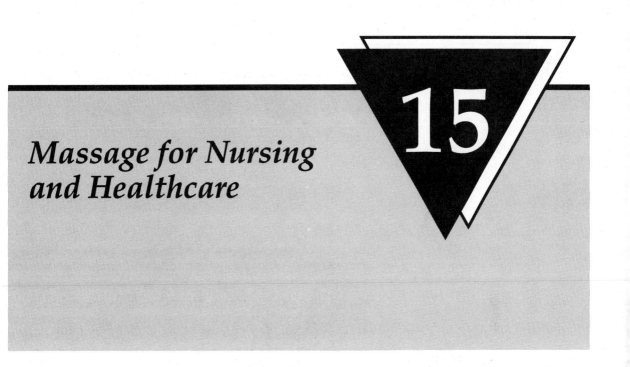

Massage for Nursing and Healthcare

Learning Objectives

After you have mastered this chapter, you will be able to:

1. *Explain the benefits of massage as given by nurses and other healthcare professionals.*

2. *Explain why a patient's physician is consulted before massage is included in a patient's care.*

3. *Explain how massage aids in healing and convalescence.*

4. *Explain the main contraindications for massage.*

5. *Demonstrate an alcohol rubdown.*

6. *Demonstrate how to take a client's or patient's medical history.*

7. *Explain when and why a mini-massage might be recommended.*

▼ INTRODUCTION

Health education is an essential component of nursing. Nurses and other healthcare professionals are involved not only in helping to restore their patients to health but also in teaching them how to live as healthy and productive a life as possible. In addition to assisting the physician, nurses and other healthcare assistants provide many other invaluable services in hospitals and healthcare facilities.

Nurses are employed in industry, research, education, private practices, and in hospitals. Although nurses work under the supervision of physicians, they are called on to assess the daily needs of their patients and to encourage them to participate in their own recovery. The mental attitude of the patient has a great deal to do with the individual's successful recovery and rehabilitation.

Patients need healing touch as much as they may need the right medication. Touching an area of the patient's body can help the nurse to note changes in body temperature and pick up other clues to the patient's state of health.

A therapeutic massage does much to help the patient, both physically and mentally.

▼ MASSAGE AS A THERAPEUTIC AID IN NURSING PRACTICE

Massage is one of the most beneficial services for patients during convalescence. Exercise and massage are often prescribed as a means of restoring the patient's fitness and sense of well-being. Swedish massage movements are most frequently used by nurses. The basic movements (manipulations) are effleurage, petrissage, and friction.

In nursing, general massage consisting of basic movements or manipulations to increase the psychological and physiological well-being of the patient may be recommended. There are also specialized treatments in which the nurse is called on to deal with some abnormal condition affecting the patient's body systems. In the case of specialized massage, the patient's physician may assign therapy procedures to a physical therapist who is trained to work with nurses and physicians. Exercise, massage, electrotherapy, hydrotherapy, and related techniques may be used in the treatment of specific diseases and injuries. For example, a sprained ankle may require special care, such as a heat or ice treatment, before massage.

Massage is valuable in the treatment of injuries to soft tissues and joints and is prescribed in a wide range of conditions. Massage is used in some cases to treat nervous fatigue, insomnia, headache, tension, stress, and other disorders.

The nurse or healthcare practitioner should have a thorough understanding of anatomy and physiology in order to determine the effects of various massage manipulations on the functions of the body's organs and systems. It is important to know when the patient will benefit from massage and when there are contraindications.

Nurses and other healthcare professionals are expected to practice the same code of ethics as other massage practitioners. They must have the same concern for the patient's comfort, privacy, and self-esteem. The main difference between nurses and massage practitioners is that nurses deal with patients who have a health problem or injury that requires hospital and physician care. The massage practitioner may also work under the supervision of a physician but may be employed in private practice, health facility, or sports complex. Many athletic organizations employ massage practitioners to travel with a team of professional athletes. Many industrial or business organizations employ a doctor, nurse, and massage practitioner as part of their staff. The massage practitioner usually works in an environment where massage is part of a client's regimen for keeping fit and healthy rather than as an aid to recovery from disease or injury.

In nursing and healthcare, massage is used as part of the physiological and psychological rehabilitation process. When a person becomes ill or is injured, it is common to feel a sense of apprehension, insecurity, and anxiety, which often leads to restlessness and insomnia. A good massage will increase the patient's comfort, induce relaxation, and help to relieve anxiety. When a patient is confined to bed for a period of convalescence, muscles lose their tone, joints become stiff, and skin develops sensitivity. Unless a patient is turned or is able to move, bedsores may develop. Massage helps to prevent these problems.

In addition to increasing the patient's comfort, massage aids healing by increasing the number of white and red blood cells and by improving circulation, which in turn nourishes the tissues. Massage, when done correctly, improves the action of lymph so that toxins are carried away. It also helps to promote blood supply to the brain and nerves so that the patient feels more in control of his or her faculties. Massage is used as an aid to preventing constipation by improving the peristaltic action of the small intestines and colon. There are numerous ways in which massage has been found to benefit patients of all ages. Many doctors recommend it as an aid to a speedier recovery.

Massage also has a place in the maintenance of good health. It acts as a stimulant or as a sedative for the nervous system and aids in the metabolic process and glandular activity. Because the skin is an organ of respiration and elimination, massage improves these functions. As the vasomotor system becomes more active, the skin is better nourished and both tone and elasticity are improved. The following is a brief review of some of the therapeutic benefits of massage to body systems.

Benefits of Massage

Massage benefits the circulatory system by:
- Helping to develop a stronger heart
- Improving oxygen supply to cells
- Improving the supply of nutrients to cells
- Elimination of metabolic wastes
- Decreasing blood pressure.

Massage benefits the digestive system by:
- Relaxing the abdominal and intestinal muscles
- Relieving tension
- Stimulating activity of liver and kidneys
- Eliminating waste material.

Massage benefits the muscular system by:
- Relaxing or stimulating muscles
- Reducing fibrosis and adhesions in muscles and connective tissue
- Helping to keep muscles flexible and pliable
- Relieving soreness, tension, and stiffness.

Massage benefits the nervous system by:
- Stimulating motor nerve points
- Relieving restlessness and insomnia
- Promoting a sense of well-being
- Relieving pain.

Massage benefits the respiratory system by:
- Developing respiratory muscles
- Assisting in proper breathing.

Massage benefits the lymph system by:
- Increasing circulation of lymph.
- Cleansing the body of metabolic wastes.

Massage benefits the integumentary system (the skin) by:
- Stimulating blood to better nourish skin
- Improving tone and elasticity of skin
- Helping to normalize glandular functions.

Massage benefits the skeletal system by:
- Improving body alignment
- Relieving stiff joints.

▼ REVIEW OF SWEDISH MASSAGE MOVEMENTS USED IN NURSING

Effleurage or stroking movements are done with slow, even pressure toward the heart. This increases lymph flow and circulation of the blood, thus increasing capillary and arterial circulation. Effleurage is called centripetal stroking because the movement is given in the direction of the lymph and venous blood flow. When effleurage is applied to reflex areas of the body, related organs are stimulated. It is important to understand which organs are principally affected by massage.

The better the circulation of blood to the extremities, the more oxygen is made available to tissues and the more efficiently wastes are removed from the cells.

Effleurage over muscles can assist in dilating blood vessels, allowing more blood to flow into the area. After surgery when movement is limited to a specific area or when there has been prolonged muscle strain, massage is beneficial in loosening tight muscles and restoring motion to the affected part.

Petrissage or kneading movements are done on the muscles by wringing, squeezing, pressing, and lifting. These movements are never done so firmly as to cause pain. The hands are used to manipulate large areas and the fingers and thumbs for small areas.

Friction movements are achieved by applying pressure with the hands or just the fingertips so that the superficial tissues move over or against the deeper tissues. Friction is used to warm tissues and is done over bony areas as well as larger groups of muscles. It is especially valuable in improving functioning of muscles and nerves. Circular friction is used to stimulate blood to the surface of the skin to nourish tissues. Cross fiber friction is used to reduce adhesion and fibrosis.

Tapotement or percussion movements include tapping, slapping, hacking, cupping, and beating. These movements should not be done so firmly as to cause pain. The movements are done on large, muscular, and fleshy areas of the body to stimulate nerves and reflex areas.

Shaking, vibrating, and jostling movements are done with a degree of pressure on the area of the body to be massaged. For example, when light pressure and vibration are applied to the abdominal region, the internal organs are affected by reflex action.

CONTRAINDICATIONS FOR MASSAGE IN NURSING AND HEALTHCARE ▼

Unlike the practitioner who deals with healthy clients, the nurse or other healthcare professional often works with people who are ill, injured, or recovering. The stage of the person's illness or injury will often determine the extent that massage might be given beneficially, or if it should be given at all. It is important to be sure that massage is approved by the patient's physician.

Massage brings more fluid, blood, nutrients, and oxygen to affected areas of the body, but there are times when massage must not be given to or near an affected part. The patient's physician will note deterioration of muscles or skin that could benefit from massage and will also be aware of contraindications for massage. The nurse or healthcare assistant does not apply massage in cases of illness or injury without the supervision or permission of the patient's physician.

The following is a general review of contraindications:
- Bleeding (internal or external)
- Skin problems such as rashes, growths, lesions

- Newly formed scar tissue, scabs, wounds, and burns
- Infections, swollen areas, pain, inflammation, heat in the area
- Nausea, vomiting, and fever
- Edema: Excessive lymph fluid often causes swelling in feet and legs, particularly in elderly people. Sometimes the physician will recommend gentle effleurage in the direction of the lymphatic flow to help relieve this condition.
- Varicose veins: Veins in the legs become dilated and lengthen due to increased blood pressure. In mild cases, massage may be done on nearby areas but not directly on the affected part.
- Inflamed joints such as arthritis and bursitis: Massage is not done on the area when it is painful and inflamed.
- Cancer: When any symptom of cancer is detected or if any condition is suspected to be cancerous, massage is avoided on or near the area.

The following are warning signs that are associated with cancer and are contraindications for massage (Clients who show any of these signs should be referred to a doctor):
- Any sore that has not healed normally
- A mole, skin tag or wort that is changing in color or size
- Lumps underneath the arms or in the breasts
- Persistent hoarseness, coughing, or sore throat
- Abnormal functioning of any internal organ, such as changes in the bladder or bowels
- Discharge or bleeding from any part of the body
- Persistant indigestion or difficulty in swallowing.

Basic Massage Procedures

Effleurage—Stroking Movements

Effleurage movements may be done in the sequence most suitable for the individual (Fig. 15.1a to g).

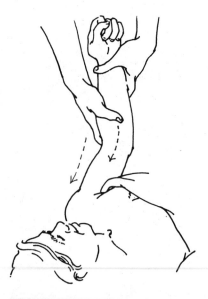

Fig. 15.1a Direction of effleurage and position of arm. The same upward movement is applied when massaging the back of the arm.

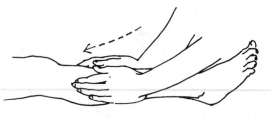

Fig. 15.1b Direction of effleurage on the lower leg. The same upward movements are applied when massaging the back of the lower leg.

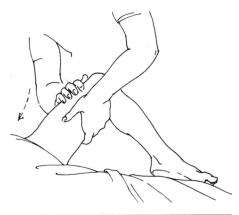

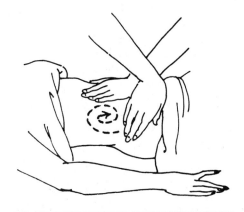

Fig. 15.1c Direction of effleurage to inner thigh and position of the hands. The same upward movements are applied when massaging the back of the leg.

Fig. 15.1d Deep circular movements are applied to the abdomen.

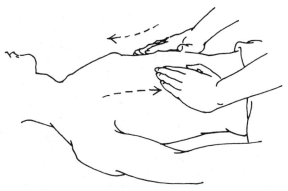

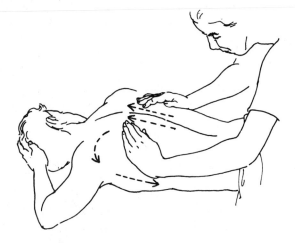

Fig. 15.1e Effleurage is applied to the center of the chest and underarms in upward and then downward strokes.

Fig. 15.1f Effleurage is applied to the back in long, continuous, soothing strokes.

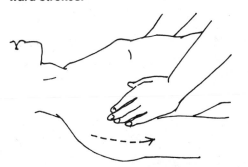

Fig. 15.1g Effleurage is applied to the shoulders, moving upward on the sides of the neck and back down the back of the shoulders and across the chest.

Petrissage—Kneading

Petrissage should be done carefully. Adjust pressure to the patient's needs. Petrissage should be done in the most suitable sequence. Painful areas of the body should be avoided (Fig. 15.2a to e).

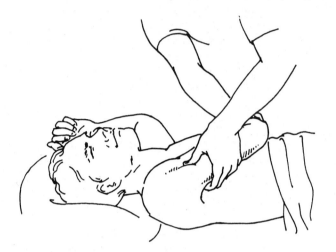

Fig. 15.2a Kneading the triceps.

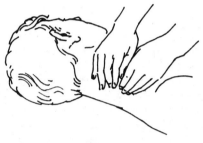

Fig. 15.2b Kneading the back of the neck and shoulder region.

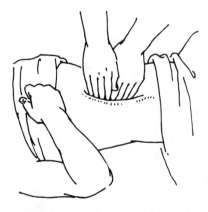

Fig. 15.2c Kneading the abdomen, applying downward kneading movements.

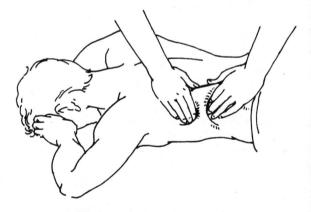

Fig. 15.2d Kneading the muscles of the back.

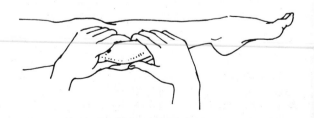

Fig. 15.2e Kneading the calf muscles.

Friction—Circular

Circular friction may be applied in the sequence most appropriate for the patient's needs (Fig. 15.3a to e).

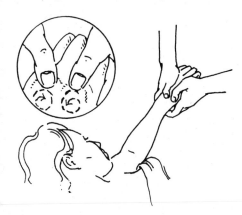
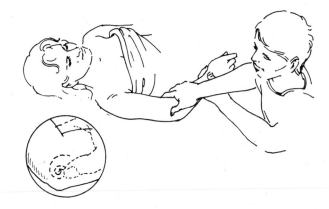

Fig. 15.3a Friction applied to the muscles and tendons of the hand.

Fig. 15.3b Friction applied to the lower arm and elbow joint.

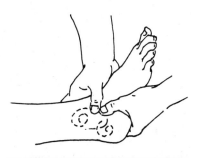
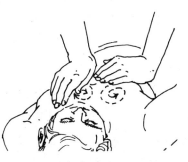

Fig. 15.3c Friction applied to the lower leg and ankle joint.

Fig. 15.3d Circular friction applied over the chest.

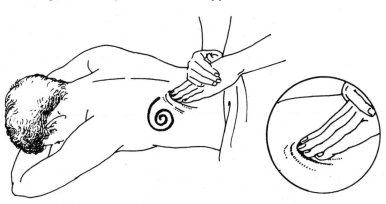

Fig. 15.3e Friction movements are applied to the spine with the fingertips of one hand held steady with the other hand. Movements are applied upward and downward along both sides of the spine.

Friction—Wringing

Circular friction may be applied in the sequence most appropriate to the patient's needs (Fig. 15.4a and b).

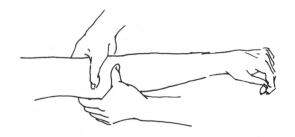

Fig. 15.4a Wringing the arm.

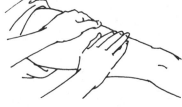

Fig. 15.4b Wringing the muscles of the anterior thigh.

Percussion

Tapping, slapping, hacking, beating, cupping, movements should be applied according to individual needs and when they will be of specific benefit to the patient (Fig. 15.5a to f).

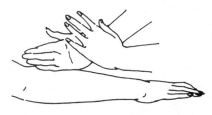

Fig. 15.5a Hacking movements are applied to the arm with alternating strikes with the ulnar sides of the hands.

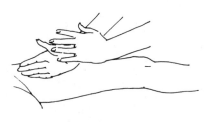

Fig. 15.5b Hacking movements are applied to the thigh muscles with alternating strikes with the ulnar sides of the hands.

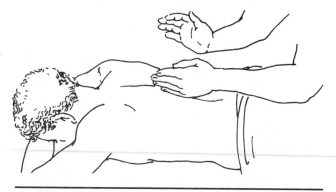

Fig. 15.5c Hacking movements are applied to the back muscles with alternating sides of the hands.

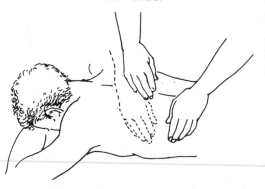

Fig. 15.5d Cupping movements are applied to the back with the hands cupped and alternating light, percussive movements over the entire back.

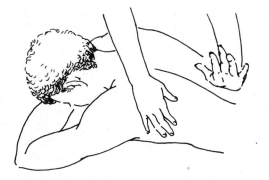

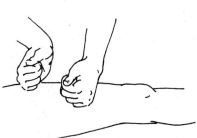

Fig. 15.5e Slapping movements are applied to the back by alternating palms of the hands.

Fig. 15.5f Beating movements are applied to the thigh muscles with alternating hands in a loose fist position.

Vibration—Shaking

Vibration or shaking movement should be applied according to individual needs and when they will be of specific benefit to the patient (Fig. 15.6a and b).

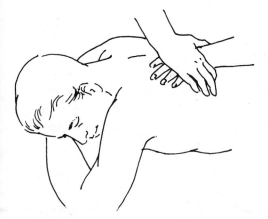

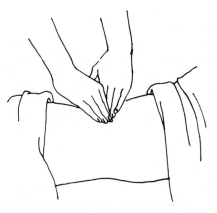

Fig. 15.6a Vibration movements are applied along each vertebra by placing one hand flat on the client's back, the other hand on top, and moving quickly back and forth.

Fig. 15.6b Vibration movements are applied over the abdominal area with the fingertips of both hands.

Joint Movements in Massage

Joint movements can be either active or passive. In active movement, the patient participates by moving joints and contracting muscles. The patient's participation can be either assistive or resistive. When the patient works with the nurse's movement it is called assistive movement. In passive movement, the patient relaxes while the nurse moves the joint. When the patient moves the joint without assistance or resistance, it is called free movement.

During the application of joint movements, the patient (or client) should be asked to express any discomfort. When extreme pain or a questionable condition exists, the patient's (or client's) physician should be consulted.

To control joint movement, the nurse places one hand above the joint to be moved and the other below the joint. This helps to control the degree of resistance or assistance on the part of the patient. Both passive and active movements improve circulation to the joints and help to prevent stiffness (Fig. 15.7a to e).

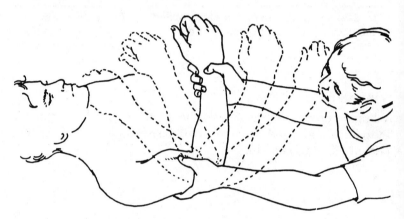

Fig. 15.7a Flexion and extension of the forearm.

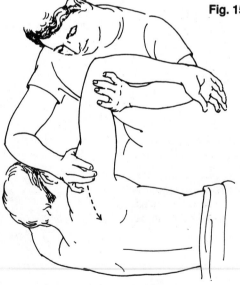

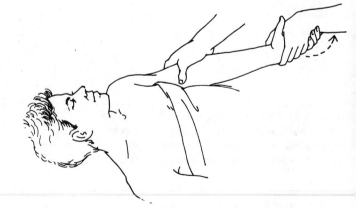

Fig. 15.7b Abduction of the arm and rotation of the shoulder. This movement involves the pectoralis major muscle, deltoid muscle, humerus bone, and the shoulder joint (ball and socket).

Fig. 15.7c Supination of the forearm. The palm of the hand is turned upward.

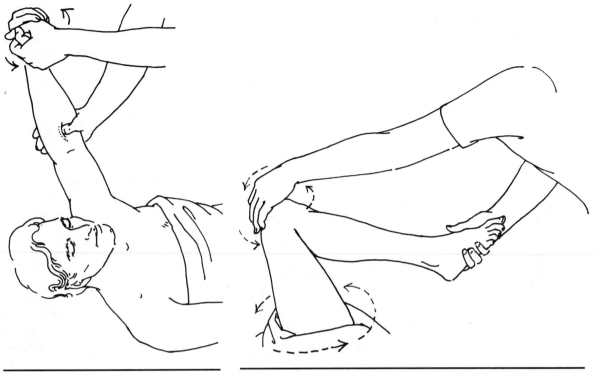

Fig. 15.7d Circumduction of the arm.   **Fig. 15.7e Circumduction of the thigh.**

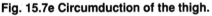

Active movements of the muscles help to prevent loss of muscle tone and strength. The following is a general guide.

The Arm

1. Begin with fingers and the thumb. Use flexion and extension, both passive and active. Follow with abduction and adduction, both passive and active.
2. Exercise the wrist. Use circumduction, passive; and radial and ulnar flexion, passive. Follow with dorsal flexion, passive.
3. Exercise the elbow. Use flexion and extension, both passive and active. Follow by both supination and pronation, passive and active.
4. Exercise the shoulder. Begin with circumduction, passive. Follow with anteflexion and retroflexion, passive and active.

The Leg

1. Begin with the toes. Exercise with flexion and extension, passive and active; and circumduction, passive.
2. Exercise the ankle. Use dorsal and plantar flexion, passive and active.
3. Exercise the knee. Use flexion and extension, passive and active.

4. Exercise the hip. Begin with circumduction, passive. Continue with extension and flexion, both passive and active. Do abduction and adduction, passive and active. Repeat exercise on upper and lower extremities.

Movements for the Head and Neck

The patient should be lying supine comfortably with arms relaxed at sides.

1. Begin with flexion forward, backward, and to the right and left, with passive response.
2. Use rotation to the right and left, passive.
3. Continue with flexion forward, backward, then to the right and left, with resistance.
4. Follow with circumduction to the right and left, passive.
5. Complete the exercise with stretching of the neck, passive.

▼ CLIENT (PATIENT) INFORMATION FORM

The form on page 497 is a basic form used to obtain information about a client or patient. Generally, this type of form would be useful in a clinic. A hospital or other healthcare facility might provide a more extensive form tailored to the records needed by the physician and the facility.

▼ STEP-BY-STEP GENERAL BODY MASSAGE

The following step-by-step procedure for general body massage is the one preferred by most nurses and other healthcare professionals because it can be adjusted to meet the needs of the patient. It is gentle yet thorough. The order of movements can be easily adjusted to combine or delete movements.

Authorities in the art of massage suggest beginning the general massage with the extremities. Massaging the extremities first tends to relax tension and helps to prepare the patient for the rest of the massage. This is particularly helpful when giving massage to the patient for the first time or to patients who are shy and withdrawn.

The use of passive and active joint movements is not described in detail in the following general massage procedures; however, they may be used when appropriate. Flexion, circumduction, and extension movements may also be included in general massage and are given before centrifugal (finishing) strokes.

Preparation

1. Check the temperature of the room to be sure it will be comfortable for the patient during the massage.
2. Assemble all the products and materials you will need.
3. Prepare the patient.

Massage Clinic
Client Information Form

Name_____ Birth Date_____

Address_____ Telephone_____

_____ Business Phone_____

     City   State   Zip   Social Security #_____

Occupation_____ Other Activities_____

General Health Condition_____ Blood Pressure_____

Have you had any serious or chronic illness, operations, chronic virus infections, or traumatic accidents? _____

Are you in recovery for addictions or abuse?_____

Are you under a doctor, chiropractor or other health practitioners care? _____

If so, for what condition/s? _____

Are you on any medication? _____ If so, what?_____

Do I have permission to contact your Doctor / Therapist?_____

Names of Doctors, Chiropractors or Health Practitioners:

Name_____ Name_____

Address_____ Address_____

Telephone_____ Telephone_____

Why did you come for our services? (relaxation, pain, therapy, etc.)_____

_____

What results would you like to achieve with our work?_____

Have you had any massage therapy before?_____ If so, by whom?_____

How did you find out about our services? _____

Were you referred to this office?_____ By whom?_____

In case of emergency notify: Name_____Phone _____

I have completed this information form to the best of my knowledge. I understand the massage services are designed to be a health aid and are in no way to take the place of a doctors care when it is indicated. Information exchanged during any massage session is educational in nature and is intended to help me become more familiar and conscious of my own health status and is to be used at my own discretion.

Our time together is precious and I agree to cancel 24 hours in advance. Unless there is an emergency, if I miss an appointment I agree to pay the full appointment fee.

Date_____ Signature_____

Fig. 15.8 Client Information Form.

When possible, it is desirable to have the patient bathe, empty the bladder. Often the massage will be given to a patient while they are in a hospital-type bed. Adjust the bed to its highest position and move it away from the wall so you will not have to bend over and will be able to move around the bed.

4. Wash your hands thoroughly.

▼ PROCEDURE

Use proper draping to assure the patient is warm and comfortable. Undrape and then redrape each part of the body as it is massaged.

To apply the lubricant, place a small amount of massage oil or cream into the palm of the hand and then rub the hands together to distribute the product evenly. Use light effleurage to apply the lubricant to the area of the body to be massaged. Use oil or cream sparingly because too much lubrication will make it difficult to perform some massage movements efficiently. Use only enough of the lubricating product to allow the hands to glide smoothly across the skin.

Massage for the Arms

1. Begin the massage with the patient's arm (either the right or left). Undrape the arm and apply the lubricant. Use both hands to apply light effleurage from the hand to the shoulder, returning with rotary movements back to the hand. Repeat the movements several times.
2. Press the metacarpals (bones of the hand) and then knead each finger from tip to knuckles. Rotate each finger.
3. Use the palm and heel of your hand to apply effleurage to the palm of the patient's hand, extending the movements several inches above the wrist. Repeat the movement on the back (dorsal surface) of the hand and wrist.
4. Bend the patient's arm so that it is resting on the elbow. Rotate the arm several times. Follow with effleurage to the forearm.
5. With palms of both hands, apply effleurage to the patient's upper arm with sweeping movements up and over the shoulder. Apply light petrissage movements to the upper arm. Repeat effleurage.
6. Use circular friction movements on the upper arm following the direction of the muscles from insertion to origin.
7. Apply circular friction to the joints of each finger, beginning with the forefinger and moving to the middle finger, the ring finger, the little finger, then back to the thumb. Alternate these movements with light effleurage to the hand and fingers.
8. Apply digital friction to elbow joints followed by effleurage. Repeat the movements several times.

9. Apply petrissage to the biceps, triceps, and deltoids. Alternate with effleurage.

10. Use both hands to apply firm, rhythmic effleurage and gentle centrifugal movements from hand to shoulder. Follow with tapotement (percussion) movements from the hand to the shoulder and back to the hand. Rotate the arm and finish this part of the massage with light centrifugal (stroking) movements.

Repeat the massage on the other arm and hand.

Massage for the Legs

1. Begin with either the right or left leg. Undrape the leg and apply the lubricant. Use the palms of both hands to apply effleurage from the upper (dorsal) surface of the foot to the knee joint, returning with large rotary movements to the foot. Repeat the effleurage movements of the feet, alternating with circular friction over the tarsals (ankle bones) and the metatarsals (bones of instep).

2. Apply effleurage to the back of the leg, followed by effleurage to the foot. Apply effleurage to the front (over the tibia) of the leg, and repeat effleurage to the foot.

3. Use both hands to apply effleurage from inner to outer thigh. Repeat the movements on the thighs, and then stroke downward to the foot.

4. Use both hands to apply circular movements from foot to hip joint, covering both the inner and outer surfaces of the leg.

5. Apply circular friction to the foot, followed by light petrissage movements. Apply circular friction to the ankle joint, followed by effleurage.

6. Use both hands to apply petrissage to calf of the leg. Follow with effleurage. Apply circular friction along the sides of the tibia, followed by effleurage.

7. Use both hands to apply petrissage to the inner surface of the thigh, followed by light effleurage. Repeat the movements on the outer surface of the thigh.

8. Use both hands to apply effleurage from the foot to the top of the thigh.

9. Apply light percussion movements such as clapping, slapping, and hacking to the thighs, moving around and down to the calf and the foot.

10. Use both hands to finish this part of the massage with light centrifugal stroking from the hip joint, down the thigh, to the foot. Repeat the movements several times with a light feathering or tapering off of movements.

Massage for the Chest

1. Undrape the chest and apply the lubricant. Use both hands to apply effleurage to the chest, sweeping from the base of the sternum, up to the median line of the chest, and outward to

the shoulders. Finish the movement with rotary movements downward on the chest. Repeat the effleurage movements from back of ears and base of neck (in direction of lymph flow), downward and outward around the breast. Repeat the movements several times.

2. Use fingers and palms of hand to apply circular friction from shoulder to sternum, circulating around the breast. Alternate the movement with effleurage several times.
3. Apply petrissage movements with thumb and fingers from neck to shoulders, alternating with effleurage.
4. Apply percussion movements (clapping, hacking, slapping) from neck and shoulders to chest, alternating with light effleurage. Do not apply movements over the breast.

Massage for the Abdomen

1. The patient should flex the knees slightly with the feet flat on the bed. Undrape the abdomen and apply the lubricant. Use the palms of both hands to apply circular, clockwise (downward and outward) movements over the abdomen. Follow by light effleurage (in direction of large intestine) to the abdomen.
2. Apply petrissage over the entire abdominal area, alternating with effleurage.
3. Place one hand flat on the abdominal area below the navel. Place the other hand on top to assist in applying pressure. With hands in place one on top of the other, apply several vibrating movements, then relax the pressure.
4. Apply effleurage (upward in direction of large intestine) to the abdomen.
5. Apply light percussion movements followed by gentle effleurage.

Massage for the Back

Have the patient lie in the prone position. Undrape the back and apply the lubricant.

1. With palms of hands, begin the stroking movements from below the waistline, sweeping up the sides of the spine, and back down in large circles. Do this several times, followed by effleurage downward over the back muscles.
2. Apply petrissage to neck and upper portion of the back, working down the spine. Use your thumbs and fingers to massage as you feel the vertebrae.
3. Apply petrissage to the gluteus maximus (buttocks), alternating the movements with effleurage.
4. Apply circular (friction) movements with the tips of your fingers working down each side of the spine.
5. Apply kneading movements to each side of the spine, beginning at the scapula and ending at the coccyx (tail bone). Follow with effleurage to the entire back.

6. Apply percussion movements along the sides of the spine moving downward; follow the movements with light effleurage.
7. Use the palms of both hands to apply effleurage to buttocks, followed by petrissage and additional effleurage movements.
8. Apply percussion movements over the entire gluteus maximus, followed by effleurage.

THE THERAPEUTIC RUBDOWN ▼

A rubdown using lotion, oil or alcohol is often a part of patient care. It is usually not as long of duration as the general body massage.

Oil Rubdown

The oil rubdown is especially good for dry skin. A mild massage oil, cocoa butter, or other mild lotion or oil can be used. The oil is applied with light effleurage (stroking) and light, circular friction movements. The oil rubdown is usually given in the following order:

1. Upper extremities
2. Lower extremities
3. Neck, chest, and shoulders
4. Abdominal region
5. Hips and back.

Preparation

The patient should be bathed and prepared with proper draping.

1. A bath blanket is placed under the patient.
2. The oil or lotion should be warmed by placing the container in a basin of hot water for a few minutes. (Do not use highly scented oil. It may be offensive or irritating to sensitive skin.)
3. Towels should be available to wipe away excess oil.

Procedure

Use effleurage and friction movements.

1. Put about a teaspoonful of oil or lotion in your cupped hand. Apply oil or lotion and then massage the hands, arms, and shoulders.
2. Apply oil or lotion to the chest and follow with massage.
3. Apply oil or lotion to the thighs and lower legs. Apply massage.
4. Have the patient turn over.
5. Apply oil or lotion to the posterior thighs and lower legs. Apply massage.
6. Apply oil or lotion to shoulders, back, and buttocks. Apply appropriate massage.
7. Stroke the spine from neck to waist, using the back of the hand in sweeping movements.

Alcohol Rubdown

The alcohol rubdown is often used to refresh the patient when a bath cannot be given, to lower body temperature when fever is present, to create a cooling effect after applications of heat.

Preparation

The patient should be prepared with proper draping. A bath blanket is placed on the bed. The bottle of isopropyl rubbing alcohol can be warmed by placing it in a basin of warm water. **Caution:** Do not use pure grain alcohol unless it has been properly diluted. Read the label to be sure it is safe for use on the skin. Alcohol can be diluted to a 70 percent solution or a solution of two parts alcohol to one part water.

Procedure

1. The patient's body should be dry.
2. Drape the patient and explain what you will do and why.
3. Place a small amount of alcohol into your cupped hand.
4. Apply the alcohol to the upper extremities first. Use light, upward strokes, returning with small, rotary movements until all the parts have been covered. Repeat if necessary. Finish with several unbroken strokes from shoulder to hand. Be sure there is no excess alcohol left on the patient's skin.
5. Apply alcohol to the chest. Use long strokes from rib cage to shoulders. Return with rotary movements to the lateral part of the chest. Repeat the movement several times.
6. Apply alcohol to both hands, and stroke the shoulder on one side with long, sweeping strokes. Repeat on the other side.
7. Apply alcohol to both hands, and use long, sweeping strokes to the anterior surface of the thigh and lower leg. Repeat on the other side.
8. Turn the patient over, and apply alcohol to the shoulders, back, and buttocks. Use long, sweeping strokes from buttocks to shoulders. Follow with light rotary movements over the shoulders, back, and buttocks.
9. Stroke the spine from neck to waist, using both hands to alternate the sweeping movements.
10. Be sure no excess alcohol is left on the patient's skin. Indicate that you have finished the alcohol rub, and assist the patient to assume a comfortable position.

QUESTIONS FOR DISCUSSION AND REVIEW

1. In addition to having technical skills that help to restore the patient's health, what is an important task of the nurse or healthcare professional?
2. How do the jobs of the general massage practitioner and the nurse differ as related to massage treatments?
3. Why do massage practitioners use the Swedish massage method along with other therapeutic aids to help restore the patient to health?
4. Why must the nurse be particularly aware of contraindications for massage?
5. Why are active movements so beneficial to muscles when the patient is convalescing?
6. Why is it necessary to obtain a medical history of a client or patient before giving a massage treatment?
7. Why is the alcohol rubdown used so frequently in patient care?
8. Why is an oil rubdown often used in patient care?

Athletic/Sports Massage

16

Learning Objectives

After you have mastered this chapter, you will be able to:

1. *Define athletic/sports massage.*
2. *Explain the purposes of athletic massage.*
3. *Explain the causes of muscle fatigue.*
4. *Explain the major benefits of athletic massage.*
5. *Explain contraindications for athletic massage.*
6. *Locate the major stress points of the body.*
7. *Explain the importance of warm-up exercises and massage to the athlete's performance.*
8. *Explain the relationship of certain athletic or sports activities to possible injuries.*
9. *Describe the four basic applications of athletic massage and the goals of each.*
10. *Demonstrate massage techniques commonly used in athletic massage.*
11. *Identify the presence of soft tissue injury.*

INTRODUCTION ▼

As far back as antiquity, massage was used to restore and to rejuvenate war-torn and weary soldiers as they returned to Rome. The Roman athletes enjoyed the benefits of restorative massage and baths.

For many years the great athletes of the European and Soviet countries included massage as part of their intensive and continuous training schedules. In 1972 Lasse Viren, sometimes called the Flying Finn, credited daily deep friction massage to enable himself to train hard enough to win gold medals in the 5000 and 10,000 meters at the Olympic games. In 1980, Jack Meagher and Pat Boughton published the first book in the United States on the subject entitled *Sportsmassage*.

In the United States, massage is recognized as a valuable asset to improve the athlete's ability to perform better with fewer physical ill effects from maximum effort. In 1984 for the first time, massage was made available for all athletes competing in the summer Olympic games in Los Angeles. Since then, massage areas have become a common sight at many athletic events across the country. Many athletes participate in regular massage as part of their training regimen. For many athletes and trainers, massage has become the therapy of choice in the rehabilitation of minor sports injuries.

Throughout the 1980s sports massage was instrumental in opening the door for the recognition of massage as a viable treatment for soft tissue injury, dysfunction, and pain. Many massage techniques used and developed for sports massage are just as applicable for soft tissue lesions and injuries suffered in the practices of day-to-day living.

PURPOSE OF ATHLETIC MASSAGE ▼

Athletic massage, also called sports massage, is the application of massage techniques that combine sound anatomical and physiological knowledge, an understanding of strength training and conditioning, and specific massage skills to enhance athletic performance. Athletic massage enables athletes to attain their highest potential by accelerating the body's natural restorative processes, enabling the athlete to participate more often in rigorous physical training and conditioning. Massage helps to reduce the chance of injury by identifying and eliminating conditions in the soft tissue that are at potential risk of injury. When injury has occurred, massage helps to restore mobility and flexibility to injured muscle tissue, while reducing recovery time. Athletic massage, when done correctly, can improve the athlete's ability to perform while reducing the incidence of lost time due to injury and fatigue. Regular athletic massage may extend the athlete's career.

Athletic massage is not reserved just for the highly competitive athlete. The same techniques are effective on any active individual for assessing and working on soft tissue conditions.

The Athletic/Sports Massage Therapist

To be an effective athletic (sports) massage therapist, a person should have a thorough understanding of anatomy, physiology, kinesiology, biomechanics, and massage technique. The massage therapist should have a sound knowledge of anatomy and be familiar with the various structures of the body. Of particular interest are the skeletal system and the muscular system. It is important also to understand the circulatory system and the nervous system, especially the neuromuscular functions. An understanding of kinesiology, which is the study of body movement, helps the therapist recognize what structures are involved in the movements of particular sports, especially when pain is present. The therapist must also understand which muscles and muscle groups the athlete is using in a particular sport.

Biomechanics refers to the integrated movement of the entire body. For instance, the manner in which the foot is placed affects what the knees, hip, back, shoulders, and head do. Tension in a particular body area also indicates tension or misalignment in other areas of the body. Because the body is used in a particular way, specific areas are going to be stressed. A deviation in the structure of one area of the body will be reflected throughout the body. Deviations often appear as patterns of structural imbalances. These deviations, when stressed, often result in injury. The more severe the deviation, the sooner an injury may occur.

Physiology is important in understanding the role each system plays in supporting the others so they function as a whole organism. The better the therapist understands the body's response to exercise, strain, and injury, the better he or she will be able to offer massage services that will benefit the athlete.

An accepted principle in sports physiology is that in order to improve either strength or endurance, appropriate stresses must be applied to **overload** the system, forcing the body to adapt to the heavier load. Proper conditioning involves overloading the system an acceptable amount, and then allowing the system time to recuperate and adapt to a new level of ability. If the intensity of the training exceeds the body's ability to recuperate, injury or breakdown will probably result.

During intense training, competition, and sometimes in everyday life, muscle strength and endurance is pushed to its limits and beyond. The result may include:
• Increased metabolic waste buildup in the tissues
• Strains in the muscle or connective tissue. These may range from microscopic microtrauma to major injury.

- Inflammation and associated fibrosis
- Spasms and pain that restrict movement.

These are negative effects of exercise. Skillfully applied athletic massage effectively counteracts each of these conditions. It normally takes a muscle that has been stressed to a point of fatigue forty-eight to seventy-two hours to rest, adapt, and recuperate. Athletic massage can reduce the recuperation time by as much as 50 percent.

Beneficial Effects of Athletic Massage

The goal of athletic massage is to enhance the athlete's performance. Performance is regulated by the efficiency, precision, and freedom with which the athlete is able to move. Efficiency is dependent on training and conditioning. Athletic massage allows for more intense training. Restrictions from pain, spasms, and tension inhibit freedom of movement. Without freedom of movement, precision is adversely affected. Athletic massage reduces many of the restrictions.

Some beneficial effects of athletic massage are:

1. Massage causes hyperemia, making more oxygen and nutrients necessary for growth and repair available to the body area being massaged.
2. Massage stimulates circulation and lymph drainage to flush out metabolic wastes of exertion quickly. It is three to five times more effective in combating fatigue than resting.
3. Massage stretches and broadens muscle, tendons, and ligaments.
4. Massage breaks down the "gluing" between fascial sheaths.
5. Massage separates fibrosis and breaks down adhesions that result from inflammation and trauma.
6. Massage helps to realign collagen fibers formed as a result of injury to produce a strong, flexible scar.
7. Massage reduces muscle spasm.
8. Massage identifies possible trouble areas and helps to eliminate them.

Special Benefits of Massage to Athletes

1. Massage allows the athlete to reach peak performance sooner and sustain it longer.
2. With massage, muscles improve in flexibility and are able to respond more quickly and powerfully.
3. Massage encourages better performance and reduces the chance of injury.
4. Massage eliminates muscle stiffness due to excess acid build-up. It rejuvenates muscles quicker after intense workouts or events.

5. Massage offers the athlete a chance to relax and recuperate more quickly.
6. Massage reduces ischemic pain and pain from spasms, splinting, and tension.
7. Athletic massage identifies and eliminates possible trouble spots, thereby preventing injury.
8. With massage, injuries heal quicker and stronger without loss of power due to transverse fibrosis.
9. Massage extends the overall span of the athlete's career.

Techniques of Athletic Massage

A thorough knowledge of the various massage techniques and their proper application makes the difference between an effective or ineffective sports massage therapist. Many of the techniques of athletic massage are identical with those of classical Swedish massage such as effleurage, petrissage, kneading, passive and active joint movements, percussion, vibration, and friction. One of the primary differences between Swedish massage and sports massage is that the movements are done two to three times more rapidly in sports massage as they are in Swedish massage. There are some therapeutic techniques in sports massage that bear special consideration.

Compression Strokes

Compression is applied with a rhythmic pumping action to the belly of the muscle. Compression strokes cause increased amounts of blood to remain in the muscle over an extended period of time. This **hyperemia** is of value in pre-event, restorative, and rehabilitative massage.

Compression strokes for athletic massage use the palm of the hand to repeatedly press the muscle against the bone. The proper way to apply compression is to start the pumping action at the origin of the muscle and proceed to the insertion of the muscle in one-half-inch to one-inch steps. This procedure may be repeated three or more times along each part of the muscle, with special attention given to the body of the muscle. Large, broad muscles require several passes to cover the entire muscle.

Compression promotes increased circulation deep in the muscle at the same time that the muscle is broadened and the fibers are separated. When the compression movement is applied with short transverse motion at the deepest pressure of the compression, it also acts to stretch the muscle and separate adhesions in the muscle fascia that result from post-edemic fibrosis in the muscle fibers and fascicles.

Usually in the process of applying compressions, specific areas of the muscle are identified that contain fibrous bands, knots, or alarm points. The stroke can be changed to a cross-fiber movement to

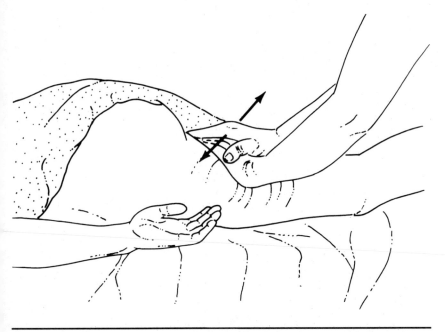

Fig. 16.1 Compression strokes are applied with the palm of the hand to the belly of the muscle.

tease and separate the muscle fibers. When done correctly, this stroke mashes the tissue and slightly stretches it, causing a broadening of the muscle and a breaking up of the binding fascia surrounding the fibers. The stroke also enhances fluid movement at the intercellular level.

The most important goal of compression is to create hyperemia in the muscle tissue. Deep compressions stretch, broaden, and separate muscle fibers and in the process release histamines (**HIS**-tah-meens) and acetylcholine (as-ee-til-**KOH**-leen). This causes the blood vessels throughout the massaged area to dilate and become more permeable to produce a lasting hyperemia (Fig. 16.1).

Deep Pressure

Deep pressure is usually applied with the thumb, a braced finger, or occasionally with the elbow. Deep pressure is used effectively to treat tender points that might be found in muscle, fascia, tendon, ligaments, joint capsules, or periosteum. If pressure on a point causes pain to radiate or refer to another area, that point is considered to be a trigger point. Trigger points are found in taut bands of muscle tissue. Pressure is used on trigger points to deactivate them and increase function to the referred area. Stress points are tender points that are usually associated with microtrauma or spasms in the muscle. They are generally located near the origin, insertion, or musculo-tendinous junction.

When a trigger point or stress point is located, pressure is applied directly into that point. The amount of pressure is determined by the tolerance of the athlete and the condition of the tissue. The pressure must not be so great as to cause the athlete to tense the muscles in a protective response. If the athlete were to rate the intensity of the discomfort on a scale of one to ten, one being very little discomfort and ten being excruciating, the discomfort level should be about five or six. After the therapist maintains the same amount of pressure for a short time, the intensity rating will decrease to about two. This is an indication that the point has been deactivated, and the therapist continues with the treatment (Fig. 16.2).

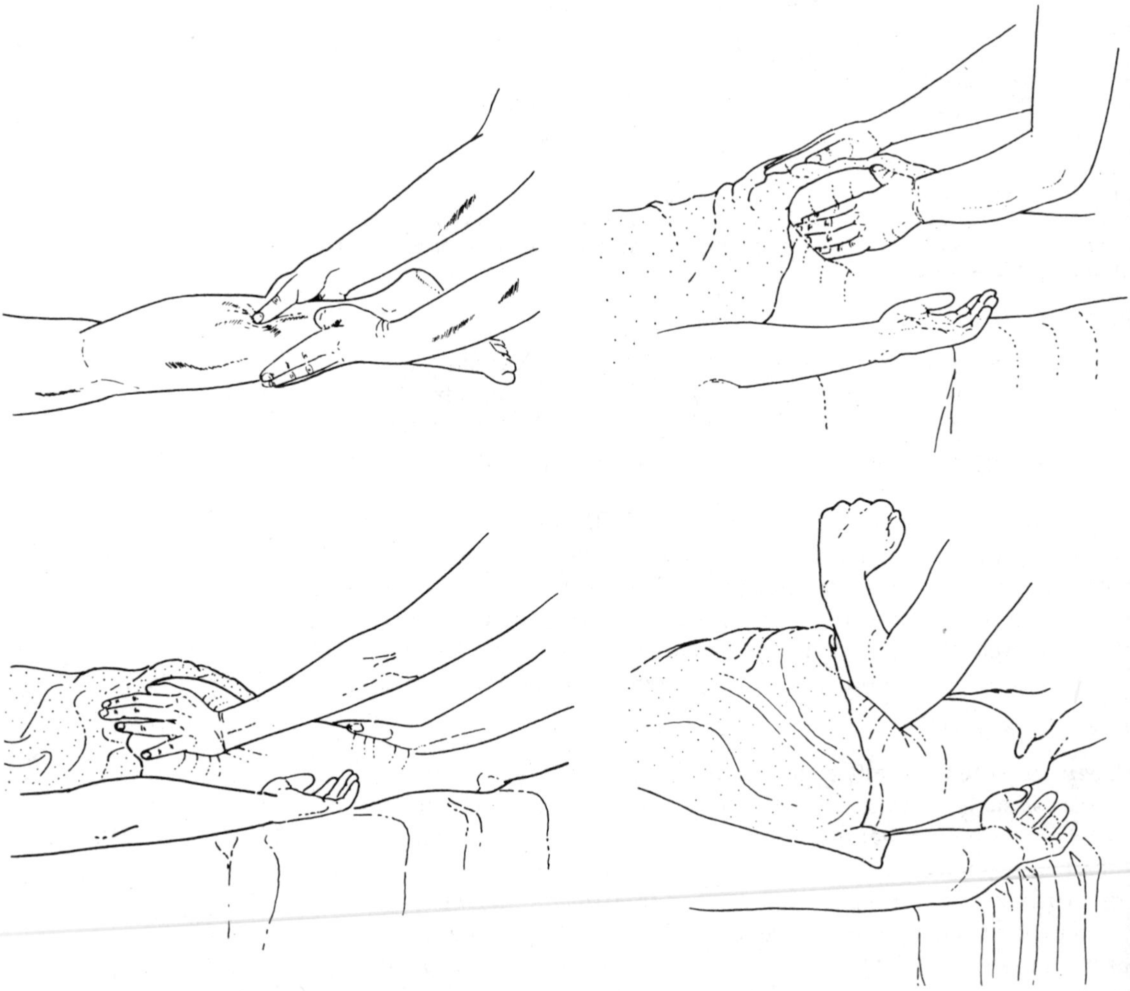

Fig. 16.2 Deep pressure can be applied with the thumb, fingers, hand, or elbow. Pressure should never be so extreme as to injure the client. Proper body mechanics assure better effects with minimal stress to the therapist.

Transverse or Cross-Fiber Friction

Transverse or cross-fiber friction is applied by rubbing across the fibers of the tendon, muscle, or ligament at a 90° angle to the fibers. The use of transverse friction massage for treatment of soft tissue lesions was popularized by the British osteopath, Dr. James Cyriax. Cross-fiber friction effectively reduces fibrosis and encourages the formation of strong, pliable scar tissue at the site of healing injuries. Cross-fiber friction is effective at reducing the crystalline roughness that forms between tendons and their sheaths that sometimes result in painful tendonitis. Cross-fiber friction can prevent or soften adhesions in fibrous tissue.

Cross-fiber massage is used during the subacute and chronic stages of strains, sprains, and contractures or any situations where scar tissue and adhesions are present.

Cross-fiber massage is generally applied with braced fingers or the thumb. As with other types of friction, the fingers, the skin, and superficial tissues move as a unit against the deeper tissues. The pressure used in cross-fiber friction is deep enough to reach the target tissue but stays within the pain tolerance of the athlete. The stroke must be applied directly at the site of the lesion and at right angles to the fibers. The stroke must be broad enough to cover the area and separate the tissue without bouncing over it. Cross-fiber friction consists of oscillating laterally across the ropy tissue, working into the fibers, and spreading them apart while working deeper into the tissue. The therapist must be careful not to pluck the constricted tissue but to work into it, teasing the fibers apart (Fig. 16.3).

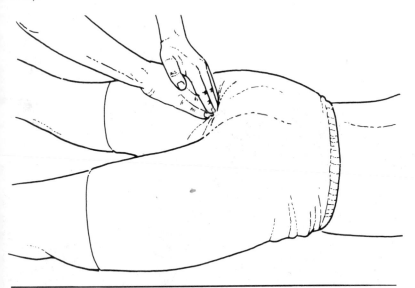

Fig. 16.3 Cross-fiber or transverse friction is applied directly to the site of a lesion. The stroke must be broad enough to cover the area and deep enough to reach the lesion.

Shaking and Jostling

A good way to relieve the intensity of deep work on the muscle is to shake or jostle the entire muscle mass or limb vigorously. This not only releases the tension that may result from the manipulations but also works to loosen fascia and improve lymph movement.

Shaking is done by grasping the body part and vigorously moving it up and down or back and forth so that the relaxed flesh flops around the bone. For example, in the supine position with the knee bent and the foot flat on the table, grasp the knee and vigorously move it laterally back and forth so the muscles of the thigh and calf are shaken. Or, grasp the wrist with both hands. Apply a slight traction to the arm and vigorously shake the entire arm and shoulder up and down. When shaking a limb, it is important not to hyperextend any joint, especially the elbow or knee.

To jostle a muscle, place the massaging hand across the muscle at the origin, and then lightly grasp and vigorously move the muscle laterally across the axis, working from origin to insertion.

Shaking and jostling requires that the muscle is relaxed as it is moved quickly back and forth (Fig. 16.4a to d).

Active Joint Movements

In the early 1950s, Dr. Herman Kabat developed a number of active movement exercises to be used in the rehabilitation of conditions such as orthopedic disabilities, spinal cord injuries, cerebral palsy,

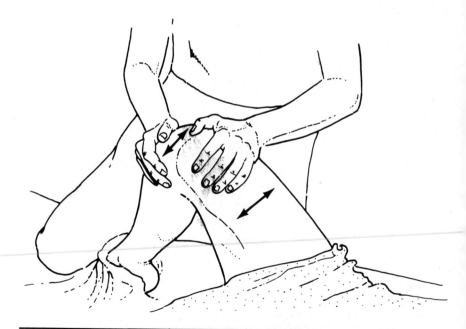

Fig. 16.4a Shaking the calf and thigh by rapidly moving the bent knee side to side.

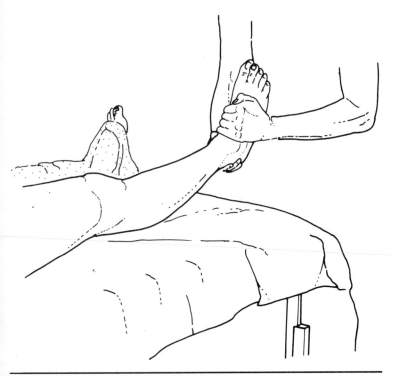

Fig. 16.4b To shake a leg, grasp the ankle as shown, apply traction, and bounce the entire leg vigorously up and down on the table. Be careful not to hyperextend the knee.

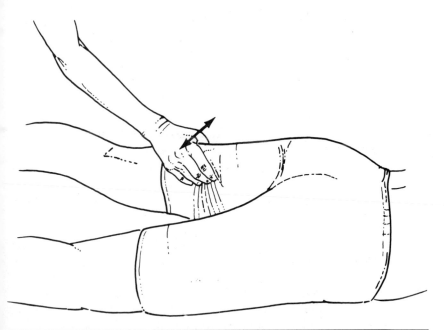

Fig. 16.4c Jostling the hamstrings. Lightly grasp the muscle and jostle it back and forth.

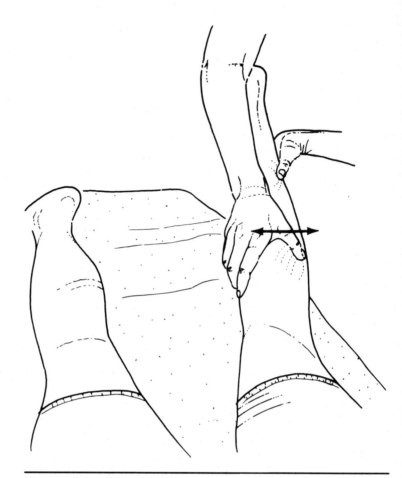

Fig. 16.4d Jostling the calf muscles.

and polio. The exercises used therapist-assisted active and resisted movement in specific patterns. Dr. Kabat based the therapy on Sherington's physiological principles of reciprocal enervation, reciprocal inhibition, post-isometric relaxation, and the process of irradiation. Following Dr. Kabot's retirement, the development of the technique was continued by physical therapists Margaret Knott and Dorothy E. Voss. In 1954 this therapy system adopted the name Proprioceptive Neuromuscular Facilitation. It is better known by the acronym PNF.

Today, PNF is still one of the widest used and most effective therapy systems for the rehabilitation of neurologic and soft tissue disorders.

Active stretching movements used in athletic massage borrow from the principles of PNF. PNF stretching is based on reciprocal inhibition and post-isometric relaxation.

Another form of active joint movements that is a modification of PNF is called Muscle Energy Technique. (MET is discussed in

Chapter 17.) MET helps to counteract muscle spasm, improve flexibility, and restore muscle strength. PNF stretching or MET is performed by moving a body part involving the affected muscle into an extended or stretched position to a point of pain or discomfort, then moving it back out of that position to a point where there is no discomfort. The therapist then supports the body part in this position while the client contracts the muscles for five to thirty seconds, and then relaxes. The process is then repeated several times as the range of motion of the affected muscle or articulation increases until flexibility is restored and spasm reduced. **Caution:** The extent of these techniques is regulated by the level of pain experienced by the client. If any movement causes the client to tense due to pain, that movement is contraindicated.

APPLICATIONS FOR ATHLETIC MASSAGE ▼

There are four basic applications for athletic massage. Each has a different goal and requires a different approach. The basic applications are:

1. Pre-event massage—Massage previous to an event to prepare the athlete for the exertion of all-out competition
2. Post-event massage—Massage after an event to normalize the tissues and relax the athlete after competition
3. Restorative or training massage—Massage during training to allow the athlete to train harder with fewer injuries
4. Rehabilitative massage—Massage during rehabilitation to recover from injury more quickly with less chance of reinjury.

Pre-Event Massage

Pre-event massage, given fifteen to forty-five minutes prior to an event, prepares the body for intense activity. The massage is short and stimulating and directed toward the parts of the body that will be involved in the exertion. The main goal of the pre-event massage is to increase circulation and flexibility in the areas of the body about to be used. Pre-event massage is fast paced and invigorating. Except for athletes who are extremely hyperactive, this is not the time for relaxing movements. Pre-event massage warms and loosens the muscles, causing increased blood supply (hyperemia) in specific muscle areas. This enables the athlete to reach his or her peak performance earlier in the event and maintain that performance longer. Increased flexibility allows the athlete more power, speed, and endurance with less possibility of injury.

Pre-event massage is not a replacement for proper warm-up before a performance, but is an adjunct to it and an aid in preparing the athlete for the all-out competition. This a not good time for the athlete to receive his or her first massage because the effects of the massage may "throw off" an athlete's timing and interfere with performance. Pre-event massage is not the time to work too deeply, to break down adhesions or work on muscle spasms.

Pre-event massage uses no oil and is usually given through the clothing. Specific techniques are compression, light cross-fiber friction, shaking, jostling, rolling, kneading, and joint movements.

Post-Event Massage

Post-event massage is given within the first hour or two after participating in an event. The goal of post-event massage is to increase circulation, clear out metabolic wastes, reduce muscle tension and spasms and quiet the nervous system. Research shows that massage of this type promotes rapid removal of metabolic wastes and is three to four times as effective as rest in recovery from muscle fatigue. These techniques enhance the movement of blood and lymph out of the most intensely worked muscles and back toward the heart and center of the body. Lactic and pyruvic acids formed as a result of oxygen depletion are flushed from the muscles. This prevents delayed onset muscle soreness and reduces the time it takes for the body to recover from exertion.

Post-event massage is given after the athlete has had a chance to warm down from the exertion of the competition or exercise. The post-event massage should stimulate circulation and at the same time calm the nervous system. It is a relaxing massage that reduces the physical and mental intensity of competition.

The most effective techniques for post-event massage are light and deep effleurage, petrissage, kneading, compression, jostling, generalized friction movements, and light stretching. All movements are aimed at "stripping out" the areas of the body that have been used during the event. The post-event massage varies from fifteen to thirty minutes in length.

Many serious athletes or teams have a massage therapist on staff to provide pre-and post-event massage. Often sports massage therapists will be available at the site of a competition. It is common for massage areas to be set up at major athletic events such as marathons, triathlons, and even the Olympic games.

After an exhaustive competition the athlete warms down, replenishes fluids, and seeks out the massage area. The first step of the post-event massage is to conduct a short interview to assess the athlete's post-race condition. The therapist should be aware of signs of hypo- or hyperthermia, cramps, spasms, or muscle strain. Questions the therapist might ask of the athlete include:

- How do you feel?
- Have you had any water or fluids since the competition?
- Do you have any problems or discomfort?
- How did you perform in the competition?
- Did you have any problems during the race?
- Are there any areas on you, body that you want me to concentrate on?
- As I work on you let me know if what I do is uncomfortable.

It is advisable to observe the athlete closely during the interview for signs of exhaustion or depression. Have the athlete sit on the table and remove his or her shoes during the conversational interview. Be aware of any blisters, abrasions, contusions, spasms, or strains and apply appropriate first aid or obtain the assistance of the attending medical personnel. It is a good idea to continue light conversation throughout the post-event massage.

The post-event massage concentrates on the muscle groups used during the exercise and includes a back massage for relaxation. The massage can be performed without oil and through the sports clothing if given on site or may include the use of some oil on the bare skin if private facilities are available.

The general procedure for each involved body area would include:

- Long effleurage strokes and kneading to flush out the area
- Light compressions to the entire area
- Jostling and traction shaking of the limb
- Range of motion and light stretching
- Repeat effleurage strokes.
- Feather, nerve strokes from proximal to distal aspect of the area being massaged.

Massage During Training

Massage during training, also called restorative massage, is the most beneficial form of massage for the athlete. Restorative massage is usually on the athlete's training schedule and is considered a regular and valuable part of his or her training. Restorative massage allows the athlete to train at a higher level of intensity, more consistently with less chance of injury. The massage routine may resemble pre-event massage if given before a workout or post-event if given after a workout. More specific therapeutic massage may be used when soft tissue conditions are encountered.

Massage during training increases blood and lymph circulation, which allows more efficient oxygen and nutrient supply to the cells as well as more efficient removal of metabolic waste. All of these benefits make more intense and frequent workouts possible, thereby improving overall performance.

Regular massage during training can locate and relieve areas of stress that carry a high risk of injury. Contractures and constricted muscle tissue containing trigger points can be released. Massage reduces minor cross-fiber adhesions resulting from microtrauma, thereby increasing muscle response and flexibility. Massage also alleviates muscle boundness (by breaking down muscle bundles) so that muscle contractions and relaxation are more efficient. This allows finer-tuned muscle response.

Another benefit of restorative massage is the breaking down of transverse adhesions that may have resulted from previous injuries. This promotes muscle power, better circulation, less chance of reinjury, increased mobility, increased flexibility, and better performance. The athlete is able to achieve maximum effort sooner, more often, and maintain it longer with fewer, if any, ill effects.

The massage process systematically involves every part of the athlete's body, concentrating on those muscle groups and body parts specifically involved in the sport and including other areas that are indirectly involved. Training massage maintains muscles in the best possible state of nutrition, flexibility, and vitality.

Restorative Massage Techniques

Techniques of restorative massage vary according to specific application. The primary techniques in this aspect of athletic massage include all of the techniques of pre-and post-event massage plus deep cross-fiber friction, trigger point therapy, active joint stretches, and neuromuscular techniques for reducing soft tissue lesions and constrictions. Effleurage and petrissage are also used, but to a lesser degree. There are a number of therapist-assisted joint movements that are very effective in this stage of massage. They include Muscle Energy Technique, strain/counter strain, and PNF stretches. See chapter 17 for more on these techniques.

There is no standard or set procedure for athletic massage due to the variety of sports situations to which it is applicable. However, there is a process to follow in choosing an effective treatment plan. When interviewing the client, it is important to find out the following:

- The sport or sports in which he or she is involved
- The location and extent of present trouble areas
- The location and extent of previous injuries
- The workout schedule and planned events
- The extent to which the athletic massage is to be incorporated in the athlete's training.

By learning the client's regular sports, the practitioner can give special consideration to related muscle areas. Trouble areas can point to particular muscle groups on which to concentrate.

Previous injuries can also target trouble areas. Often an injury occurs as a result of a muscle not being flexible enough or not being able to let go. Trouble areas may also indicate fascia that is stuck or bound together. Injuries, especially when muscle spasm or tears exist, also point to synergistic, or opposing, muscles as being primary or potential problems.

Workout schedules indicate how serious a person is about a particular sport and can also reveal injury-prone weekend warriors. How much or how often the athlete wants to include massage in his or her training program helps the practitioner to determine the frequency and intensity of treatments. If the plan is to include only one or two sessions, the massage should be limited. However, if several regular sessions are planned, a thorough preliminary massage can be given. Work can then be done systematically on trouble areas or areas that receive continuous and intense use.

The first massage is primarily a hunt-and-search process using compression and deep stroking to seek out muscle bundles, spasms, and tender points as well as constrictions and areas of fibrosis. These bands or bundles of muscles usually feel like cords or lumpy growths that roll around or snap under the skin. Healthy, pliable muscle is smooth and evenly textured across its whole breadth and length. To the client such trouble areas are generally painful when palpated.

Muscles often contain alarm (stress) points that are either located in taut bands in the muscle body or where the muscle ends and joins the tendon or tendon sheath. Points located in taut bands are trigger points. Stress points are often located at the musculo-tendinous junction. This is where fascia and connective tissue are more prevalent. Because many muscle fibers terminate here, the area is vulnerable to strain and microtrauma. This is also where the ratio of blood vessels to tissue is less, and therefore where fatigue occurs first. Often when a muscle is headed for trouble, the first indication appears in this area (Fig. 16.5).

Deep pressure on alarm points and trigger points gives the first clue to future problems. Early treatment of the muscles associated with the alarm points can stop an injury long before it begins to affect the athlete's performance adversely . Once the trouble areas have been identified, the procedure for working on them is to deactivate the trigger point and then stretch, broaden, and strengthen the associated muscle while encouraging increased blood and lymph circulation.

Some applications of restorative massage tend to be deep and intense. Deep techniques do not mean painful techniques. *All* manipulations must stay within the pain tolerance of the athlete. The athlete must understand that a certain amount of discomfort may be a part of a treatment and be willing to work with the therapist on deep breathing and relaxation techniques. The practitioner must not persist if in the process of working the muscle it becomes tighter. If muscle tightening occurs and the practitioner continues to "dig," there is a chance of actual injury; the condition could worsen instead of improve. The athlete and practitioner should work together for the improvement of the athlete's ability to train and condition his or her body.

If the restorative massage is deep and intense, it is like an intense workout and should be done on days when training is light or on days the athlete is off training. Intense restorative massage should not be given just before a competition. It is preferable to allow at least a couple of practice days between a deep massage and an event so that the athlete can become familiar with how his or her newly released muscles respond.

Massage During Rehabilitation

Rehabilitative massage focuses on the restoration of tissue function following injury. The best way to treat an injury is to prevent it. Restorative massage during training is invaluable for locating

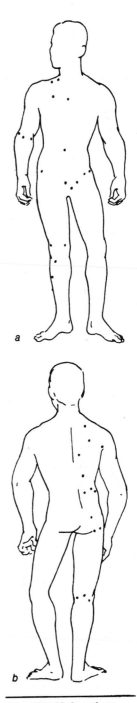

Fig. 16.5 Major alarm (stress) points of the body; (a) anterior and (b) posterior views.

potential trouble spots and relieving them before they progress into debilitating injuries. When injury does occur, massage can be an important part of the rehabilitation program. Treatment strategy varies depending on the nature of the injury. Rehabilitative athletic massage

- Shortens the time it takes for an injury to heal
- Helps to reduce swelling and edema
- Helps to form strong, pliable scar tissue
- Maintains or increases range of motion
- Eliminates splinting in associated muscle tissue
- Locates and deactivates trigger points that form as a result of the trauma
- Helps get the athlete back into training sooner with less chance of reinjury.

A great number of therapeutic techniques are valuable in treating injuries in any of their progressive stages of healing and/or degrees of severity. The application of proper techniques to the type of injury is important. Improper use of movement and pressure can aggravate a condition and possibly cause more permanent damage.

The massage practitioner should practice therapy at this level only after receiving proper training under the supervision of a qualified instructor who is familiar with sports injuries and the practice of therapeutic athletic massage. Before attempting rehabilitative massage, the therapist must be well trained in sound evaluation and treatment techniques. When skilfully applied, massage will reduce the healing time with return to full function; improper application of techniques may prolong healing time and result in more severe injury.

Some general rules for the application of rehabilitative massage are:

- Do not massage directly on the site of an injury or trauma during the acute stage or when it is inflamed.
- Do not stretch muscles or fibrous tissue that is in the acute stage of injury.
- Never cause pain! Pain is the guide for proper application of all techniques. The less pain, the more the gain.
- Apply deep cross-fiber friction and stretching only after inflammation is gone and the healing process is well established.
- When in doubt—Don't.

The advantages of massage therapy are numerous. Prompt application of the appropriate therapy can reduce much swelling and pain caused by an injury. Proper therapy allows the injured tissues to remain in close proximity so that healing progresses faster and with less need for the body to produce excess scar tissue. When massage is administered, the quality of healed tissue is far superior than if an injury is left to heal on its own.

Proper massage therapy improves circulation, enabling excess fluid and damaged tissue to be carried away. With improved circulation, more nutrients are brought to the rebuilding tissue so that it becomes strong and pliable and heals more quickly. Research has also shown that with massage therapy fibrosis caused by muscle injury is reduced and the presence of transverse adhesions is almost nonexistent.

Proper therapy and accelerated healing of injuries means that the athlete's "down time" is cut to a minimum. With continued treatment during the rehabilitation period, there will also be fewer ill effects on performance.

Therapy may be given at the rate of once or twice a day during the time the athlete is out of training and every other day or every third day until he or she is back to a full training schedule. Massage for new or fresh injuries should only be given by properly trained therapists in conjunction with a physician's approval.

Athletic Injuries

It is the nature of athletes to push their abilities to their limits and beyond in order to excel at their particular sport. Because of the rigorous training and participation in competition, athletes' bodies are continuously exposed to stress, strain, fatigue, and sometimes microtrauma or more serious injury. Maximum athletic effort is physical abuse.

Most athletic injuries are either the result of trauma (contact with another athlete or in a fall) or the result of excessive and/or repeated stress to an area of the body due to extreme exertion. Injuries of the traumatic sort are often in the form of broken bones, dislocated joints, and torn ligaments. Such injuries are generally accidental and nonpreventable. Injuries of the second type are far more common and generally affect the soft tissue in the form of muscle strains, pulls and tears, or inflammation of tendons and ligaments. These are usually the result of fatigue, overtraining, poor tissue integrity, muscular weakness, imbalance, or biomechanical deviation. The majority of these injuries are preventable and treatable by massage and proper training.

Athletic injuries are categorized according to the onset and duration of the injury. Acute injuries have a sudden and definite onset and are usually of relatively short duration. Examples of acute injuries include dislocations, sprains, strains, lacerations, fractures, and contusions. Strains and sprains and their side effects respond well to massage therapy. Strains involve the tearing of muscle tissue or tendons. Sprains involve ligaments. The severity of strains and sprains is graded as follows:

Grade I: Mild pain
Severe overstretching of the fibrous tissue with little or no damage
Full range of motion and full strength available

Grade II: Moderate to severe pain
Swelling and possible discoloration
Some tearing of the fibrous tissue
Reduced range of motion and strength.

Grade III: Immediate pain
Severe or complete tissue rupture.
Extensive swelling and tissue deformity
No strength or range of motion (Fig. 16.6a–c).

Massage on acute injuries is contraindicated; however, prompt first aid measures greatly reduce secondary injury that is the result of swelling and therefore reduce the rehabilitation time for the injury. First aid for acute soft tissue injuries involves RICE. As noted earlier, RICE is the acronym for Rest, Ice, Compression, and Elevation. Frequent applications of RICE for the first twenty-four to forty-eight hours will reduce the pain, swelling, and spasm significantly.

After one or two days of rest, the injury enters the subacute stage. The majority of the swelling and inflammation has subsided and the tissues are beginning the healing process. Massage treatments are begun to stimulate circulation to and away from the area and to begin to mobilize the tissue so that as the tissue regenerates, scar tissue forms that is strong, pliable, and flexible. Extreme caution is used not to aggravate the injury or cause more damage to the tissues. Pain is the indicator to the athlete and therapist as to the intensity of the techniques. As the tissues continue to mend and get stronger, the aggressiveness of the therapy increases until the athlete returns to full participation.

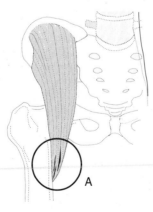 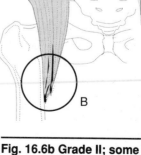 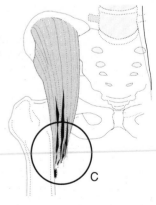

Fig. 16.6a Grade I; over stretched fibrous tissue with some microtrama.

Fig. 16.6b Grade II; some tearing of the fibrous tissue.

Fig. 16.6c. Grade III; severe tearing of the fibrous tissue with loss of function.

Chronic injuries have a gradual onset, tend to last for a long time, or reoccur often. Often they are the result of repetitive stressful activity and are sometimes labeled overuse syndrome. Repeated or extreme stresses cause microscopic lesions in the connective tissue of the tendons, muscles, the musculo-tendinous junction, or the tendinoperiosteo junction. This in turn causes local, low-grade inflammation, selected muscle spasms (taut bands), reduced circulation to the area, pain, and dysfunction. Examples of chronic injury include chronic muscle spasm, tennis elbow, shin splints, tendonitis, fasciitis, and iliotibial band syndrome.

When working with chronic injuries, it is important to relieve the injury and identify and eliminate, if possible, the predisposing cause of the injury.

Soft Tissue Lesions and Injury

Skeletal muscles contain several tissues including muscle tissue, blood and other fluids, nerve tissue, and a variety of connective tissues. The structure of skeletal muscle is unique with its arrangement of contractile fibers aligned and supported in such a way that by contracting, they exert a force on the bony levers of the skeleton, producing movement.

Muscle tissue consists of contractile fibrous tissue arranged in separate parallel bundles (fascicles) which, in turn, consist of a number of parallel muscle fibers that are held in place by an extensive and intricate connective tissue system. The connective tissue supports the muscle fibers in such a way that when the fibers contract, a force is exerted on whatever structure the muscle is attached to, causing movement.

Connective tissues form a continuous net-like framework throughout the body. Connective tissue consists largely of a fluid matrix (ground substance) and collagen fibers that support, bind, and connect the wide range of body structures. Collagen fibers provide the tensile strength in connective tissue. Depending on the consistency of the connective tissue and the varying proportions of fluid to fibers, a wide array of fibrous connective tissues are formed. Some examples are the fluid intercellular environment, the fascia of the muscles, the tendons and ligaments, and even bone.

The muscular system is a highly organized system of compartmentalized contractile fibrous tissues that work together to produce movement. The fibrous tissue is organized and supported by an intricate network of connective tissue. Connective tissue organizes muscles into functional groups, it surrounds each individual muscle, it extends inward throughout the muscle-creating muscle bundles, and eventually houses each muscle fiber. Connective tissue also creates the supporting structure for the intricate network of blood vessels and nerves. The connective tissue projects beyond the ends of the muscle to become tendons which connect the muscles to the bones and other structures (Fig. 16.7).

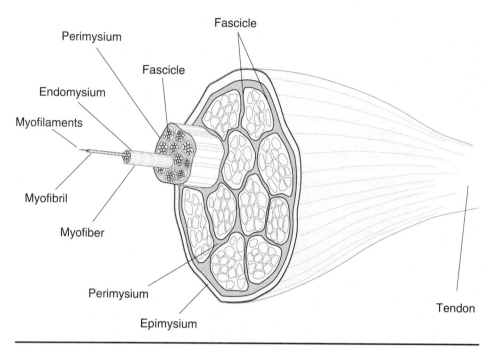

Perimysium

Fascicle

Fascicle

Endomysium

Myofilaments

Myofibril

Myofiber

Perimysium

Epimysium

Tendon

Fig. 16.7 Muscles are contractile organs that are compartmentalized, organized, and supported by intricate layers of connective tissue or fascia.

The layer of connective tissue that closely covers an individual muscle is the **epimysium** (ep-ih-**MIS**-ee-um). The **perimysium** per-ih-**MIS**-ee-um) extends inward from the epimysium and separates the muscle into bundles of muscle fibers or **fascicles** (**Fas**-ih-kis). Within the fascicle, each muscle fiber is covered by a delicate connective tissue covering called the **endomysium** (en-do-MIS-ee-ium). The sarcolemma (cell wall) of the muscle cell and the endomysium are intimately connected and act as a unit so when the muscle fiber contracts and shortens, the connective tissue covering moves right along with it.

The connective tissue organizes the muscle fibers, connects the muscle to tendons, tendons to bones, and even bones to bone. Without this complicated system of connecting sheets, hinges, and ropes that transfer the action of the muscle fibers to the levers of the skeleton, motion and postural stability would not be possible.

Soft tissue injuries are the result of over stretching and eventual breaking of the collagen fibers in one or more layers of the connective tissue. Whether it is micro trauma in or between the muscle fibers, strained muscles or torn ligaments, stresses to the connective tissue exceed their tensile strength resulting in the tearing of collagen fibers in the connective tissue (Fig. 16.8).

The healing process in all soft tissue injuries is essentially the same. The cell damage initiates an inflammatory response. Extra fluid is infused into the area (swelling). The positive effects of swelling are to immobilize the area and supply an environment rich in leukocytes and fibroblasts so the natural healing process of the body can start to repair the injury. The negative effect is that the swelling creates pressure in the tissue that causes further tissue damage and separates the ends of the injury and the connective tissue layers, slowing healing. Inflammation and swelling are accompanied by pain.

The fluid carries an abundance of fibroblasts that within a couple of hours of the injury begin to lay down new collagen fibers to secure the injured tissue. Within two to three days collagen formation is at its maximum. Fibroblasts generate collagen fibers that extend in random directions, forming a cobweb-like network that adheres to any structure in the vicinity. Collagen formation that reconnects the injured tissue forms scar tissue. The criss-cross formation of fibers that connect to structures other than the injured tissue forms undesirable adhesions that restrict mobility and flexibility in the healed tissues.

The swelling that takes place when tissue is injured also creates space between the various layers of fascia. Wherever swelling has

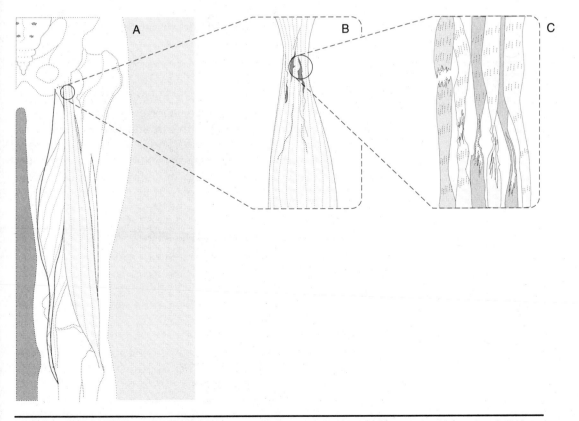

Fig. 16.8 Soft tissue injuries occur when the tissue is pulled and stretched to the point that the integrity of the collagen fibers is broken.

separated tissues, collagen fibers form to adhere the separated tissue. The more extensive the swelling, the more extensive the formation of fibrosis and adhesions. Also, the more severe the injury and the greater the separation in the injured tissue, the more extensive the formation of scar tissue. As long-term swelling is reduced, the fibrosis left behind sticks or glues the adjoining layers of fascia together. This type of gluing may also be the result of stressed and confined muscle movement over a long period of time. The resulting fibrosis reduces mobility and flexibility, leaving a reduction of power and a greater chance of reinjury. Both of these conditions can be greatly reduced with proper first aid and athletic massage therapy.

Proper first aid greatly reduces swelling, and the accompanying secondary trauma. With reduced swelling the space between the ends of the injured tissue and between associated connective tissue layers is minimized. This minimizes the formation of scar tissue, fibrosis, and adhesions.

As the tissue heals, proper therapy including massage encourages new fibers to form along appropriate lines of stress. Properly applied transverse friction massage helps to organize and align collagen fibers to produce strong, pliable tissue at the same time as it breaks down unwanted interfiber cross links and adhesions.

▼ CONTRAINDICATIONS

The athlete's physician (employed by the organization or school) takes case histories and is responsible for pre-season evaluations and for advising the athlete on health-care and care of injuries. The physician treats illnesses and injuries and is responsible for rehabilitation of the athlete. The massage practitioner or trainer works under the direction of the physician and follows his or her guidelines when massage is to be a part of treatment or rehabilitation of injuries.

The physician or practitioner avoids doing anything that might make him or her liable or subject to malpractice. Negligence is defined as imprudent action or failure to act properly or failure to take reasonable precautions. Athletes understand that there are always some risks involved and that a physician or therapist is not held liable for poor judgment on the part of the athlete. Athletic massage is contraindicated in any abnormal condition, acute injury, illness, or disease except as advised by the athlete's physician.

There are times when an amateur or school athlete will request the services of the massage practitioner. The same contraindications for massage apply for this client as for the professional. The client must take responsibility for his or her own health and provide a physician's report if deemed necessary. Any heart condition, anemia, diabetes, thyroid disorders, liver and lung conditions, cancer, skin disease, varicose veins, hypertension, internal injuries, wounds, or like conditions are contraindications for massage. In these cases, massage would be only done upon the recommendation of the client's physician and at the request of the client.

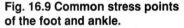

GENERAL PROBLEM AREAS AND SUGGESTED MASSAGE

The following are common areas of potential stress that may be addressed during restorative massage.

The Foot and Ankle

The heels take a lot of shock in sports such as jogging and running, and muscles can become painful to pressure (Fig. 16.9).

Massage: To apply general massage to the foot, have the athlete lie face down with feet over the edge of the table, You may sit on a stool if you are more comfortable. Use your finger or thumb to apply deep friction to sore spots. Apply cross-fiber friction for about ten counts, pause, then repeat the movement. Flex and rotate the foot.

Achilles' Tendon

The Achilles' tendon, located just above the heel, is a sheathed tendon that may become swollen and painful if the ankle has been strained or if the tendon has been pulled at its attachment to the heel. Stress points may have formed at the attachment to the calf muscle.

Massage: At the musculo-tendinous junction, use your thumbs to apply ten or more direct pressure movements, followed by cross-fiber friction. Repeat direct pressure to the tendon, followed by compression with your thumb. Search the calf muscle for related fibrosis or knots. **Caution:** It is contraindicated to do deep strokes along a fibrous tendon like the Achilles' tendon because it tends to aggravate abnormal conditions such as pulls and tears. Since the Achilles' is a sheathed tendon, it is necessary to stretch the tendon before applying cross-fiber friction. To do this, with the athlete lying prone, dorsal flex the ankle. With one thumb, move the tendon to the side and with a braced finger of the other hand apply transverse friction massage to the site of tendonitis (Fig. 16.10).

Metatarsal Cramp or Fatigue

An athlete often suffers muscle cramps, tightening, and spasms of the muscles in the foot.

Massage: Hold the foot steady as you use the tip of your thumb to apply pressure to the stress point near the big toe. Follow pressure with deep cross-fiber friction for ten to twenty counts, then release and repeat the movement. Move your thumb to the stress point near the little toe, and repeat the same movements. Check for stress points near the heel. Apply deep strokes from toes to heel, and gently stretch the plantar tendon.

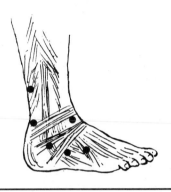

Fig. 16.9 Common stress points of the foot and ankle.

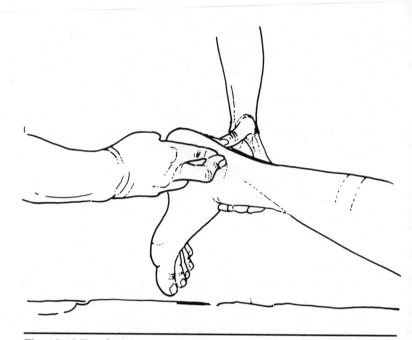

Fig. 16.10 To apply transverse friction to a lesion on a sheathed tendon, like the Achilles, the tendon must be stretched while friction is applied. The foot is dorsal flexed. The tendon is displaced to one side with the thumb of one hand. Transverse friction is applied with a braced finger directly to the site of the lesion.

Ankle Strains and Twists

The feet and ankles play an important part in sports and, due to the varied and stressful movements, are prime targets for injury and fatigue.

Massage: Use your thumb and forefinger to apply pressure and cross-fiber friction to the stress points near the ankle bone. Continue for twenty counts. Release and repeat. This must be done gently, as the area may be painful. Apply friction to the instep, working gently and from the toes to the heel. Move to the stress point of the outer ankle, and apply direct pressure for ten counts. Release and repeat the movement. Shake and rotate the foot, then gently stretch it in every direction. Finish the massage with friction.

The Thigh, Calf, and Knee

Sports such as skiing, skating, ice hockey, surfing, horseback riding, and cycling all require quick reflexes and muscle power. While the neck, shoulders, and back are under stress in these sports, the muscles of the lower back and hips also undergo stress and strain. Often there is pain in the knee area and thigh after a day of heavy exertion.

Massage: Use the tips of your fingers to apply direct pressure to the stress points of the knee, and then follow with cross-fiber friction. Repeat the sequence several times. Use your fingertips to apply circular friction over the knee. Use your fist to finish with circular friction movements. Locate the stress areas in the thighs above the knee and in the groin and inguinal fold. With your thumb, apply pressure for ten counts; release and repeat the movement several times. Apply cross-fiber friction for ten counts. Apply compressions to the entire thigh. Finish the massage by applying deep strokes from knee to hip, shaking, jostling, and rolling the thigh (Fig. 16.11).

Golf Knee

In golf the twisting movements of the torso cause the knee to rotate until the ligaments are sometimes strained. Golf appears to be a mild enough game, but injuries to the knees (and back) do occur.

Massage: Locate the stress points. Use the middle finger or thumb to apply direct pressure. Hold for twenty counts. Release and repeat the movement. Apply cross-fiber friction for twenty counts; release and repeat the movement. Apply friction around the patella. Movements should be gentle.

Calf

Tennis and similar games place stress on the muscles of the calves and ankles, often causing spasms.

Massage: Have the athlete lie face down. Bend the knee and flex the ankle several times. Locate the stress points at the outside of the knee joint. Use your thumbs to apply direct pressure, holding for ten counts. Release and repeat the movement. Follow with cross-fiber friction on the stress points. Repeat the direct pressure and friction on the lower stress points of the ankle. Use the palm of your hand to apply deep compression all over the calf muscles. Apply cross-fiber friction along fibrous bands in the muscle. Apply deep strokes from heel to knee, followed with shaking and jostling of the muscle and effleurage.

Runner's Cramp

The runner will often suffer muscle cramps, spasm, muscle tightening, and calf pull. Ice may be applied to the spasmed area. Have the athlete tighten and relax the antagonist muscle to the one in spasm several times while slightly stretching the spasmed muscles between contractions (reciprocal enervation).

Massage: To massage the leg, have the athlete lie face down on the table. After the spasm subsides, bend and flex the knee several times. Flex the ankle, and rotate it several times. Locate the stress points below the knee joint, then with your thumb, apply pressure for ten counts, release, and repeat the movements. Find the stress point on the ankle, and repeat the same movements. Apply steady, firm compression movements to the calf. Compress stress points for ten counts, release, and follow with cross-fiber friction. Repeat the compression. Apply several deep strokes from heel to knee.

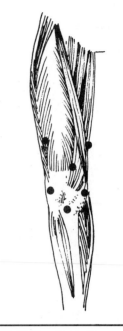

Fig. 16.11 Common stress points around the knee.

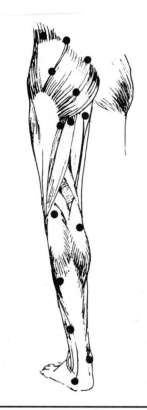

Fig. 16.12 Common stress points of the posterior leg and buttock.

Shake and jostle the calf muscle from knee to ankle, and apply effleurage to the area.

Strain to Hamstrings

Sports requiring sustained leg tension for some time can lead to strain. Examples of such sports are dance and distance running. Generally, the strain will be in the back mid-thigh extending to the back of the knee.

Massage: Use your thumb to locate the stress point behind the knee and in the gluteal crease. Apply direct pressure for ten counts. Release and repeat. Apply cross-fiber friction for ten counts. Release and repeat. Slightly flex the knee while supporting the ankle. Use the palm of your hand to apply compression over the entire back of the thigh from the buttock to the knee. Release and repeat. Finish the massage with deep strokes along the hamstring from knee to hip for ten counts (Fig. 16.12).

Hip, Leg, Buttock, and Groin

Sports such as golf cause strain to the back because of the twisting and swinging motions.

In the hip area there are four main stress points with which you need to be concerned: the side of the hip, the leg, the buttock, and the groin area.

Massage: Have the athlete lie face down on the table. Use the point of your thumb to apply direct pressure all over the buttock area. Locate tight stress areas. Apply pressure for ten counts, release, and repeat the movement several times. Controlled use of the elbow is very effective in this area. Apply cross-fiber friction for twenty counts. Release and repeat the movement. Use the thumb to apply direct pressure to the lateral side of the leg to ten counts. Release and repeat. Apply direct pressure to the lateral side of the midcalf. Find the pressure point in the buttock and along the iliac crest. Apply deep direct pressure for ten counts; release and repeat the movement. Apply cross-fiber friction for ten counts to each affected area; release and repeat the movement. Repeat the cross-fiber friction for ten counts; release and repeat the movement. Apply direct pressure again using the thumb or elbow. Apply for ten counts; release and repeat the movement. Repeat the cross-fiber friction, and finish with deep shaking and vibration movements.

The Elbow and Arm

The muscles in the arm and shoulder may be weakened by overuse or strain from an activity such as tennis. Muscles can become stiff and sore. Generally, the extensor muscles of the forearm will be affected. In the acute state this condition is characterized by inflammation, swelling, and intense pain near the lateral epicondyle of the elbow.

Massage: Using the heel of your hand, apply compression to the wrist for ten counts. From the wrist, work up to the elbow, the shoulder, and then back down to the wrist so that the entire arm is covered. Find the pressure point at the side of the elbow, and with your thumb apply direct pressure for about ten counts. Release and repeat the pressure three or more times. Using cross-fiber friction, move to the next pressure point. Follow along the length of the muscle, repeating the cross-fiber friction where the muscle fibers seem stuck together. Follow this with several more compressions along the muscle. Apply deep stroking movements along the muscle from insertion to origin, and follow these with shaking and jostling movements. Repeat the same procedure to other stress points, and finish with general compression on the entire arm, gentle passive-joint movements, stretching, and soothing effleurage. Instruct the athlete to rest the arm, and repeat the treatment daily until all symptoms are gone (Fig. 16.13).

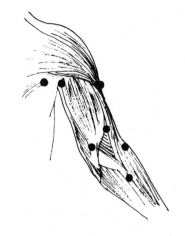

Fig. 16.13 Common stress points of the elbow and arm.

The Wrist

The ligament, tendons, and muscles of the wrist can be affected by tension caused by grasping and tensing for long periods of time. Examples are grasping the handlebars of a bicycle and lifting weights.

Massage: Find the pressure point. Use your fingertips to apply direct pressure to the stress point, holding for ten counts. Release and then repeat the movements several times. Apply cross-fiber friction for ten counts; release and repeat. Use your thumb to apply cross-fiber friction all around the wrist and back again. Do this for about fifteen to twenty counts; release and repeat the movement. Follow with a series of compressions using the heel of your hand. Apply compression up the forearm from wrist to elbow going all around the arm. Repeat these movements several times. Finish the massage by applying direct pressure to the stress points for ten to twenty counts; release and repeat the movement (Fig. 16.14).

Back, Shoulder, and Neck

The back and shoulder muscles are often strained during weightlifting, bowling, golf, and other sports. Shoulder joint injuries are due to such sports as baseball, bowling, basketball, and other sports requiring exertion of the arm and shoulder. These usually result in injury to the rotator cuff or associated muscles.

Massage: Have the athlete lie face down on the table. Use the thumb to apply deep pressure and cross-fiber friction at high stress areas for ten counts. Release and repeat the movement. Do this sequence about four times. Apply cross-fiber friction to the side of the neck and downward on the shoulder. Apply for ten counts; release and repeat until the area has been covered. Find the stress points on the shoulder blade. Apply direct pressure for ten counts;

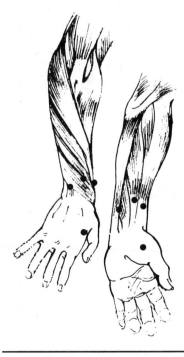

Fig. 16.14 Common stress points of the wrist.

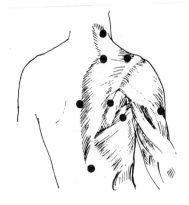

Fig. 16.15 Common stress points of the back and shoulder.

release and repeat the action. Apply cross-fiber friction for ten counts; release and repeat the movement. Do this sequence several times. Find the stress points around the shoulder blade and repeat the direct pressure for ten counts. Release and repeat the cross-fiber movements for ten counts. Finish the massage with compression done with the palm (Fig. 16.15).

Midback and Lower Back

Massage: Have the athlete lie on the table face down. Find the stress points in the muscular bands along each side of the spine. With your thumb, apply direct pressure for ten counts. Release and repeat the movement all the way down the back. Do the sequence down the back several times. Work with the client's breathing. Apply pressure on the exhale and release on the inhale. Apply cross-fiber friction with your thumb for ten counts. Release and repeat the movement moving an inch or so down the back. Use the palm of your hand to apply several compressions on the muscle. Use your thumb to apply cross-fiber friction on the outside of the muscle. Return to cross-fiber friction with your thumbs for ten counts. Release and repeat the movement. Do this sequence several times. Apply deep strokes with the thumbs from the top of the shoulders down to the tailbone, and then shake and vibrate the muscles back up to the shoulders. Apply compressions to the buttock with the heel of your hand, and finish by flushing out the area with effleurage.

Racquetball Shoulder

This is somewhat like tennis elbow but can be more severe. It affects the trapezius and deltoid muscles.

Massage: Begin with direct pressure on the stress points, holding for ten counts. Apply friction over the back, including the neck, for about twenty counts. Use compression movement on the shoulders. Release and repeat the movements. Massage the entire back from the waist upward over the shoulders. Massage over the deltoid muscle. Find the pressure points of the shoulders and apply deep compression for ten counts and release. Continue with cross-fiber friction for ten counts and release, and then finish with compression, using deep stroking to stretch the fibers. Shake the involved areas to release tension. Apply repeated pressure to the stress points once more, and then apply effleurage to the entire area.

Triceps Strain

This is a condition usually occurring when the muscle is overused and stressed.

Massage: Find the stress point. Use your thumb or fingertip to apply direct pressure for ten counts. Release and repeat the movements. Apply cross-fiber friction for ten counts. Release and repeat the movements. Do this sequence (gently) several times. Apply deep strokes from elbow to shoulder; then shake and flush out the area.

The Groin

The groin is more likely to be pulled in sports such as horseback riding, gymnastics, and soccer. This is a painful condition caused by overstretching of the gracilis and adductor muscle located high on the inner thigh.

Massage: Have the athlete lie on his or her side with the affected leg on the bottom. The knee of the top leg is bent and the bottom leg remains fairly straight. Stand behind the athlete and apply compressions to the inner thigh with the palm of the hand. Use your thumb to apply pressure and cross-fiber friction for 20 counts. Release and repeat the movement. This area will be quite tender, so it is necessary to be gentle. Find the spasm area, and apply compression with your fingertips. Release and repeat the movement.

The Chest and Abdomen

During some sports and especially weight-lifting, the pectorals and the intercostal muscles may be strained. There may be spasm, soreness, and tenderness (Fig. 16.16).

Massage: The athlete should lie on his or her back with the body relaxed. Apply circular compressions using the palm of your hand to the pectoral muscles, moving from the breastbone to collarbone across the chest and shoulders. Avoid doing movements over or near the nipples because this is a sensitive area. Follow compression movements with effleurage. Apply light percussion (hacking movements) with the little finger sides of your hand over the pectoral muscles. Finish with a few light strokes over the entire chest area.

The Abdomen

The rectus abdominis is often affected by sports that involve bending and twisting movements. Tension, soreness, and spasm may develop in the area around the navel. Keep in mind that the abdominal region of the body is sensitive to pressure. The athlete should lie on his or her back with knees slightly raised and feet flat on the table. Raising the knees helps to relax the abdominal area. Use gentle movements and direct pressure downward (never upward) from the waistline toward the pubic bone.

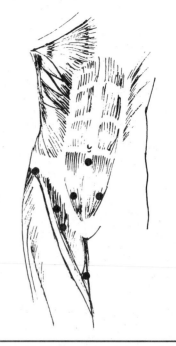

Fig. 16.16 Common stress points of the groin and abdomen.

STEP-BY-STEP PROCEDURE FOR ATHLETIC MASSAGE ▼

Preparation and draping for athletic massage is the same as for regular massage. The athlete lies face up on the table, and a slight amount of oil is applied to the part to be massaged first. Some therapists use no oil. The following routine may be varied as necessary or desirable.

Foot Massage

1. Grasp the foot so that your fingers are on the sole and your thumb is on top of the foot to hold it firmly.
2. Use deep strokes with the tips of your fingers from toes across the instep and to the heel and back again. Apply about ten strokes.
3. Hold the foot firmly around the toes while pressing the knuckles of the other hand into the ball of the foot, moving down to the instep and heel. Repeat the movements several times.
4. Apply compression with the tips of your thumbs over the sole of the foot, moving across and down the foot.
5. Rotate the ankle clockwise and counterclockwise.
6. Rotate each toe.
7. Use circular friction movements with the fingers and thumbs to massage tendons and ligaments and to massage over the foot and the ankle bone.
8. Repeat rotation and combine with flexing.

Lower Leg Massage

1. With the heel of your hand, apply deep compression movements from the outside of the knee to the ankle, concentrating on the muscle mass. This movement is done by making a dozen or so compressive movements to a pass and about three to five passes.
2. Finish this part of the massage by using the palm of your hand or fingers in circular friction movements across the front of the leg. Apply deep strokes from ankle to knee.

Thigh Massage

1. Use your palms to apply firm compression movements to the front of the leg, beginning with the knee. Make about five or six passes applying compression movements over the thigh from the hip area to the knee joint.
2. Apply circular friction to the knee joint.
3. Apply kneading movements, working from the knee to the groin and then down again.
4. Apply compression movements.
5. Apply percussion movements to the entire thigh area (use hacking and beating movements).
6. Finish with deep effleurage strokes and flexing of the knee and hip.

7. Bend the knee toward the chest and extend it several times. Rotate the femur in its socket, and then make circles with the knee while flexing it.
8. Massage the other foot and leg.

Arm Massage

1. Use the fingers, pad of your thumb, or the heel of your hand to apply compression to the entire length of the arm, from wrist to shoulder.
2. Apply circular friction to the back of the hand.
3. Use the tips of your fingers to apply friction to the palm of the hand and around the wrists.
4. Finish with deep effleurage and flexing of the elbow.
5. Shake the arm vigorously.
6. Massage the other arm.

Abdominal Massage

For massage of the abdomen, the athlete should raise his or her knees slightly, keeping the feet flat on the table. This tends to relax the abdominals.

1. Begin with kneading movements over the entire abdominal area, graduating from gentle to stronger movements.
2. Use the thumbs to apply direct pressure to stress areas along the pubic bone, pelvis, and ribs.

Chest Massage

1. Use the palm of your hand to apply circular compression to the pectoral muscles of the chest, over the breastbone, collarbone, and shoulders. Avoid any movement over the sensitive area of the nipples.
2. With the palm of your hand, apply circular friction movements over the rib cage.
3. Use the outer edge of your hands to apply percussion (hacking) movements to the pectorals. This should not be so brisk as to cause discomfort.

Back of the Leg Massage

1. The athlete turns over to a prone position. It is advisable to place a bolster or support under the ankles.
2. Use the palm of your hand to apply compression to the entire calf and posterior thigh.
3. Use kneading movement from the ankle, up the thigh, and over the buttock.
4. Use your fist or the heel of your hand to apply compressions down to the inner side of the leg to the knee, and then repeat

the movements to the middle and outside portions of the leg. Do three to six passes for each section.

5. Use the fist or palm to apply compression movements to the buttock. Begin with the gluteus maximus, and move upward to cover the entire buttock. The number of compressions depends on the size of the person being massaged. Generally, fifty compressions for each section will be sufficient.
6. Use your thumbs to apply direct pressure to stress points.
7. Apply percussion movements from the knee to the buttocks.
8. Finish the massage by bending the knee several times. Grasp the foot and bend the knee by pushing the foot toward the buttocks.

Back Massage

1. Use your palm to apply petrissage movements, beginning with the shoulder blades and covering the entire back to the knees. Make six or eight circles in the same place, and then move on to another area. Do three to four passes.
2. Apply friction to the muscles along both sides of the spine.
3. Apply direct compression (with palms) to the shoulders, about twenty to fifty compressions.
4. Use thumbs to apply pressure to stress points across shoulders, around the scapula, along spine above and below the iliac crest.
5. Apply cross-fiber friction to "tight" areas.
6. Apply deep compression to the buttock.
7. Use the thumbs or heel of the hand to apply gentle circular friction movements to the muscles along the spine.
8. Apply slow compression with the heel of the hand to the muscles along the sides of the spine, moving upward from the waistline to the neck.
9. Apply compression with the tips of your fingers to the entire upper back and across the shoulder blades to the base of the neck.
10. Apply kneading movements to the trapezius and base of the neck.
11. Apply percussion with your fist, using hacking and beating movements over the shoulders.
12. To finish the massage, do light percussion over the entire back.

Neck Massage

Have the athlete fold his or her hands palms down and rest the forehead on them.

1. Apply compression movements from the base of the neck to the base of the skull. Cover the entire area of the back of the neck.

2. Apply compression movements to shoulders with the palms of the hands.
3. Apply effleurage to the shoulders and neck. Revisit areas and repeat massage movements as necessary, especially in heavily used or tight areas of the body.

QUESTIONS FOR DISCUSSION AND REVIEW ▼

1. What is athletic massage?
2. In addition to thorough understanding of human anatomy and physiology, which four major body systems and their functions must the therapist know?
3. What is the overload principle?
4. What are negative effects of exercise?
5. What techniques are commonly used in athletic massage?
6. What is the primary goal of compression?
7. In athletic massage, what does the term *hyperemia* refer to?
8. In athletic massage, how is deep pressure used?
9. Who popularized the use of transverse friction massage for treating soft tissue lesions?
10. What is the objective of using cross-fiber friction in athletic massage?
11. What are the four basic applications for athletic massage?
12. What is the goal of each athletic massage application?
13. When is massage considered to be the most beneficial to the athlete?
14. What are stress points and where are they generally located?
15. Why must the therapist be sure to apply proper techniques at all times?
16. What is the best way to treat an athletic injury?
17. What are some beneficial advantages of rehabilitative massage?
18. How does massage therapy affect the healing time of injuries?
19. Who is qualified to give athletic massage to new or fresh injuries?
20. What is RICE?
21. How often should rehabilitative massage be administered?
22. Differentiate between acute and chronic injuries.
23. What massage techniques should be used at the site of acute muscle injuries?
24. Differentiate between a strain and a sprain.
25. When is athletic massage contraindicated?

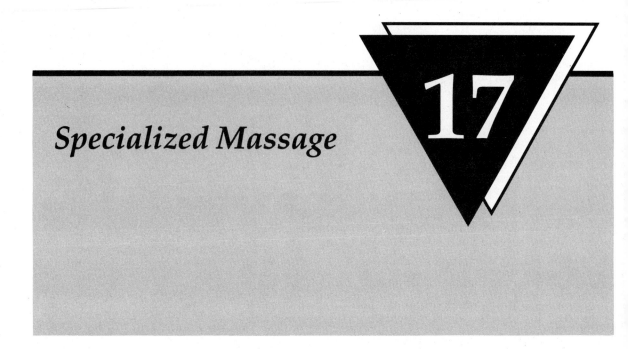

Specialized Massage

Learning Objectives

After you have mastered this chapter, you will be able to:

1. Explain the benefits of prenatal massage.
2. Explain contraindications for prenatal massage.
3. Explain the benefits of lymph massage.
4. Describe the basic functions of the lymphatic system.
5. Explain the purpose of structural integration.
6. Define a trigger point and describe its location.
7. Describe how to treat trigger points.
8. Describe techniques used in neuromuscular therapy.
9. Describe the techniques used in Muscle Energy Technique.
10. Define passive positioning and the bodywork styles that incorporate passive positioning.
11. Explain the basic philosophy of acupressure and acupuncture.
12. Describe shiatsu as related to pressure points of the body.
13. Define reflexology.

INTRODUCTION ▼

In recent years there has been a resurgence of interest in various massage therapies that relate to the maintenance of physical, mental, and emotional health. Many of these techniques are related to or are descendants of Swedish massage in that they encourage relaxation, increase the movement of body fluids, and soothe the nervous system. Others have origins in the far Eastern philosophies of Japan and China. Some touch techniques are referred to as bodywork.

It is not within the scope of this book to cover in detail every therapy style. However, serious students or practitioners are encouraged to continue their training by exploring various styles and sharpening their skills to better serve their clientele. Continuing education through advanced programs at schools or in workshops is necessary to stay current regarding new developments and techniques available to the massage professional. There is a wealth of reference material listed in this book's bibliography. The brief discussions in this chapter will acquaint the practitioner with the basic concepts of a variety of techniques.

PRENATAL MASSAGE ▼

In normal, healthy pregnancies, massage has proved to be beneficial to both mother and unborn child. Properly applied massage can aid relaxation, benefit circulation, and soothe nerves. Prenatal massage is applied like any regular massage except for the following considerations:

Positioning: The client may take any of several positions depending on which is more comfortable. If the client takes a supine position, arrange pillows under her back to support her in a semi-reclining position. Also place a pillow or a small bolster (six or eight inches) under the bend of her knees to take the strain off her abdominal muscles. During the second half of the pregnancy, use the supine position with great caution because in this position the weight of the fetus may press on the descending aorta and impede the flow of blood to the placenta.

The mother may prefer lying on her side, especially during the final months of pregnancy. Use plenty of pillows to comfortably support the head, womb, and between the knees. Ask the client to indicate if at anytime during the treatment she becomes uncomfortable.

During the first two to three months of pregnancy, the prone position may be used. However, as the abdomen becomes larger, pillows placed underneath the client's head, chest, abdomen, and legs will add to her comfort. During the second and third trimester, a preg-pillow can be used for a safe and comfortable prone position.

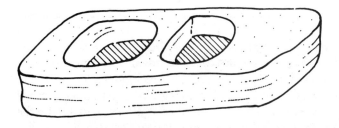

Fig. 17.1 A preg-pillow is a special supporting cushion with cutouts for the womb and breasts that can be used to allow even a full-term mother to lie safely and comfortably in the prone position.

A preg-pillow is a cushion, six to eight inches thick, with space cut out for the enlarged abdomen and breasts. There are commercially available cushions and bolsters specifically designed for pre-natal massage that safely and comfortably support the mother in side lying and prone positions (Fig. 17.1).

Body Areas Subject to Discomfort

The lower back is a common area of strain during pregnancy due to the extra weight of the growing fetus. Lateral and abdominal muscles are also under strain from carrying the extra weight and from stretching to accommodate the growing fetus. Effleurage and light petrissage are soothing and will relieve tension in the muscles. The main aim of prenatal massage is to help the expectant mother to relax.

Strokes on and around the abdomen should be done in a clockwise manner, the same as for any abdominal massage. However, the strokes must be light, using very gentle pressure. Women often comment on how pleasant and soothing they find massage to be during pregnancy because of its calming and reassuring effects.

Plan on a relatively short massage. Most pregnant women will not remain comfortable lying down for more than forty-five or fifty minutes.

Contraindications for Prenatal Massage

Before beginning a prenatal massage, it is important to ask the expectant mother if there is any reason why massage would not be advisable. High blood pressure and excess edema are contra-indications and should be referred to a physician.

During pregnancy, do not give massages when contraindications are present. Problems can occur during pregnancy, and the expectant mother should be under her physician's care regarding diet, exercise, and massage. However, many physicians recommend massage for its therapeutic effects.

Preeclampsia, a type of toxemia, is a condition sometimes occurring in the latter half of pregnancy and is characterized by high blood pressure, edema (swelling of hands, feet, and face), and sodium retention. Indications of this condition include excessive weight gain or protein in the urine. The expectant mother may suffer headaches and dizziness and, in serious cases, convulsions. When toxemia is suspected, the expectant mother should see her physician without delay.

If edema is minimal, it is acceptable to massage (effleurage) the legs and arms. If the edema is serious, massage should not be done and the client should be referred to her physician.

Varicose veins are often a problem during pregnancy due to the effects of progesterone on the blood vessels and to the increased pressure on the main blood vessels that return blood from the legs. Light effleurage can be done around, but not on, affected areas.

MASSAGE DURING LABOR ▼

A physician may recommend light effleurage on the patient's abdomen and upper legs as a means of obtaining relief between contractions. Lower back pains can also be relieved by the application of firm continuous counterpressure. During a contraction, counterpressure can be applied to both sides of the spine in the area of the sacrum.

MASSAGE FOLLOWING BIRTH ▼

Often a mother will request massage throughout her pregnancy and after the child is born. Massage helps to relieve neck, shoulder, and lower back discomfort and is an aid in the relief of tension. When combined with proper exercise and diet, massage will be of value in regaining normal weight and firming slack muscles.

LYMPH MASSAGE ▼

Lymph or lymphatic massage is a descendant of Swedish massage. Dr. Emil Vodder, Ph.D, of Copenhagen, Denmark, pioneered the practice of manual lymph drainage massage in the 1930s. He is credited with having discovered the benefits of lymphatic massage and for the development of massage techniques widely used today. Dr. Vodder's method of manual lymph drainage massages uses light, rhythmical, spiral-like movements to accelerate the movement of lymphatic fluids in the body.

Before beginning the study of lymph massage, the practitioner or student must have a thorough knowledge of anatomy, particularly of the lymphatic system. Lymph drainage massage requires careful training procedures; therefore the student must be guided by the instructor at all times.

The following overview will be helpful to understanding the basic functions of the lymphatic system and the principles of the lymph massage.

The Lymphatic System

The lymphatic system is a system of vessels and nodes supplementary to the blood vascular system. The spleen, tonsils, and thymus are related organs. Lymph capillaries are small, thin-walled tubes that collect lymph from interstitial fluid in the tissues and join to form other lymphatic vessels. In structure the larger vessels are like veins but have thinner walls and more numerous valves. The larger vessels converge to form the right lymphatic duct, which carries the lymph from the right arm, the right side of the thorax, the right side of the head and neck, and empties into the right brachiocephalic vein. The thoracic duct collects lymph from the rest of the body and empties into the left brachiocephalic vein.

Lymph is interstitial fluid that is absorbed into the lymphatic system. Interstitial fluid is derived from blood plasma and continuously bathes the cells and connective tissues. It is through this fluid that tissues receive their nourishment and building materials. Without it, tissues would soon dry out and degenerate. Ninety percent of this fluid, containing dissolved gasses, waste products of metabolism, and water is reabsorbed into the blood vessels. The other 10 percent, containing excess water, cellular debris, bacteria, viruses and other inorganic materials, is absorbed into the lymphatic system.

Lymph circulation is vital to life; When it slows down, waste products can accumulate and stagnate. This affects normal metabolism and produces a feeling of fatigue. The movement of lymph is maintained by the difference in the pressure within the lymphatic system, by normal respiration, and by muscular movements of the body in general.

Specialized lymph vessels in the walls of the small intestine called lacteals carry away fat that is absorbed in the digestive tract.

The immune system, of which the lymphatic system is an important part, produces lymphocytes and other cells in response to the presence of inflammation, antigens, bacteria, viruses, and other cellular debris in the body. A lymphocyte, or leukocyte, is a white blood corpuscle found in the lymphatic tissue, blood, and lymph. Lymphocytes are active in the immune responses of the body and play a major role in the healing of wounds and fighting of infections. They penetrate all tissues and are abundant in lymph tissue, blood, bone barrow, mucous membranes, connective tissue, skin, and all body organs.

Lymph Nodes

Lymph nodes, are small masses of lymphatic tissue. They vary in size and shape but are usually less than one inch (2.5 cm) in length.

They are often bead-like or bean-shaped compact structures that lie in groups along the course of lymphatic vessels. When inflamed and swollen, lymph nodes can be felt beneath the skin. The chief function of lymph nodes is to produce lymphocytes and serve as a filtering system.

Lymph enters the lymph nodes by way of the afferent (inward) lymph vessels. Contaminants that may be harmful if left to circulate freely through the vascular system are carried by the lymph and deposited in the nodes. Here, antigens, damaged cells, and toxins are acted on, broken down, or devoured by the lymphocytes. They are turned into harmless substances and passed out of the lymph nodes through efferent (outward) vessels. Eventually they pass through the lymph ducts and back into the blood system to be eliminated.

Lymph nodes are usually distributed in groups. Regional lymph nodes include:

- Submaxillary nodes, located beneath the mandible
- Pre-auricular nodes, located in front of the ear
- Post-auricular nodes, located behind the ear in the region of the mastoid process
- Occipital nodes, located at the base of the skull
- Superficial cervical nodes, located at the side of and over the sternocleido mastoid muscle
- Deep cervical nodes, located along the carotid artery and internal jugular vein
- Axillary nodes are located in the armpit. Constituting the main group of the upper extremity, axillary nodes receive lymph from vessels that drain the wall of the thorax, mammary glands, and upper wall of the abdomen.
- Supratrochlear nodes, located in the elbows
- Inguinal nodes, located in the groin and constituting the most important group of the lower extremity, receive lymph from the leg, external genitalia, and lower abdominal wall.
- Popliteal nodes, located behind the knee
- Abdominal and pelvic cavities also contain numerous lymph nodes.

Influence of Massage on Body Fluids

It is important to understand the influence of massage on circulation of fluids in the human body. Both the lymphatic and venous circulation are accelerated by massage movements. These movements are applied from the extremities toward the heart, stimulating lymphatic circulation. The lymph capillaries, which end in the tissues, absorb lymph and assist its flow into the lymphatic vessels. While blood is being returned to the heart by way of the veins, the lymphatics are draining the tissues of excess and contaminated interstitial fluid. Lymph massage stimulates the activity of the lymph centers, increases the production of lymphocytes and improves body metabolism. The natural movements of the body such as walking, breathing, and exercising aid this process. Skillfully applied massage more fully augments the circulation of lymph.

Correct lymph massage accelerates the flow of lymph, helping to rid the body of toxins and waste materials. Lymph drainage massage promotes balance of the body's internal chemistry, purifies and regenerates tissues, helps to normalize the functions of organs, and enhances the function of the immune system.

Techniques of Lymph Massage

The techniques of lymph massage are based on alternate pressure and release movements and light stroking. Light compression movements create a pumping action that encourages the movement of lymph through the lymph vessels. Decreased pressure opens lymph valves, while increased pressure closes them. Light stroking promotes the movement of superficial lymph, while deeper stroking moves lymph through the deeper channels.

Lymphatic compression massage is a light pumping motion done with the palm of the hand pressing into the tissue and directed toward the center of the body. Attention should be paid to muscle tissue, with concentration on the proximal areas of the limb where there is a higher concentration of lymph tissue. Successful lymph drainage massage depends on the expertise of the practitioner. He or she must consider the effects to be achieved by various movements. For example, body fluids can be displaced intravascularly (within vessels) or extravascularly (in the interstitial spaces). This displacement of fluid is achieved by manual strokes.

Lymph movement is also increased in the muscles and organs by stimulation of neurolymphatic reflexes located primarily on the front and back of the trunk and on the medial and lateral aspects of the thigh. Affected points may be massaged with strong, deep friction massage for twenty to thirty seconds. These points may be quite tender and more evident on the front of the body (Fig. 17.2).

Before attempting lymph massage, the practitioner should be thoroughly familiar with the functions of the lymphatic system. Lymph massage is done to encourage, but not force, the movement of lymph through the lymphatic system. The procedure begins at the junction of the right thoracic lymph duct and vein adjacent to the junction of the jugular veins, and just behind the clavicle near its articulation to the sternum. This is where the lymph system dumps into the venous blood.

The practitioner uses a pumping action in this area of the neck first on one side and then on the other side. Pressure should not be applied to both sides at once because the junction of the lymphatic ducts and the brachiocephalic vein are very near the jugular vein and the junction of the carotid artery and the aorta. Simultaneous stimulation and/or pressure to both sides could adversely affect

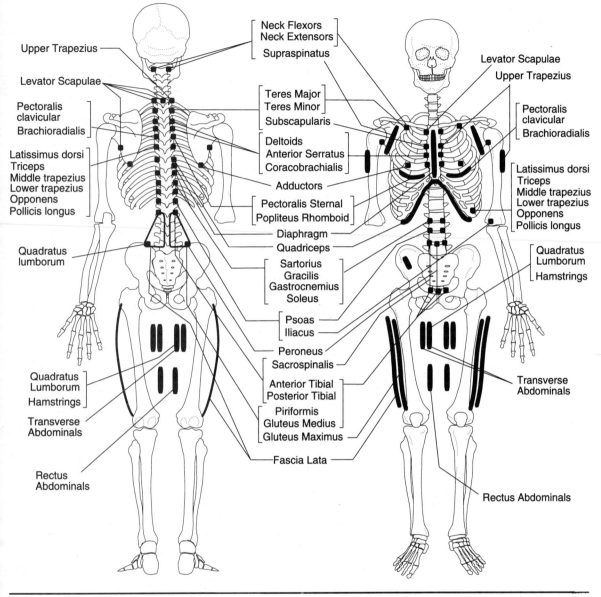

Fig. 17.2 Neurolymphatic reflex areas.

the blood flow to the brain. The practitioner may want to do one side of the lymph drainage area before proceeding to the other. For example, begin the massage with the right lymphatic duct and the part of the body drained by it, and then proceed to the thoracic duct and the rest of the body.

Procedure for a Lymph Massage

The following procedure should be done only under the supervision of an instructor.

1. **Base of neck:** Begin with the right side of the neck just superior to the clavicle. Apply light compression movements toward the clavicular-sternal sinus, and then proceed up the side of the neck to include the entire area from the occiput to the submandibular area and to the cervical spinous process with light compression. Continue to include the sternocleidomastoid muscle. Finish with superficial effleurage in a downward direction on the entire side of the head and neck.

2. **Pectoral and axillary area:** Right side compressions and strokes begin along the sternal and clavicular borders and are directed toward the center of the body, continuing down and out to cover the entire chest area. If the client is a woman, avoid pressure directly on the mammary glands or breast tissue. Finish with light brushing and superficial effleurage directed from the clavicle and sternum toward the axillary area.

3. **Right arm:** Support the arm abducted and elevated to expose the underside of the arm and axillary area. Do compression movements to the entire arm beginning in the axillary area (proceeding distally) while directing the compression toward the bone and up the arm toward the shoulder. Finish with light brushing and superficial effleurage to encourage lymph movement toward the axillary area.

4. **Axillary area:** Abduct and extend the arm to expose the axillary area. Apply gentle compressions directed toward the axillary fold. Finish with light effleurage directed toward the axillary from all directions.

   Left side: Proceed with steps 1 through 4 on the left side of the body.

5. **Abdomen:** The lymph from the abdomen, lower extremities, and the digestive system empties into the cisterna chyli located at the inferior end of the thoracic duct, at a level just inferior to the umbilicus (the navel). Direct all compression movements toward this area. Begin compressions on the upper abdomen near the costal border, directing the compression upward and toward the center while proceeding down the inguinal crease in the groin area. Movements are more effective if the knees are elevated so the feet remain flat on the table. Finish with effleurage. Repeat the movements on the other side of the abdomen.

6. **Legs:** Begin in the groin area of the right leg and continue light compression movements on down the medial aspect of the leg. Direct force of the compressions into the leg and upward. Pay special attention to the medial portion of the thigh. Finish the massage with light brushing and superficial effleurage, continuing up to the abdomen. Repeat the massage on the left leg.

7. **Back of legs:** The client should assume a prone position. Begin in the gluteal area around the iliac crest, and apply compression movements covering the entire buttock and posterior leg, proceeding from the hip to the heel. Use light pressure in the popliteal space behind the knee. Finish the massage with light brushing and superficial effleurage. Do the other leg and buttock.

8. **Back:** In lymph massage little effect is achieved over a large portion of the back. However, there are neurolymphatic reflexes along both sides of the spine that may be stimulated with deep friction. Continue with compression massage in the area of the latissimus dorsi, teres, and upper trapezius area. Deep effleurage over the entire back concludes the massage.

Lymphatic massage is very stimulating and invigorating, so the client should be encouraged to rest for a few minutes before getting off the massage table.

Lymphatic Pump Manipulation

The lymphatic pump manipulation enhances the flow of lymph through the entire system and may be done in conjunction with a lymph drainage massage at the beginning or end of the massage or as a separate manipulation (Fig. 17.3).

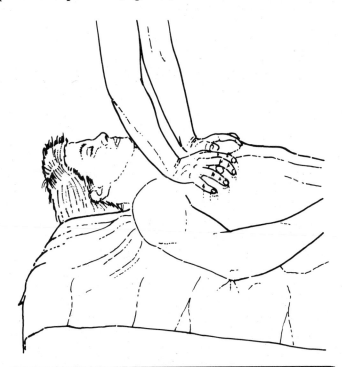

Fig. 17.3 Positioning for the application of the lymphatic pump maneuver.

Procedure

The client lies supine. The practitioner stands at the head of the massage table and places his or her hands to cover as much of the client's rib cage as possible. This enables the practitioner to press his or her weight into the client's ribs. The practitioner encourages the client to breathe deeply for five or more deep breaths, forcing the ribs up under the pressure of the practitioner's hands. As the client breathes deeply, the practitioner begins to bounce at the rate of about 150 bounces per minute using the weight of his or her upper body. Pressure should be sufficient to force complete expulsion of the breath but not so heavy as to prevent inhalation. The client should lie quietly for a few minutes following this procedure.

This process is contraindicated for persons with high blood pressure, heart condition, osteoporosis, or broken or cracked ribs.

▼ DEEP TISSUE MASSAGE

The term **deep tissue massage** refers to various regimens or massage styles that are directed toward the deeper tissue structures of the muscle and fascia. Some of the techniques focus just on the physiological release of tension or bonds in the tissues, while others use bodywork in conjunction with or as a means of psychological release. In most deep tissue massage techniques the aim is to affect the various layers of fascia that support muscle tissues and loosen bonds between the layers of connective tissues. Some deep tissue massage techniques are named after the person who developed or specialized them, such as Rolfing, after Ida Rolf; Trager after Milton Trager; Hellerwork after Joseph Heller; and Feldenkrais after Moshe Feldenkrais. The following are brief explanations of some of these techniques.

Structural Integration

As the name implies, structural integration attempts to bring the physical structure of the body into alignment around a central axis. This is done by manipulating the fascia of the structural muscles. After structural integration sessions, both physical and psychological balance are often experienced by the client.

Throughout life, traumas, both physical and emotional, may cause a reduction of movement that results in a shortening or binding together of the connective tissue surrounding muscles. Restriction may affect fibers, bundles, and whole muscles. This condition can also come about as a result of habitual postures while sitting, walking, and standing. Poor posture can be learned by imitating parents, from environmental factors, or as a reaction to some forms of punishment and emotionally charged situations. Structural integration can be beneficial when given by a practitioner who knows the methods and understands how to achieve the desired results.

Rolfing

Rolfing, a method of structural integration, is a deep connective tissue massage originated by Dr. Ida Rolf, a biochemist and massage practitioner. Dr. Rolf discovered that in a normal, healthy body the spine and body segments are correctly aligned, allowing the organs to function properly. However, during childhood and in early adult formative years, poor posture habits are often formed, throwing the body off center or out of its normal, healthy alignment. This in turn causes structural problems. Incorrect body alignment can also cause tension in muscles and connective tissues that may interfere with normal functioning of internal organs. Dr. Rolf originated a series of treatments called Rolfing to bring the body into proper structural alignment.

The goal of Rolfing treatments is to reshape the body's physical posture and to realign the muscular and connective tissue. The benefits of Rolfing also include increased suppleness of the muscles, improved appearance, and a renewed sense of well-being.

Rolfing techniques involve the use of heavy pressure applied carefully to the client's body with the fingers, a knuckle, a fist, or sometimes an elbow. Rolfing is usually done in a series of ten treatments of one-hour duration each. During this time, the practitioner (Rolfer) works on various portions of the body.

Contraindications for Rolfing are the same as for any other type of massage. When in doubt about the use of this type of treatment, the client's physician should be consulted. The practitioner who wishes to pursue Rolfing techniques should study under the supervision of a qualified instructor.

NEUROPHYSIOLOGICAL THERAPIES

Several therapy systems are emerging that are directed toward neurophysiological processes that effect the musculo-skeletal system. These systems recognize the importance of neurological feedback between the central nervous system and the musculo-skeletal system in maintaining proper tone and function. Alterations or disturbances in the neuromuscular relationship often result in dysfunction and pain. Neurophysiological therapies utilize methods of assessing tissues and delivering soft tissue manipulative techniques to normalize the tissues and reprogram the neurological loop to reduce pain and improve function. These neurophysiological therapies include trigger-point therapy, neuromuscular therapy, and passive positioning therapies.

TRIGGER-POINT THERAPY

A trigger point is a hyperirritable spot that is painful when compressed. Trigger points are so called because stimulating the point triggers a painful response. Dr. Janet Travell, author of *Myofascial Pain and Dysfunction,* classifies trigger points as latent and active. Active trigger points cause the client pain. When stimulated, active trigger points refer pain and tenderness to another area of the body that is usually not associated by nerve or dermatomal segment. The pattern of referred pain is generally characteristic of a specific point. Latent trigger points only exhibit pain when compressed, do not refer pain, and may or may not radiate pain around the point. Trigger points, whether latent or active, result in dysfunction.

Trigger points are associated with dysfunctional neurological reflex circuits. A **physiopathological reflex arc** is a self-perpetuating neurological phenomenon that affects not only the muscle where the trigger point is located but also will have referred effects in tissues supplied by associated nerves of both the peripheral and autonomic nervous system. In other words, a trigger point is more than a tender nodule. A trigger point is an indication of physiological dysfunction. The trigger point may be reflexively related to:

- Contracture in the muscle
- Increased muscle tonus
- Constriction and hypersensitivity in the skin in local or referred areas
- Increased pressure in the joints associated with the muscle
- Decreased activity in visceral organs associated through depressed autonomic nerve activity
- Constriction in local circulation resulting from hypertonus and constriction in the muscle
- Vasoconstriction in referred areas from effects in the autonomic nervous system
- Development of secondary and associated trigger points due to compensating from the effects of the primary trigger point.

Research and practice indicates that deactivating the trigger point reflexively improves the function of the associated referred phenomena. When an active trigger point is successfully quieted, the referred pain and dysfunction will decrease.

A myofascial trigger point is found in muscle tissue or its associated fascia. It is located in a taut band of muscle fibers. Normal muscles do not contain taut bands of muscle fibers and do not contain trigger points. Taut bands in muscle are responsible for muscle shortening and the resultant impaired mobility and pain. The taut band is located by stroking across the muscle. A palpable band will be apparent to the sensitive fingers. Palpating the full length of the band will locate one or more highly sensitive points. Trigger points may be found in the belly of the muscle, at the musculo-tendinous junction, or at the tendinoperiosteal junction (Fig. 17.4a to c).

Locating and deactivating trigger points are valuable for reducing pain and improving function in the location of the trigger point and in the referral areas. Procedures for deactivating trigger points

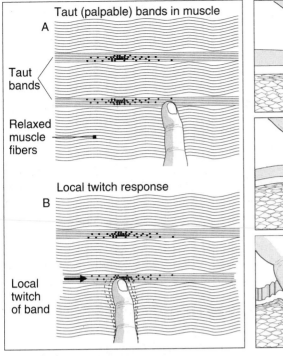

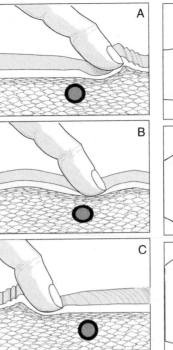

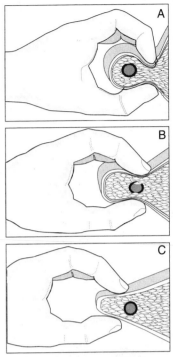

Fig. 17.4a Taut bands, myofascial trigger points, and a local twitch response seen in longitudinal view of the muscle. (a) Palpation of a taut band (straight lines) among normally slack, relaxed muscle fibers (wavy lines). The density of stippling corresponds to the degree of tenderness of the taut band pressure. The trigger point is the most tender spot in the band. (b) Rolling the band quickly under the fingertip (snapping palpation) at the trigger point often produces a local twitch response that is most clearly seen toward the end of the muscle, close to its attachment.

Fig. 17.4b Flat palpation of a taut band and its trigger point. Flat palpation is used for muscles that are accessible only from one direction, such as infraspinatus. (a) Skin pushed to one side to begin palpation. (b) Fingertip slid across muscle fibers to feel the cord-like texture of the taut band rolling beneath it. (c) Skin pushed to other side at completion of snapping palpation.

Fig. 17.4c Pincer palpation of a taut band at a trigger point. Pincer palpation is used for muscles that can be picked up between the digits, such as the sternocleidomastoid, pectoralis major, and latissimus dorsi. (a) Muscle fibers surrounded by the thumb and fingers in a pincer grip. (b) Hardness of a taut band felt clearly as it is rolled between the digits. The change in the angle of the distal phalanges produces a rocking motion that improves discrimination of the fine detail. (c) Edge of the taut band sharply defined, as it escapes from between the fingertips, often with a local twitch response.
(Courtesy Janet G. Travell, *Myofascial Pain and Dysfunction, The Trigger Point Manual.* Baltimore: Williams and Wilkins, 1983.)

include injections, stretch and spray technique, active stretching and ischemic compression. Injections using saline solution or procaine are beyond the scope of the massage therapist. Stretch and spray techniques are very effective however the sprays are either very volatile or contain fluorocarbons and are not recommended by this author.

Ischemic compression and stretching are the methods of choice for the massage therapist when working with trigger points. Ischemic compression involves digital pressure directly into the trigger point. The pressure must be deep enough and held long enough to deactivate the trigger point. Too much pressure will cause the client to react by tightening muscles in a protective response that defeats the purpose of the treatment. Pressure on a trigger point will cause pain. The deeper the pressure, the more intense the pain. The amount of pressure must be regulated to stay within the tolerance of the individual client. In other words, on a pain scale from 1 to 10, where 0 is no pain and 10 is excruciating, the target level is 5 or 6. Pressure is increased until the client begins to elicit a pain reaction. As the pressure is maintained, the pain intensity usually decreases. As this happens, the pressure can be increased to maintain the level of intensity. When the point has been inactivated, the pain level will reduce to an intensity rating of 1 or 2.

Following the inactivation of the trigger point, the associated muscle should be stretched to return to its normal functioning length.

Other methods of treating hypersensitive or trigger points will be discussed in the following sections on neuromuscular therapy and passive positioning.

▼ NEUROMUSCULAR THERAPY

Neuromuscular Therapy (NMT) was originally developed in the 1930s by Stanley Leif in England. Dr. Stanley Leif was born in Latvia, one of the Baltic States, and was raised in South Africa. He received training as a chiropractor and naturopath in the United States before the First World War. He established a healing resort in England and there, along with a cousin, Boris Chaitow, developed the system of soft tissue manipulation called neuromuscular therapy. More recently in the United States, Paul St. John has popularized and advanced a method of neuromuscular therapy that is taught through a series of seminars.

The body continuously endures stresses from trauma, improper body mechanics, poor posture, as well as tensions of a psychological or emotional nature. Regardless of the nature of the stress, be it mechanical, postural, or emotional, the adaptive tendencies of the body will attempt to compensate for the stress by producing neuromuscular changes. Many of the changes result in reduced mobility, pain, fatigue, and depression. Neuro-muscular dysfunctions become apparent in the soft tissues of the musculo-skeletal system as contractures, hypersensitive areas and tissue restriction. Neuromuscular dysfunction is self-perpetuating. When an area of the body is restricted from pain or mobility impairments, other areas of the body compensate, resulting in further physiological dysfunction.

NMT identifies soft tissue abnormalities and at the same time manipulates the soft tissue to normalize its function. In so doing, the perpetuating cycle is broken, much of the referred pathologic activity is reversed, and overall function is improved.

NMT depends on anatomical knowledge and palpatory skills to assess the tissue condition and treat neuromuscular lesions. Careful and systematic examination of the muscle and associated soft tissue identifies abnormal signs, including:

- Postural and biomechanical deviation
- Congestion in the tissues
- Contracted tissue or taut, fibrous bands
- Nodules or lumps
- Trigger points
- Restrictions between the skin and underlying tissues
- Variations in temperature (warmer or cooler than surrounding tissues)
- Swelling or edema
- General tenderness.

Neuromuscular lesions are always hypersensitive to pressure and often associated with trigger points. NMT recognizes the importance of trigger points and their relation to local and referred dysfunction and pain. Besides trigger points, NMT also takes into account other natural and physiologic laws that account for hypersensitive or painful spots on the body. For example, acupuncture points and neurolymphatic reflexes not associated with trigger points are often tender. Tenderness usually means some degree of dysfunction in the associated tissues or organs. General NMT treatment often stimulates the reflex improvement of the associated or referred function.

NMT treatment involves assessment and soft tissue manipulation. Postural assessment is important to determine any postural distortion. Postural distortion indicates an imbalance in the tone of structural muscles and is an indicator of chronic stress patterns. Palpating the tissues with initial light strokes and progressively deeper strokes reveals areas of tension, contracted tissue, and hypersensitivity.

Treatment manipulations are similar to the gliding and pressure techniques used to palpate and assess the tissue. Many NMT treatment techniques are incorporated from other modalities. They include but are not limited to:

- **Gliding:** The primary technique of NMT generally uses the thumb to move across, along, and through the tissues. Gliding strokes are applied to the tissue in one direction at a time using varying amounts of pressure. Light pressure assesses the superficial tissues and stimulates circulation of lymph and blood. Deeper stroking assesses deeper structures and stretches the fascia, releasing fibrotic adhesions.
- **Ischemic compression:** When painful spots and trigger points are located, pressure is held directly on these points. The depth of the pressure is determined by the tolerance of the client. The pressure

should be deep enough to illicit a mild amount of discomfort in the client. Pressure that is too deep causes the client to tense up and is counterproductive. Pressure that is too light is usually ineffective. Duration of the pressure, according to St. John, is from eight to twelve seconds and is repeated.

- **Skin rolling:** When there is tightness between the skin and the underlying tissues, the skin is picked up and rolled between the thumb and fingers of both hands in several directions across the area. This tends to loosen the superficial fascia and improve nerve and fluid circulation to the underlying structures.

- **Stretching:** After hypersensitive spots have been quieted and trigger points inactivated, the involved muscle and connective tissue must be stretched to achieve its normal resting length. This is accomplished with passive and active stretching. Slow, sustained passive stretching is encouraged to regain and maintain length of the connective and muscle tissues. Active stretching is valuable in overcoming contractures and neuromuscular programming that restricts mobility. Active stretching, also known as Muscle Energy Technique (MET), is discussed in the following section.

To maintain improvements achieved with NMT, the stresses that precipitated the soft tissue dysfunctions must be addressed and, if possible, eliminated. It is also helpful to monitor the areas of dysfunction with follow-up NMT sessions and incorporate a program of regular exercise to improve strength, endurance, posture, and stamina.

MUSCLE ENERGY TECHNIQUE

Muscle Energy Technique (MET), sometimes known as PNF stretching, utilizes neurophysiological muscle reflexes to improve functional mobility of the joints. By employing active joint movements, muscle activity that restricts movement is inhibited, allowing for better mobility. MET uses active muscle contraction followed by relaxation and subsequent passive stretching to increase range of motion of the related joints.

There are two basic inhibitory reflexes produced during MET manipulations:

- **Post-isometric relaxation:** Following an isometric contraction, there is a brief period of relaxation during which impulses to the muscle are inhibited.

- **Reciprocal inhibition**: When a muscle acting on a joint is contracted, the muscle responsible for the opposite action on that joint is inhibited.

MET involves the contraction of a muscle by the client against the resistance provided by a therapist. The direction of the contraction and the position of the muscle and the limb previous to the contraction are determined by the condition and movement restrictions of the joint and target muscle or muscle groups. Range of motion and palpation assessment techniques are used to determine the nature of the restriction and the direction of maximum limitation. Often the limitation is due to hypertonic muscles that are shortened and incapable of attaining their normal resting length. These situations respond well to MET.

There are three main variations of muscle energy technique that are effective in lengthening tense and shortened muscles:
- Contract relax or hold relax
- Antagonist contract
- Contract-relax-contract the opposite.

Contract Relax

The **contract-relax** technique incorporates the **post-isometric relaxation** theory that as soon as a strong muscle contraction releases, the muscle is inhibited and relaxes.

To perform the contract-relax technique:
1. Position the limb so that the target muscle is in a lengthened but comfortable position. This can be done by moving the limb to the point of resistance or pain and then backing off slightly.
2. Support the limb in that position securely and have the client contract the target muscle isometrically against the resistance for five to ten seconds. It is not necessary for the client to perform a maximal contraction. A contraction of 30 to 50 percent is adequate for this procedure. The contraction should not cause acute pain. If the contraction is painful, try the antagonist-contraction procedure discussed next.
3. Instruct the client to relax the muscle.
4. As soon as the client relaxes, move the limb farther into the stretch until resistance is encountered.
5. Back off of the resistance slightly and repeat the procedure. The procedure may be repeated three or five times.

Antagonist Contraction

Antagonist contraction takes advantage of a physiological process known as **reciprocal inhibition.** When a muscle acting on a joint contracts, the muscle that causes the opposite action is reflexively inhibited. To perform the antagonist contraction technique:
1. Position the limb so that the target muscle is in a lengthened but comfortable position. This can be done by moving the limb to the point of resistance or pain and then backing off slightly.
2. Support the limb securely in that position and instruct the client to attempt to continue the movement. Resist the movement for a couple of seconds and then allow the movement to continue slowly. The contraction should not cause acute pain. If there is acute pain on both contract-relax and

antagonist-contract techniques, pathologies may be present that contraindicate MET.

3. After about ten seconds, instruct the client to relax.
4. When the client relaxes, gently resume the stretch until resistance is encountered.
5. Back off of the resistance slightly and repeat the procedure. The procedure may be repeated three to five times.

Contract-Relax-Contract the Opposite

This technique, sometimes called Contract-Relax-Antagonist-Contract (CRAC), essentially combines the two previous techniques. To perform Contract-relax-contract the opposite technique:

1. Position the limb so that the target muscle is in a lengthened but comfortable position. This can be done by moving the limb to the point of resistance or pain and then backing off slightly.
2. Support the limb in that position securely and have the client contract the target muscle isometrically against the resistance for five to ten seconds.
3. Instruct the client to relax the muscle and then contract the muscle opposite the tight muscle (the antagonist). In so doing the client actively moves the limb in the direction of the intended stretch. The therapist may or may not assist in the final stretch.
4. After a short rest, repeat the procedure.

A number of factors determine the effectiveness of MET. It is essential to identify the contractile tissue involved in the movement limitation and direct the resistance to the contraction directly toward or away from those restrictions. Generally, pathological changes to structures of the joint other than contractile tissues will not respond to MET. The success of MET is dependent on the skill of the therapist in:

• Assessing the muscles involved
• Determining the direction of maximum limitation
• Determining when the joint movement is approaching its limitation
• Choosing a post-isometric relaxation or reciprocal inhibition technique
• Instructing the client in the direction, duration and intensity of the contraction.

MET is a valuable tool when addressing soft tissue conditions that involve tense or shortened muscles. Muscle spasms are effectively quieted. Joint mobility can be improved and lengthened or weak antagonistic muscles can be toned.

MET for Improving Strength or Reducing Fibrosis

There are two other variations of MET that are valuable for toning weak muscles or reducing fibrosis in the muscle fascia.

To improve tone or strengthen a weakened muscle, the client is instructed to move the limb through the full available range of motion as the therapist provides resistance directed against the target muscle. For maximum effect movement through the full range of motion should take about three to four seconds. During the first repetition, the client uses approximately 20 percent effort. On subsequent repetitions the resistance is increased until maximum resistance is achieved. The resistance is continuous during concentric and eccentric contractions. That is, the therapist provides resistance while the client shortens the target muscle and as the client lengthens the muscle. Rapid gains in strength are experienced with this type of exercise. The use of this technique may be limited depending on the strength of the therapist relative to the strength of the target muscle. The therapist may not be able to provide enough resistance for large muscles or muscle groups such as the hip flexors. The therapist must be aware of positioning and body mechanics to avoid injury to self, or the client.

Fibrosis in the muscle fascia may be the result of trauma, inflammation, strain, or aging. Fibrosis causes contractures and loss of mobility. A MET manipulation that may be effective in reducing fibrosis involves a resistance that overpowers a muscle contraction. As the client contracts the target muscle, the therapist provides a resistance greater than the force of the contraction and forces the muscle to lengthen. Fibrotic muscle may be quite painful when stretched. When using this technique, a maximum contraction is most effective, but the client must be instructed to contract the muscle to the extent that is within the comfort level. The therapist must not use ballistic movements against the contractions. The resistance must be steady and forceful enough to overcome the client effort.

Extreme caution must be used by the therapist to avoid further injury to the muscle tissue.

PASSIVE POSITIONING TECHNIQUES

Passive positioning techniques are perhaps the gentlest of soft tissue manipulations when addressing mobility restrictions due to pain and soft tissue dysfunction. As the name implies, passive positioning involves the gentle, passive movement of a joint into a position of maximum comfort, holding it there for an appropriate time and then very slowly returning it to its normal resting position.

Three bodywork systems that incorporate this technique are strain-counterstrain, orthobionomy and structural muscular balancing. Although each system utilizes passive positioning, each determines the appropriate position for maximum release in a different manner and will be discussed individually.

Strain-Counterstrain

The strain-counterstrain (tender point) technique was developed by Lawrence Jones, D.C. Dr. Jones happened upon the basis of the technique by accident when a patient came into his office in a great deal of pain. At the time Dr. Jones was very busy and was not able to treat the patient immediately. He instructed his assistant to take the person into the next room, lay him down, and make him as comfortable as possible. The assistant did as instructed. The patient lay down, and using various cushions and pillows the assistant positioned the patient's body so that he was virtually out of pain and then left him there until the doctor was able to see him. When the doctor finally came in, he carefully removed the pillows and gently positioned the client flat on the table and asked where the pain was. It was then that the patient realized the pain had disappeared.

Dr. Jones was able to produce similar results with other patients by positioning and supporting them in pain-free comfortable positions. Through his own research he developed the technique he calls strain-counterstrain.

Dr. Jones postulated that impaired joint mobility is often due to protective proprioceptive reflexes that fire when the muscle is shorter than its resting length. In other words, as the body attempts to move through its normal range of motion, a premature myotatic reflex (stretch reflex) causes the muscle to contract, thereby limiting movement. Often the contraction is accompanied by spasm and pain. Jones theorizes that this pathologic reflex may have been initiated when the joint was in a stretched position and a panic reaction to return to a normal position caused the muscles opposite the stretched muscles to spasm. For example, a person bends over for a short time. When he or she attempts to stand up, there is a sharp pain and the person is not able to stand up without pain. There is a position, however, somewhere between the bent-over position and an erect position that is pain free. An overcontraction of the antagonist of the stretched muscle resists any attempt to return to a normal position.

Jones feels that a quick stretch of the shortened antagonist muscle caused the spindle cells to report to the central nervous system (CNS) that the muscle was being strained. A physiopathologic reflex circuit is created that maintains the antagonist muscle in a hypertonic state. This phenomenon can also result from muscle splinting following trauma. Once the reflex has been initiated, the body has no way to reset it.

Jones found that by positioning the joint in a position of comfort, which was usually close to the position where the spasm occurred, the pain ceases. By holding that position, which is usually a more exaggerated angle than the painful posture, then very slowly and passively returning to a normal position, the muscle shortening and the pain and spasm are eliminated.

Jones also noted that most joint problems have associated tender spots. When movement of a joint is restricted, pressure on the associated myofascial tender point will be painful. As the joint is moved into the position of maximum comfort, the pain in the tender point will diminish. By monitoring the sensitivity of the associated tender points while positioning the joint, the ideal angle for maximum benefit can be determined. When the client indicates that the pain in the point is reduced and there is a noticeable "letting go" in the palpated tissues, the pain or discomfort in the joint is also reduced and the client is in a comfortable position. Hold that position about a minute and a half (ninety seconds), and then slowly return the body to a neutral position. The pain and restriction are often eliminated and the pain in the associated tender spot has disappeared.

Orthobionomy

Orthobionomy was developed by an English osteopath named Arthur Lincoln Pauls. After reading of the work of Dr. Lawrence Jones, Dr. Pauls began to develop a healing system based on the body's self-correcting reflexes. *Ortho* means to correct or to straighten. Bionomy is the study of life processes. Dr. Pauls defines the term *orthobionomy* as the correct application of the natural laws of life.

Dr. Pauls feels that disease and injury are often the result of the body's inappropriate response or reaction to some stimulus or situation. The inappropriate reaction is a misinterpretation or a misunderstanding brought on by fear or habit. Orthobionomy works to restore the body's natural understanding by safely and slowly moving the body into and through those places where fear or habit is holding it in patterns that block vital energy, restrict movement, or cause pain.

Techniques include both methods that use physical contact and those that address energy systems of the body (*chi*, aura, etheric energy). The hands-on manipulations used in orthobionomy are passive positioning methods that relax tense ligaments and muscles by moving them into their position of greatest comfort and gently supporting them there. Techniques combine contact of trigger points with passive movement of the joint to produce the release of pain and tension in the related muscles. There are movements to release every joint of the body that increase circulation and relaxation throughout the body. The client experiences movement through a wider range of motion with less pain and tension.

Because of the gentle, caring, and loving way orthobionomy is done, the release of muscular tension is often accompanied by mental and emotional release. As areas of the body begin to unwind, especially in areas where there has been trauma (physical or emotional), the stored body memories will also release. The release of physical and emotional restrictions along with the restoration of circulation and energy flow provides an environment in which the self-healing powers of the person can function.

Structural/Muscular Balancing

Structural/muscular balancing integrates techniques from several bodywork systems including those of Drs. Lawrence Jones and Arthur Pauls. Dr. Ray Lichtman incorporated the passive positioning techniques of Pauls and Jones with precision muscle testing into a system he called Positional Release. Mark Beck and Marcia Hart further adapted the techniques of Positional Release to include tools to identify and balance the body-mind or psychophysical aspects which are intimately related to physical dysfunction.

Structural/muscular balancing (SMB) is a method of:
• Gently moving the body away from pain and toward more comfort
• Improving neuromuscular communication in the body
• Rebalancing the energy flow in the muscles
• Releasing tension which limits body range of motion.
(from *Structural Muscular Balancing*: Hart, 1992)

SMB provides an extremely gentle, noninvasive method of working with a client's unique self-knowledge to locate and release constricted tissues that cause pain and rigidness. SMB uses a variety of techniques to address the physical, neuromuscular, energetic, and psychoemotional aspects of an individual's dysfunctional patterns. The main physical techniques used in SMB include precision muscle testing, passive positioning, directional massage, and deep pressure. The aim of SMB is to release tension in the structural muscles and reset the neuromuscular reflexes that perpetuate tension, spasms, and the associated pain.

Precision Muscle Testing

Precision muscle testing is a type of specialized kinesiology that is used to evaluate energetic imbalances in the body and determine exactly what remedies will work best for the individual at that particular time. Whenever there is a dysfunction in a muscle, organ, tissue, or mental or emotional process, it will cause an energetic imbalance that can be revealed through muscle testing even before it becomes symptomatic.

Precision muscle testing evolved from the original work of Dr. George Goodhart, D.C., a Michigan chiropractor, who since the 1960s has guided research in the development of a system called Applied Kinesiology for detecting imbalances in the body. The system was simplified and popularized by Dr. John Thie, D.C. with the publication of Touch for Health and the development of Touch for Health seminars. Specialized muscle testing has been adapted to several alternative health practices as a way to determine physical or emotional imbalances and the effects of corrective measures or stresses on the systems of the mind or body. Precision muscle testing as it is used in SMB was refined by the work of Gordon Stokes and Daniel Whiteside of Three in One Concepts, Burbank, California.

In SMB precision muscle testing is used to indicate:

- Where imbalances or lesions are in the body
- What parts of the body will be worked on
- What techniques will be used on each part
- Priorities as to what needs to be done in what order
- Relationships between two or more dysfunctional patterns.

Precision muscle testing is the information-gathering tool that directly accesses the body's wisdom and self-knowledge. Through muscle testing the body reveals where tension or imbalances exist and what corrective techniques it prefers.

Positional Release

Position release addresses muscle tissue that is tense, hypertonic, overcontracted, or in spasm. Muscles in a hypertonic state generally are ischemic, contain trigger points, have a high level of nerve activity, and may be painful. The presence of tight muscles in one area of the body usually is an indication of muscle imbalance in other areas as well. This is especially true with structural muscles of the pelvis and trunk.

The tense muscle is attempting in vain to bring its ends closer together. The tension may be the result of a protective reflex, muscle splinting, or strain. Tension is often self-perpetuating. The static tension of tight muscles restricts the flow of blood and fluids in those tissues. Tension causes increased metabolic activity, requiring more nutrients and producing more metabolic wastes. This ischemia and congestion impede the function of the muscle and may cause pain. Pain causes spasm, muscle splinting, and protective posturing, which further perpetuate the dysfunction.

Neuromuscular activity is increased. Proprioceptive feedback maintains the local tension and facilitates imbalances in the immediate area and in other related areas of the body. A viscous cycle of tension-pain-dysfunction builds on itself to a point that activity becomes restricted or stopped.

Positional release breaks the tension cycle by gently allowing the body to achieve the exaggerated positions it has been attempting without straining or initiating protective reflexes.

Contracted tissues are gently moved into their direction of contraction (preferred position). The body part is slowly and passively positioned so the ends of the hypercontracted muscle tissue are brought closer together. When the right position for release is achieved, a slight compression into the joint is applied. The proprioceptive information created during the positioning resets the pathophysiologic reflex circuits that have held the joint and associated tissues in a state of tension. After holding the position for thirty to ninety seconds, the body part is slowly and passively returned to its normal position. Muscle tension is reduced and associated trigger points are inactivated.

Directional Massage

Directional massage uses a short "hook and stretch" or J stroke on a specified body area or muscle. As the name implies the stroke is done in one direction either up, down, or across the muscle. The area of the body and the direction of the stroke are determined with precision muscle testing. Tension and pain in the tissue are reduced and energy flow is improved.

Deep Pressure

Occasionally deep pressure is applied to specific hypersensitive spots. Deep pressure as it is used in SMB is similar to the ischemic compression used in trigger-point techniques. Deep pressure is used when passive positioning to release the affected tissues is not possible or does not completely inactivate the points.

Advanced Techniques

Techniques of advanced SMB are adapted from the work of Gorden Stokes and Daniel Whiteside of Three and One Concepts. They address the psychological and emotional aspects of how what we know and feel affects the way our body functions. The tools used in advanced structural/muscular balancing include:
• Emotional Stress difussion
• The Behavioral Barometer
• Age Recession
• Transformational Guided Imagery
• Reactive Circuits.

It is beyond the scope of this text to discuss these techniques in detail. Emotions and psychophysical reactions the body has adopted to protect itself from real or imagined danger do affect the way each individual reacts to a given situation. When those reactions become unhealthy or restrictive, advanced SMB techniques provide tools to identify and gently defuse the emotional charge related to the dysfunctional reactions.

▼ ENERGETIC MANIPULATION

Throughout the philosophies of Eastern countries is the premise that there is a force, or vibration, common to all living matter. It is believed that the smooth flow of this force is the predeterminator of good health.

When this flow is out of balance in the body, the person experiences physical illness and a sense of uneasiness. Techniques have been developed that detect imbalances in the flow of the force in the body and affect it in such a way as to bring it back into balance, or homeostasis.

Some techniques based on these theories are acupuncture (a traditional medical procedure rather than a massage technique), acupressure, *shiatsu*, polarity, *Reiki*, and reflexology. The following is a brief explanation of some of these techniques.

Acupuncture

Acupuncture is said to have originated in China more than 5000 years ago. It is recognized around the world today as a remedial and medical technique. Throughout history, more people have been treated with acupuncture than all other therapies combined. Acupuncture is not a massage technique, but the basic philosophy underlies to some degree many of the energetic massage techniques. Touch is an integral part of acupuncture treatment. Acupuncture is a traditional Chinese medical practice whereby the skin is punctured with needles at specific points for therapeutic purposes. Acupuncture must be done only by highly trained practitioners.

It is not within the scope of this book to cover the philosophy that supports such therapies as acupuncture and *shiatsu* but the following information will help the beginning practitioner or student gain a better understanding of the therapies that originated in the ancient cultures of China and Japan.

Eastern Thought

Religious philosophies of the Far East speak of *Tao* or "the way" and refer to the law of the universe or "that which is all there is." The belief is that *tao* was split into two parts, and those two parts became opposed and dynamically in motion, thus creating the energy that sustains the whole. These two parts are represented by *yin* and *yang*.

Yin and *Yang*

The *yin* and *yang* theory demonstrates the natural process of continuous change where nothing is of itself, but is seen as aspects of the whole or as two opposite, yet complementary, aspects of existence. Therefore, *yin* and *yang* are seen as opposites of the same phenomenon and exist only in relation to one another (Fig. 17.5). The following list of words shows *yin* and *yang* contrasts:

Aspects of *Yin* and *Yang*

YIN	YANG
dark or night	light or day
low	high
cold	hot
inside	outside
contracting	expanding
passive	active
deficient	excessive

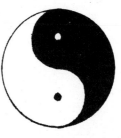

Fig. 17.5 Yin yang symbol depicting balance and change.

Yin and *Yang* on the Body

YIN	YANG
front of the body	back of the body
inner body	outer body
lower body	upper body
underactive	overactive
coldness	hotness
weak	forceful

Although *yin* and *yang* are diametrically opposed, one has no meaning without the other. There is continuous and constant vying as one creates and transforms into the other while at the same time holding the other in check. It is said that when *yin* and *yang* are in balance, there is harmony and well-being. The outcome of long-term disharmony is disease. If *yang* is too strong or excessive, *yin* will appear to be too weak. If *yang* is weak, *yin* will be overbearing. If the imbalance becomes too severe, *yin* and *yang* will separate, and the result is death of the organism. Breathing, digestion, metabolic rest and activity, and even the seasons are examples of this interaction. This relationship is considered to be the source of all change and movement.

Chi or Bioforce

In the constant interplay of *yin* and *yang*, a subtle vibratory substance or a force or energy existing in all life forms is created. Many philosophers recognize this force as the vital force of growth and change. **Chi** (China) and **ki** (Japan) are two of the words used to describe this concept, while **bioenergy** and **bioforce** are terms in current usage that reflect similar ideas. There is no one word in English that adequately translates the *yin* and *yang* concept of *chi* (ki).

In discussing *chi* as it relates to health, it is much clearer to speak in terms of function. *Chi* in the body comes from three major sources: heredity from parents, the food we eat, and the air we breathe. These three sources combine and permeate our beings. According to ancient philosophy, *chi* (or *ki*) manifests itself as five interrelated aspects of energy, which are the five elements. These are fire, earth, metal, water, and wood. Everything is created from one or more of these elements. Humans are said to be combinations of all five (Fig. 17.6).

Meridian *chi* refers to the energy that circulates in a network of meridians, channels, and collaterals in the body. Channels and meridians are like rivers of *chi* (energy) that course along the extremities into the body and through related organs. There are twelve bilateral meridians, or channels, that are associated with organs, and eight extra meridians that have regulatory effect. The extra meridians or collaterals flow from meridian to meridian and allow for regulation and harmonization of *chi*.

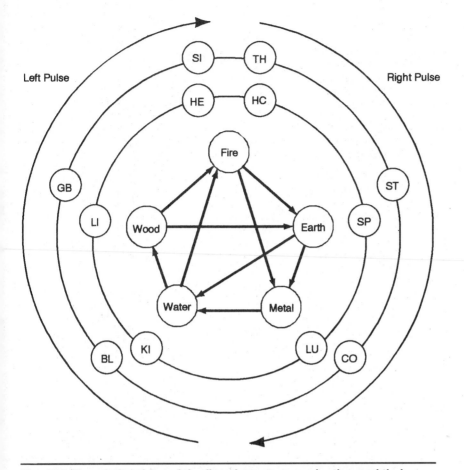

Fig. 17.6 The relationships of the five elements to each other and their related organs are depicted in this diagram. The arrows in the center that look like a star depict the *ko* or control cycle: Wood controls earth by covering it or holding it in place with roots. Earth controls water by damming it or containing it. Water controls fire by dousing or extinguishing it. Fire controls metal by melting it. Metal controls wood by cutting it. The next arrows that form a pentagram depict the *sheng* or creative cycle: Water engenders wood. Wood fuels fire. Fire creates earth (ashes). Earth engenders metal. Metal engenders water. The two rings indicate the solid (yin) and hollow (yang) organs that are associated with the elements. The outer arrowed circle indicates the location of the pulse points that are used for diagnosis.

Along these meridians are small areas of high conductivity called acupoints (acupuncture points), where *chi* can be affected by a number of modalities such as pressure, heat, electricity, needles, and touch. There are 365 acupoints located on the meridians where the *chi* (or *ki*) flow can most easily be influenced. A number of extra acupoints are not located on a specific meridian. It is at these points that the acupuncturist will insert needles or the therapist will apply pressure.

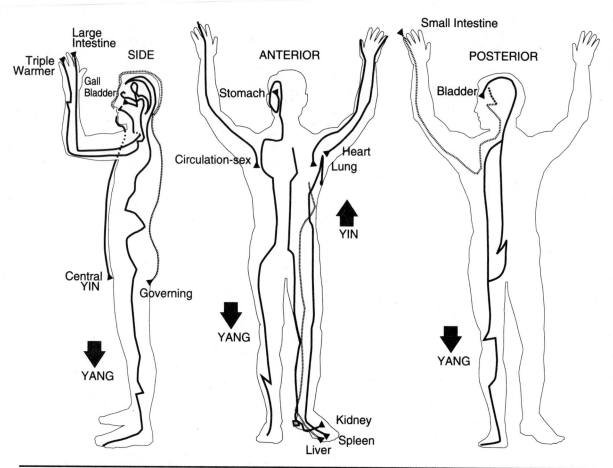

Fig. 17.7 The twelve organ meridians are located bilaterally on the body.

Meridians have been mapped on the body very specifically in terms of location and direction of energy flow. The practitioner who is seriously interested in pursuing the mastery of the subject must learn the location of each meridian, the direction of *ki* flow within the meridian, and the commonly used meridian points (Fig. 17.7).

Organ Meridians According to *Yin* and *Yang*

Organ Meridian	*Yin* or *Yang*	Element	Location
Lung	*Yin*	Metal	Chest to end of thumb.
Large intestine	*Yang*	Metal	Index finger to face
Stomach	*Yang*	Earth	Face to front of body to end of second toe
Spleen	*Yin*	Earth	Middle side of large toe to inside of leg to chest
Heart	*Yin*	Fire	Chest to inside of arm to end of little finger
Small intestine	*Yang*	Fire	Small finger to back of arm to side of face
Bladder	*Yang*	Water	Medial side of eye, over the head, and down the back and back of leg to little toe

Organ Meridian	*Yin* or *Yang*	Element	Location
Kidney	*Yin*	Water	Bottom of foot and along inside of leg to upper chest
Pericardium	*Yin*	Fire	Chest to end of middle finger
Triple heater	*Yang*	Fire	End of ring finger back to side of head
Gall bladder	*Yang*	Wood	Side of head and body and along side of leg to the fourth toe
Liver	*Yin*	Wood	Big toe and along inside of leg to chest
Governing vessel	*Yang*		Tip of tailbone, up midline of back, and over the heart to upper lip
Conception vessel	*Yin*		Perineum and up front of midline to bottom lip and chin

The eight meridians that have a regulatory effect are:

Conception vessel	Governing vessel
Regulatory channel of *yin*	Regulatory channel of *Yang*
Connecting channel of *yin*	Connecting channel of *Yang*
Belt channel	Vital or penetrating channel

Achieving the balance of *yin* and *Yang* is the aim of most energy therapists. Imbalance in the body is recognized by a number of signs and symptoms. Various therapists have differing means of recognizing imbalances and offering techniques for affecting and regulating energy flow so that a more healthful condition might be achieved.

Acupressure

Acupressure refers to any of a number of treatment systems that incorporate various manipulations of acupoints. The basic philosophy comes from the traditional Chinese. Most Eastern societies incorporate some touch pressure in their traditional touch remedies. A number of acupressure techniques have been developed in Western societies.

Acupressure is often used to facilitate better circulation of blood and *chi* to an affected area and to relieve pain. Techniques usually include touching, pressing, or rubbing one or more points, depending on what is to be achieved. Acupressure as well as many of the health practices of oriental origin are used in conjunction with diet, exercise, and meditation. The goal is to balance the physical and psychological aspects of a person's being into a holistic (wholesome) way of life.

Shiatsu

The Japanese word **shiatsu** (composed of *shi*, [finger], and *atsu* [pressure]), means pressure of the fingers or digits. In a sense it is like acupuncture without the use of needles. The purpose of *shiatsu* is to increase circulation and restore energy balances in the body. It is also an aid in soothing the nervous system and is said to be particularly effective in relieving headache, fatigue, insomnia, nervous tension, sore and stiff muscles, and such disorders as constipation and high blood pressure.

Like acupuncture, *shiatsu* recognizes strategic points (called *tsubo*) or energy pathways situated on the meridians, but which do not correspond entirely to the Chinese method. Instead of using needles, the *shiatsu* expert uses the ball of the thumb to apply pressure. The treatment can be given to the entire body to restore complete harmony or according to specific needs. By applying pressure to the points, the natural recuperative powers of the body are generated, toxins are dispersed, muscles are relaxed, circulation of blood and lymph are improved, energy is released or balanced, and the entire body is revitalized.

To be effective, the practitioner must build strength and dexterity of the fingers, thumb, and entire hand. Pressure is applied with only the tips of the fingers pointing straight into the point. One finger with another finger placed over it as a brace is used. The palm of the hand is sometimes used to apply pressure over a larger area. Three fingers held together may be used generally for the face, abdomen, and adjacent areas. The thumbs are used most often in *shiatsu*. Only the ball of the thumb is used to press straight down (no rubbing motions) on the pressure points. Pressure is exerted perpendicularly to the surface of the skin with the pads of the fingers or thumb, for two to five seconds or more, depending on the area being treated.

Pressure Points

To become better acquainted with pressure points, study Figs. 17.8 and 17.9 then note the basic benefits attributed to pressure points on specific areas of the body. The practitioner who wishes to become proficient in the art and science of *shiatsu* must study the philosophy and techniques under the direction of a skilled teacher. *Shiatsu* is not exceptionally difficult to learn, but it is an art that cannot be learned correctly by hit-or-miss methods or experimentation. Certain contraindications, as with other massage techniques, must be observed.

Shiatsu need not be applied in the order listed next. Judge the area to be treated, and then determine the duration of pressure and procedure to follow for maximum benefit to the individual.

Anterior View of Pressure Points

The following list refers to points indicated on Fig. 17.8 reading clockwise from the head.

1. Frontal crown of the head, forehead, temple, and mastoid process. Use the thumbs on pressure points to relieve headache and tension.

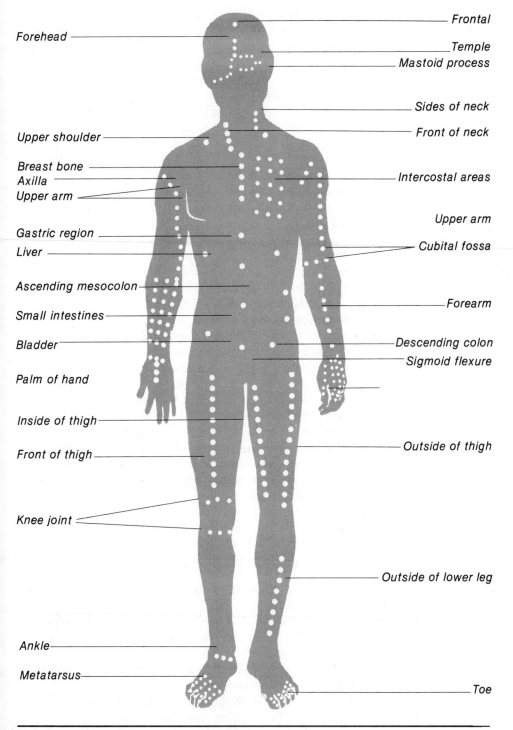

Fig. 17.8 Anterior view of pressure points.

2. Sides and front of the neck. Use the thumbs to press first the right and then the left carotid artery. Pressure here relieves stiff neck and fatigue.
3. Intercostal area. Gentle pressure with thumbs encourages relaxation.
4. Upper arm, cubital fossa forearm, elbow joint. People who use their arms a lot enjoy relief from fatigue when this technique is used. Apply pressure to points using the thumbs.
5. Descending colon and sigmoid flexure. Use the palms of the hands and the fingertips on pressure points. Pressure here relaxes tension, and improves metabolism.
6. Outside of thigh and outside of lower leg. Use the fingers on the pressure points to relieve fatigue and sore muscles.
7. Toes, metatarsus, and ankle. Use the thumbs to press the toes several times each. Repeat on the metatarsus and ankle. This relieves fatigue, tension, and soreness.
8. Knee joint, front, and inside of the thigh. Use the thumbs to work down the front and inside of the thigh. Apply pressure above and below the kneecap. Relieves strained muscles and prevents soreness.
9. Palm of the hand. Use the thumbs on the pressure points to relieve strained muscles, stiffness, and soreness.
10. Bladder, small intestines, ascending colon. Use fingertips to apply pressure to the points, and use the palm of the hand to apply pressure to the abdomen. This stimulates the flow of blood to the area and relieves constipation.
11. Gastric region and liver. Use the tips of the fingers to apply pressure. This relaxes nerves and promotes good digestion.
12. Inside upper arm and axilla. Use the thumbs on the pressure points to relieve strain and soreness.
13. Breastbone. Use the fingertips to apply pressure. This stimulates the endocrine gland.
14. Shoulder. Use the fingertips on pressure points to relieve soreness, strain, and fatigue of muscles.

Posterior View of Pressure Points

The following list refers to points indicated on Fig. 17.9 reading clockwise from the head.

1. Medulla oblongata. Use the fingertips on the pressure points to relieve fatigue, restore energy, soothe headaches, and promote alertness.
2. Back of upper arm. Use the thumbs on the pressure points to relieve fatigue, soreness, and stiffness.
3. Dorsum (back). Use thumbs on pressure points to increase circulation, relieve tension, relax muscles, and soothe anxieties.
4. Lumbar vertebrae and upper end of thigh bone. Use thumbs on the pressure points to stimulate circulation to the area, relieve fatigue, and impart a sense of well-being.

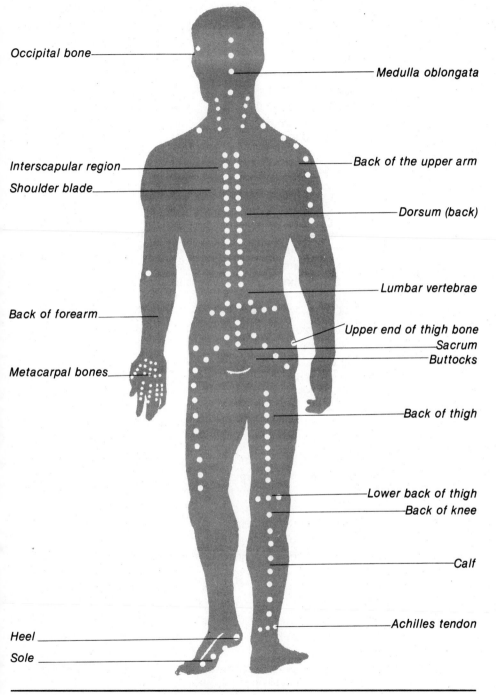

Fig. 17.9 Posterior view of pressure points.

5. Buttocks and sacrum. Use thumbs on the pressure points to relieve aching lower back, fatigue, and feelings of anxiety.
6. Back of thigh, lower back of thigh, and back of knee. Use the tips of the fingers on pressure points to relieve soreness, fatigue, and strain in muscles.
7. Calf and Achilles' tendon. Use the fingers to pinch the calves, and use the thumbs to press the points from calf to ankle. This relieves soreness, strain, and fatigue in muscles.
8. Heel and sole of the foot. Use the thumbs on the pressure points of the instep and the plantar arch (sole). Pressure here relieves strain and soreness, relaxes nerves, and strengthens muscles of the foot.
9. Metacarpal bones, hand, and fingers. Press the tips of all the fingers on the surfaces of the hand. Move pressure until all fingers have been treated. This technique adds strength and flexibility and improves general well-being.
10. Back of forearm. Use the thumbs on the pressure points from wrist to elbow to relieve muscles that are fatigued, strained, and sore.
11. Shoulder blade and interscapular region. Use the thumbs on the pressure points to improve circulation to the area, soothe nerves, and relieve anxieties.
12. Occipital. Use the thumbs on the pressure points to help regulate blood pressure and relieve fatigue, insomnia, and headache.

▼ REFLEXOLOGY

Reflexology is the art and science of stimulating the body's own healing forces by locating and stimulating certain points on the body that affect organs or functions in distant parts of the body. A form of compression massage, reflexology is based on the principles that reflex points in the hands and feet are related to every organ in the body. By applying pressure to a reflex point, the practitioner can effect certain beneficial changes. For example, when reflex massage is given on the big toe, it is said to relieve headache and tension. Various parts of the hands and feet are linked with specific glands, organs, and muscles. Activating these links through reflex massage can relieve tension, improve the blood supply to certain regions of the body, and help to normalize body functions.

In recent years public interest in reflexology has been aroused. Some people are skeptical whether this form of massage is beneficial while others credit the method with remarkable success.

Practitioners do not claim reflexology to be a major cure-all. They encourage those who are interested to be sure to master the techniques well before attempting to use them.

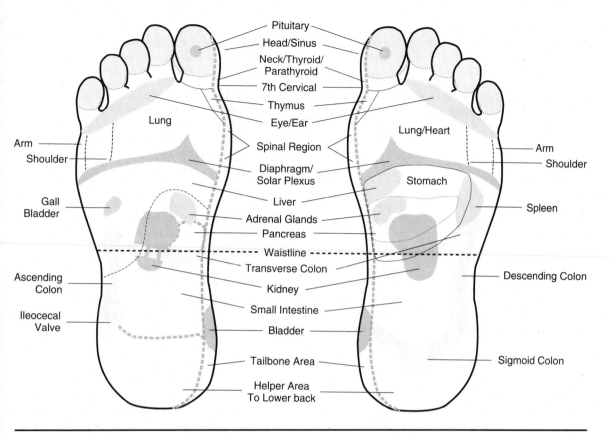

Pituitary
Head/Sinus
Neck/Thyroid/
Parathyroid
7th Cervical
Thymus
Eye/Ear
Lung
Lung/Heart
Arm
Shoulder
Arm
Shoulder
Spinal Region
Diaphragm/
Solar Plexus
Stomach
Gall
Bladder
Liver
Spleen
Adrenal Glands
Pancreas
Waistline
Transverse Colon
Ascending
Colon
Descending Colon
Kidney
Small Intestine
Ileocecal
Valve
Bladder
Tailbone Area
Sigmoid Colon
Helper Area
To Lower back

Fig. 17.10 Foot reflexology chart indicates points on the foot that reflexively correspond to other areas of the body.

For further sources of study in the art and science of body, hand and foot reflexology, see the massage reference list (Fig. 17.10).

STRESS THERAPY AND RELAXATION MASSAGE

Stress is a condition that affects both the body and the mind. Originally it was caused by certain physical reactions in humans and animals that served as life-saving signals to enable the organism to react quickly when danger threatened. This became known as the "flight or fight" response. Today, we face different kinds of stress situations, but the body still reacts in somewhat the same manner. To prepare the body to flee or to confront a problem, the sympathetic nervous system increases blood pressure and elevates the pulse rate. Hormones (adrenaline and noradrenalin) are released, and energy reserves are mobilized.

In cases of extreme fright or certain forms of nervous tension, a person may perspire profusely. The skin may become affected by the contraction of the erector pilorum muscles around a hair follicle. This condition, resembling a profusion of small bumps with erect hairs, is referred to as gooseflesh.

A certain amount of stress is normal and desirable, but there is a difference between positive and negative stress. Stress is an involuntary response. Whether it is positive or negative, the body deals with it in the same way. Positive stress expels excess energy, stimulates motivation, and is advantageous, while negative stress can cause adverse responses. For example, when under stress the body's metabolism changes, and, if prolonged, body systems begin to react. A person may develop internal problems such as ulcers or skin problems such as psoriasis, hives, and problem blemishes. The great danger of stress is that when it becomes a chronic condition rather than an occasional reaction, it can eventually lead to serious health problems. Continued anxiety, tension, or hypertension can lead to allergies, arthritis, indigestion, constipation, high blood pressure, heart disease, insomnia, and many other conditions.

Stress-related illnesses account for most of the reasons for nonproductivity on the job as well as for problems that affect people personally and socially. When a person is suffering from negative stress, incidents that are normally accepted as minor or inconvenient are blown out of proportion as to their actual seriousness. Often the affected person will react by exhibiting excessive anger and frustration. Stress tends to deplete the body's supply of vitamins and minerals; therefore, people under stress should pay attention to their dietary habits. When under stress, there is a tendency to eat too fast and to eat meals lacking essential nutrients. Sometimes stress stimulates a craving for food or causes a feeling of fullness without satisfaction. Also it is not uncommon for the stressed individual to lose his or her appetite .

A sense of hopelessness is often associated with stress. When depression sets in, a person may turn to drugs or alcohol or both, hoping to find relief. However, alcohol and drugs only compound the problem. The most effective way to deal with stress when it becomes unmanageable is to seek counseling and treatment. It is important to identify causes and look for a solution. For example, when stress is work related, making a list of daily, weekly, and monthly activities may be helpful in pinpointing stress-producing activities that can be rescheduled or eliminated.

Individuals respond differently to the same stressful situations. For example, major life changes, a new job, illness, or financial setback may be devastating to one person while another will be able to handle such events with less distress. Those individuals who have stressful life experiences should make an effort to balance their lives with some type of enjoyable recreation such as a hobby or special interest. A good balance of work and relaxation helps to combat stress.

Doctors often recommend massage for the relief of tension, anxiety, worry, and anger—all causes of stress. Many practitioners create a restful environment with relaxing background music for clients who are experiencing stress and for those who want to prevent stress-related illnesses. The goal is to induce complete mental and physical relaxation. When working with clients who are highly stressed, the practitioner should be aware of the effects of pressure, rhythm, and duration of each movement as well as the client's response. In some cases the client may experience deep relaxation that is somewhat like a hypnotic state.

A great deal can be determined during the consultation, so the client should be encouraged to express his or her feelings. Also, the practitioner will want to know how long the beneficial effects of the massage lasted; clients often experience renewed energy and relief from stress for several days or longer.

When giving relaxation massage, the practitioner's hands are much better than any machine. In stress therapy and relaxation massage, human contact is most important. The massage practitioner is not expected to serve as the client's personal psychologist or counselor, but he or she should have an instinct for what is right for the client and an understanding of human feelings in order to apply a therapeutic healing touch.

CORPORATE MASSAGE—THE SEATED MASSAGE ▼

In the last several years, massage in the work-place has become a common occurrence. On-site massage was popularized by David Palmer of the Amma Institute. This stress-reducing, rejuvenating massage is done in a supported, seated position with the clothes on. Several manufacturers produce massage chairs or other devices that fasten to the top of a desk. The massage chair allows the recipient to relax as the therapist massages the back, neck, shoulders, and arms. The techniques used resemble shiatsu or acupressure but also include kneading and shaking (Fig. 17.11).

Seated massage is an abbreviated massage usually lasting ten to twenty minutes and is well suited to a short, relaxing break in a busy, hectic day. It has been shown that corporate massage increases productivity, raises employee morale, and reduces sick leave. Today many corporations are finding corporate massage to be good business.

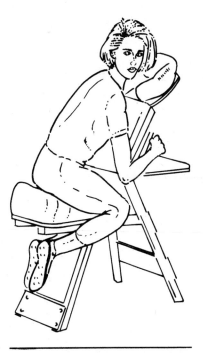

Fig. 17.11 Seated massage uses a massage chair or face rest that attaches to the top of a desk.

▼ QUESTIONS FOR DISCUSSION AND REVIEW

1. How does prenatal massage benefit the expectant mother?
2. What are the major benefits of lymph massage?
3. What are lymphocytes?
4. What is lymph?
5. What is deep tissue massage?
6. What is the purpose of structural integration?
7. What is the basis for neurophysiological massage therapies?
8. What is a trigger point?
9. Where are myofascial trigger points located?
10. What techniques deactivate trigger points?
11. Who developed the system known as neuromuscular therapy?
12. What are the abnormal tissue signs that indicate neuro-muscular lesions?
13. What are the primary treatment techniques used in neuro-muscular therapy?
14. Name the two inhibitory reflexes utilized in Muscle Energy Technique.
15. What are the three primary active joint movements used in MET?
16. What are passive positioning techniques?
17. What are three important considerations when using passive positioning techniques?
18. Who developed the technique known as Strain Counter-strain?
19. How is the preferred position determined in strain-counter-strain?
20. What are the primary tools used in structural/muscular balancing?
21. What is precision muscle testing?
22. Where is acupuncture said to have originated?
23. In Eastern thought there are two parts that contrast or exist as opposites of the same phenomenon. What are these two parts called?
24. What are the three main techniques used in acupressure?
25. What is the meaning of the Japanese word *shiatsu*?
26. Why do doctors often recommend massage to people who are suffering from stressful life experiences?
27. What is the main purpose of reflexology?

Therapeutic Exercise

18

Learning Objectives

After you have mastered this chapter, you will be able to:

1. *Explain the benefits of a regular exercise program.*
2. *Define therapeutic exercise.*
3. *Describe the benefits of exercise.*
4. *State the goals of an exercise program.*
5. *Define strength, endurance, flexibility, coordination, and relaxation and describe how they can be improved through an exercise program.*
6. *Describe warm-up and cooling-off exercises.*
7. *Explain the relationship of aerobic exercise to cardiorespiratory fitness.*
8. *Perform basic stretching exercises.*
9. *Explain the differences between passive and active flexibility exercises.*
10. *Explain how to improve coordination and skill.*
11. *Instruct a client in proper breathing techniques.*
12. *Instruct a client in relaxation exercises.*
13. *Explain the importance of good posture.*

▼ INTRODUCTION

Exercise is an important factor in maintaining wellness. It is also an effective therapeutic agent for the maintenance and rehabilitation of musculo-skeletal, cardiovascular, and neurological disorders. Therapeutic massage and exercise have many of the same goals and benefits. An individual may incorporate both massage and exercise to improve health or enhance wellness. Even though the massage therapist may not be an exercise specialist, a basic understanding of the effects and benefits of therapeutic exercises will be helpful to better serve the needs of the client. It is beyond the scope of this text to provide instruction in therapeutic exercise or personal training programs. What is offered here is a brief overview of techniques and benefits of various kinds of exercise.

Since ancient times, physical fitness has gone hand in hand with concepts of mental alertness, a strong, healthy, well-proportioned body, and personal pride. The ancient Greeks were known for their athletic contests, which are still a part of modern athletics. In recent decades there has been an increased interest in physical fitness. Millions of people of all ages have made some type of sport or other workout a part of their daily lives.

Regular exercise enhances the level of health by maintaining the physical body and at the same time relieving mental stress.

While exercise is a must for optimum health, it can be harmful if done improperly. A person may decide to trim, slim, and develop a well-muscled body and enthusiastically begin workouts with weights and various kinds of apparatus without understanding either the benefits or dangers. At first there may be some improvement, but unsupervised exercise can lead to strain on the muscles, nerves, the heart, and other organs of the body. Also, improper exercise can cause muscles to become hard and stiff and can result in injury. It is recommended that an individual who is interested in beginning a fitness program first visit his or her doctor for a physical check up and then seek the advice of a personal trainer or other exercise professional in order to develop an exercise program to best fit his or her needs and interests.

The major benefits of exercise are:
- Improvement in appearance
- Improvement in body functions
- Maintenance of normal weight
- Relief of tension and stress
- Prevention of fatigue
- Improvement of coordination
- Increased mental alertness
- Increased strength
- Increased endurance
- Improved posture
- Enhanced sense of well-being.

THERAPEUTIC EXERCISE ▼

Therapeutic exercise includes any exercise done with the intent of improving some physical condition. The goal of therapeutic exercise is to regain, improve, or maintain the function of the body or a part of the body. The effects of therapeutic exercise focus on strength, endurance, mobility, flexibility, and coordination. Therapeutic exercise may be performed with or without the assistance of a therapist or the use of exercise equipment. Before suggesting any exercises to a client, the therapist must know the physiological implications and effects of the exercises used and fully understand the client's conditions, limitations, precautions, and contraindications.

CONSULTATION FOR AN EXERCISE PROGRAM ▼

Before beginning an exercise program, a careful assessment should be made to determine the physical abilities and needs of the client. If there are any questionable medical conditions, the client must have a physical checkup by a physician as a precautionary step.

Consultation Card

Name Telephone _____

Address _____

City _____ State _____ Zip _____

Birthdate Height Weight _____

Posture: ☐ good ☐ fair ☐ poor

Exercise recommended _____

Results desired _____

Exercises recommended

1. _____
2. _____
3. _____
4. _____

Restrictions (the client should not do certain exercises)

General goals _____

Date (to begin program) _____

Statement of health

    I have no health problems that prevent normal exercising with or without machines or apparatus. I hereby release (name of business) and its employees from responsibility for injuries I may incur as the result of participation in a program of health-related exercises.

Client's signature _____

▼ **BEGINNING AN EXERCISE PROGRAM**

Exercising gradually and building up to more strenuous routines will help to prevent sore, stiff muscles. Each exercise should be done correctly. It is best to exercise regularly to promote progressive improvement. Some people enjoy a brisk workout in the morning or the evening, while others prefer different times. The individual can choose the time that is most suitable to his or her daily schedule.

Stresses on the body cause physiological change. Therapeutic exercise applies progressive stresses to the body in a controlled manner in order to effect positive change. Any effective exercise is based on what physiologists call the **overload principle.** That is, regardless of whether it is strength training, endurance training, or flexibility training, the participant applies stresses to the body that are greater than what the body is accustomed too. Through the process of **adaptation** the body changes to tolerate the increased load.

The goal of therapeutic exercise is to maintain or improve:
• Strength
• Endurance
• Flexibility
• Coordination or skill
• Relaxation.

▼ **STRENGTH**

Strength is the ability of a muscle or muscle group to contract and produce tension with a resultant maximum force exerted on some resistance. Strength is usually measured as the ability of a muscle or group of muscles to exert a maximum force one time. For example, the strength of the biceps would be measured by determining the maximum weight that could be lifted with a biceps curl for one repetition. Factors that determine relative strength include muscle size and the number of motor units involved in the contraction. Other factors are the position of the muscle at the time of the contraction and the type of contraction (isometric or isotonic).

The larger the cross-sectional size of the muscle, the greater the strength. Exercises designed to increase strength also increase muscle bulk. The increased bulk is the result of an increase in the thickness of myofibrils (actin and myosin filaments) in the muscle fiber and an increase in the density of the capillary bed within the muscle. This is called **hypertrophy** (hi-**PUR**-troh-fee). Another ingredient that determines the force of a muscle contraction is the recruitment of motor units. A **motor unit** is all of the muscle fibers controlled by a single motor neuron. When a neuron fires, the fibers affected by that neuron contract maximally (the all or none response). The greater the number of neurons firing at the same time, the more motor units are recruited and the greater the force of the contraction.

Exercises to increase strength use the overload principle. In order for adaptive increases in strength to occur, the muscles must contract against a force that is greater than that to which it is accustomed. To increase strength, a weight that is at least 75 percent of the maximum capacity for the involved muscle is lifted a number of times (repetitions). In a strengthening program the relationship between resistance (weight) and repetitions progressively increases. More repetitions at a lesser load or fewer repetitions at a higher load both increase muscle function. In either case the muscle must be exercised to a point of fatigue for adaptive increases to occur. Maximum resistance with low reps tend to build strength and muscle bulk. Lighter resistance with high reps builds endurance. Most strengthening exercises tend to increase endurance, and vice versa.

Strength gained as a result of strength training is the result of adaptations that take place in the muscle tissue, the connective tissue, and the nervous system. Muscle hypertrophy is an increase in the size of the muscle due to an increase in the actin and myosin in the myofibrils. The connective tissue associated with the muscles becomes thicker and stronger to support the stronger contractions of the muscles.

The nervous system responds by recruiting motor units for a given activity that may have been inactive. The early gains in a strengthening program are often the result of better nerve recruitment.

There is also a decrease in nervous inhibition. The Golgi tendon organ (GTO) is part of the sensory system that acts as a protection against the muscle generating too much force and causing injury. When the GTO is stimulated by too forceful of a contraction, a neurological reflex causes the muscle to relax, thereby preventing injury to the muscle or connective tissues. Strength training raises the threshold at which the GTO reacts so that more tension can be exerted on the tendons.

Types of Muscle Contractions

When a muscle contracts, tension is created that applies a force against a resistance. The action that force has on the resistance defines the type of muscle contraction that takes place.

Isometric contraction: If the force of the contraction is equal to the resistance, there is no perceivable movement and the muscle length remains the same. This is known as an isometric contraction. The force generated during an isometric contraction varies depending on the position of the muscle. Maximum force is generally achieved when the muscle is stretched slightly beyond its resting length when contracted.

Isotonic contraction: If the force of the contraction is different from the resistance and movement occurs, this is known as an isotonic contraction. There are two types of isotonic contraction: concentric and eccentric.

Concentric contraction: When the force of contraction is greater than the resistance and the muscle shortens during the contraction this is known as a concentric contraction.

Eccentric contraction: When the force of the contraction is less than the resistance and the muscle lengthens during the contraction, this is known as an eccentric contraction.

A maximum isometric contraction will generate approximately 20 percent more force than a maximum concentric contraction and about 20 percent less force than a maximum eccentric contraction. For example, a person performing a biceps curl can hold a maximum 100 pounds with the elbows at 90 degrees (isometric contraction). He or she should be able to lift a weight of 80 pounds (concentric contraction) and slowly lower a weight of 120 pounds (eccentric contraction).

▼ TYPES OF STRENGTHENING EXERCISES

Types of strength training exercises may be classified according to the type of muscle contraction employed. Each type has advantages and disadvantages.

Isometric Resistance Exercises

During isometric exercise there is no joint movement. Although isometric exercise will increase strength, the strength will only increase in the position in which the exercise is performed. To increase strength throughout a range of motion, isometric contractions would have to be done with the limb in several positions.

Isotonic Resistance Exercises

During isotonic resistance exercise the muscles contract against either a constant or variable resistance as the body part moves through a full range of motion. The resistance for isotonic exercise can be supplied manually by a therapist, by the participant's body weight, or from a variety of weight equipment.

Muscle contractions during isotonic exercise may be concentric, eccentric, or both. Most programs use both concentric and eccentric contractions. As a weight is lifted, the muscle is contracted. It is important to shorten the muscle into a full contraction to get the maximum effect from the exercise. As the weight is lowered the muscle lengthens in an eccentric contraction. Since an eccentric contraction generates more force than a concentric contraction, in order to get the most benefit from an exercise the timing of the

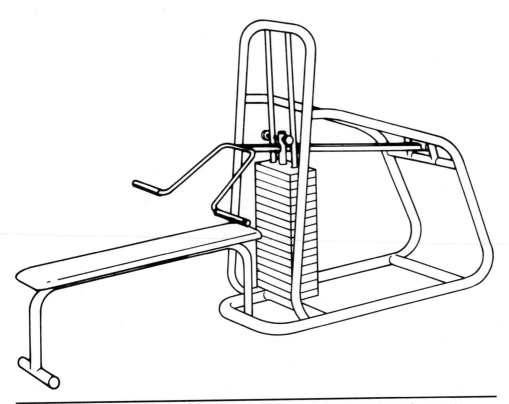

Fig. 18.1a A bench press weight machine uses a lever with a sliding resistance to provide variable resistance.

movement can be considered. The speed of a contraction has an influence on the force of the contraction. Slower contractions may incorporate more motor units and require more metabolic activity. To maximize the effect of the exercise, the concentric contraction should be smooth and deliberate (one to two seconds) and the eccentric contraction slightly slower (two to four seconds).

Variable or Constant Resistance

Isotonic exercise may be done against a variable or a constant resistance. As a muscle contracts through its available range of motion, the force it generates varies. When exercising against a constant weight the muscle exerts maximum force at only very small portion of its available range. When a **variable resistance** is used to provide maximum load at several points during the muscle contraction, the exercise is much more effective. Variable resistance may be applied when a therapist uses manual resistance techniques or by specially designed exercise equipment. Variable resistance weight equipment uses a system of cams or levers so the resistance varies in relation to the force generated by the muscle at different points throughout its range of motion (Fig. 18.1a and b).

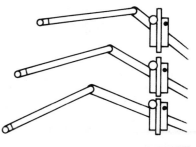

Fig. 18.1b As the lever is raised the attachment for the weight slides along the lever to increase resistance.

Isokinetic Exercise

Isokinetic exercise is done on special machines that maintain a constant speed of the exercise through the full range of motion. The equipment supplies a varying resistance equal to the force of the contraction. By limiting the speed of the movement and varying the resistance, maximal force can be applied throughout the range of motion. Many exercise specialists believe isokinetic exercise strengthens muscles more efficiently than any other form of resistive exercise.

▼ METHODS OF RESISTANCE FOR ISOTONIC EXERCISE

There are several methods of providing resistance for strength training exercises. Each has advantages and disadvantages. The following are various types of resistive exercises and examples of each.

Manual Resistance Exercises

In manual resistance exercises, the resistance is provided by a therapist. This is a valuable technique in rehabilitation or when a muscle is recovering from injury. If possible, resistance is provided through the full range of motion of the joint involved. The therapist regulates the speed and amount of resistance so that the client supplies maximum pain-free effort throughout the movement. The therapist's point of contact should be near the end of the body segment that the target muscle activates. The resistance is applied in the opposite direction of the desired motion. In controlling the resistance, the therapist can provide either an isometric, eccentric, or concentric exercise. The therapist must stabilize the client's body so that the target muscle is exercised with minimal substitute motion (Fig. 18.2a to c).

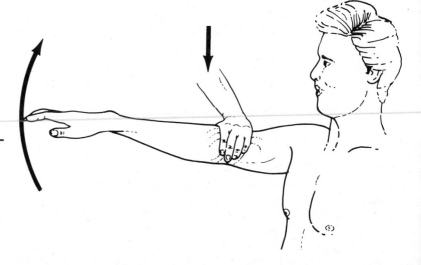

Fig. 18.2a In manual resistance exercises, the therapist applies a resistance near the distal end of the body segment being exercised. The resistance is applied in the opposite direction to the intended movement.

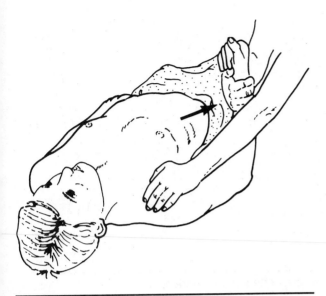

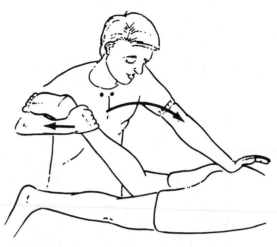
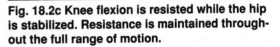

Fig. 18.2b Elbow flexion is resisted while the shoulder is stabilized.

Fig. 18.2c Knee flexion is resisted while the hip is stabilized. Resistance is maintained throughout the full range of motion.

Body Weight Exercises

Exercises that use the weight of the body as resistance are excellent for building or maintaining muscle strength and endurance. Body weight exercises require no equipment and can be done virtually anywhere. The major disadvantage of body weight exercises is that the amount of resistance remains essentially the same. The only variables to increase the load are to increase the repetitions or change body position. Examples of body weight exercises are push-ups, pull-ups, sit-ups, leg lifts, and squats (Fig. 18.3a to c).

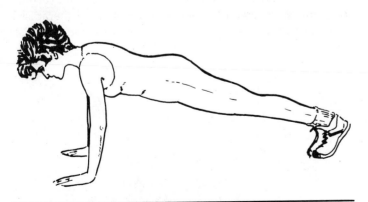

Fig. 18.3a In body weight exercises, the resistance is provided by the weight of the body. Pushups strengthen the triceps and shoulders.

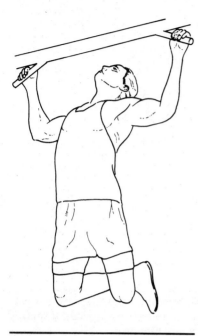

Fig. 18.3b Pullups strengthen the biceps if the hands are turned inward and the latissimus dorsi if the hands are turned outward.

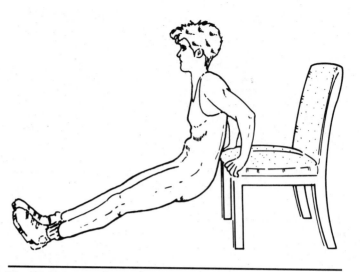

Fig. 18.3c Letdowns strengthen the triceps.

Mechanical Resistance Exercises

Mechanical resistance exercises are any form of resistance exercise in which the resistance is supplied by some type of equipment. Examples of mechanical resistance equipment include free weights (dumbbells, barbells), elastic bands, pulley weights, and weight machines. Using mechanical resistance equipment simplifies the process of progressively overloading the muscle to increase strength. When several repetitions of a particular weight can be lifted, more weight is added to the stack and the maximum number of repetitions is reduced.

There are several variables to the safe and effective planning and implementation of a strength training program. It is beyond the scope of this text to cover the subject in depth. The practitioner and client are encouraged to consult with a trained and certified personal trainer, exercise physiologist, or physical therapist before engaging in any rigorous strength training program (Fig. 18.4a to c).

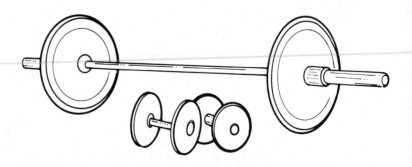

Fig. 18.4a Free weights include barbells and dumbbells.

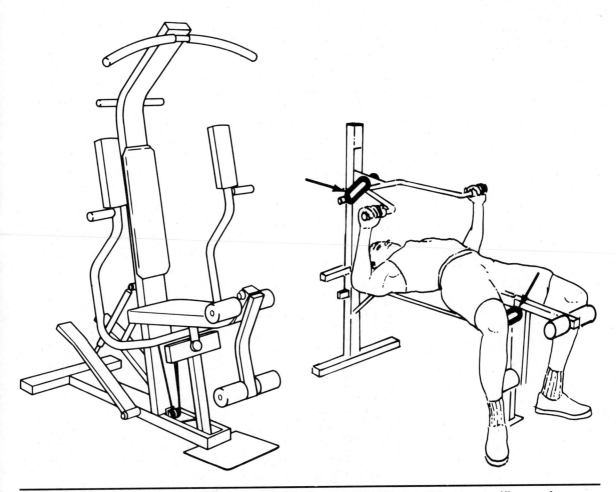

Fig. 18.4b There are a variety of weight machines that provide strength training to specific muscle groups.

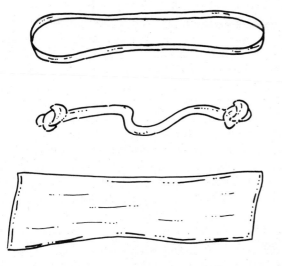

Fig. 4c Large rubberbands, rubber surgical tubing and Theraband® can provide resistance for strength training exercises.

▼ ENDURANCE

Endurance is the ability to carry on an activity over a prolonged period of time and resist fatigue. Endurance relates to the development of the cardiovascular and pulmonary systems.

Endurance can pertain to general body endurance or muscular endurance. A muscle or muscle group is said to have endurance when it can hold a contraction for an extended period of time or perform a great number of contractions without becoming fatigued. General endurance or **cardiorespiratory endurance** is the ability of an individual to continue a general exercise over an extended period of time. Cardiorespiratory fitness is the ability of the cardiovascular and cardiopulmonary systems to deliver an adequate supply of oxygen to the exercising muscles and the muscles' ability to extract and convert the oxygen to energy efficiently.

To improve endurance for a particular muscle or muscle group, the muscle is contracted against a moderate resistance repeatedly to the point of fatigue. With regular exercise, the endurance and the strength of the muscle will improve.

General endurance can be improved with regular **aerobic exercise.** Aerobic exercise improves cardiorespiratory fitness. Factors that determine the effectiveness of an aerobic exercise program are type, intensity, duration, and frequency of aerobic exercise.

The **type** of exercise is often determined by the preference of the client. To be effective, the exercise should involve large muscle groups and be continuous and rhythmic. Popular aerobic activities include walking, jogging, running, aerobic dancing, swimming, hiking, cycling, skating, and cross country skiing. A variety of mechanical devices have been designed for developing cardiorespiratory fitness. They include the stationary bicycle, the treadmill, the rowing machine, and the stair climber. Some of the more sophisticated equipment is computerized to regulate the intensity and monitor the individual's pulse and output (Fig. 18.5a to c).

Exercises set to dance rhythms (generally called dance exercise or aerobics) have become popular. This type of exercise has been the answer for millions of people who are unable to participate in regular sports, but who can join an exercise class or do the exercise using an instructional cassette tape or video.

Frequency refers to the number of exercise sessions per week. To maintain or improve cardiorespiratory fitness, it is recommended that a person exercise at least three to five times a week with no more than two days off in between. Frequency is somewhat dependent on duration and intensity of the workout. Workouts of low intensity and short duration may occur more frequently, while intense workouts once or twice a week can be interspersed with lighter sessions.

The **intensity** of exercise refers to the amount of stress or overload put on the body, especially the cardiovascular system, by the

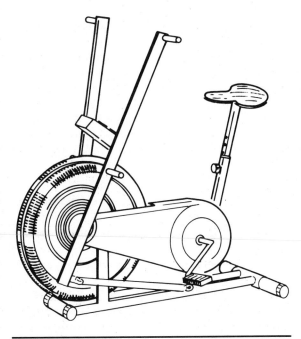

Fig. 18.5a The stationary bicycle is used to provide aerobic exercise. Note that this model exercises the lower and upper extremities.

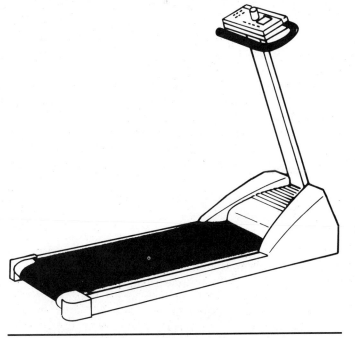

Fig. 18.5b Most treadmills have adjustments for speed and elevation so the intensity of the workout can be controlled.

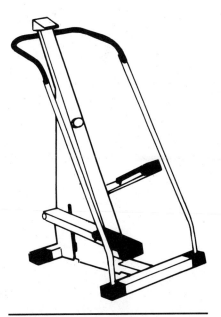

Fig. 18.5c The stair climbing machine provides aerobic exercise similar to climbing up several flights of stairs.

exercise. This may be the most important factor in regulating the exercise program.

There are a number of ways to monitor exercise intensity. According to the American College of Sports Medicine, the optimum benefits of cardiovascular training are obtained when the heart rate is sustained at between 60 and 90 percent of an individual's maximal heart rate. The maximal heart rate can be approximated by the formula 220 minus your age. To determine if an exercise is of aerobic benefit, monitor the pulse. For example, for a person 40 years old:

220 minus 40 equals 180

180 multiplied by .60 equals 108 low limit for cardiovascular benefit

180 multiplied by .90 equals 162 high limit for cardiovascular benefit

The range of pulse to obtain aerobic benefit would be between 108 and 162 beats per minute.

Another way to monitor the intensity of aerobic exercise is the **talk test.** A client should be able to breath comfortably and rhythmically at any time during a workout. During the workout, they should be able to talk and carry on a conversation. The talk test is a subjective indicator that a person is staying within the limits of aerobic intensity. Gasping for breath or breathing extremely deeply is an indication that the activity has become anaerobic in nature.

Exercise **duration** is the length of an exercise session. To gain cardiorespiratory benefits, an exercise session may be from twenty to sixty minutes in length. The relationship between the duration and the intensity of an exercise determines the cardiorespiratory effects. An intense workout of shorter duration may have similar benefits as a light workout of longer duration. For example, running three miles in twenty minutes has similar benefits to walking three miles in thirty-five minutes.

Components of an Aerobic Workout

An aerobic workout has three basic components;
1. The warm-up
2. The primary exercise
3. The cool-down.

The warm-up is done just previous to the primary exercise. The goal of the warm-up is gradually to increase the heart rate, blood pressure, and elasticity of the muscles. The warm-up consists of activities similar to the primary exercise that are done at a slower pace. After five to seven minutes of movement to warm up the tissues, a number of flexibility exercises that include the muscle and joints of the primary activity should be performed.

The cool-down follows the primary exercise activity and includes a slowing down of the primary aerobic activity followed by stretching the muscle groups used in the active phase. The goal of the cool-down is to reduce slowly the elevated metabolism and heart rate achieved during the exercise. The cool-down allows the blood circulation to normalize, preventing the lightheadedness, cramps, or delayed stiffness that sometimes follows intense exercise.

Benefits of Cardiorespiratory Fitness

There are numerous benefits to cardiorespiratory fitness that are commensurate with the physiological adaptations and conditioning that result from regular aerobic exercise. Some of the physiological adaptations resulting from aerobic exercise include:

- A lower resting heart rate, and increased maximum cardiac stroke volume and output
- Denser capillary beds in muscles with more blood flow
- Improved respiration both in the lungs and at the cellular level
- More oxygen taken into the blood
- Increased oxygen consumption by the cells.

Benefits of Cardiorespiratory Fitness include:

- Increased heart function
- Reduced blood pressure
- Reduced total cholesterol
- Increased high-density lipoprotein (HDL)-cholesterol.
- Reduced overall body fat.
- Noticeable reduction in the symptoms of depression, tension, and anxiety.

    Aerobic fitness is a primary ingredient in the safe practice of any sporting activity. Aerobic activity has proven effective in reducing the risk of cardiovascular disease and in the treatment of conditions such as sleep disorders, pulmonary and cardiac reconditioning, and anxiety and stress disorders.

FLEXIBILITY ▼

Flexibility refers to the ability of a joint to move freely and painlessly through its range of motion (ROM). A certain suppleness in the soft tissues (muscles, fascia, tendons, and skin) and joints provides the flexibility and mobility necessary for an individual to perform the movements of everyday life. Flexibility may be restricted because of prolonged immobility or positioning, trauma, disease, inflammation, or genetic tendencies. If full motion is restricted, the adaptive tendencies of the body will cause the soft tissues or joints to tighten and mobility becomes reduced. When joint mobility is reduced by decreased extensibility of muscle or other tissues crossing the joint, it is termed **contracture.** There are several types of contractures depending on the soft tissues they affect. Soft tissues include muscle, connective tissues, and the skin. Muscle contracture is the adaptive shortening of the musculotendinous unit resulting in "tight" muscles. Contractures in the connective tissues are the result of fibrosis from chronic inflammation. Fibrotic adhesions between the layers of fascia greatly reduce motion. Contractures also develop from scar tissue and related adhesions that can affect the mobility of muscles, tendons, joint capsules, or the skin.

Elasticity and Plasticity

Two important properties of contractile and noncontractile tissue that relate to flexibility are plasticity and elasticity. **Elasticity** refers to the tissue's ability to return to normal resting length when a stress that has been placed on it is removed. **Plasticity** refers to the tissue's ability to adapt to ongoing stresses and conditions. It is the plastic property of tissues that cause reduced flexibility with immobility and increased flexibility with a program of maintained stretching.

Muscle tissue has the ability to contract when stimulated, relax and return to its resting length when the stimulation ceases, and to be passively stretched. Muscle has a high degree of elasticity. When a muscle is immobile or used only through a shortened range of movement, adaptive changes will restrict the muscle's ability to lengthen beyond its accustomed range. This is due to the plastic property of muscle tissue.

Connective tissue is a fibrous noncontractile tissue made up of collagen fibers, elastin fibers, and reticulin fibers in a ground substance matrix. Collagen fibers give connective tissue its tensile strength. Elastin fibers provide the elastic properties. Reticulin fibers mostly provide bulk. In various forms and proportions, connective tissue makes up tendons, ligaments, fascia, scar tissue, and bones. The organization of the collagen and elastin fibers and the ratio of fibers to matrix relate directly to the plastic and elastic properties of the connective tissue.

Bone has a highly organized structure impregnated with minerals. It is the least plastic or elastic of the structures of the body. Long-term stresses, however, will cause deformation. For example, long-term imbalance in the muscles supporting the spine will result in a curvature of the spine and changes in the shape of the vertebrae.

The fibers in ligaments and tendons are dense and highly organized. They have a very high tensile strength but are supple and will elongate minimally with a maintained stretch or shorten if immobilized.

Fascia has an elaborate network of fibers in a loose matrix of ground substance that permeates every level of the muscle tissue. The fascia supplies the supportive structure that organizes the muscle fibers and connects them to the tendons and bones so that the contraction of the muscle fiber translates into the resultant action. Because of its multilayered and relatively loose structure, fascia has the highest elastic and plastic properties.

The normal suppleness of the skin allows for unrestricted range of motion. Scar tissue from severe burns or lacerations may result in tightness and a limitation of motion.

Scar tissue forms as injured tissue heals. Collagen fibers in scar tissue are abundant and random. Scar tissue that forms in immobilized tissue is thick and has little plasticity or elasticity. Studies indicate that if soft tissues are mobilized as scar tissue is forming, the healed tissue will be stronger, more pliable, and resilient.

FLEXIBILITY EXERCISES ▼

Exercises that maintain or increase flexibility are important whether an individual is immobile and recuperating from injury or illness or is a highly trained athlete. Flexibility exercises vary depending on the situation and condition of the user. Types of flexibility exercises include:
• Range of motion
  Passive ROM
  Active ROM

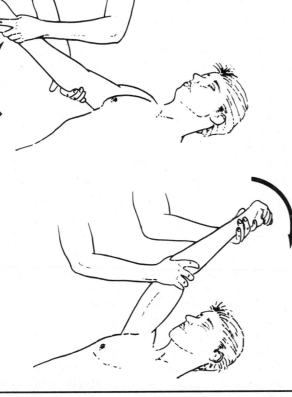

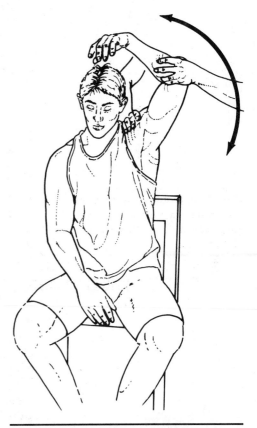

Fig. 18.6a Apply passive range of motion to the shoulder by supporting the arm and moving it without any assistance from the client.

Fig. 18.6b Passively circumduct the arm through its full range of motion.

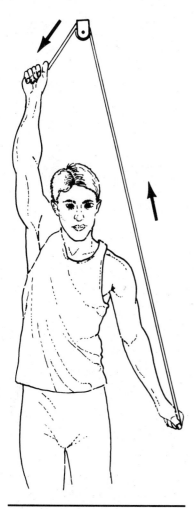

Fig. 18.6c A pulley and rope can be used to move one arm passively by actively moving the other.

- Stretching exercises
    Passive stretching
    Therapist-assisted stretching
    Mechanical-assisted stretching
    Self-stretching
    Active stretching.

Range of Motion

Range of motion exercises are carried out by moving the affected segment of the body through its available movement. The intent of ROM exercise is to maintain existing soft tissue and joint mobility and prevent the formation of contractures or restrictions that tend to form as the result of immobility or trauma. Range of motion exercises may be used to determine where limitations of movement exist but do not challenge those limitations in order to increase ROM. ROM exercises that travel beyond movement limits in order to increase ROM are technically stretching exercises and will be discussed later.

Passive range of motion is the movement of a body segment through its available ROM by some external force without the voluntary contractions of the muscles acting on that segment. The external force may be mechanical, from a therapist or another part of the individual's body. During passive range of motion exercises, the client neither assists nor resists as the body part is moved through its free range of motion. The free range of motion is the available movement that is not forced and is pain free (Fig. 18.6a to c, beginning page 593).

Active range of motion exercises are performed when the individual voluntarily contracts the muscles to move the body segment through its range. If the individual's muscles are unable to move the body part, assistance may be provided by a therapist. Active range of motion helps to maintain muscle contractility and elasticity, circulation, and neuromuscular coordination (Fig. 18.7).

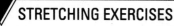

STRETCHING EXERCISES

Stretching exercises are effective in overcoming limitations of movement, especially if those limitations are the result of soft tissue shortening or tightness. The goal of stretching exercise is the elongation of soft tissue in order to maintain or increase full range of motion. Most stretching occurs in the muscle either as a result of neuromuscular changes or plastic changes in the connective tissue.

Neurologic changes are the result of the resetting of the myotatic **stretch reflex.** Sensory receptors responsible for the myotatic reflex are the **spindle cells** in the muscle and the **Golgi tendon organs** (GTO) near the musculo-tendinous junction. Muscle spindle cells monitor the velocity and extent of muscle movement. If a muscle is lengthening too far or too fast, a reflex contraction of the muscle will stop the movement to protect the muscle. The GTO senses the amount of tension placed on the tendon. Excessive tension on a tendon causes a reflex that inhibits the muscle, thereby unloading the tension and protecting the muscle and tendon from injury.

Ballistic Stretching versus Sustained Stretching

Ballistic stretches employ rapid, bouncing movements against the end of the normal ROM. They are high-velocity, high-intensity movements of low duration. These movements tend to fire the myotatic reflex, causing muscle contraction, and may force connective tissue structures beyond their elastic limits. The firing of the stretch reflex actually increases muscle tension and increases the possibility of injury to the muscle. Moving beyond the elastic limits of the connective tissue may result in injury to tendons, ligaments, or fascia. Whereas this type of activity might be appropriate for a specific sport that requires dynamic, explosive movement, it is not recommended for general stretching activities. Except for the highly trained athlete, ballistic stretches are the least beneficial form of stretching. They are counter-productive for muscle lengthening and because of the potential of tissue damage are unsafe.

Sustained stretching uses slow, gradual movement to challenge gently the limitations at the edge of the range of motion. The low-intensity, long-duration technique allows for adaptive changes to take place within the tissues and results in better flexibility. Sustained stretching suppresses the stretch reflex. The discharge from the spindle cells is reduced due to the slow movement. The gentle stretch to the GTO causes the muscle to be inhibited and relax even more. Stretching in this manner encourages the plastic elongation of connective tissue with less chance of injury.

Passive Stretching

Passive stretching is applied to move body segments beyond their free range of motion while the muscles that act on that segment remain as relaxed as possible. Passive stretching may be done by an individual alone, using the weight of gravity or another body part to produce the stretch, or the stretching may be applied by another individual.

In manual passive stretching, another person or therapist moves the client's body into the stretching positions. The therapist controls the force, direction, speed, and duration of the stretch. To perform this type of stretching safely, the therapist must be knowledgeable of the physiology and kinesthetics of the involved structures. The therapist must maintain close communication with the client and stay within the client's pain and comfort tolerances. The client should remain as relaxed as possible as the body part is moved through its range to the point of tightness and then just

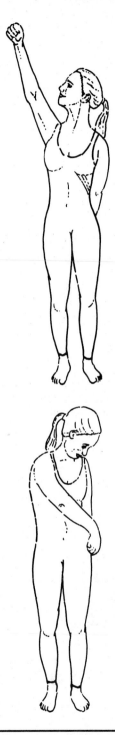

Fig. 18.7 During active range of motion, the client participates by contracting the muscles associated with the involved body part.

beyond. The force used must be enough to put tension on the structures but not enough to cause pain or injury. The client should feel a sense of pulling or tightness in the tissues that are being stretched, but not pain. Manual stretches are generally held for fifteen to thirty seconds and repeated several times (Fig. 18.8a to f).

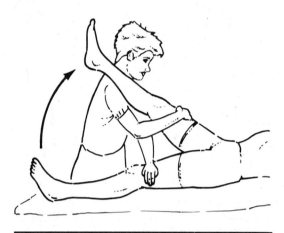

Fig. 18.8a In passive manual stretching, the therapist moves the body part into a stretching position while the client remains relaxed.

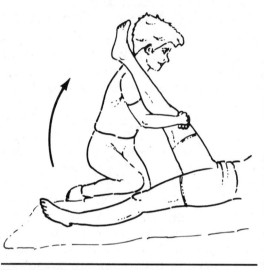

Fig. 18.8b Positioning to stretch the hamstrings and increase hip flexion.

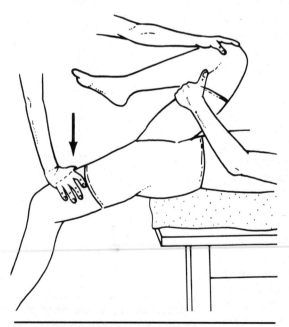

Fig. 18.8c Positioning to stretch the iliopsoas muscle and increase hip exertion.

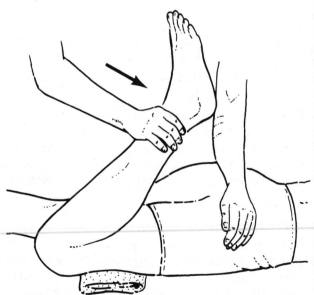

Fig. 18.8d Positioning to stretch the quadriceps and increase knee flexion.

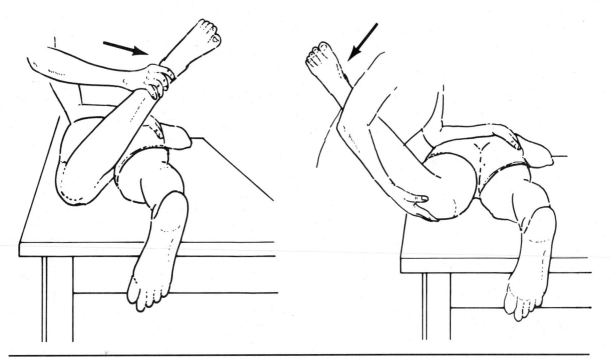

Fig. 18.8e Positioning to increase internal and external rotation of the hip.

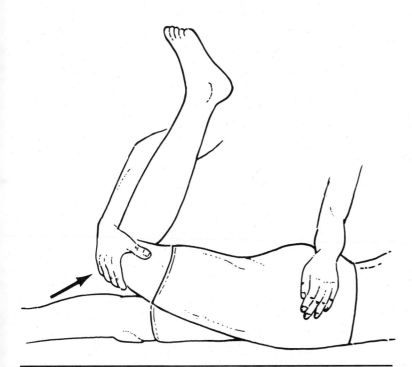

Fig. 18.8f Positioning to increase hip hyperextension with client lying prone.

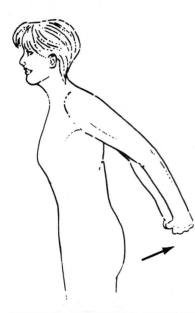

Fig. 18.9a Self-stretching of the anterior shoulder.

Self-Stretching Exercises

Self-stretching exercises are flexibility exercises the client does on his or her own. By using positioning, gravity, or other parts of the body to supply an external force, the client is able to stretch different parts of the body. The same guidelines concerning intensity, duration, and pain apply to self-stretching as apply to manual stretching exercises (Fig. 18.9a to h).

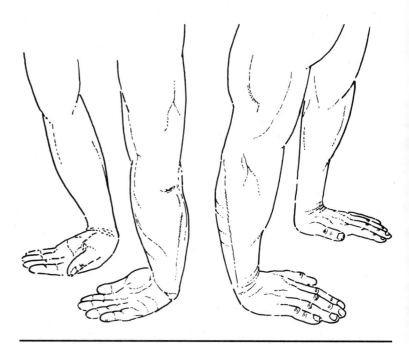

Fig. 18.9c The wrists are stretched in flexion and extension by putting them on a flat surface and increasing the angle to the point of a gentle stretch.

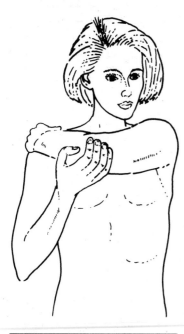

Fig. 18.9b Stretching the posterior shoulder by using the other hand to increase the stretch.

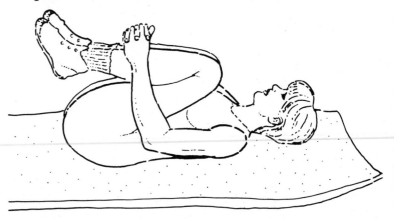

Fig. 18.9d The low back is stretching by pulling both legs gently to the chest.

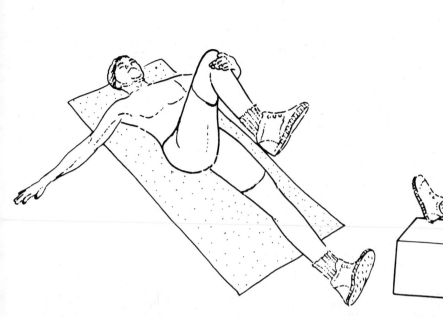

Fig. 18.9e Pulling one knee to the chest stretches the muscles of the low back and hips.

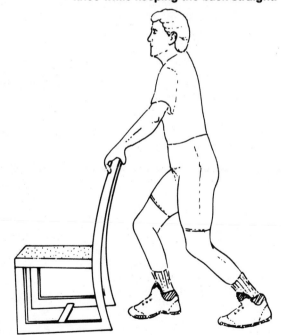

Fig. 18.9f The hamstrings are stretched by raising a straight leg and bringing the chest toward the knee while keeping the back straight.

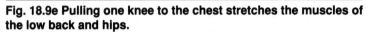

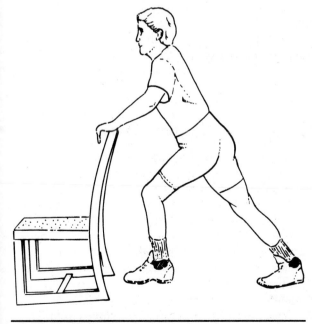

Fig. 18.9g Dorsal flexing the ankle with a straight knee stretches the gastrocnemius.

Fig. 18.9h Dorsal flexing the ankle while flexing the knee stretches the soleus muscle.

Active Stretching

Active stretching refers to techniques that utilize neuromuscular reflexes to enhance the elongation of muscles when they are stretched. These techniques reflexively inhibit the tension in the contractile tissue just previous to its being stretched. The techniques were originally associated with proprioceptive neuromuscular facilitation.

Contract-relax

There are three variations of the reflexive inhibition technique. They are contract-relax, antagonist contract, and contract-relax-contract the opposite,

The **contract-relax** technique works on the premise that as soon as a strong muscle contraction releases, the muscle is inhibited and relaxes.

To perform the contract-relax technique:

1. Position the limb so that the target muscle is in a lengthened but comfortable position. This can be done by moving the limb to the point of resistance and then backing off slightly.
2. Support the limb in that position securely and have the client contract the target muscle isometrically against the resistance for five to ten seconds. It is not necessary for the client to perform a maximal contraction. A contraction of 30 to 50 percent is adequate for this procedure. The contraction should not be painful. If the contraction is painful, try the antagonist-contraction procedure discussed next.
3. Instruct the client to relax the muscle.
4. As soon as the client relaxes, move the limb farther into the stretch until resistance is encountered.
5. Back off of the resistance slightly and repeat the procedure.

Antagonist Contraction

Antagonist contraction takes advantage of a physiological process known as **reciprocal inhibition.** When a muscle acting on a joint contracts, the muscle that causes the opposite action is reflexively inhibited. To perform the antagonist contraction technique:

1. Position the limb so that the target muscle is in a lengthened but comfortable position. This can be done by moving the limb to the point of resistance and then backing off slightly.
2. Support the limb securely in that position and instruct the client to attempt to continue the movement. Resist the movement for a couple of seconds and then allow the movement to continue slowly.
3. After about ten seconds, instruct the client to relax.
4. When the client relaxes, gently resume the stretch until resistance is encountered.
5. Back off of the resistance slightly and repeat the procedure.

Contract-Relax-Contract the Opposite

This technique essentially combines the two previous techniques. To perform **contract-relax-contract the opposite** technique:

1. Position the limb so that the target muscle is in a lengthened but comfortable position. This can be done by moving the limb to the point of resistance and then backing off slightly.
2. Support the limb in that position securely and have the client contract the target muscle isometrically against the resistance for five to ten seconds.
3. Instruct the client to relax the muscle and then contract the muscle opposite the tight muscle (the antagonist). In so doing the client actively moves the limb in the direction of the intended stretch. The therapist may or may not assist in the final stretch.
4. After a short rest, repeat the procedure.

COORDINATION EXERCISES

Coordination refers to the complex neuromuscular process of using the correct sequence of muscular movements with the right timing and force. Motor patterns are organized through the central nervous system to produce smooth and efficient movement. Coordination is necessary to perform skills of daily living (walking, eating, etc.) as well as the most complicated learned physical procedures (gymnastics, skiing, typing, etc.). Skills become more automatic as they are practiced repeatedly with positive reinforcement. Improving coordination and skill requires practice and repetition. To learn or improve a skill, or to become more coordinated in the practice of a skill,

• Break the skill into its component parts.
• Slowly practice each part.
• Repeat the skill component, thinking it through each time and then performing it.
• Increase the speed.
• As you become proficient, add more components or practice their components and add them together.
• Repetitively practice the skill until proficient.

Many skills that initially required close concentration become automatic after extensive practice.

RELAXATION

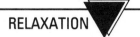

Relaxation is the process of relieving physiologic (muscular) and mental tension. Physical exercise is beneficial for general relaxation because the muscular and mental activity relieves built-up tension. Therapeutic relaxation exercise is a conscious effort of becoming aware of and controlling mental and muscular tension. Conscious relaxation is often coupled with deep breathing to facilitate and enhance the state of relaxation.

One effective relaxation technique utilizes the post-contraction inhibition theory that a muscle will relax after a muscle contraction. To practice the technique:

1. Assume a comfortable position (either a reclining or a supported seated position).
2. Take two or three deep releasing breaths.
3. Contract the muscles of the foot for two to three seconds and then relax those muscles. As you contract and relax the muscles, continue to breath in a deep relaxed manner. *Do not hold the breath.*
4. Contract the muscles of the lower leg for two to three seconds and then relax those muscles.
5. Contract the muscles of the thigh for two to three seconds and then relax those muscles.
6. Repeat the procedure for the other leg.
7. Repeat a similar process for the hand, forearm, upper arm, and shoulder.
8. Continue to systematically contract and relax the muscles of the upper, mid, and low back, and the muscles of the abdomen, chest, neck.
9. Contract and relax the muscles of the jaw, cheeks, and around the eyes and the forehead.
10. After systematically contracting and relaxing all the muscles of the body, continue breathing deeply and be consciously aware of the relaxed state of the entire body.

This exercise takes ten to twenty minutes. It can be used as a relaxing break in a busy day or as an exercise to induce sleep for those who have difficulty winding down at bedtime.

Relaxation is an important part of a healthy life style. Physical exercise, recreation activities, and relaxation techniques can be incorporated into everyone's agenda to balance out life's stress and tension and provide for a better quality of life.

Stress-Reducing Exercises

An excellent way to reduce stress is to have a vigorous daily workout, but are times when it is just as important to take a few minutes to do relaxing exercises. Many executives have found relaxation exercises the best way to combat stress and tensions when they are required to maintain a stressful schedule with few opportunities for relaxation. The following exercises can be done while sitting at a desk or standing. The exercises release tension and revitalize the body.

1. Deep breathing. Inhale slowly for ten counts. Hold the breath for 5 counts. Exhale slowly for ten counts. Hold the breath out for five counts. Repeat the exercise at least ten times.

2. Toe to head relaxation. Sit in a comfortable chair and concentrate on relaxing the feet and ankles. Systematically relax adjacent parts of the body from the toes to the head.

3. Remove shoes and then rotate the feet inward for ten counts, then outward for ten counts. Point the toes and stretch the arches for five counts. Bring the toes toward the knees, and hold for five counts. Repeat the exercise several times.

4. Sit erect with shoulders thrown back. Rotate the shoulders forward and back several times.

5. Rotate the head first to the right and then to the left several times.

6. Close the eyes and massage the temples with the fingertips. Make circular movements for ten counts.

YOGA FOR BALANCE AND RELAXATION ▼

Hatha yoga is a form of exercise that combines mental concentration, muscular control, breathing, and relaxation in the performance of a series of postures and body positions. A yoga routine is effective in stretching and balancing the muscles of the body. When practiced regularly, yoga improves the posture, relaxes and tones the muscles, and relieves mental and physiological stress. It increases stamina and imparts a sense of physical and mental balance. Teachers of yoga recommend that a person practice moderation in eating and drinking. Western culture has borrowed many of these exercises from India (their point of origin), where they are practiced as a way of life with spiritual overtones.

It is important for the person seriously interested in yoga to study the postures with a proficient teacher. Some postures are very strenuous and may cause strain or bodily damage if not practiced correctly.

The following are just a few yoga exercises the average person may include in his or her daily exercise routine.

1. **Posterior stretching pose:** Sit on the floor with the feet extended. Catch hold of or touch the right big toe with the right hand and the left big toe with the left hand. Bring the chest forward and toward the knees to stretch and tone the back and leg muscles. While breathing deeply, fall forward over the knees (Fig. 18.10).

2. **Cobra pose:** Lie on the floor face down. Place the palms of the hands flat on the floor under the shoulders and raise the chest while bending the back as much as possible. Hold the pose, while breathing evenly, for about ten seconds. Relax, and then repeat the exercise several times. *Caution*: The spine should not be forced and the pubic bone should stay on the floor (Fig. 18.11).

3. **Bow pose:** Lie face down on the floor and then reach back and grasp the ankles, curving the back. While breathing

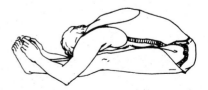

Fig. 18.10 Posterior stretching pose.

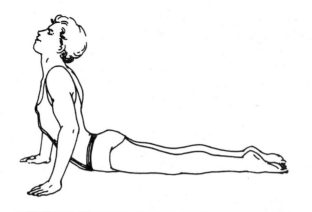

Fig. 18.11 Cobra pose.

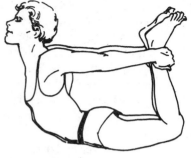

Fig. 18.12 Bow pose.

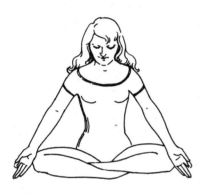

Fig. 18.13 The easy sitting pose.

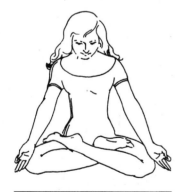

Fig. 18.14 The lotus pose.

evenly, hold the position for five to ten counts. Relax and repeat several times. This exercise is excellent for strengthening the back, chest, and abdominal muscles (Fig. 18.12).

4. **The easy sitting pose:** Sit on the floor with the right leg bent at the knee and the right foot placed under the left thigh. The left leg is bent at the knee and the left foot is placed under the right thigh. The arms are extended, palms up. The spine is held erect. Breathe deeply from the diaphragm, making inhalations and exhalations the same length. This pose is used for concentration and meditation (Fig. 18.13).

5. **The lotus pose:** This pose should not be attempted unless the body is quite supple. The right leg is bent and the right foot placed on the left thigh close to the hip joint. The sole of the foot is turned upward. The other foot is placed on the right thigh with the ankles crossed. The arms are extended, palms up at the sides of the body. Again, breathing should be deep and from the diaphragm. This pose is used for concentration and meditation. There are a number of yoga poses and positions the client may want to learn. With all yoga exercises, proper, controlled breathing is encouraged (Fig. 18.14).

▼ BREATHING EXERCISES

By means of respiration, oxygen, which is essential to life, is taken into the system, and carbon dioxide is given off. A healthy person breathes approximately 12,000 to 20,000 times in a 24-hour period. The following is a brief description of the respiratory forces.

Inspiration is the act of inhaling, or breathing inward, while expiration is the act of exhaling, or breathing outward. Ordinary inspiration takes place because of the contraction of a muscle called the diaphragm. When the diaphragm contracts, its sides collapse, and it flattens into the abdominal cavity. This contracting motion causes the thorax to enlarge downward and the abdominal walls to expand during inspiration. During deep or forced inspiration, other muscles work to increase the chest capacity by expanding and elevating the rib cage. The muscles that elevate the ribs and enlarge the thorax are the intercostals, the scaleni, and the levatores costarum.

Ordinary expiration is brought about by the elastic recoil of the diaphragm and lung tissue, the stretching of the costal cartilages, and the action of the abdominal muscles.

The main benefits of deep breathing exercises are:

1. To keep the lungs healthy by maintaining their natural elasticity
2. To increase the intake of oxygen and the giving off of carbon dioxide
3. To improve the function of all internal organs
4. To benefit circulation and nourishment of the body.

The client will find deep-breathing exercises beneficial and should observe the following rules for proper breathing:

1. It is important to breathe with the mouth closed. The nasal cavities warm the air as it enters. Also, the small hairs and mucous membrane are constructed to catch any small, impure particles of dust in the air and prevent them from entering the lungs. If the client has an obstruction that prevents normal breathing through the nasal passages, he or she should consult a physician without delay.
2. Deep-breathing exercises should be done in the fresh air (out doors) when possible. Deep breathing is most beneficial when done with active exercises. An example is raising the arms and inhaling, then exhaling while lowering the arms to the sides.
3. The client may not understand the meaning of diaphragmatic (deep) breathing and may be breathing in a shallow manner. Have the client place a hand just above the waistline and inhale deeply. The abdominal region should expand as the lungs are filled with air. The client should then exhale slowly to feel the abdominal region contract as air is expelled from the lungs.

Proper breathing is an asset in developing a speaking and singing voice and is an aid to relaxation of tension. The following exercises can be done lying down or standing:

1. Inhale slowly while raising the arms forward, with palms down, to a straight position directly overhead. Exhale slowly as the arms are returned to the sides of the body. Repeat the exercise five to ten times.
2. Inhale while lifting the shoulders as high as possible toward the ears. Exhale slowly while rolling the shoulders backward

and down to a normal relaxed position. Repeat five to ten times.

3. Place a hand on the diaphragm (area above the abdomen), and pant quickly five to ten times.
4. Use the forefinger to close one nostril, inhale slowly and deeply, and then exhale. Repeat the exercise on the other nostril. Continue breathing in this manner for several minutes.

▼ POSTURE IMPROVEMENT

Posture refers to the relationship and alignment of body parts to one another and is usually observed in the standing position. Normal posture is different for different people depending on their personalities, environmental situations, and many other genetic and physiological conditions.

Good posture is observable when the body is balanced between left and right, back and front, and the segments of the axial skeleton are properly aligned. When the posture is in equilibrium, the line of gravity will pass through the center of each segment and the base. The farther the line is from the center of each, the more strain will be generated in the muscles and connective tissue in order to maintain the faulty posture (Fig. 18.15a and b).

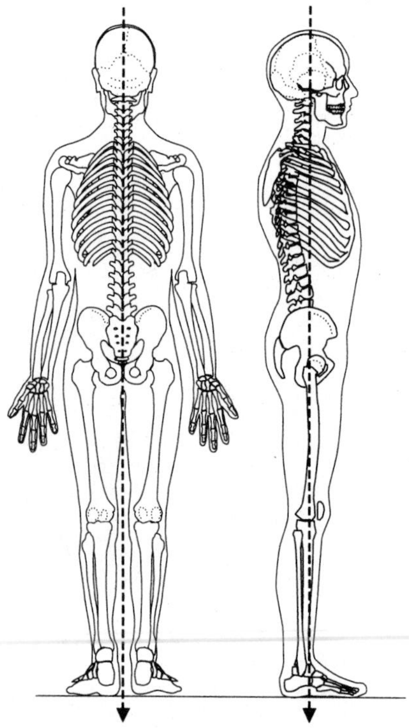

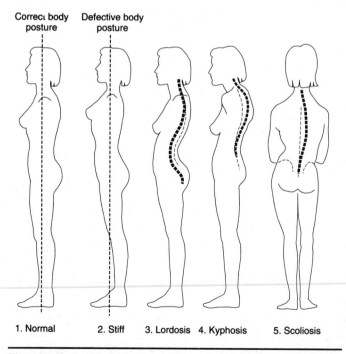

Fig. 18.15a Good posture is indicated if a plumb line passes through the middle of each body segment and the base.

Fig. 18.15b Body postures. 1. Normal erect posture. 2. Stiff rigid posture. 3. Swayback (lordosis). 4. Humped shoulders (kyphosis). 5. Deviation of the spine (scoliosis).

Poor posture habits cause fatigue and strain on the muscles, joints, and spinal column. In addition, they cause the figure of a man or woman to appear older. Good posture helps to prevent backaches, fatigue, sagging muscles, and internal problems such as constipation and poor circulation. Good posture also improves appearance in clothes and imparts a sense of well-being.

The client will welcome a few lessons in posture improvement. These basic instructions can be given before the beginning of regular exercises. Posture problems can be detected better if the client is wearing close-fitting garments such as leotards or shorts and T-shirt. The following are indications of poor posture:

- The shoulders are tense and held high and the arms appear stiff.
- Knees are locked, causing the back to sway and the shoulders to droop.
- The back sways into an inward curving, causing the hips to protrude. The head is held forward, causing the shoulders to be rounded.

Any lateral deviation of the spine may indicate scoliosis and should be brought to the attention of a physician.

Posture Correction Exercises

When teaching posture correction, have the client stand before a full-length mirror with a side view of the body. While looking over the shoulder into the mirror, the client should be able to detect posture faults that need attention. Normal erect posture does not mean stiff, rigid positions, whether standing, sitting, or walking. Good posture is relaxed, yet controlled. Check the following points:

1. When standing and walking, the weight should be distributed evenly on the feet and not excessively on the heels or the toes.
2. When walking or standing, the knees should be kept slightly flexed. Stiff knees throw the body off balance.
3. To align the body properly, the head should be lifted up from the waistline and the upper body balanced over the pelvic area. There should be no sagging of the shoulders or midsection of the body, nor should the shoulders be held too high or thrust back.

The client should be encouraged to practice walking, standing, and sitting with correct body alignment until the correct posture feels natural and comfortable.

Exercises for Strength, Balance, and Coordination

Among the factors that affect posture is the stability and position of the pelvis. The angle and tilt of the pelvis is reflected in the stability and curvature of the spine. Deviations in the position of the pelvis may be due to pathologhical conditions (short leg, trauma, deformities, etc.). More often they are due to imbalances or weaknesses in the musculature that acts on or stabilizes the pelvis (that is, the muscles of the hips and trunk) (Fig. 18.16).

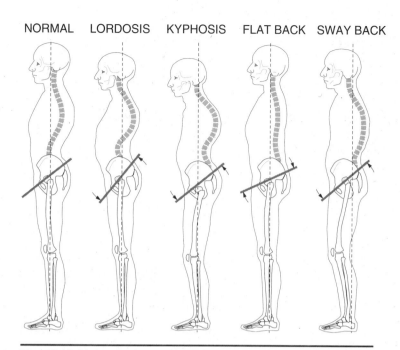

NORMAL   LORDOSIS   KYPHOSIS   FLAT BACK   SWAY BACK

Fig. 18.16 Abdominal postural deviations in relation to the tilt of the pelvis.

The best exercises for correcting faulty posture and for strengthening the back are exercises that stretch and strengthen the hip and trunk muscles. The following exercises will improve coordination and will strengthen the legs and trunk (Figs. 18.17 to 18.28).

Exercise 1—The Demi-Knee-Bend Exercise for Posture

Fig. 18.17a Starting position— Place a hand on the back of a chair or side of a door for balance (ballet dancers use a barre). The feet are placed in a comfortable stride slightly apart. The hips are kept tucked under as the pelvic area is lifted up and forward.

Fig. 18.17b The body is slowly lowered as if to sit on the heels. This takes about 4 to 6 counts. The body is raised slowly back to a standing position. The exercise should be repeated about 4 times then increased as client becomes more comfortable and the muscles of the legs and back becomes stronger.

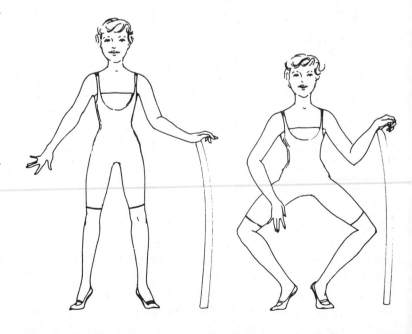

Exercise 2—Wall slide

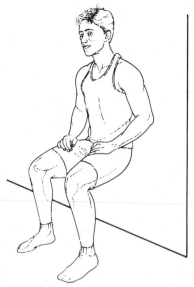

Fig. 18.18 Lean back against a wall with the feet about 14 to 16 inches from the baseboard. Slide down the wall, keeping the back flat against the wall until the thighs are about parallel to the floor. Hold the position for three to five minutes. This exercise strengthens the muscles of the thighs and hips to improve support of the spine.

Exercise 3—Rotating arm swing

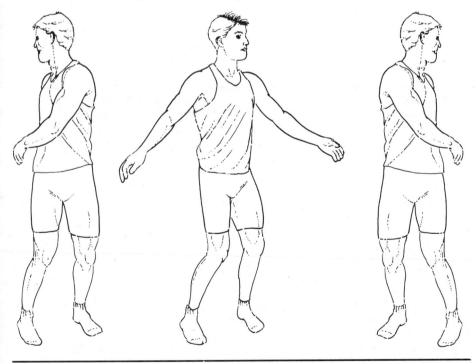

Fig. 18.19 Stand with the feet about hip width apart and the knees slightly flexed. Rotate the head and shoulders rhythmically to the right, then to the left as far as possible, while keeping the knees slightly flexed and the hips facing forward. Keep the arms relaxed as they swing all the way around the body, first to one side then the other. This exercise stretches the ligaments and rotating muscles of the spine.

Exercise 4—Exercise for Stretching the Waist and Back

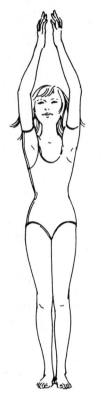

Fig. 18.20a Starting position: Stand erect with the feet in a comfortable stride with both hands overhead.

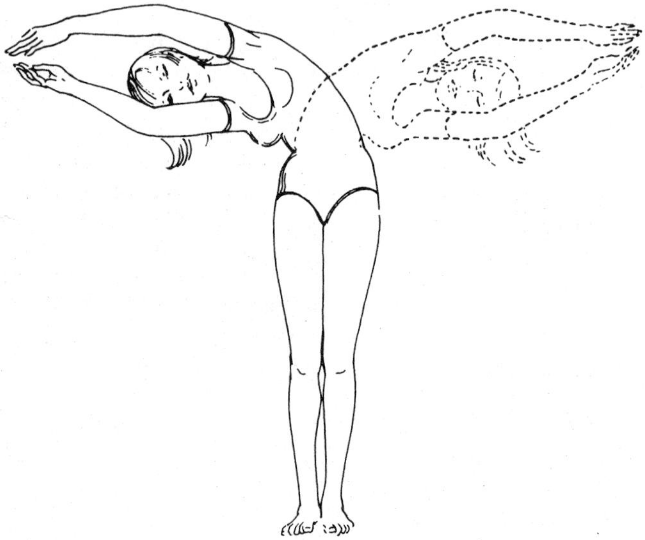

Fig. 18.20b First count: Keeping the hands together, twist the upper body toward the right. Second count: return to the erect position. Third count: Lean the upper body to the left. Fourth count: Return to the erect position. Repeat this exercise combination five to ten times or more as strength increases.

Exercise 5—Abdominal Curls

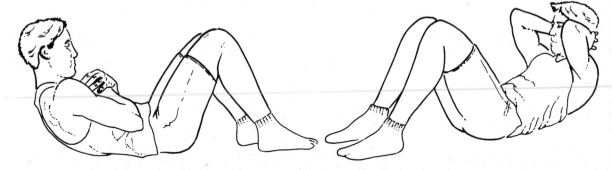

Fig. 18.21 Increased strength in the abdominal muscles help stabilize the spine. Abdominal curls can be done with the arms folded across the chest or behind the head. Lift the head until the shoulders are lifted from the floor. Hold the position for a second and relax to the floor. Repeat.

Exercise 6—Diagonal Curls

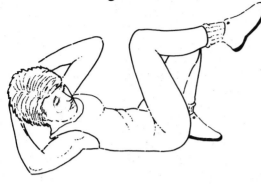

Fig. 18.22 Diagonal abdominal curls increase the strength in the abdominal oblique muscles. The exercise is the same as abdominal curls except that when lifting the shoulders from the floor, one shoulder is pulled toward the opposite knee. On the next repetition, the other shoulder is pulled toward the opposite knee.

Exercise 7—Leg Swings

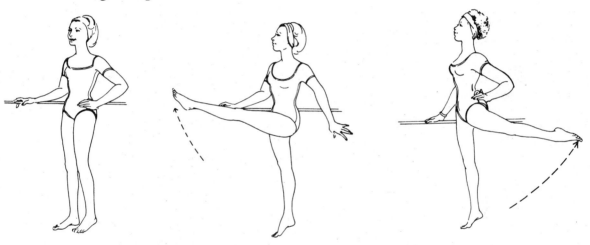

Fig. 18.23 Leg swings lengthen and strengthen the hip flexors and extensors while increasing hip flexibility. Place one hand on the back of a chair or the wall for support. Lift the opposite leg as far up in front as possible. Swing that leg down and up in back as far as possible. Swing the leg backward and forward several times. Turn around and repeat the exercise on the other leg.

Exercise 8— All-Fours Leg and Arm Extensions

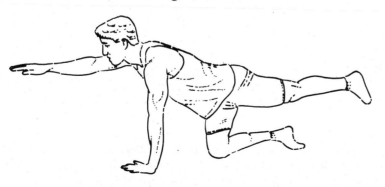

Fig. 18.24 This exercise tones postural muscles, improves balance, and helps stabilize the spine. Starting position: hands and knees. First count, extend one arm above the head and parallel to the floor and at the same time extend the opposite leg straight back and parallel to the floor. Keep the hips level. Hold the position for a count of five. Return to a hands and knees position and follow the same procedure with the opposite arm and leg. Repeat several times.

Exercise 9—Bicycle on the Back

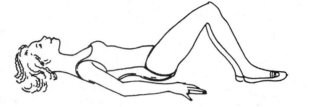

Fig. 18.25a Starting position: Lie flat on the back, with knees bent and feet flat on the floor. Keep arms down at sides.

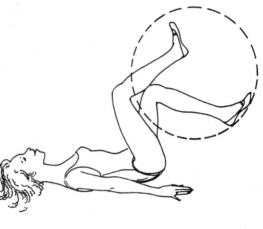

Fig. 18.25b First count. Lift both legs and perform a bicycling movement with both legs, making larger circles. Continue this exercise for fifty counts. Reverse the movement, making larger and larger circles with both legs. Repeat for fifty counts.

Exercise 10—Back Extensions

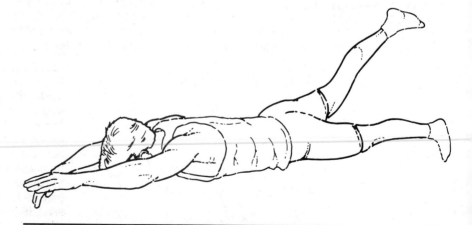

Fig. 18.26 Lie face down with both hands extended above the head. Lift one arm and the opposite leg off the floor as far as possible and hold for a count of five. Relax, then do the other arm and leg. Repeat several times.

Exercise 11—Lumbar Twist

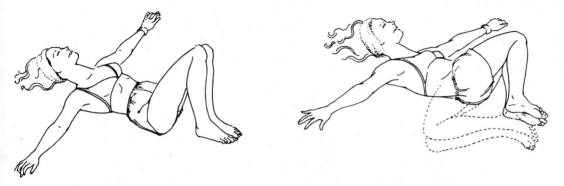

Fig. 18.27 Lie flat on the back with the arms down to the sides and the knees bent so the feet are flat on the floor. Exhale as both knees drop to the floor to one side. Inhale and bring the knees back to the center. (Make sure the small of the back is pressed toward the floor.) Exhale as the knees drop the other side. Inhale and bring the knees back to center. Repeat moving the knees to one side and then the other in time with the breath. As the exercise is repeated, slowly move the extended arms out to the sides until they are extended above the head.

Exercise 12—Knee to Chest and Leg Extension

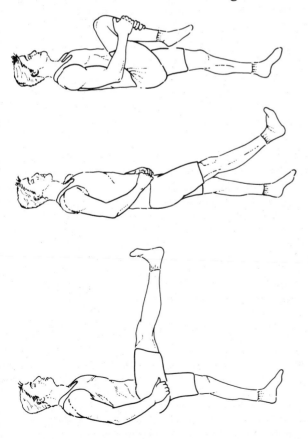

Fig. 18.28 Lie on the back and relax, taking several deep breaths. First count: Inhale deeply. Second count: Exhale and flex one knee and hip, grasping the knee and pulling it into the chest. Third count: Tense the muscles of the flexed leg, dorsal flex the foot. Inhale deeply as the tensed leg is extended to a position where the foot is about 16 to 18 inches above the floor. Count four: Exhale and relax the foot and leg to the table. Follow the same procedure on the other leg. Repeat the procedure 10 times. A variation is to extend the leg straight up toward the ceiling on the third count.

▼ PLANNING A PERSONAL FITNESS PROGRAM

There are numerous reasons to exercise. When planning an exercise program, the individual must look at the desired goals for exercising and develop a program that will result in meeting those goals. A well-rounded program will include all aspects of exercise with emphasis on those that best meet the needs of the individual. In review, the aspects of exercise are:

• Strength
• Endurance
• Flexibility
• Skill or coordination
• Relaxation.

It is important to begin the exercise routine with specific exercises that warm up the muscles and speed up the action of the heart and lungs. This is done to prepare the body for more strenuous exercises. It is important to wear appropriate exercise clothing and to prime the muscles before a workout.

Following warm-up exercises, circulatory exercises may be done to stimulate and strengthen the circulatory and respiratory systems. They are done at a fairly fast pace and include such exercises as running, dancing, jumping, and skipping rope. Strengthening exercises might follow to tone and strengthen the abdomen, back, leg, arms, and other major muscle groups. Strengthening exercises are those that contract muscles against sufficient resistance to overload the muscle. They are usually done slowly as in isotonic exercises or presses and lifts.

Cooling-down exercises are important in preventing sore, stiff muscles. Such exercises might include walking, stretching, and slow dancing exercises.

Basic rules for exercise:

1. All machines and apparatus used in the exercise program should be in safe condition and the client should be instructed in how to use them correctly.
2. A clean towel or mat should be used to sit or lie on the floor for exercises.
3. Wear the appropriate clothing and shoes.
4. The instructor or trainer should question the client about his or her health before determining a specific exercise routine.
5. Do not to eat a heavy meal directly before exercising.
6. Use proper breathing techniques.
7. Types of exercises and benefits should be understood before beginning the exercise routine.
8. Allow short rest periods between exercises.
9. Warm up before strenuous exercises and cool down following them.

10. Regulate the exercise period according to the your strength and endurance.
11. Keep a record of the exercise program in order to monitor progress.

QUESTIONS FOR DISCUSSION AND REVIEW

1. Why should the individual consult with a physician and an exercise specialist before beginning an exercise program?
2. List the major benefits of exercise.
3. Define therapeutic exercise.
4. List the major goals of therapeutic exercise.
5. Why is it necessary to have a consultation with the client before suggesting an exercise regimen?
6. Describe the overload principle.
7. What is strength and how is it measured?
8. What are two main factors that determine the strength of a muscle?
9. What is hypertrophy?
10. What is an isometric contraction?
11. What is an isotonic contraction?
12. What is an eccentric contraction?
13. What is a concentric contraction?
14. What is the advantage of variable resistance exercises?
15. List six methods of providing resistance for strength training exercises.
16. What is muscle endurance?
17. What is cardiorespiratory fitness?
18. What factors determine the effectiveness of an aerobic exercise program?
19. What are two methods for monitoring the intensity of an aerobic workout?
20. List the components of an aerobic workout.
21. Why is it important to do warm-up exercises before doing more strenuous ones?
22. Why are cooling exercises recommended following a brisk workout?
23. What is flexibility?
24. What is a contracture?
25. Define elasticity as it refers to soft tissue.
26. Define plasticity as it refers to soft tissue.
27. What is the difference between range of motion exercises and stretching exercises?
28. Why are ballistic stretches unsafe?
29. What type of exercises improve coordination and skill?
30. What is yoga?
31. How does yoga enhance well-being?
32. What are the differences between the posture problems lordosis, kyphosis, and scoliosis?

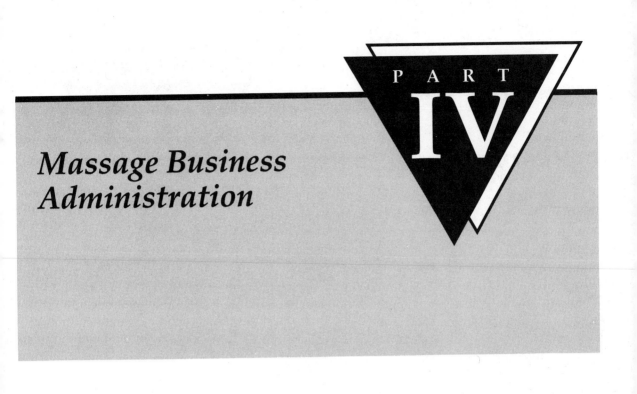

Massage Business Administration

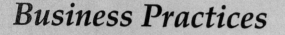

Business Practices

19

Learning Objectives

After you have mastered this chapter, you will be able to:

1. *Explain the relationship between attitude, self-image, and business success.*

2. *List the major expenses related to starting a massage business.*

3. *Explain the difference between a partnership, a corporation, and a sole proprietorship.*

4. *Explain the advantages and disadvantages of operating your own business.*

5. *List the various permits and licenses required to operate a massage business and where to obtain them.*

6. *List the types of insurance a massage business owner should carry to protect his or her business.*

7. *Describe a physical layout for a beginning business operation.*

8. *Explain the importance of business location to the success of a personal service business.*

9. *Explain why careful planning is important before opening a business.*

10. *Explain the application of rules of professionalism to business practice.*

11. *Explain why keeping accurate records is necessary in a successful business.*

12. *List the major ingredients of a basic bookkeeping system.*

13. *Explain the importance of marketing to business success.*

14. *Define target market.*

15. *Make a checklist of factors to consider before opening a business.*

INTRODUCTION ▼

As the emphasis on wellness and physical fitness continues to grow, there will be more business opportunities for ethical and well-trained massage practitioners. Whether the practitioner is self-employed, works as an employee, or aspires to managing a business, it is important to understand the responsibilities associated with doing business. The practitioner who understands business procedures is more likely to succeed because he or she will be more aware of the importance of good customer relations, more involved in the overall operation of the business, and more profit oriented.

The practitioner who wishes to gain valuable experience may look for employment in a health spa, on a cruise ship, in conjunction with a health facility, or as a freelance professional. An ambitious practitioner may choose to open his or her own business or occupy space within an established salon, clinic, or studio. Regardless of the environment in which the practitioner works, it is important to know something about business procedures. This includes keeping records for tax purposes, understanding laws and regulations, being familiar with insurance requirements, and much more.

ATTITUDE/SELF-IMAGE/PUBLIC IMAGE ▼

As a massage therapist, you are not only a healthcare practitioner, you are also a businessperson. To be a successful businessperson, a positive self image is essential. A positive self image means you feel good about who you are and what you are doing. A good self-image is a positive attitude reflected in the enthusiasm and quality exhibited in your work and other activities. There is a sense of excitement about what you are doing. Often this is accompanied by a desire to be involved and to learn more. A positive attitude and an inner knowledge that "I will attain my goals" is a major advantage in being successful.

A good self-image and a positive attitude are the foundation for creating a good public image. Your public image is the way you are perceived through your appearance, the way you do business, and how you interact with your clients and associates. Your public image relates to your reputation and the degree of professionalism with which you operate. Success is dependent on a good reputation, a good public image, and a high degree of professionalism.

▼ BUSINESS PLANNING

Business planning starts when a business is first conceived and continues throughout the life of the business. Planning is the first step in setting the stage for the development of the business. Planning involves clarifying your purpose, stating a mission, setting goals, and determining priorities.

A **mission statement** is a short general statement of the main focus of the business. Developing a mission statement requires careful consideration. The mission statement expresses the intent of the business and can be used on promotional material as a reflection of the business's public image.

A **purpose** is a theme that is derived from your dreams and ideals. You may have several purposes for doing business. Clarifying those purposes allows you to direct your energies toward those purposes.

Some examples of a purpose might be:

To provide a pleasant, environmentally friendly working environment

To make a positive difference for my clientele

To prosper and enjoy

Goals are specific, attainable, measurable things or accomplishments that you set and make a commitment to achieve. The business goals you set support your mission and reinforce your purpose. Setting goals clarifies your intentions and directs your creative energy toward realizing your dreams, toward success.

Goals may be short term or long term. You can have life-long goals, five-year goals, one-year goals, 6-month goals, goals for next week, goals for tomorrow, or goals for today. Although it is helpful to include a deadline with a goal, it is not necessary. Keep your goals personalized and in the present tense. Make your goals realistic and attainable but don't hesitate to think big. The more specific the goals are the better.

The following are some examples of goals:

- I will see twenty clients per week.
- I will attend the next National Convention.
- I will spend at least three evenings a week at home with my family.
- I will increase my income by 20 percent this year.

Develop a Strategic Plan

It is helpful to write your goals. Refer to them often to see how you are progressing. Setting goals is only a clarification of where you are heading. Once you set goals, it takes planning and commitment to realize them. Some goals are simple: "I will maintain my client files daily." Others are more complicated and have many subgoals contained within them. "I will increase my income be 20 percent this year." To accomplish the larger goal, it helps to break it into doable chunks, examine them, and develop a course of action.

List the benefits of attaining the goal. Brainstorm possible steps needed to reach the goal. Note potential obstacles or conflicts and solutions to those problems. Then develop a step-by-step plan of how to reach the goal. Include in the plan resources and timetables of what actions to take. Once the plan is formulated, *do it*!!

BEGINNING IN BUSINESS

As a business owner and manager, you must have knowledge of your field, good business sense, a sense of diplomacy, and clear business goals. In addition, you must keep accurate records and understand all business procedures involved in your kind of business. You can hire tax consultants and bookkeepers to do some of the more extensive work, but it is the owner who is responsible for the success of the business.

Most people who succeed in the personal service business gain experience by learning while working for someone else. They learn efficiency of management, motivating employees, promoting good customer relations, and numerous other business procedures. Once a practitioner has gained experience and knowledge, he or she may decide to start a business or look for an established business to buy or manage.

If you are beginning a new business, there are several things you must consider. What type of a business operation will it be? How will you finance the costs of equipment and other start-up costs before you can begin to generate income? Other considerations in starting a business are choosing a location, acquiring permits and licenses, and selecting adequate insurance coverage.

TYPES OF BUSINESS OPERATIONS

A business may be organized as a sole proprietor, a partnership, or a corporation. Each has advantages and disadvantages.

As a **sole proprietor** you are an individual owner and carry all expenses, obligations, liabilities, and assets. You would receive all profits from your business and be responsible for all losses. Business obligations and debts are the owner's personal responsibility. Legally as a sole proprietor, you and the business are one and the same in the eyes of the law. If the business gets too far into debt, or in legal trouble, you as an individual are liable. There is the potential for numerous tax advantages, but you must comply with all tax responsibilities including self-employment taxes. Many people prefer being a sole proprietor if they can handle the financial and personal responsibilities involved.

Most massage therapists are self-employed and are sole proprietors. Being self-employed means being your own boss and setting your own schedule. It also means you are responsible for the success or failure of your business. Being self-employed requires you to be self-motivated and disciplined. You are solely responsible for not only working with clients but also all promotional and operational activities.

A **partnership** may be the answer if you know someone who wants to invest and who is qualified to carry his or her share of the responsibility. The combined ability and experience of two people can make a business easier to operate. While a partnership can relieve a sole proprietor of the pressures of doing everything himself or herself, there are some drawbacks. A partnership is a relationship wrought with all the bonuses and misunderstanding of any interpersonal association.

One key to a good working partnership is a clear **partnership agreement**. Though it is not a legal requirement, a written partnership agreement will clarify the rights and responsibilities of each partner and strengthen the relationship. A partnership agreement should include the business goals, what each partner will contribute (money, material, and time), how the profits will be divided, and how the business will continue should one partner want out.

Legally in a partnership each partner carries the same responsibilities as a sole proprietor in the case of debt and liability. There are also certain tax regulations specific to partnerships. An accountant and a lawyer may be helpful if you are considering setting up a partnership.

A **corporation** has advantages and disadvantages. It is subject to regulation and taxation by the state, and a charter must be obtained from the state in which the business operates. Management of the corporation is in the hands of a board of directors who determine policies and make decisions in accordance with the charter. Stockholders share in profits but are not legally responsible for the actions of the corporation. Stockholders and corporate owners are not directly liable for lawsuits and debts against the corporation. However, as a professional, the corporation will not shield you from the liability of actions of gross negligence that result in a malpractice suit. If you are considering incorporating, consult with knowledgeable authorities to determine if it is worth the time, money, and effort it will take.

▼ START-UP COSTS AND NEEDS

The start up costs for beginning a business include all the expenses incurred before any revenues are collected. Those costs vary according to the size and complexity of the operation. Start-up costs are out-of-pocket expenses that must be considered during the planning stage and recovered before a profit is realized.

The two main reasons small businesses fail are undercapitalization and poor management. Most massage practitioners are self-employed. They work out of their home, a small office space, a space shared with another practitioner, or in conjunction with another healthcare provider (doctor, chiropractor, etc.). Regardless of where you locate your practice, there will be certain expenses in setting up your practice.

Start-up expenses may include:

- Rent or Lease: May include first and last month's rent and a cleaning/damage deposit

- Utilities: Hook-up charges and deposits for electric, gas, telephone; telephone answering service

- Equipment and supplies: Table, bolsters, therapy equipment, linens, massage oils, etc.

- Furniture: Desks, chairs, supply cabinets, music system, file cabinet, lighting, etc.

- Decorating supplies: Paint, curtains, plants, etc.

- Office supplies: Calculator, typewriter or computer, pens, staple gun, writing paper, filing supplies, appointment and receipt books, etc.

- Advertising expense: Ads and announcements, etc.

- Printing expense: Business cards, stationery, information forms, brochures, etc.

- Insurance and license costs

- Initial operating expense: Opening business checking account with enough capital to cover miscellaneous expenses until the business is up and running.

When planning a business operation, it is important to establish good credit and banking relations. Many businesspeople rely on getting business loans when necessary in order to have sufficient working capital. It usually takes time to build clientele, so money must be available to take care of necessary expenses. Always know where your money is being spent and operate with sufficient cash flow. A major cause of small business failure is the owner's inexperience in judging overhead expenses and having inadequate capital to carry the business through slow periods. As income and profits grow, the budget may be increased for expansion of facilities, advertising, and other areas of growth.

▼ BUSINESS LOCATION

Finding the right location for your massage practice will affect its success. A frequent cause of business failure is locating in an area that is wrong for that particular type of business. The building in which a personal service business is located should be in good condition and in a fairly prosperous location.

Choose a site that will accommodate your business needs, be pleasing to your clients, fit your image, and is properly zoned and within your budget. The office location must be easy to locate, with the address clearly visible from the street. It should be easily accessible and relatively quiet. An ideal space would have one or more massage rooms, a reception/waiting area, an office, and bathroom facilities with a shower.

If a business is large enough to support a consistent advertising program, it may be located in an out-of-the-way, prestigious location. However, the smaller, less affluent business should be located near other active places of business in order to attract the attention of potential clients. Being near public transportation and having adequate parking facilities are important considerations.

Before signing a rental agreement or lease on a location, make certain that it fits your needs. If remodeling is necessary or if the building must be "brought up to code," the costs may be overwhelming. If you plan to lease a location or business, be sure you insert into the lease agreement any options for removing or replacing fixtures, making repairs, changing specific structures, or installing equipment, plumbing, and electrical work.

Many therapists choose to work independently out of their homes. This is an inexpensive alternative but may require a special use permit because of local zoning regulations. When working out of your home, it is imperative that the portion of the home that is used for an office is kept clean and neat. A clean bathroom, preferably with a shower, should be available for your clients. There are certain tax deductions that can be claimed for having an office in the home (check with your tax accountant).

▼ BUYING AN ESTABLISHED BUSINESS

You may have an opportunity to buy an established business, in which case you must weigh the advantages or disadvantages. Be sure the business has a good reputation, that it is worth the price being asked, and that it has an established clientele. It is a good idea to question customers as well as other business owners in the vicinity regarding the reputation of the business. Of course, you will want to know why the present owner is selling. It will not be to your advantage to buy a business that is being sold because it is failing. Generally, the owner is moving, retiring, or changing occupations.

It is important to consult a lawyer who can handle all legal aspects of the transaction to the satisfaction of everyone involved. A written purchase and sale agreement will be needed. You will also need a complete inventory of all fixtures, equipment, supplies, and materials as well as the value of each article that is to be part of the agreement. To avoid future misunderstandings, it is advisable to take photographs of furnishings and equipment. This will help to assure that you receive the exact items listed. It is also necessary to examine all records to understand the assets and liabilities of the business you are buying. An investigation should be made to determine any outstanding debts or obligations that may be held against the business.

LICENSES AND PERMITS ▼

There are local, state, and federal regulations that must be considered when beginning, locating, or relocating a business. It is to the advantage of the business owner to be aware of and comply with all regulations in the process of organizing the business rather than to be surprised after the fact and have to pay heavy penalties or restructure or relocate the business. Following is a partial list of permits and licenses that may be required and who to contact to determine how to comply.

Fictitious name statement (DBA): Required if the business name is different from the owner's name. A fictitious name statement, also called DBA (Doing Business As), is filed with the county to ensure that no other business uses the same name when doing business. *Contact:* County clerk's office.

Business License: May be required to operate a business in the city. *Contact:* City government, business licensing department.

Massage license: May be a city, county, or state requirement to perform massage services for a fee. *Contact:* County / city licensing bureau or the state agency in charge of occupational licensing.

Sales tax permit: Required if you sell products or if services are taxed. Provides information and materials to collect and file sales tax. *Contact:* State department of revenue.

Planning and zoning permits: Required to assure that the operation and location of the business is in compliance with local zoning requirements. This may especially affect those who operate a business out of their home. *Contact:* County or city planning and zoning board.

Building safety permit: May be required to obtain a business or professional license. May be issued after the place of business has been inspected and found to comply with building and fire codes and be free of conditions that may pose a hazard to you or your clients. *Contact:* Local fire department.

Employers Identification Number (EIN): This is the federal tax identification number issued to businesses and is used on all tax related forms. An EIN is required of partnerships and businesses that hire employees. *Contact*: Internal Revenue Service.

Provider's Number: This is an identification number issued to licensed healthcare providers. It is used and required when submitting claims to and receiving payment from medical insurance companies for services rendered. Massage practitioners in most states are not eligible to hold a provider's number but do receive third-party payments (insurance payments) by contracting with, billing through, or being an employee of a licensed provider (doctor, chiropractor, physical therapist, etc.).

▼ PROTECTING YOUR BUSINESS

You will need to have adequate insurance against fire, theft, and liability. To determine the specific types and amounts of coverage to cover your business and yourself, consult with one or more insurance agents. If you work out of your home, review your homeowner's policy concerning the liability of operating a business out of your home. If you lease an office, check the lease to determine which liability responsibilities are yours and which are the landlord's.

Following is a list of some types of insurance you may want to obtain.

Liability insurance covers costs of injuries and litigation resulting from injuries sustained on your property. This is usually a part of a homeowner's policy but may not cover business-related occurrences. Check your policy.

Malpractice liability insurance protects the therapist from lawsuits filed by a client because of injury or loss that results from negligence or substandard performance of a professional skill. Malpractice insurance can be purchased reasonably through some professional organizations such as the American Massage Therapy Association and the Associated Bodywork and Massage Professionals.

Automobile insurance full coverage provides medical and liability insurance to the driver and any passengers, and covers the vehicle and its contents regardless of who is at fault.

Fire and theft insurance covers fixtures, furniture, equipment, products, and supplies. If you rent or lease an office, the landlord may carry this insurance. Make sure it is adequate. If you have an office in the home, be sure your homeowner's policy is adequate to cover your office.

Medical/health insurance helps cover the cost of medical bills, especially hospitalization, serious injury, or illness.

Disability insurance protects the individual from loss of income because he or she are unable to work due to long-term illness or injury.

Worker's compensation insurance is required if you have employees. It covers the medical costs for employees if they are injured on the job.

PLANNING THE PHYSICAL LAYOUT OF A BUSINESS

The layout of a business takes careful planning in order to achieve efficiency and economy of operation. Once the building or space within a building has been decided, the interior must be designed. An efficient salon, studio, or clinic offering massage should have the following:

1. Air conditioning and heating systems that will provide warmth and comfort to your clients
2. Appropriate plumbing for showers and restrooms
3. Adequate and appropriate lighting for the entire operation, including indirect lighting in the massage rooms
4. An adequate dispensary
5. Proper equipment and adequate space for its use
6. Accessibility to all areas
7. Furniture that is appropriate, attractive, durable, and in keeping with the dignity of the business
8. An attractive and comfortable private consultation area
9. An attractive and comfortable reception area

Clients form either a positive or negative first impression of a business operation by the appearance of the office facility. The decor and appointments need not cost a fortune, but should give the impression that the business and the people employed there are highly professional. Your office can be one of your best promotional tools if the client is favorably impressed. Design the office so it is comfortable, uncluttered, and professional.

Massage Business Floor Plans

When planning a massage business, all facilities must be considered. A business may be located within another business such as a

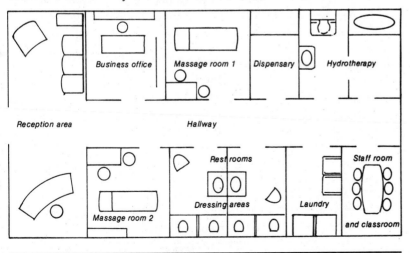

Fig. 19.1 Floor plan A—ideal space 28' × 50'.

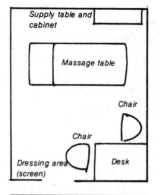

Fig. 19.2 Floor plan B—basic space 10' × 12'.

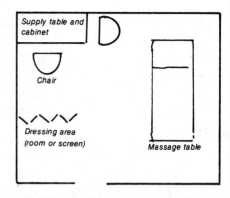

Fig. 19.3 Floor plan C—functional space 12' × 16'.

hairdressing and skin care salon, athletic club, or chiropractic office. The reception area, storage, restrooms, and other facilities might be shared between the office, club, or salon. The basic floor plan B and the functional floor plan C show only essential furnishings of a massage room. This is often the ideal plan for the beginning practitioner and to maintain a low operational cost.

Floor plan A shows adequate space for a larger business with room for several practitioners (Figs. 19.1, page 627 to 19.3).

▼ OFFICE MANAGEMENT

Establishing business practices and office procedures may be the farthest thing from a massage practitioner's mind or desires. Most people who become massage therapists do so for the personal contact and the chance to enhance their intuitive and creative abilities through healing touch. Generally they have a limited background at best about office management or bookkeeping and may consider it an unsavory or even incomprehensible task.

▼ BUSINESS ETHICS FOR THE MASSAGE PRACTITIONER

A massage practitioner must always practice according to a professional code of ethics. Ethics are standards of acceptable and professional behavior by which a person or business conducts business. Chapter 3 discusses ethics. Good ethics provide guidelines for professional conduct. The following guidelines reflect ethical behavior for the massage practitioner.

1. Always present a professional appearance.
2. Maintain a sense of dignity and professionalism in your work.
3. Project a pleasant, optimistic personality.
4. Treat each client with courtesy.
5. Maintain good health habits.

6. Keep surroundings neat, clean, and attractive.
7. Follow a systematic plan and organize your work properly.
8. Space appointments so that sufficient time is allowed.
9. Keep clients' records and conversations confidential.
10. Keep accurate records of all treatments.
11. Keep an active card file and mailing list of regular and prospective clients.
12. Use professional business cards and stationery.
13. Make periodic mailings of services that are offered.
14. Be sure that all advertising represents your business in the most professional manner.
15. Let physicians and other professional people know about your work and how you may be of valuable assistance to them.
16. Make every effort to eliminate negative concepts of your business by speaking before groups and educating the public about your work.
17. Join professional organizations that strive to upgrade, improve, and set high standards for your business.
18. Continue to promote your own personal and professional growth.
19. Work to eliminate any activities that cast unfavorable light on your business and profession.
20. Be responsible in keeping your word and meeting your obligations.
21. Obey all laws and legal requirements regulating the practice of massage and your business operation.
22. Charge a fair price for services rendered.
23. Continue to build a good reputation by your own work and conduct.
24. Recommend massage treatments only as the client requires and desires them.
25. Be loyal to your employers, associates, and clients.
26. Keep your professional and private lives separate by not discussing your personal problems with your clients.

SETTING YOUR FEES ▼

As a businessperson offering a personal service, your income is dependent of the fees you charge for your services. In determining your fee structure, there are several factors to consider. There are various strategies you may use to set your fees.

You are a professional massage therapist selling a valuable service. Set a fee that compensates you fairly and reflects your credibility. Consider the market and your competition. A little research will tell you what services are offered by other practitioners in the area and what they charge for those services. Set your fees in accordance with others in your area.

If you offer a unique service in high demand, your fee may be higher. If you are just beginning and want to attract more of the market, you may set a lower fee or offer special introductory rates.

If you are self-employed and massage is your sole source of income, you must consider all the costs of operating your business and determine how many sessions you must do at what rate in order to earn a living. If you are working for someone else, you may work for an hourly wage or for a percentage for each massage you perform. You must determine what you are willing to receive for each massage you do. The percentage you receive may depend on who furnishes the equipment, supplies, and services such as telephone, receptionist, advertising, etc.

▼ YOUR BUSINESS TELEPHONE

The business telephone is a powerful advertising tool. It is your contact with potential and steady clients. Anyone placing or receiving calls must know and use proper telephone techniques and courtesies. Your telephone number will accompany your business ads in telephone directories or newspapers and will be printed on your business cards. Therefore, the person answering your telephone should know how to do the following:

- Give accurate information and encourage a potential client to make an appointment.
- Make or change appointments for clients when necessary.
- Take messages accurately.
- Return all calls promptly.
- Place orders for supplies and other items when needed.
- Handle any complaints tactfully.
- Remind clients of appointments or needed services.
- Build goodwill and new business.
- Screen calls.

In addition to the foregoing, your business telephone serves as a security instrument in calling for help in case of emergency. For the protection of your employees and clients, the following phone numbers should be displayed near your business telephone:

- Nearest fire station
- Nearest ambulance service and hospital emergency service
- Police, local and state
- Taxi service
- Companies that provide needed services such as telephone, utilities, etc.
- Names and telephone numbers of owners, managers, custodians, and employees
- Names, addresses, and telephone numbers of all clients, which are kept in a private file but available in case of emergency

If you work out of your home and use your personal telephone for business purposes, there are a few special considerations. Business telephone expenses are tax deductible. If you use your home telephone for business purposes, the portion of your home telephone bill that is business related (i.e., long-distance business phone calls) is tax deductible if you maintain a telephone log book with the date, destination, and purpose for the call. (The base charges for your personal home phone are not deductible.) If you use your home phone number on your business cards and other advertising, it is considered a business phone and is subject to higher business telephone rates. If your phone is a business telephone (you pay business rates), the entire bill is tax deductible.

BASICS OF BOOKKEEPING ▼

A good recordkeeping system is essential to the success of a business. You will need to keep client records as well as records of income from both services and sales of products. Receipts, canceled checks, and invoices should be kept in appropriate files for tax purposes. Even though businesses hire accountants, it is still important for the self-employed practitioner, business manager, or owner to understand the basics of the system. It is more difficult to manage a business if you don't understand the principles of sound business administration and management. It is a plus for an inexperienced person to have some training in business administration before opening a business.

Without a proper bookkeeping system and accurate records, the owner or manager of a business would not be able to determine the progress of the business, especially the cost of doing business in relation to income. Business records are necessary to meet the requirements of local, state, and federal laws pertaining to taxes and employees. The manager of the business should see that records are kept properly for social security and taxes (state, local, federal taxes). If employees are involved, the manager should also be aware of recording payroll, wage and hour laws, worker's compensation, and any other laws or regulations that apply to hiring (or firing) employees.

A bookkeeping system should only be as complicated as the business requires. For a self-employed individual, a simple system that records income and disbursements is sufficient. Once a good system is set up and kept current, it reduces the year-end tax preparation drudgery and offers an accurate accounting of the business's financial position. Consulting an accountant is helpful when setting up a bookkeeping system and advisable when preparing taxes. A good accountant knows the changing tax laws and can often find many deductions you may otherwise miss.

Accounting packages have been designed specifically for the massage therapist. They may be advertised in one of the massage industry's journals or magazines. Make sure they are updated and meet your needs.

There are several ingredients to a workable bookkeeping system. The following are some of the basics.

Business Checking Account

A business checking account enables you to separate personal and business expenses. Open a separate account under the name of the business. Deposit all business income into the account. Use it whenever making cash disbursements. Pay all business bills by check. Do not use the business account to pay personal or nonbusiness expenses. An updated checkbook ledger is a good way to register disbursements and income. More complete ledgers are necessary to track a business's financial standing.

Petty Cash Account

A **petty cash fund** can be maintained to pay small disbursements for incidentals. Receipts should be kept for each transaction, which should be properly recorded in the ledger. Occasionally a check should be written from the business checking account to bring the petty cash fund back to a desired level.

Bank Statements and Reconciliations

Each month the bank will send a **bank statement** listing the deposits you have made for the month, the checks that have been processed through your account, and the balance left in the account. Be prompt in reconciling the statement with your checkbook. Note any errors, omissions, or miscalculations. Correct your mistakes and notify the bank immediately of any problems. Keep all bank statements, reconciliations, and canceled checks in your files a minimum of three years as proof of expenditures.

Income Records

These include daily receipts and a ledger sheet of all income with information as to the source, type and amount of income. A receipt or invoice should be prepared for each business transaction.
The invoice should include:
• Your business name
• The date
• The client's name (and address)
• A description of services given
• Amount charged for services
• A description of goods sold
• Amount charged for the goods sold
• Amount of sales tax
• The total
• A space to indicate the date paid

If you extend credit, you must include on the invoice your credit terms and finance charge. Keep a copy of the invoice for your records and give a copy to the client.

The **income ledger** is a summary of all sales and cash receipts. It is a record of the business income. There are different ways to set up the income ledger. You may record every income transaction, daily income, or weekly income. Income may be categorized as massage services, gift certificates, retail services, nontaxable sales, sales tax, and totals. There is a column on the ledger for each category. Each month the columns are totaled. The monthly summaries are totaled at the end of the year.

The income ledger is invaluable in preparing sales and income tax. It also allows you to forecast business activity, such as specials and vacations, according to slow or busy times (Fig. 19.4a and b, pages 634 and 635).

Disbursement Record

The disbursement record is a ledger that separates and classifies every business expenditure. Each column of the ledger is for a different category of expenditure. Occasionally more than one seldom used category may share the same column. Nearly all the information posted in the disbursement ledger comes from the checkbook register. All currency expenditures should also be recorded.

Each entry in the ledger includes the date, check number (or cash indicated), the payee, and total amount with the appropriate amount entered in the appropriate column. Each month, total the columns. The combined total of all the expenditure columns should equal the total of the total amount column. If it does not, go back and find the mistake. Note: If you use a computer, a variety of software companies have accounting programs that include checking, income, and disbursement functions (Fig. 19.5, page 636).

List of Business Expenses

Business expenses are partially or totally deductible from the business income when determining the profit or loss of the business. These categories can be used when writing checks and on the disbursement ledger.

The following are possible expenses:
- Accounting expense
- Advertising
- Automobile expense
  Fuel
  Maintenance
  Payments
  License fees

(text continues on page 637)

Daily Income Ledger for Month of _____ 19 ___

Date	Massage Income	Gift Certificates	Other Income	Non Taxable Retail	Taxable Retail	Sales Tax	Total Income
Total							
YTD							

Fig. 19.4a Sample income ledger.

Yearly Summary Income Ledger for 19 ___

Month	Massage Income	Gift Certificates	Other Income	Non Taxable Retail	Taxable Retail	Sales Tax	Total Income
January							
February							
March							
1st Quarter							
April							
May							
June							
2nd Quarter							
July							
August							
September							
3rd Quarter							
October							
November							
December							
4th Quarter							
Yearly Total							

Fig. 19.4b Sample yearly income summary ledger.

Expenditures From _____ 19 __ To _____ 19 __ Page ____

Date	Check No.	Payee Description	Check Amount	Advertise Insurance	Inventory Education	Cleaning Labor	Tax, Lic. Dues	Postage Supplies	Rent Repair	Utilities Tele	Misc	Owners Draw
Total Line A												
Total Line B												
GRAND TOTALS												

Fig. 19.5 Sample disbursement ledger.

- Bad debts
- Bank fees
- Cleaning and janitorial
- Contract labor
- Convention costs
- Cost of products to be sold
- Depreciation
- Donations to charity
- Dues to business and professional associations
- Education expense
    Seminars, professional journals, books, etc.
- Entertainment
- Equipment expense
- Furnishings and fixtures
- Insurance premiums
    Auto, liability, malpractice, fire, theft
- Interest paid on loans
- License and permit fees
- Office supplies
- Payroll, wages, and withholdings
- Postage, freight, and shipping
- Professional, legal, or consulting fees
- Refunds for services or products
- Rent
- Repair and maintenance
- Supplies
- Taxes
    Sales, property, state, federal
- Telephone
- Travel, business related
- Utilities.

An expenditure that is not considered an expense is the owner's expense or salary paid to yourself.

Business-Related Receipts

Keep all receipts for every purchase or expenditure related in any way to the business. After recording transactions, file the receipts. Each month create a new file so the receipts are separated to reflect and support the entries in the monthly disbursement ledger. For tax reasons, keep all receipts for a minimum of three years.

Accounts Receivable

If you extend credit and bill your clients, you will have to keep an ongoing record of each transaction. This does complicate the book-keeping process considerably. To keep it simple, require cash payments at the time of service for everything except gift certifi-cates, advance payments, insurance billings, and credit card pay-ments (i.e., Visa and Mastercard). **Accounts receivable** is a record of moneys owed to you by other persons or businesses. Record each charge and payment, including the date of the transaction and current balance.

Accounts Payable

If you buy supplies or services on credit, keep a file for each account or business that extends you credit. **Accounts payable** records the moneys you owe other persons or businesses. File statements and purchase orders so that you have an accurate record when it is time to pay the bills. Trades and barters should be recorded on a separate record.

Assets and Depreciation Records

Items and equipment purchased to be used in your business for an extended period of time (more than a year) are considered business assets. Supplies and inventory are not considered assets. Maintain a current record of business assets that includes an item description, date of purchase, and purchase price. Add new items when purchased and remove items when they are sold or retired from use.

Depending on the purchase price of a durable item and the business's financial situation, you may choose to declare it, for tax purposes, as a one-time business expense or depreciate its cost over a number of years. Methods and schedules for depreciating different items vary according to the length of the useful life of the item. It is not within the scope of this book to discuss depreciation methods. Consult with your accountant or refer to *The Tax Guide for Small Business* published by the IRS for detailed instructions. Maintain a depreciation record for all depreciable assets.

Keep a file on all major items and equipment including purchase records, instruction manuals, service records, warranties, and guarantees.

Inventory

A good inventory system helps to assure that you will not run out of supplies or be overstocked on items that do not move well. Supplies to be used are classified as consumption supplies, and those to be sold are classified as retail supplies. You may need to keep records of sales tax on supplies sold.

Mileage Log

All business-related travel should be recorded for tax purposes. Expenses for operating a vehicle for business are deductible from taxable income. This does not include travel from home to the place of business. There are two ways of determining this deduction: the standard mileage allowance or actual automobile expense.

When an automobile is used in the course of the business, keep a mileage log and record all business travel. For each trip, record the destination, beginning and ending odometer readings, total miles traveled, and purpose of the trip. An allowance of twenty-two cents per mile may be deducted. (This figure may vary. Check with an accountant or the IRS for the current rate.)

If you deduct the actual auto expense, keep an itemized record of all expenses (fuel, service, insurance, license fees, parking, and depreciation records of actual purchase price). The auto expense is prorated between business use and personal use. For example, if you drove the vehicle 12,000 miles in a year and 4000 miles was business related, you would deduct 33.3 percent of the total auto expenses from the business income.

Updated Client Files

The client file is the mechanism practitioners use to record pertinent client information and document the work they have done with clients. The information a practitioner keeps in the client files varies as much as the massage routines of different practitioners. Updated client files helps the practitioner render prompt and efficient service and ensures access to current information regarding the client. Information that is often found in a client file includes intake information, a treatment plan, session documentation, and a record of payment. Intake information includes name, address, phone, and medical information and history. A treatment plan provides a kind of a blueprint for the sessions that is updated periodically. Each session is documented with the type of service given, the date given, the products used, and the results obtained. A payment record lists the amount charged and received for each item and service. Keeping accurate and updated records is a tedious but essential part of a professional operation (Fig. 19.6a and b, page 652 and 653).

Appointment Book

The appointment book is possibly the most important document for organizing a successful and prosperous business. It is an important tool in time management. A well-kept appointment book assures that appointments are not missed and are scheduled so that you can be prompt and on time. There is nothing more embarrassing than to have two people show up for a massage at the same time. Keep your appointment book handy and always up to date. If you carry an appointment book with you, it can become a portable file to record mileage, important phone numbers, business expenses, as well as appointments. It is still advisable to maintain a client appointment book at your office. Be sure to transfer information from your portable appointment book to your office book to avoid double bookings.

The appointment book should have enough space to record each client's appointment time, name, phone number (address and directions if it is an outcall), and possibly the amount you receive from each client.

Massage Clinic
Client Information Form

Name_____ Birth Date_____

Address_____ Telephone_____

_____ Business Phone_____

City   State   Zip   Social Security #_____

Occupation_____ Other Activities_____

General Health Condition_____ Blood Pressure_____

Have you had any serious or chronic illness, operations, chronic virus infections, or traumatic accidents? _____

Are you in recovery for addictions or abuse?_____

Are you under a doctor, chiropractor or other health practitioners care? _____

If so, for what condition/s? _____

Are you on any medication? _____ If so, what?_____

Do I have permission to contact your Doctor / Therapist?_____

Names of Doctors, Chiropractors or Health Practitioners:

Name_____ Name_____

Address_____ Address_____

Telephone_____ Telephone_____

Why did you come for our services? (relaxation, pain, therapy, etc.)_____

_____

What results would you like to achieve with our work?_____

Have you had any massage therapy before?_____ If so, by whom?_____

How did you find out about our services? _____

Were you referred to this office?_____ By whom?_____

In case of emergency notify: Name_____Phone_____

I have completed this information form to the best of my knowledge. I understand the massage services are designed to be a health aid and are in no way to take the place of a doctors care when it is indicated. Information exchanged during any massage session is educational in nature and is intended to help me become more familiar and conscious of my own health status and is to be used at my own discretion.

Our time together is precious and I agree to cancel 24 hours in advance. Unless there is an emergency, if I miss an appointment I agree to pay the full appointment fee.

Date_____ Signature_____

Fig. 19.6a Sample intake form.

Client Name _____ Date 1st Session _____

Address _____ City _____ St _____ ZIP _____

Phone (h) _____ (w)_____ Insurance _____

Date	Service	Products	Tax	Charges	Credits	Balance	Comments

REFERRAL RECORD

Client Referred By _____ Date _____

New Clients Referred by This Client

Name	Date 1st Session	Acknowledged

Fig. 19.6b Sample payment record.

Some clients will book the same time on a regular basis. These regular customers are the mainstay of many businesses because they can be counted on for a certain amount of regular income.

Bookkeeping Tips

Recordkeeping is an essential part of maintaining a successful business. Once a filing and bookkeeping system is established, be persistent by continually updating the files. Here are a few tips that will simplify the task:

- Keep all records current.
- Review client files before each session and document each session promptly after the session.
- When writing checks, record the amount and expenditure category in the check register.
- Keep and file all business-related receipts.
- Update income and disbursement ledgers regularly.
- Reconcile bank statements promptly.
- Keep all tax-related records:

Receipts	at least three years)
Ledgers, canceled checks, etc.	(at least seven years)
Tax Returns	(at least ten years)
Real estate and business contracts	(indefinitely)

▼ MARKETING

Marketing is all the business activity done to promote and increase your business. Some marketing activities include advertising, promotion, public relations, referrals, and client retention. Marketing is an educational process of getting yourself and what you do known. It is the enticement that encourages an individual to seek your services. Marketing is an ongoing activity in your business. The goal of marketing is to create and maintain a thriving practice. When developing marketing materials and practices in the field of massage, be certain that they reflect the image you want to portray.

Assess Marketing Needs

Your particular marketing needs are determined by several factors including the amount of time or money you can afford, your target market, and the size of your practice. If you are starting out in your practice, you may not have a large clientele and therefore have a lot of time and not a lot of money. More time can be spent on making contacts, giving presentations, writing articles, and making personal appearances. Concentrate on activities that are low cost but may be more time consuming. Actively educate the public as to what you do and how it will benefit them.

If you have a fairly busy practice already, time may be limited but you have a larger advertising budget. You may concentrate more on client retention, developing referrals, direct mail, and targeted advertising to announce special services.

There are many marketing techniques to choose from that can be selected and designed to best suit your personal marketing needs.

Analyze Target Markets

Massage is a service that tends to appeal to specific segments of the population. Target groups are various segments of the population that have similar characteristics. Your target market consists of those target groups that you prefer to attract to your services. Selecting a target market enables you to modify your advertising and promotional activities to appeal to the specific group.

The parameters of target groups are innumerable. They may be very broad (i.e., women or athletes or the elderly or professional people). They can be specific (i.e., low birth weight infants, female runners, accountants, or abuse survivors). Several attributes that depict groups are age, gender, income, occupation, interests, and location.

There are at least two ways to determine your particular target market. One is to consider what type of clientele you want to attract. When you have made your choices, contact clubs and organizations in your area that cater to individuals from that group. Offer to be a speaker or do a demonstration. Create brochures highlighting benefits of massage for the specific conditions common to that group. Place ads and articles in magazines and newsletters. Make personal contact with individuals and participate in activities common to your target market.

Another way to determine your target market is to assess your client files to determine who is presently using your services and what they have in common. Then design promotional activities that reach that segment of the population.

It is wise to have more than one or even several target markets. The number depends of your preference, your expertise, and the size of your practice.

Business Promotion

The objective of promotion is to become known, to be visible to those in the community that may seek your service. It is also to create the desire in potential clients to use your services. Promotional activities, especially in a service industry such as massage, are largely educational in nature. They let your target population know who you are, what you do, and how your services will benefit them.

Common methods of business promotion include public speaking and appearances, articles in newspapers and professional magazines, and booths at health fairs and other public functions. These provide excellent opportunities to educate prospective client groups.

Developing Promotional Material

An important part of your promotional activity is having appropriate printed materials to distribute when you come in contact with potential customers. Printed materials include business cards, brochures, stationery, and newsletters. Your printed material should appeal to your target market and reflect your professionalism. Always include your name, address, and phone number on every piece of promotional material.

Whenever you speak to a group or an individual about your services, be sure to leave them with a card or brochure. Even though you will not generally get a new client directly from your printed material, it serves as a reminder and contains information about how to contact you.

Advertising

Advertising is generally the marketing activity that is done in return for direct payment. This includes magazine and newspaper ads and listings, signs, embossed pens and calendars etc.

Advertising is important to business success because it notifies the public about your services and how to contact you. When giving personal services such as massage, it is particularly important that your advertising not be misunderstood and that it creates a favorable impression to the public. Advertising should always reflect your professional status and the quality of your services. Keeping your name before the public will be important to building your business and reminding clients to use your services.

Plan your advertising budget. You must try to obtain the most effective media for the amount of money you have budgeted for advertising purposes. Newspaper advertising is generally the most economical way to reach the most people when you are opening a new business. By placing your ad in a specific section of the newspaper, such as the health or sports section, you can target the ad to the market you want to reach. The people in the advertising department of the paper will help you determine cost, size, and style of your ad.

A classified ad in the yellow pages of your local telephone directory is a fairly inexpensive and effective method of advertising for personal service businesses. Make sure to list your service under Massage—Therapeutic, with your credentials and association affiliations.

Direct mail is effective advertising for certain target markets. You may want to obtain a mailing list from a company that sells specifically targeted consumer lists.

Advertising consultants are expensive, but if you have a flexible advertising budget, you may find that a professional consultant can save you both time and money. A good consultant will be able to help you with creative ideas for logos, letterheads, and advertising that gets your message across in the most professional, tasteful, and dramatic way (Fig. 19.7).

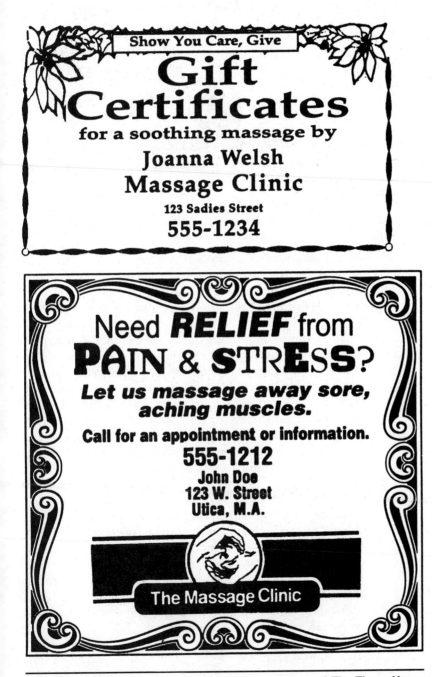

Fig. 19.7 Effective advertising. Advertising courtesy of *The Times News*, Twin Falls, ID.

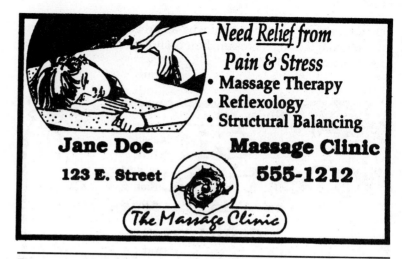

Fig. 19.7 continued

Public Relations

Some of the best advertising you can get is free. A feature article in a local newspaper is an excellent way to gain recognition in your community. News releases that announce classes you offer or awards and certifications you receive are also ways of promoting your business.

Offer to make personal appearances to give talks and demonstrations to various groups. You may offer to speak at social meetings, health clubs, sports events, schools, or as a guest on a radio or television talk show. You could act as guest instructor at a school or health facility where your type of personal services could be taught.

An essential aspect in developing good public relations is networking. Networking is developing personal and professional contacts for the purpose of giving and receiving support and sharing resources and information. Become involved in networking groups such as the Chamber of Commerce or other business groups. Participate in seminars or functions to meet others with whom you may develop networking relationships. Always keep business cards handy when attending these functions and freely distribute them. It is a good practice to give two or three cards at a time so the recipient can pass one along to someone else. When you receive a business card from someone, make a note on the card as to what that person may provide for you. Keep a professional card file or a Rolodex® with those cards and refer to it when needs arise or when you are mailing out information.

Encouraging Referrals

One of the most effective and inexpensive methods of creating new business is through referrals. The two main sources of referrals are current clients and other healthcare professionals.

Satisfied customers are one of your most effective means of advertising. Remember, in word-of-mouth advertising, the most important mouth is yours. Encourage referrals. Let your clients know that you not only appreciate their business, but that if they appreciate what you do they should tell others. Give them extra business cards and encourage them to tell their friends and associates about your service.

To promote referrals from other professionals, make yourself and what you do known to them. Explain how your services would benefit them and their clients. Write letters, and then follow up the letter with a phone call. Set up a personal meeting or take them to lunch. Give them a treatment so they can experience firsthand what you have to offer. Always present yourself in a professional manner. When other health care professionals send referrals, confer with them to determine their reasons and goals for sending the client to you. Report back to them about the client's progress as a result of massage. A good working relationship between healthcare professionals will generate more referrals. It will also initiate more holistic client care by promoting interdisciplinary treatment plans.

Whenever a new client comes in that has been referred, be sure to acknowledge the person who referred him or her with a thank-you note. Extend a special discount or even an occasional extra no charge product or service to individuals who make multiple referrals.

When you do get referrals from someone, return the courtesy by referring people back to him or her or using the person's services yourself.

Remember the three R's of referrals: request, reward, and reciprocate. Request referrals from satisfied clients and professionals. Reward those who send you referrals with prompt thank-you cards or personal phone calls. Reciprocate by sending referrals or using the services of those who send you referrals.

Client Retention

Your clients are your most valuable asset. Clients who return on a regular basis are the mainstay of your practice. According to Cherie Sohnen-Moe (Business Mastery, 1991), "On the average it costs six times as much money and takes three times the effort getting new clients as retaining current ones." Encourage clients to return for regular appointments. A weekly massage is a healthy investment. Before a client leaves your office, be sure he or she has scheduled the next appointment.

Treat your clients with courtesy and respect. Give them the service for which they will want to return. This requires more than just being a skilled massage technician to retain clients. Besides giving a good massage, make sure your client feels appreciated and cared for. Document each session, paying attention to the client's personal interests, likes, and dislikes. Refer to your records before each visit to remind you of their idiosyncrasies. Avoid their dislikes, discuss their interests, and do those special little things they like. Thank them for coming in.

Follow-up especially intense sessions with a phone call to ask how the client is. Send cards for important occasions such as birthdays and holidays. Always send thank-you notes when a client sends a referral. If a client is deserving, send him or her a certificate for a free massage. Many personal service businesses offer gift certificates or special prices to loyal customers.

Keep your clientele on a mailing list, send them newsletters, periodic flyers, birthday or holiday greetings, or offer special discounts during slow times.

Remember, the clients are your reason for practicing, they are the source of your income, and they deserve the best service you can give.

▼ BUSINESS LAW

In conducting business and employing help, it is necessary to comply with local, state, and federal laws and regulations. Federal laws cover social security, unemployment compensation or insurance, and tax payments on income as well as a number of other taxes. Income tax laws are covered by both the state and federal governments. State laws cover sales taxes, licenses, worker's compensation, employment regulations, and the like. Business owners and managers may hire a lawyer or a tax accountant, but they should also be familiar with these laws and regulations.

▼ HIRING EMPLOYEES

Hiring employees increases your potential to provide services to more people. It also increases the employer's responsibility regarding recordkeeping and tax regulations. An employer is required to maintain separate payroll records for each employee, withhold state and federal taxes and social security, prepare quarterly payroll tax returns, pay the employer's portion of social security and unemployment taxes and purchase worker's compensation insurance.

Many businesses will want to hire massage therapists as **contract labor.** When doing so a person is an **independent contractor** and is hired on as his or her own boss for a per client fee or a percentage without taxes, worker's compensation, or social security being deducted from wages. An independent contractor is self-employed and is responsible for his or her own taxes. If you hire an independent contractor and pay him or her more than $600 in the course of a year, you are required to file tax forms 1099 and 1096. There are federal IRS guideline which must be followed closely when dealing with contract labor. Be sure to check with the state employment office or the IRS for a copy of these guidelines before hiring contract labor.

If you are an employer, you are expected to be fair and honorable in dealing with employees and you have a right to expect the same consideration from those you hire. Employees can make the difference between success and failure of a personal service business. Clients often return to a place of business because they like the people who serve them as much, if not more, than the products and services. The following are important considerations when hiring someone to represent your place of business. The potential employee should:

1. Have the necessary licenses or other credentials required by law.
2. Set a good example by having clean, healthy personal habits.
3. Be profit conscious and willing to work hard to achieve business goals.
4. Be courteous and professional when dealing with all clients.
5. Obey all rules, regulations, and laws pertaining to the business.
6. Be willing to learn new techniques and to grow both personally and professionally.
7. Be self-motivated and industrious.
8. Be honest and ethical.

CHECKLIST

In summary, there is more to being successful in a massage business than being able to perform a good massage. A positive attitude, clear goals, and some understanding of business practices are essential for success.

The following is a checklist of important basics to consider before opening a business of your own. Use this checklist as a guide to important factors before opening a business.

- Capital
  Amount available
  Amount required
- Organization
  Sole proprietor, partnership, corporation
- Banking
  Opening a business account
  Deposits, drawing checks
  Monthly statements
  Establishing credit
  Business loans
- Selecting a Location
  Population
  Transportation facilities

Quiet enough to induce relaxation
Space required
Zoning ordinances
Parking
Accessibility
Surrounding neighborhood
- Decorating and Floor Plan
  Interior decorating
  Installing telephones
  Exterior decorating
- Bookkeeping System
  Record of appointments
  Receipts and disbursements
  Petty cash
  Profit and loss
  Inventory
  Client files
- Cost of Operation
  Supplies, depreciation
  Rent, lights, utilities
  Cleaning service, laundry
  Salaries
  Products for services
  Telephone
  Taxes, insurance
- Management
  Methods of building goodwill
  Client courtesies, gifts
  Adjusting complaints
  Personnel relations
  Public relations
  Selling merchandise
- Equipment and Supplies
  Selecting equipment
  Installation of equipment
- Advertising
  Planning
  Business cards and brochures
  Direct mail
  Newspaper
  Radio
  Television
  Personal appearances
- Legal
  Lease, contracts
  Compliance with state, local, and government laws
  Licensing of business
  Licensing of managers and practitioners

- Ethics and Professional Growth
    Setting goals
    Courtesy
    Observation of professional practices
    Interaction with professional groups
- Insurance
    Public liability and malpractice
    Compensation, unemployment
    Automobile
    Fire and theft
- Methods of Payment
    Cash
    In advance
    Open account
    Time payments
    Charge cards

QUESTIONS FOR DISCUSSION AND REVIEW

1. How do attitude and self-image relate to business success?
2. Explain the difference between a partnership, a corporation, and a sole proprietorship.
3. What start-up costs may you expect when beginning a massage business?
4. List five important considerations when choosing a location for a massage business.
5. List the various permits and licenses that may be required to operate a massage business.
6. List the types of insurance a massage business owner should carry to protect the business.
7. Why is keeping accurate records necessary in a successful business?
8. List the major ingredients of a basic bookkeeping system.
9. What is marketing?
10. What are the main marketing techniques used in the massage industry?
11. Define target market.
12. What are the three R's of referrals?

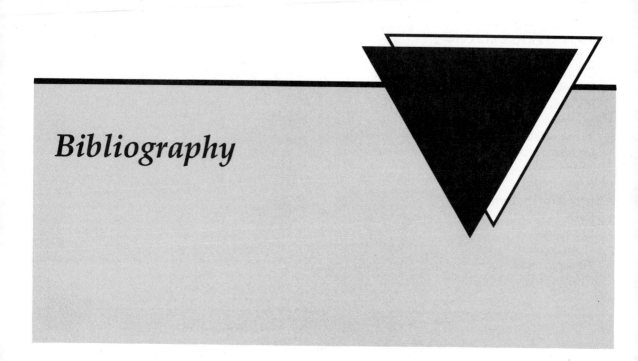

Bibliography

Chiatow, Leon. *Soft Tissue Manipulation*. Rochester, VT: Healing Arts Press, 1988.

Clemente, Carmine D. *Anatomy, A Regional Atlas of the Human Body*, 3rd ed. Baltimore: Urban & Schwarzenberg, 1987.

Fong, Elizabeth; Ferris, Elvira B.; Skelley, Esther G. *Body Structures & Function*, 7th ed. Albany, NY: Delmar Publishers, 1989.

Hoppenfeld, Stanley. *Physical Examination of the Spine and Extremities*. New York: Appleton Century Crofts, 1976.

Hungerford, Dr. Myk. *Beyond Sports Medicine*. Costa Mesa, CA: Sports Massage Training Inst., 1991.

Hungerford, Dr. Myk. *The Professional's Guide to Massage Therapy*. Costa Mesa, CA: Sports Massage Training Inst., 1988.

Jones, Lawrence D. O. *Strain and Counterstrain*. Colorado Springs, CO: American Academy of Osteopathy, 1981.

Juhan, Deane. *Job's Body, A Handbook for Bodyworkers*. Barrington, NY: Station Hill Press, 1987.

Hart, Marcia. *Structural/Muscular Balancing*. Carson City, NV: Thoth Inc., 1992.

Kamoroff, Bernard. *Small Time Operator*. Laytonville, CA: Bell Springs Publishing, 1987.

Kapit, Wynn and Elson. *The Anatomy Coloring Book*. New York: Harper & Row, 1977.

Kendall, Florence; McCreary, Elizabeth. *Muscles: Testing and Function 3rd ed*. Baltimore: Williams & Wilkins, 1983.

Knapp, Joan E., Antonucci, Eileen J. *A National Study of the Profession of Massage Therapy and Bodywork*. Princeton, NJ: Knapp & Associates, 1990.

Lillis, Carol A. *Brady's Introduction to Medical Terminology*. Bowie, MD: Robert J. Brady Co., 1983.

Lindner, Harold H. *Clinical Anatomy*. Norwalk, CT: Appleton & Lange, 1989.

Magee, David. *Orthopedic Physical Assessment*. Philadelphia: W. B. Saunders, 1987.

Memmler, Ruth L.; Wood, Dena Lin. *The Human Body in Health and Disease, 5th ed*. Philadelphia: J. B. Lippincott, 1983.

Michlovitz, Susan L., Wolf, Steven L. *Thermal Agents in Rehabilitation*. Philadelphia: F. A. Davis Company, 1986.

Moor, Peterson, Manwell, Noble, Meunch. *Manual of Hydrotherapy and Massage*. Oshawa, Ontario, Canada. Pacific Press Publishing Assn., 1964.

Mulvihill, Mary Lou. *Human Diseases, A Systematic Approach, 2nd ed*. Norwalk, CT: Appleton & Lange, 1987.

Prudden, Bonnie. *Pain Erasure*. New York: M. Evans & Co., 1980.

Sieg, Kay M.; Adams, Sandra P. *Illustrated Essentials of Musculoskeletal Anatomy*. Gainesville, FL: Megabooks, 1985.

Smith, Genevieve Love; Davis, Phyllis E. *Medical Terminology, 4th ed*. New York: John Wiley & Sons, 1981.

Smith, Irene. *Guidelines for the Massage of AIDS Patients*. San Francisco, CA: Service Through Touch, 1992.

Sohnen-Moe, Cherie. *Business Mastery, 2nd ed*. Tuscon, AZ: Sohnen-Moe Associates, 1991.

St. John, Paul. *St. John Neuromuscular Therapy Seminars Manuals 1 & 4*. Largo, FL: 1990.

Tappan, Frances M. *Healing Massage Technique, Holistic, Classical and Emerging Methods*. Norwalk, CT: Appleton & Lange, 1988.

Thompson, A.; Skinner, A.; Piercy, J. *Tidy's Physiotherapy, 12th ed*. Oxford, England: Butterworth & Heinmann, 1990.

Travell, Janet G., M.D.; Simons, David G, M.D. *Myofascial Pain and Dysfunction, The Trigger Point Manual.* Baltimore: Williams & Wilkins, 1983.

van Why, Richard. *The Bodywork Knowledgebase, Lectures on the History of Massage.* New York: Self Published, 1991.

Voss, Dorthy E., Ionta, Marjorie K., Myers, Beverly J. *Proprioceptive Neuromuscular Facilitation.* Philadelphia: Harper & Row, 1985.

Williams, Ruth E. *The Road to Radiant Health.* College Place, WA: Color Press, 1977.

Wood, Elizabeth; Becker, Paul. *Beard's Massage, 3rd ed.* Philadelphia: W. B. Saunders, 1981.

Yates, John. *A Physician's Guide to Therapeutic Massage.* Vancouver, B.C.: Massage Therapists' Association of British Columbia, 1990.

Ylinen, Jari; Cash, Mel. *Sports Massage.* London: Stanley Paul & Co. Ltd., 1988.

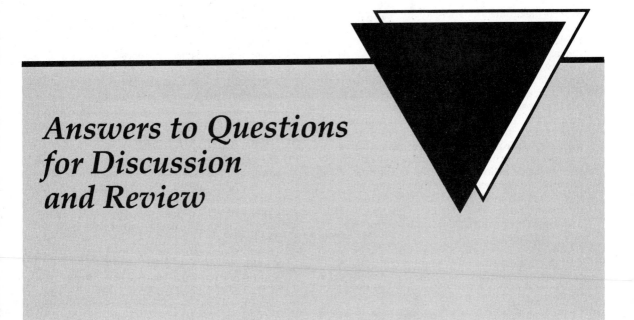

Answers to Questions for Discussion and Review

CHAPTER 1 HISTORICAL OVERVIEW

1. Massage is the manual (use of hands) or mechanical (use of machines or apparatus) manipulation of a part of the body by rubbing, kneading, pressing, rolling, slapping, and like movements for the purpose of improving circulation of the blood, relaxation of muscles, and other benefits to body systems.

2. Various artifacts show evidence that ancient civilizations used massage and exercise in their social, personal, and religious practices.

3. Massage is said to be the most effective and most natural means of obtaining relief from pain or discomfort, because a person can use his or her hands to rub, touch, or exercise a part of the body to obtain immediate relief.

4. The Chinese called their massage system *amma*. This method grew from various pressing and rubbing of parts of the body to produce therapeutic effects.

5. The Greeks and Romans were health and beauty conscious. Both men and women believed that exercise improved the body and the mind. Exercise and massage were utilized in the training and rehabilitation of gladiators. Both Greek and Roman physicians prescribed various kinds of exercise and massage movements as aids to the healing of diseases and wounds.

6. Hippocrates, the Greek physician, became known as the father of medicine and originator of the Hippocratic oath, which is still used as the ethical guide to the medical professions. The Hippocratic oath can be found in its entirety in most modern dictionaries.

7. The Middle Ages were called the Dark Ages because the arts and sciences were allowed to deteriorate, leading to the decline of learning.

8. As the Greco-Roman culture fell into the decay of the Middle Ages, many of the important teachings of the great physicians and philosophers were carried on by the Persians of the Arabic Empire. The Islamic Persian philosopher/physicians, Rhazes or Razi and Avicenna, who followed the teachings of Hippocrates and Galan, authored important books that eventually returned to the West by way of trade and conquest and paved the way for the Renaissance.

9. The Renaissance, meaning "rebirth," revived interest in the arts and sciences and renewed interest in health and personal hygiene practices.

10. The invention of the printing press in the latter part of the fifteenth century led to the publishing of more writings in the arts and sciences. This improved circulation of educational materials led to a better understanding of the value of massage and exercise as therapeutic aids.

11. Per Henrik Ling based the Swedish Movement Cure on the developing science of physiology applied to the treatment of disease. The system's primary focus was on gymnastics, which consisted of movements classified as active, duplicated, and passive.

12. In 1858, the brothers Charles Fayette Taylor and George Henry Taylor started an orthopedic practice in New York. They specialized in the Swedish movements.
13. There were several reasons for the decline of the scientific and medical use of massage at the turn of the twentieth century. An inquiry by the British Medical Association in 1894 revealed numerous abuses in the education and practice of massage practitioners, including unscrupulous recruitment practices, inadequate training, deceptive advertising, and false certification. Technical innovations, such as the invention of electricity and various electrical apparatuses (such as the vibrator) and intellectual advances in medicine that led to new treatment strategies based more on pharmacology and surgical procedures, also had a detrimental affect on massage.
14. Because there were more diseases and injuries during wartime, physicians employed therapeutic massage and exercise more often. The good results led to wider acceptance of massage and exercise as aids to healing.
15. Manual massage became a secondary treatment following World War II because new mechanical and electrical devices were designed to take over some of the manipulative movements.
16. The increased awareness of physical and mental fitness as well as the increasing cost of traditional medicine opened the way for viable alternatives in healthcare. The development of the wellness model, which placed more emphasis on prevention and recognized the importance of controlling stress, has caused a renewed interest in massage.
17. Passive exercise of muscles incorporates massage and is done by the practitioner on the client. Active exercise of muscles is movement done by the individual, as in sports or gymnastics.
18. The Japanese use a system called *shiatsu* (*shi*, fingers; *atsu*, pressure). It is the finger pressure method based on the Oriental concept that the body has a series of energy points. When pressure is properly applied to these points, circulation is improved and nerves are stimulated. This system is said to improve body metabolism and to relieve a number of physical disorders.
19. Athletes often have injuries and sore muscles that can be relieved by massage. Massage and proper exercise also help to prevent fatigue and contribute to the maintenance of optimum fitness.
20. A person contemplating a career in any important field should have some understanding of problems of the past and the progress that has been made over a period of time. Understanding the past helps us to measure our own progress in the development of the art and practice of therapeutic body massage.
21. The Swedish massage system is still the most widely used and is most frequently incorporated into other systems.
22. The points of stimulation in Japanese massage (tsubo) are much the same as points used in Chinese traditional medicine.
23. Sports massage is used in sports medicine as an aid to treating injuries that have occurred during sports activities. It is also used as a means of keeping the athlete's muscles supple and strong.

CHAPTER 2 REQUIREMENTS FOR THE PRACTICE OF THERAPEUTIC MASSAGE

1. The practitioner must be concerned about the laws, rules, regulations, and obligations concerning the practice of therapeutic body massage because the practitioner has a responsibility to the public and to individual clients. Massage is a personal, health-related service, and, as such, strict rules must be observed.
2. The scope of practice defines the rights and activities legally acceptable according to the licenses of a particular practice or profession. Scope of practice is defined legally and determines the educational focus and requirements that become the national standards of a given profession.
3. Laws governing the practice of massage often differ because there are no national standards and some states have fewer complaints, or problems, while others have found it necessary to establish state boards and stringent guidelines for licensing practitioners, schools, and establishments.
4. Being licensed in one locality does not guarantee that the same license will be valid or recognized in another locality. Since laws and regulations vary greatly from state to state and city to city, a practitioner who has a license and wishes to practice in another city or state should contact the proper agency in the area where he or she wishes to practice, provide proof of ability to meet any requirements, and make any applications that are required.
5. The general educational requirements to practice massage vary depending on discipline or techniques and the licensing requirements of the city or state where the practice is located. Because there is not a national standard for massage therapy, educational requirements in licensing laws may contain no educational requirement or may require as much as 1000 hours of training. The educational requirements to enroll in a program of instruction at a certificate-granting school or institute of massage may differ, but generally a high school diploma or equivalency diploma is required.
6. A person may receive a certificate in recognition of an accomplishment or achieving or maintaining some kind of standard. Certificates are awarded by schools and institutions to show the successful completion of a course of study and by professional organizations to indicate that the recipient has met the qualifications to become a member or in

recognition of achievements in the recipient's chosen profession.

7. The grounds upon which the practitioner's license may be revoked, canceled, or suspended are:
   1. Practicing fraud or deceit in obtaining a license
   2. Being convicted of a felony
   3. Being engaged in any act of prostitution
   4. Practicing under a false or assumed name
   5. Being addicted to drugs, alcohol, etc.
   6. Being willfully negligent of the health of a client
   7. Prescribing drugs or medicine
   8. Being guilty of fraudulent or deceptive advertising.

CHAPTER 3 PROFESSIONAL ETHICS FOR MASSAGE PRACTITIONERS

1. It is important to have a code of ethics for your business in order to protect the public and your reputation.
2. A satisfied client is your best means of advertising because he or she will recommend you, your business, and your services.
3. Successful business managers know that employees who practice sound personal and professional ethics will help them to build their business and keep their customers.
4. It is necessary for the massage practitioner to be concerned with personal hygiene and health habits because his or her own good health inspires confidence on the part of clients. Good health is also a form of protection for the practitioner and the client.
5. Professional projection in attitude and appearance means that the practitioner acts, speaks, and dresses to project a professional image.
6. Human relations is defined as the art of being able to work successfully with others and to give excellent service.
7. The practice of good human relations is important because it helps the practitioner interact successfully with different personalities.
8. When building your business image, pay attention to the use of appropriate wording in your business name and in advertising so that potential clients get the right message.

CHAPTER 4 HUMAN ANATOMY AND PHYSIOLOGY OVERVIEW

1. Anatomy is defined as the study of the gross structure or morphology of the body or the study of an organism and the interrelations of its parts.
2. Physiology is the science and study of the vital processes, mechanisms, and functions performed by the various systems of the body.
3. Histology is the branch of biology concerned with the microscopic structure of tissues of a living organism.

4. Pathology is the study of the structural and functional changes caused by disease.
5. Disease is an abnormal and unhealthy state of all or part of the body wherein it is not capable of carrying on its normal function.
6. A symptom is caused by the disease and is perceived by the victim, such as dizziness, chills, nausea, or pain. A symptom is a clear message to the individual that something is wrong. Signs of a disease are observable indications such as abnormal pulse rate, fever, abnormal skin color, or physical irregularities.
7. Regardless of the source or nature of stress, the physiological reaction of the body is essentially the same. When we encounter high levels of stress, our bodies respond with the "fight or flight " reactions. The adrenal secretions, adrenaline and cortisol, give us a physical and mental boost that heightens our senses, sharpens our reflexes, and strengthens our muscles.
8. There are two responses to pain: psychological and physical. The physical response to pain is very similar to the body's response to stress. Blood pressure and pulse increase, blood flow is shifted from the intestines and brain to the muscles, and mental alertness intensifies, readying the body for a fight or flight. The physical experience also informs us of the location, intensity, and duration of the pain.
9. The pain-spasm-pain cycle is associated with muscle spasms. The natural reflex reaction to the tissue damage and pain is a contraction of the muscles that surround the injury. Contracted muscles pinch the blood vessel and capillaries in the muscles, restricting blood flow and causing ischemia. Metabolic activity of the muscles increases as oxygen and nutrients are burned, producing increased amounts of metabolic wastes. Lactic acid and other toxins collect in the tissues and soon ischemic pain appears. Reflex reactions to the ischemic pain mirror and perpetuate the reaction to the original injury to become a vicious cycle.
10. In the case of the pain-spasm-pain cycle wherein pain is intensified because of ischemia, skillfully applied massage therapy diverts some attention away from the acute intensity of the pain. By massaging the contracted ischemic tissues, chronic spasms can be relieved and circulation restored. As oxygen and nutrients flood the area and lactic acid and other irritants are removed, the pain disappears and mobility is restored.
11. Infection is the result of the invasion of the body by disease-producing micro-organisms such as bacteria, viruses, fungi, or protozoa. If micro-organisms enter the body in sufficient numbers to multiply and become harmful and are capable of destroying healthy tissue, the body reacts by developing an infection. Inflammation is a protective and healing response that happens when tissue

is damaged. Blood vessels in the area of the damaged tissues dilate, increasing blood flow to the area; capillary walls become more permeable, allowing large quantities of blood plasma and white blood cells to enter the tissue spaces; and leukocytes flood the area to engulf and digest the invading organisms and the damaged tissue debris.

12. The four principal signs and symptoms of inflammation are swelling, redness, heat, and pain.

13. Fever is a warning sign that usually accompanies infectious diseases or infected burns and cuts. A disturbance of the body's heat-regulating system causes an elevated body temperature.

14. Extreme or prolonged fever may be dangerous or even fatal. Prolonged fever will cause dehydration so fluids must be replaced. Fevers above 106 to 108 °F may cause damage to the tissues of the kidneys, liver, or other organs or may cause irreparable brain damage, possibly resulting in death.

15. Medical terms are usually compound words constructed of root words, or stems, prefixes, and suffixes. Anatomical terms often include more than one word. Generally the first word acts as an adjective and will indicate the region or location of the structure. The second word is the noun and names the structure.

16. The stem, or root word, generally indicates the body part or structure involved. A prefix is added in front of the stem to further its meaning. Suffixes often denote a diagnosis, symptom, or surgical procedure or identify a word as a noun or adjective.

CHAPTER 5 HISTOLOGY

1. All living matter consists of various cells.
2. Nucleus, centrosome, cytoplasm, and the cell membrane or wall.
3. The nucleus and the centrosome control cell reproduction.
4. As long as the cell receives an adequate supply of food, oxygen, and water, eliminates waste products, and is surrounded by a favorable environment (proper temperature, and the absence of waste products, toxins, and pressure), it will continue to grow and function. When these requirements are not provided, the cell will stop growing and will eventually die.
5. Cell reproduction in human tissue occurs by the process called mitosis, the indirect division of cells.
6. The five phases of mitosis are interphase, prophase, metaphase, anaphase, and telophase.
7. Catabolism and anabolism.
8. Anabolism is the process of building up of larger molecules from smaller ones.
9. Catabolism is the process of breaking down of larger molecules into smaller ones.
10. Enzymes are protein substances that act as organic catalysts to initiate, accelerate, or control specific

chemical reactions in the metabolic process, while they themselves remain unchanged.

11. All tissues are composed of specialized cells.
12. The five main categories of tissues are epithelial, connective, muscular, nervous, and liquid tissue.
13. Endoderm, mesoderm, and ectoderm are the cell layers of the embryo that form the primary germ layers that, in turn, form all the tissues and organs of the body.
14. Epithelial tissues cover all surfaces of the body, both inside and out, and function in the process of absorption, excretion, secretion, and protection.
15. Two main types of membranes are epithelial and connective.
16. The main function of connective tissue is to bind structures, to create a framework, and to provide support.
17. The main function of areolar (loose) tissue is to bind the skin to underlying tissues and to fill spaces between the muscles.
18. Adipose tissue is areolar tissue with an abundance of fat-containing cells.
19. Three types of cartilage are fibrous, hyaline, and elastic.
20. Bone tissue is made hard by mineral salts, calcium phosphate, and calcium carbonate.
21. Dentine is the hard, dense, calcareous tissue that forms the body of a tooth beneath the enamel.
22. Three types of muscle tissue are skeletal, smooth, and cardiac muscle tissue.
23. Striated muscle tissue is made of cylindrical fibers, is found in voluntary muscles, and appears striated if observed under a microscope. Smooth muscle tissue fibers are not striated and are found in involuntary muscles.
24. Cardiac muscle tissue is found only in the heart.
25. The main function of nervous tissue proper is to initiate, control, and coordinate the body's adaptations to its surroundings and environment.
26. Liquid tissue is found in blood and lymph.

CHAPTER 5 ORGANIZATION

1. Anatomic position shows a person from the front standing upright with the palms of the hands facing forward.
2. The three imaginary planes are called the sagittal (vertical), the coronal (frontal), and the transverse (horizontal) planes.
3. When studying anatomy, it is important to know the anatomical position and the regions and planes of the human body to describe the position of a structure or to locate one structure in relation to another. Once you know the body planes, you will understand the location of body cavities and which organs are located in a particular cavity.
4. The subdivisions of the ventral cavity are the thoracic cavity, containing the heart and lungs, the

abdominal cavity, containing the liver, stomach, spleen, pancreas, small and large intestines; and the pelvic cavity, containing the bladder, rectum, and some of the reproductive organs. The dorsal cavity is divided into the cranial cavity, containing the brain; and the spinal or vertebral cavity, containing the spinal cord.

5. The four main anatomic parts of the body are the head consisting of the cranium and the face; the spine, including the vertebrae and the sacrum; the trunk, including the chest or thorax and the abdomen and the organs they contain; the upper extremities, including the shoulders, arms, and hands; and the lower extremities, including the hips, legs, and feet.

6. The ten most important systems of the body are the integumentary (skin), skeletal, muscular, nervous, endocrine, circulatory (blood and lymph vascular), digestive, excretory, respiratory, and reproductive systems.

Answers to Matching I
1. g; 2. j; 3. i; 4. k; 5. h; 6. e; 7. c; 8. b; 9. d; 10. a; 11. f

Answers to Matching II
1. f; 2. c; 3. i; 4. g; 5. a; 6. d; 7. j; 8. b; 9. e; 10. h

CHAPTER 5 THE SKIN

1. The skin (integumentary system) is the external covering and largest organ of the body.
2. The skin protects the parts of the body situated beneath its surface, regulates body temperature, and functions as an organ of secretion and excretion, absorption, and respiration.
3. The two main layers of the skin are the epidermis and the dermis.
4. The layers of the epidermis are the stratum corneum, lucidum, granulosum, and mucosum.
5. Keratin is both hard and soft. Soft keratin is found in the skin, and hard keratin is found in hair and nails.
6. Subcutaneous tissue is a layer of fatty tissue found below the dermis. It contains a network of arteries and a superficial and deep layer of lymphatics.
7. The color of the skin depends partly on the blood supply but more on melanin, the pigment or coloring matter deposited in the deepest layer of the epidermis and the superficial layer of the dermis.
8. The layers of the dermis are the papillary and the reticular layers.
9. A gland is an organ of either excretion or secretion, taking materials from the blood and forming new substances.
10. The two major glands in the skin are the sudoriferous glands, which excrete sweat, and the sebaceous glands, which secrete sebum.
11. Sebum is an oily substance of the sebaceous glands. A pore is a minute opening of the sweat glands on the surface of the skin and is also referred to as a follicle. A duct is a passage or canal for fluids.
12. Appendages of the skin include hair and nails. In addition, the oil and sweat glands are appendages.
13. A lesion is a structural change in tissues caused by injury or disease.
14. An occupational disorder is a skin condition or reaction caused by some substance a worker uses in his or her occupation.
15. The massage practitioner should observe the client's skin condition because the skin often given clues as to whether massage would be beneficial or potentially harmful.

CHAPTER 5 THE SKELETAL SYSTEM

1. The skeletal system is composed of bones, cartilage, and ligaments.
2. The function of the skeletal system are:
1. To offer a framework that supports body structures and gives shape to the body
2. To protect delicate internal organs and tissues
3. To provide attachments for muscles and act as levers in conjunction with muscles to produce movement
4. To manufacture blood cells in the red bone marrow
5. To store minerals such as calcium phosphate, calcium carbonate, magnesium, and sodium
3. Organic matter of bones consists of bone cells, blood vessels, connective tissue, and marrow. Inorganic matter consists of calcium phosphate and calcium carbonate.
4. Two types of bone tissue are cancellous (spongy) tissue and dense (compact) tissue. Dense bone tissue is found on the outer portion of the bone just under the periosteum. Cancellous tissue is found on the interior of flat bones and in the ends of long bones.
5. The periosteum covers and protects bone.
6. Bones receive their nourishment through blood vessels that enter through the periosteum into the interior of the bone. Bone marrow also aids in the nutrition of the bone.
7. Flat bones, such as the skull; long bones, such as the legs; short bones, such as the fingers; and irregular bones, such as the vertebrae of the spine.
8. Yellow bone marrow is found in the medullary cavity of the long bones. Red bone marrow is located in the ends of the long bones and in flat bones. In infants and young children, red marrow also occupies the cavities of long bones.
9. Red bone marrow is the site of blood cell synthesis.
10. The main parts of the skeleton are the axial skeleton and the appendicular skeleton.
11. The three classifications of joints are synarthrotic joints such as those in the skull, which are immovable; amphiarthrotic joints, which have limited motion; and diarthrotic joints, which are freely movable.

12. Articular cartilage cushions bones at the joints.
13. Bones are supported at the joints by ligaments.
14. Joints are lubricated by synovial fluid or synovium.
15. There are approximately 206 bones in the adult human body.
16. The form or outline of the bones must be carefully followed and the limitations of the range of movements be considered when practicing massage therapy. Knowing the names of bones serves as a guide in recalling the names of related structures connected with the body part being massaged.
17. Pivot joints, as in the neck between the atlas and the axis. Hinge joints, as in the elbow, knees, and two distal joints of the fingers. Ball and socket joints, as in the hips and shoulders. Gliding joints, as in the spine or hand. Saddle joints, as in the wrist, thumb, and ankle.
18. A fracture is a break or rupture of a bone.
19. A sprain is an injury to a joint that results in the stretching or tearing of the ligaments. In a class I sprain there is a stretch in the ligament, some discomfort and minimal loss of function. In a class II sprain, the ligament is torn with some loss of function. In a class III sprain, the ligaments are torn, and there is internal bleeding and severe loss of function.
20. Arthritis is an inflammatory condition of the joints often accompanied by pain and changes of bone structure. The three most common types of arthritis are rheumatoid arthritis, osteoarthritis, and gouty arthritis.
21. Osteoporosis literally means porous bones and is a condition where minerals are drawn out of the bones, leaving them brittle and weak. When massaging a person with osteoporosis, the therapist must not use heavy pressure or forceful joint movements, either of which may fracture the weakened bones.
22. Three abnormal curves of the spine are as follows: Kyphosis is an exaggerated convex curve usually associated with the thoracic spine. Lordosis is an exaggerated concave curve usually associated with the lumbar spine. Scoliosis is an abnormal lateral curve of the spine.

Answers to Matching I
1. i; 2. g; 3. b; 4. e; 5. h; 6. f; 7. j; 8. c; 9. a; 10. d

Answers to True or False Test
1. F; 2. T; 3. T; 4. F; 5. F; 6. T; 7. T; 8. T; 9. T; 10. F

Answers to Matching II
1. c; 2. e; 3. h; 4. j; 5. b; 6. a; 7. d; 8. i; 9. f; 10. g

CHAPTER 5 MUSCULAR SYSTEM

Matching Test I 1. c; 2. e; 3. a; 4. b; 5. d
True or False Test I 1. F; 2. F; 3. T; 4. T; 5. F

Matching Test II 1. c; 2. d; 3. b; 4. e; 5. a
True or False Test II 1. T; 2. F; 3. F; 4. T; 5. T

Matching Test III 1. b; 2. c; 3. d; 4. e; 5. a
True or False Test III 1. T; 2. F; 3. T; 4. F; 5. T

Matching Test IV 1. e; 2. a; 3. d; 4. c; 5. b
True or False Test IV 1. F; 2. F; 3. T; 4. T; 5. T

Matching Test V 1. b; 2. c; 3. d; 4. e; 5. a
True or False Test V 1. T; 2. T; 3. F; 4. T; 5. F

1. Muscles are contractile fibrous tissue that produce various movements of the body.
2. There are approximately 600 muscles in the human body.
3. Voluntary (striated) muscle is found in the muscles that attach to the skeleton; involuntary (nonstriated) muscle is found in the hollow muscular organs such as the stomach, intestines, bladder, and blood vessels; heart (cardiac) muscle is found only in the heart.
4. Voluntary muscles can be controlled by the will; involuntary muscles are not controlled by the will and receive nerve stimulation from the autonomic nervous system.
5. The characteristics that enable muscles to produce movement are irritability, contractility, and elasticity.
6. Skeletal muscles are striated muscles attached to the bones of the skeleton.
7. The functional unit of skeletal muscle is the muscle cell or muscle fiber.
8. The striated appearance of voluntary muscle is due to the arrangement of the actin and myosin in the myofibrils.
9. Besides the muscle fibers, muscle contains a variety of connective tissue, blood and other fluids, blood and lymph vessels, and nerves.
10. Muscles are attached to bones, cartilage, ligaments, tendons, skin, and sometimes to each other.
11. Origin of a muscle refers to the more fixed attachments, such as muscles attached to bones, that act as anchors for movements.
12. Insertion of a muscle refers to the attachments that perform the action, such as muscles attached to skin, other muscles, or the more distal and movable attachment.
13. Tendon or sinew attaches muscles to the bone.
14. The function of fibrous connective tissue is to organize and support muscle tissue, blood vessels, and nerves. Connective tissue anchors the muscle fibers and connects them to the structures they act on.
15. Fascia is a delicate membrane of connective tissue covering muscles and separating their several layers or groups of layers.
16. Three layers of connective muscle are the epimysium that covers the muscle, the perimysium that separates the muscle bundles, and the endomyseum that surrounds each muscle cell.
17. A motor unit is all of the muscle fibers that are controlled by a single motor neuron.

18. Acetylcholine is a chemical neurotransmitter found at the myoneural junction. When a nerve impulse travels to the end of a motor neuron, acetylcholine is released and travels across the gap to excite the muscle cell to contract.
19. Muscles receive energy from the breaking down of adenosine triphosphate (ATP) into adenosine diphosphate (ADP).
20. Oxygen debt results from the muscles expending energy faster than the body can supply the oxygen needed to produce the energy. When oxygen debt becomes extreme, the muscles will stop functioning in a condition known as muscle fatigue.
21. A muscle has tone if it is firm and responds readily to stimulation.
22. A muscle lacks tone if it is flabby.
23. When massage practitioners understand how muscles function, they are better able to apply massage techniques that will relax tense muscles and rejuvenate tired muscles.
24. Extensibility is the ability of muscle fibers to lengthen and stretch.
25. An isometric muscle contraction is a static contraction wherein the distance between the ends of the muscle does not change so there is no movement. With an isotonic muscle contraction, the distance between the ends of the muscle changes and there is movement.
26. Eccentric and concentric muscle contractions are both isotonic contractions. In a concentric contraction, the ends of the contracting muscle are coming closer. In an eccentric contraction, the ends of the contracting are moving farther apart.
27. Prime mover and agonist both refer to the primary muscle that is responsible for a specific movement.
28. When flexing the elbow, the triceps become the antagonist.
29. The three components of motion are flexion/extension, adduction/abduction, and rotation.
30. Diarthrotic joints are freely movable.
31. There are three degrees or grades of muscle strain. Grade I is an overstretching of a few of the muscle fibers with a minimal tearing of the fibers. Grade II involves a partial tear of between 10 and 50 percent of the muscle fibers. Grade III is the most severe injury with between 50 and 100 percent muscle tearing.
32. Muscle atrophy is a degenerative process due to muscle disuse. The muscle fibers reduce in size, blood supply is reduced, and the muscle weakens.
33. Ampiarthrotic joints have limited motion.
34. Synarthrotic joints, as in the skull, are immovable.

CHAPTER 5 THE CIRCULATORY SYSTEM

Matching Test I   **True or False Test I**
1. b; 2. c; 3. d; 4. e; 5. a   1. T; 2. F; 3. T; 4. F; 5. T

Matching Test II   **True or False Test II**
1. d; 2. a; 3. e; 4. c; 5. b   1. T; 2. F; 3. T; 4. F; 5. F

1. The heart, blood vessels (arteries, veins, and capillaries), lymph vessels, and the fluids that circulate through them are the main parts of the circulatory system.
2. The two divisions of the circulatory system are the blood-vascular system and the lymph-vascular system.
3. The heart is an efficient pump that keeps the blood moving in a steady stream through a closed system of blood vessels.
4. The pericardium is a protective sac surrounding and supporting the heart in position and at the same time allowed to move frictionlessly as it continually pulsates.
5. The chambers of the heart are the right atrium (or auricle), the right ventricle, the left atrium and the left ventricle.
6. Two sets of nerves, the vagus and sympathetic nerves, regulate the heart beat.
7. The arteries carry blood away from the heart to the capillaries.
8. An arteriole is the microscopic final division of the arteries before the capillaries.
9. Movements of the arterial walls are controlled by vasomotor nerves from the autonomic nervous system consisting of the vasoconstrictor nerves and the vasodilator nerves.
10. The capillaries connect the smaller arteries with the veins. The permeable walls of the capillaries allow a two-way diffusion of substances between the blood and the tissue fluid, thereby bringing nourishment to the cells and removing waste products.
11. The veins carry blood from the various capillaries back toward the heart. Veins of general circulation carry waste-laden, oxygen-poor blood from the body while pulmonary veins carry freshly oxygenated blood from the lungs.
12. A venule is the smallest vessel of the venous system that collects blood from the capillaries.
13. The purpose of the venous pump is to assist in moving the blood through the veins and toward the heart.
14. The main artery is the aorta.
15. Two portions of the blood vascular system are the pulmonary circulatory system and the general or systemic circulatory system.
16. The pulmonary veins carry freshly oxygenated blood.
17. The constituents of blood include plasma, red corpuscles, white corpuscles, and platelets.
18. The red blood cells primarily carry oxygen from the lungs to the cells and carbon dioxide from the cells to the lungs.
19. The primary function of white blood cells is to protect the body against disease by combating

different infectious and toxic agents that may invade the body.

20. Blood carries water, oxygen, food, and secretions to the body cells.
21. Blood carries carbon dioxide gas and metabolic waste products away from the body cells.
22. The blood protects the body against extreme heat or cold, harmful bacteria, and the excessive loss of blood by forming an external clot.
23. Normal body temperature is 98.6 °F (37° C).
24. The lymph system includes the lymph, lymphatics, lymph ducts, lymph nodes, glands, and lacteals. Also considered a part of the lymph system are the tonsils, the spleen, and the thymus gland.
25. The function of the lymph-vascular system is to collect excess tissue fluid, invading micro-organisms, damaged cells, and protein molecules. The lymphoid tissue also produces lymphocytes, a white blood cell that is an important element of the body's immune system.
26. The lymph nodes filter harmful bacteria and toxic matter from the lymph and are the site of production of lymphocytes.
27. The parts of the body containing lymph nodes are the back of the head, around the neck muscles, under the armpit, under the pectoral muscles, along the blood vessels of the abdomen and pelvis, the back of the knees, and the groin.
28. Lymph is derived from interstitial or extracellular fluid.
29. Lymph returns to venous blood through the brachiocephalic veins.
30. Lymph drainage is draining of lymph fluids from various areas of the body.
31. The lacteals are lymphatic vessels that carry chyle from the small intestine to the thoracic duct.
32. Massage increases flow of lymph and prevents stagnation.
33. Lymphatics are named according to their location in the body.
34. The lymphatic pump is similar to the venous pump. A system of valves in the lymph vessels operates so that external pressure on the walls of the vessel force the movement of lymph through the vessel in one direction.
35. Tissue fluid becomes lymph when it enters through the wall of a lymph capillary. From there lymph flows into larger lymphatics and into the first of possibly several lymph nodes. Eventually the lymph flows out of the nodes, through another lymph vessel, and into either the right or thoracic lymph duct. From the lymph duct, lymph flows into the brachiocephalic vein.

CHAPTER 5 THE NERVOUS SYSTEM

Matching Test I
1. c; 2. d; 3. e; 4. b; 5. a

True or False Test I
1. F; 2. T; 3. F; 4. T; 5. T

Matching Test II
1. e; 2. d; 3. a; 4. c; 5. b

True or False Test II
1. F; 2. T; 3. T; 4. F; 5. T

Matching Test III
1. b; 2. e; 3. a; 4. c; 5. d

True or False Test III
1. T; 2. F; 3. F; 4. T; 5. T

Matching Test IV
1. b; 2. e; 3. d; 4. c; 5. a

True or False Test IV
1. F; 2. T; 3. T; 4. F; 5. T

Matching Test V
1. e; 2. c; 3. b; 4. a; 5. d

True or False Test V
1. T; 2. F; 3. T; 4. F; 5. T

1. The nervous system controls and coordinates the functions of other systems of the body so they work harmoniously and efficiently. The primary function of the nervous system is to collect a multitude of sensory information, process, interpret, and integrate that information, and initiate appropriate responses throughout the body.
2. The main parts of the nervous system include the brain, spinal cord, and the peripheral nerves.
3. A nerve cell is called a neuron and consists of a cell body, a single axon, and numerous dendrites.
4. Neurons have the ability to react to certain stimuli (irritability) and to transmit an impulse generated by that stimulus over a distance or to another neuron (conductability).
5. A synapse is the junction between two nerve cells where a nerve impulse is transmitted from one nerve cell to another.
6. A sensory neuron or afferent neuron carries impulses from the sense organs in the periphery of the body toward the central nervous system. A motor or efferent neuron carries impulses away from the central nervous system to the muscles or glands that they control. Interneurons, located in the spinal cord or brain, transmit impulses from one nerve cell to another.
7. A nerve is a bundle of nerve fibers held together by connective tissue that extends from the central nervous system to the tissue that the neurons enervate.
8. An efferent nerve or motor nerve is composed of motor neurons.
9. An afferent nerve or sensory nerve is composed of sensory neurons.
10. A mixed nerve is composed of both sensory and motor nerves. Most nerves in the body are mixed nerves.
11. The two divisions of the nervous system are the central nervous system (CNS) and the peripheral nervous system.
12. The central nervous system consists of the brain, which is located in the cranium, and the spinal cord, which is located in the vertebral canal of the spine.
13. The meninges is a fibrous connective tissue covering of the CNS consisting of the dura mater, the arachnoid mater, and the pia mater.
14. Cerebrospinal fluid is a clear fluid derived from the blood and secreted into the inner cavities or ventricles

of the brain. Cerebrospinal fluid carries some nutrients to the nerve tissue and carries wastes away; however, its main function is to protect the CNS by acting as a shock absorber for the delicate tissue.

15. The main parts of the brain are the cerebrum, the cerebellum, and the brain stem consisting of the midbrain, the pons, and the medulla oblongata.

16. The peripheral nervous system consists of all of the nerves that connect the central nervous system to the rest of the body and therefore is located throughout all the enervated tissues of the body.

17. The two divisions of the peripheral nervous system are the somatic nervous system and the autonomic nervous system.

18. There are twelve pairs of cranial nerves.

19. The twelve cranial nerves are the I olfactory nerve, II optic nerve, III oculomotor nerve, IV trochlear nerve, V trigeminal or trifacial nerve, VI abducent nerve, VII facial nerve, VIII acoustic or auditory nerve, IX glossopharyngeal nerve, X vagus or pneumogastric nerve, XI spinal accessory nerve, and XII hypoglossal nerve.

20. There are thirty-one pairs of spinal nerves.

21. The spinal nerves are numbered according to the vertebral level where they exit the spinal column. They are numbered as follows: Cervical nerves—C1 through 8 Thoracic nerves —T1 through 12 Lumbar nerves —L1 through 5 Sacral nerves —S1 through 5 One pair of coccygeal nerves.

22. A nerve plexus is a network or gathering of nerves located outside of the CNS

23. The important nerve plexuses are: The cervical plexus formed by the spinal nerves C 1–4, serving the structures in the region of the neck; The brachial plexus formed by the spinal nerves C 5–T1, serving the shoulder, arm and part of the chest; The lumbar plexus formed by the spinal nerves T12–L4, serving the muscles and organs of the abdomen, hip and upper leg; The sacral plexus formed by the spinal nerves L4–S4 creating the sciatic nerve and serving the legs; The coccygeal plexus formed by part of S4 and S5, serve the area around the coccyx.

24. The autonomic nervous system regulates action of glands, smooth muscles, and the heart.

25. The parasympathetic and sympathetic are the two divisions of the autonomic nervous system. The activity of the sympathetic system is primarily to prepare the organism for energy-expending, stressful, or emergency situations. Stimulation of the sympathetic nerves can bring about rapid responses, such as increased respiration, dilated pupils, and increased heart rate and cardiac output. Blood vessels dilate, the skin constricts, and the liver increases conversion of glycogen to glucose for more energy. There is increased mental activity and production of adrenal hormones. The parasympathetic nervous system balances the action of the sympathetic system. The general function of the parasympathetic division is to conserve energy and reverse the action of the sympathetic division.

26. The involuntary muscles, heart, lungs, stomach, intestines, and blood vessels are supplied by the sympathetic nervous system. Also the adrenal and salivary glands, the bladder and reproductive organs.

27. Reflex action is the involuntary response of a muscle to a stimulus.

28. Proprioception is a system of sensory and motor nerve activity that provides information as to the position and rate of movement of different body parts to the central nervous system. Proprioception provides information as to the state of contraction and position of the muscles.

29. Two categories of proprioceptors are spindle cells and golgi tendon organs. Spindle cells located mostly in the belly of the muscle record changes in the length and stretch of the muscle as well as how far and fast the muscle is moving. The golgi tendon organs are located in the tendon near its connection to the muscle and record the amount of tension produced in muscle cells that occurs as a result of the muscle stretching and contracting and the amount of force pulling on the bone to which the tendon attaches.

CHAPTER 5 THE ENDOCRINE SYSTEM

1. The endocrine system is composed of a group of glands whose functions are vital to the maintenance of health.

2. The major function of the endocrine system is to assist the nervous system in regulating body processes.

3. A duct gland possesses a duct or canal that carries its secretions to their destination, whereas a ductless gland has no duct and therefore must depend on the circulatory system to carry its secretions to various affected tissues.

4. The blood supplies the raw materials that glands use to produce secretions. The nerves control many of the functional activities of the glands.

5. Sebaceous glands are duct glands that provide sebum (oil) to lubricate the skin.

6. A ductless or endocrine gland has no duct but delivers its secretion directly into the bloodstream, affecting the growth, development, sexual activity, and health of the entire body, depending on the gland's target organs and the quality and quantity of its secretions.

7. The pancreas and sex glands (gonads) function as both duct and ductless glands.

8. The ductless or endocrine glands produce hormones.

9. Hormones are specialized to act on specific tissues (target organs) or influence certain processes in the body. Some have a profound effect on physical or sexual development. Others regulate metabolism or

body chemistry. Some hormones stimulate or restrain the activity of another gland. The endocrine glands operate cooperatively with one another and the nervous system to maintain a state of homeostasis within the organism.

10. The important endocrine glands are the pituitary gland, thyroid gland, parathyroid glands, adrenal glands, sex glands (gonads), and pancreas. Other organs that have hormone-producing tissue include the pineal gland, the hypothalamus, the kidneys, the placenta, and intestinal mucosa.

11. Most diseases or dysfunctions of the endocrine system are the result of overactivity or underactivity of one or more glands. Overactive or hyperactive glands oversecrete hormones due to lack of regulation or glandular tumors. Underactive or hypoactive glands secrete insufficient amounts of their perspective hormones.

12. The pituitary gland is often called the master gland because many of the hormones it secretes stimulate or regulate other endocrine glands.

13. The hormone-producing parts of the adrenal glands are the adrenal cortex and the medulla.

14. The male sex glands produce testosterone and the female sex glands produce estrogen and progesterone.

Answers to Matching I

1. a; 2. f; 3. g; 4. a; 5. b; 6. i; 7. a; 8. e; 9. h; 10. e; 11. a; 12. g; 13. f; 14. c; 15. a

Answers to Matching II

1. j; 2. a; 3. h; 4. d; 5. g; 6. f; 7. b; 8. i; 9. e; 10. c

CHAPTER 5 THE RESPIRATORY SYSTEM

1. The major respiratory organs include the nose, nasal cavity, pharynx, larynx, trachea, bronchial tubes, and the lungs.

2. The respiratory system is responsible for the vital exchange of oxygen and carbon dioxide.

3. The lungs are two sacs composed of spongy tissue, blood vessels, connective tissue, and microscopic air sacs called alveoli.

4. The three levels of respiration are external respiration, internal respiration, and cellular respiration or oxidation. External respiration takes place in the lungs. Internal respiration takes place between the blood stream and the cells of the body. Cellular respiration or oxidation takes place within the cells.

5. The alveoli are microscopic air sacs at the terminal ends of the bronchioles that are surrounded by the pulmonary capillaries, where the exchange of carbon dioxide for oxygen takes place.

6. Breathing or ventilation is the process of inhaling and exhaling air.

7. The natural rate of breathing is fourteen to twenty times a minute.

8. The diaphragm is a muscular sheet separating the thorax from the abdominal cavity. It is the major muscle used in breathing.

CHAPTER 5 THE DIGESTIVE SYSTEM

1. Structures of the digestive system include the alimentary canal and accessory digestive organs. The alimentary canal consists of the mouth, pharynx, esophagus, stomach, small intestine, and large intestine. The accessory organs include the teeth, tongue, salivary glands, pancreas, liver, and gall bladder.

2. The main functions of the digestive system are digestion and absorption. Digestion is the process of converting food into substances capable of being used by the cells for nourishment.

3. Absorption is the process in which the digested nutrients are transferred from the intestines to the blood or lymph vessels so that they can be transported to the cells.

4. The physical process of digestion involves the teeth, which tear and grind the food, and the action of the muscles, which churn and mix the food as well as push it through the digestive tract.

5. Enzymes aid digestion.

6. In the mouth food is chewed and mixed with saliva, and carbohydrates begin to be digested to the sugar stage.

7. The alimentary canal is a muscular tube about thirty feet in length that extends from the mouth to the anus. The wall of the alimentary canal consists of four distinct layers: The mucosa or mucous membrane is made up of epithelial cells, connective tissue, and a variety of digestive glands. This layer protects the underlying tissues and carries on secretion and absorption. The submucosa consists of connective tissue, nerves, and blood and lymph vessels that serve to nourish the surrounding tissues and carry away the absorbed material. The muscular layer has two layers of smooth muscle that churn the contents and propel it through the canal. The serous layer is the outer covering of the tube.

8. Peristaltic action is a rhythmic, wave-like muscular action of the smooth muscles of the alimentary canal that propels and churns the food throughout the length of the canal.

9. In the stomach food is mixed with gastric juice. Protein digestion begins.

10. The parts of the small intestine are the duodenum, the jejunum, and the ileum.

11. Digestive secretions in the small intestines are supplied by the liver, pancreas, and glands in the small intestine.

12. In the small intestine, food is completely digested.

13. The blood vessels and lacteals in villi in the walls of the small intestine absorb the end products of digestion.

14. The rectum of the large intestine eliminates undigested food waste from the body.

CHAPTER 5 THE EXCRETORY SYSTEM

1. The organs that comprise the excretory system are the lungs, kidneys, skin, liver, and large intestine.
2. The body will become poisoned by its own waste products.
3. The excretory system eliminates metabolic waste and undigested foods from the body.
4. The urinary system includes two kidneys, two ureters, the bladder, and a urethra.
5. The functional unit of the kidney is the nephron.
6. A urinalysis will indicate the presence of white blood cells, blood, glucose, or other chemicals in the urine that may be an indication of metabolic imbalance, infection, or numerous other conditions.
7. A change in the color of the urine, such as cloudiness or a reddish or brownish color, can indicate infection or other health problems.
8. The liver secretes bile.
9. The main excretory function of the liver is the production of urea, which is returned to the blood to be excreted by the kidneys. The liver also excretes bile into the small intestines.

CHAPTER 5 THE REPRODUCTIVE SYSTEM

1. The reproductive system is the generative apparatus necessary for organisms to reproduce organisms of the same kind or species.
2. Asexual reproduction as in some one-celled organisms means that no partner is needed to reproduce. In humans and animals reproduction is sexual and requires a male and female to reproduce.
3. A gonad is a sex gland—the ovary in the female and the testes in the male.
4. A zygote is the fertilized ovum, the cell formed by the union of a spermatozoon (sperm) with the ovum (egg).
5. The reproductive system in males includes two testes, two vas deferens, two seminal vesicles, a prostate gland, the bulbourethral glands (Cowper's glands), and the penis.
6. The functions of the male reproductive system are the production of sperm, the production of the male hormones, and the performance of the sex act.
7. The reproductive system in females includes two ovaries, two fallopian tubes (oviducts), a uterus, a vagina, and the vulva or external genitalia.
8. The functions of the female reproductive system are to produce the ovum and female hormones, to receive the sperm during the sex act, and to carry the growing fetus during pregnancy.
9. From the beginning of conception until approximately the third month of pregnancy, the developing child is called an embryo. After that time it is called a fetus.
10. Ovulation is the discharge of a mature egg cell from the follicle of the ovary.
11. Pregnancy lasts approximately forty weeks or 280 days.

CHAPTER 6 EFFECTS, BENEFITS, INDICATIONS AND CONTRAINDICATIONS OF MASSAGE

1. The main physiological benefits of massage are stimulation of the muscular, vascular, and glandular activities of the body. Circulation is increased and soreness and stiffness of the muscles relieved.
2. The psychological benefits of massage result from the reduction of tension and relief from stress and anxiety. Massage can also promote a sense of renewed energy and well-being. Massage helps the client to feel healthier, invigorated, and more energetic.
3. Massage has direct mechanical effects and indirect reflex effects on the body.
4. Massage is beneficial to all body systems including the circulatory, nervous, skeletal, muscular, digestive, glandular, integumentary (skin), respiratory, and excretory systems.
5. Massage benefits the development of the muscular system by way of stimulation of its circulation, nerve supply, and cell activity. Massage is also an effective means of relaxing tense muscles and releasing muscle spasms. Massage prevents and relieves stiffness and soreness of muscles. Muscle tissue that has suffered injury heals more quickly with less connective tissue build-up and scarring when therapeutic massage is applied regularly.
6. Nearly all massage movements enhance circulation; however, stroking, kneading, and compression most effectively promote circulation.
7. Massage relieves stiff, sore muscles by improving circulation of the blood through the body part. It helps in the removal of waste products and supplies the cells with oxygen and nourishment.
8. Cross-fiber friction and compression movements prevent the formation of adhesions and fibrosis in muscles.
9. The immediate effects of massage on the skin include increased circulation of the blood, which nourishes the skin, improves tone, and helps to normalize the functioning of the sebaceous (oil) glands.
10. Depending on the type of massage movement applied, the nervous system can be stimulated or toned.
11. Friction, vibration, and light percussion movements produce a stimulating effect on the nervous system.
12. Gentle stroking, light friction, and petrissage produce a sedative effect on the nervous system.
13. Massage affects the quality and rate of blood flowing through the circulatory system. Direct and

reflex effects of massage increase circulation and stimulate the production of red and white blood cells.

14. Massage movements are directed toward the heart to facilitate the flow of blood and lymph back toward the heart.

15. Light stroking, deep stroking, light percussion, friction, petrissage, and compression are all useful in increasing the flow of blood and lymph.

16. Massage improves the circulation of the blood, which in turn supplies beneficial nutrients to the skin.

17. When the client has a condition that appears to be a contraindication to massage, massage should be avoided.

18. Contraindication means the expected treatment or process is inadvisable. In massage it refers to any condition in which massage is not advisable, as it would not be beneficial or might be dangerous.

19. It is important to take a client medical history to help determine potential indications and contraindications for the massage.

20. The practitioner should have a thermometer in order to take a client's temperature if a fever is suspected. Massage is not recommended when the client's temperature is abnormally high. An abnormally high temperature is an indication of illness or other health problems.

21. Massage should be avoided when there is a contraindication, such as a physical or mental condition that needs medical attention or when there is doubt of its benefits. The therapist should refer the client to an appropriate health professional.

22. The signs of inflammation are heat, swelling, pain, and redness.

23. In the case of local inflammation, massage must be avoided on the inflamed area and applied to the area of the body proximal to the inflammation in order to promote circulation toward and away from the area.

24. The practitioner will recognize varicose veins as bluish, protruding, thick, bulbous, distended superficial veins usually found in the lower legs.

25. A hematoma is a mass of blood trapped in some tissue or cavity of the body and is the result of internal bleeding. When the hematoma is in the acute phase, massage is contraindicated because of the risk of reinjuring the tissue. Once the bruise has changed colors, light massage will enhance circulation to the area and actually assist the healing.

26. Massage benefits a woman during a normal, healthy pregnancy by promoting relaxation, soothing nerves, relieving strained back and leg muscles, and instilling a sense of well-being.

27. Massage for the critically ill helps to control discomfort and pain, improve mobility, helps reduce disorientation and confusion by bringing person back to a more positive body awareness, reduces isolation and fear, helps to ease the emotional and physical discomfort of the individual.

28. The virus that causes AIDS is transmitted from person to person only through the exchange of body fluid that contains the virus.

29. Certain areas of the body warrant consideration while being massaged because of the underlying anatomical structure and the possibility of injury to the structure by certain massage manipulations.

CHAPTER 7 EQUIPMENT AND PRODUCTS

1. The massage practitioner should project a professional image of relaxed confidence.

2. A massage space should be comfortable, clean, and free of distractions and safety hazards.

3. A room that is ten by twelve feet allows ample space for a massage table, desk, dressing area, and other equipment and supplies necessary to perform massage.

4. Equipment should be checked for safety and sanitation. Supplies must be checked to assure an adequate supply and to see that they are clean and stored properly.

5. Preparation is essential to good service, and it shows that you are professional.

6. Oils, creams, and powders are products used for body massage.

7. The massage room is usually most comfortable for clients when the temperature is around 75° F.

8. The height of the massage table should be adjusted to give the practitioner more leverage to do the massage efficiently. Correct height also prevents the practitioner from becoming fatigued.

9. Soft, natural, indirect lighting is best in the massage room.

10. Some people find music distracting and prefer absolute quiet.

CHAPTER 8 SANITARY AND SAFETY PROCEDURES

1. All states have laws pertaining to sanitation for the protection of the public. These laws protect both clients and practitioners.

2. The practitioner should practice the rules of sanitation because he or she is responsible for safeguarding the client's health as well as his or her own health.

3. The practitioner should have some knowledge of bacteria in order to understand the importance of preventing the spread of disease.

4. Pathogenic bacteria are harmful, while nonpathogenic bacteria are harmless and sometimes helpful.

5. The body produces antibodies to inhibit or destroy harmful bacteria.

6. Three forms of pathogenic (harmful) bacteria are cocci, bacilli, and spirilla.
7. The strict practice of sanitation is the best prevention against the spread of harmful bacteria.
8. Before using any disinfectant or antiseptic product, you should read the manufacturer's instructions and follow them.
9. Disinfectants are used in the practice of massage to keep all equipment and the premises in a clean, sanitary condition.
10. The best method for keeping the hands and nails clean is to scrub them with a brush in warm, soapy water, rinse with mild alcohol, and then pat them dry.
11. Suitable strengths for Creosol and Lysol used to clean floors, sinks, and restrooms are 5 to 10 percent.
12. Sterilization is the procedure for making an object germ free by destroying bacteria, both the harmful and harmless kinds.
13. Safety is an attitude put into practice that is concerned with the prevention of situations and elimination of conditions that may lead to injury of the massage practitioner or client.
14. Safety considerations in a massage practice need to focus on (1.) the facility, (2.) the equipment, (3.) the massage practitioner, and (4.) the client.

CHAPTER 9 THE CONSULTATION

1. The consultation is important to obtain certain data regarding the client's conditions and to determine the most effective treatments.
2. An assessment includes taking the client's medical history, observing the client's actions, and performing verbal and manipulative tests that may indicate the client's conditions.
3. A preliminary assessment is advisable when doing massage therapy because it clarifies the client's conditions, reveals indications and contraindications, determines if referral to another health professional is advisable, and indicates which therapeutic techniques to use.
4. The treatment plan is an outline the practitioner can follow when giving massage treatments.
5. The treatment plan is formulated using information from the intake and medical history forms, the interview, and preliminary assessment to formulate session goals and choose massage techniques.
6. Accurate records are important to both the practitioner and client because special information may be needed for reference. Well-kept records also help the practitioner to determine and render the most effective treatments.
7. Information that is often found in a client file includes intake information (name, address, phone, etc.), medical information and history, treatment plan and recorded notes, and financial and billing information.

8. The client may not understand why pre-massage procedures are necessary or may feel uneasy and not know what is expected of him or her.
9. Being able to anticipate and answer questions the client may ask gives the practitioner more credibility.
10. An abnormally high temperature or pulse rate may indicate conditions where massage is not advisable.

CHAPTER 10 CLASSIFICATION OF MASSAGE MOVEMENTS

1. The six basic classifications of movements are touch, stroking, kneading, friction, percussion, and joint movements.
2. The practitioner should regulate the intensity of pressure, direction of movement, and duration of each type of manipulation to meet the client's needs.
3. Light movements should be applied over thin tissues and bony parts.
4. Heavier movements should be applied over thick tissues and muscular parts.
5. Massage is generally applied in a centripetal direction, or toward the heart.
6. Massage strokes directed away from the heart should be light enough that they do not affect fluid flow.
7. The approximate duration of a full-body massage is about one hour.
8. When referring to massage technique, touch is the stationary contact of the practitioner's hand and the client's body.
9. Light or superficial touch is purposeful contact in which the natural and evenly distributed weight of the practitioner's finger, fingers, or hand is applied on a given area of the client's body. The main objective of light touch is to soothe and to provide a comforting connection that is calming and allows the powerful healing mechanisms of the body to function. Touch is effective in the reduction of pain, lowering of blood pressure, control of nervous irritability, or reassurance for a nervous, tense client.
10. Deep touch is performed with one finger, thumb, several fingers, or the entire hand. The heel of the hand, knuckles, or elbow can be used according to desired results. Deep touch is used when calming, anesthetizing, or stimulating effects are desired. Deep pressure is useful in soothing muscle spasms and relieving pain at reflex areas, stress points in tendons, and trigger points in muscle.
11. Aura stroking is done with long, smooth strokes where the practitioner's hands glide the length of the client's entire body or body part, coming very close to but not actually touching the body surface.
12. Another name for feather stroking is nerve strokes. These are usually used as the final stroke to the individual areas of the body.
13. Effleurage is a succession of strokes applied by gliding of the hand over a somewhat extended portion of the body.

14. Superficial stroking is a kind of effleurage that requires the lightest possible touch.
15. Deep gliding strokes require firm pressure.
16. Superficial gliding strokes produce soothing effects and overcomes tiredness or restlessness.
17. Deep gliding strokes have a stretching and broadening effect on muscle tissue and fascia. It also enhances and stimulates the venous and lymphatic flow.
18. Kneading movements are applied by grasping muscular tissue with one or both hands, then squeezing, rolling, or pinching with a firm pressure.
19. Kneading enhances the fluid movement in the superficial as well as the deeper tissues.
20. The classical term that means the same as kneading is *petrissage*.
21. Fulling is recommended for the muscular areas of the arms and legs.
22. Friction movements are applied to the body by moving more superficial layers of flesh against the deeper tissues in order to flatten, broaden, or stretch the tissue.
23. Heat created during friction movements affects the connective tissues surrounding the muscles, making them more pliable so they function more efficiently.
24. Cross-fiber friction uses short, deep strokes transverse to the direction of muscle, tendon, or ligament fibers. The fingers do not move over the skin but move the skin and superficial tissues across the target tissue.
25. Compression movements are rhythmic pressing movements directed into muscle tissue perpendicular to the body part by either the hand or fingers.
26. Compression movement invigorates the body, stimulates the flow of blood and lymph, and prevents muscular stiffness following exercise. Compression movements cause increased circulation and a lasting hyperemia in the tissue.
27. Vibratory movements are applied with a continuous shaking or trembling movement by means of the practitioner's hands or an electrical vibrator.
28. Vibration is safe at a rate of five to ten times per second by hand, 10 to 100 times per second by electric vibrators.
29. The practitioner can control the effects of vibratory movements by controlling the rate of vibration, intensity of pressure, and duration of treatment.
30. Excessive vibration produces a numbing effect.
31. Percussion movements are applied with quick striking movements performed with both hands simultaneously or alternately.
32. Percussion movements are slapping, beating, hacking, cupping, and tapping.
33. Percussion movements tone the muscles, stimulate the nervous and circulatory systems.
34. Joint movements can be used to manipulate any joint in the body, including joints of the toes, knees, hips, arms, the vertebrae, or even the less movable joints of the pelvis and cranium.
35. Two types of joint movements are active joint movements and passive joint movements.
36. During an active assistive joint movement the client is instructed to perform a motion at the same time the practitioner assists the movement. During an active resistive movement, the client is instructed to make a motion while the limb is held to resist movement.
37. Range of motion is the movement of a joint from one extreme of the articulation to the other.
38. End feel is the change in the quality of the feeling the therapist senses as the end of a joint movement is approached.
39. Pressure regulated during a massage according to the technique used and according to the intended outcome. The rule is to begin with a light and sensitive touch, increase the pressure as you work into an area and then gradually reduce pressure as you leave the area.
40. A person's pain threshold is the amount of discomfort or pain he or she can tolerate without adverse reactions. When the pain threshold is violated, the client will tense up and the massage work will become less effective or even be counterproductive.

CHAPTER 11 APPLICATION OF MASSAGE TECHNIQUE

1. The massage practitioner must develop strong, flexible hands in order to deliver massage manipulations to the body over an extended period of time and to control the pressure and rhythm while working over the contours of the body.
2. Body mechanics is the observation of body postures in relation to safe and efficient movement in daily living activities.
3. Using good body mechanics increases the strength and power available in a movement while at the same time reducing the risk of potential injury to the individual.
4. To increase the power and strength in a movement and at the same time conserve energy, the practitioner must use the muscles in the legs and the movement of the whole body to deliver the strokes. Keeping the hands in good alignment and close to the practitioner's body and moving the whole body conserves energy and increases the power and strength when performing massage.
5. Correct posture and stances aid balance, allow the delivery of firmer, more powerful massage strokes, conserve strength, and sustain energy when it is necessary to work long hours.

CHAPTER 12 PROCEDURES FOR COMPLETE BODY MASSAGES

1. The practitioner should wash his or her hands before and after each treatment.
2. For reasons of safety and liability, it is advisable that the practitioner assist the client onto the table at the beginning of a massage and into a sitting position and off the table at the end of the massage.
3. Chilling of the client's body can be prevented by keeping the room warm and by using proper draping.
4. Three common methods of draping are: Diaper draping, which uses a folded towel to cover the client's private areas Top cover method, which uses a table covering and a separate sheet or towel to cover the client. Full sheet draping, which uses a double-size sheet to cover the table and wrap the client.
5. Besides draping, the therapist can ensure the client's warmth by keeping the room at a comfortable temperature or using an electric mattress pad or supplying extra coverings.
6. Scratching the client can be avoided by filing the nails short and smooth and removing jewelry.
7. Heavy pressure, rapid movement, or jarring contact cause fear and should be avoided.
8. It is better for the client to receive a massage before eating a meal.
9. The average duration of a massage is about an hour.
10. Massage should never be applied to an area where there is injury or abrasion of the skin, fever, inflammation of joints or veins, or when other contraindications are present.
11. Before a body massage, check facilities for readiness, obtain and arrange supplies, and check self for readiness. Obtain necessary information regarding client's needs and wishes, advise the client regarding preparation procedures and assist as necessary, record the client's pulse and body temperature when necessary.
12. The position the client assumes first for a massage depends on the treatment to be given and the preference of the therapist and the client; however, generally the massage begins with the client in supine (face-up) position.
13. The order of massage movements is determined by the purpose of the massage and the preference of the therapist. Movements should follow a logical sequence such as:
    a. Begin with the hands and arms, left then right.
    b. Proceed to front of the legs and feet, left then right.
    c. Continue movements over chest, neck, and abdomen.
    d. The client will turn over to assume a prone (face-down) position.
    e. Begin with the back of the legs, right then left.
    f. Finish the massage with the back of the body.
14. The final considerations of massage involve completing the client's record card, suggesting supplementary services, placing supplies in their proper places, discarding refuse, and arranging the massage table and bath for the next client.
15. Undesirable aftereffects may include a slight headache, upset stomach and nausea, or the feeling that comes with the onset of a cold. Such reactions are due to an increase in metabolic waste material in the circulatory system. This waste material puts an extra burden on the excretory system. If this waste is not flushed out of the tissues, it will be re-absorbed into the tissues. The particular symptom the client experiences depends on the organs that are being overtaxed.
16. The client should drink plenty of water to keep the system flushed out following a massage.
17. The four steps of the therapeutic procedure are assessment, planning, performance, and evaluation.
18. The purpose of assessment is to review any information available at the onset of the process in order to best understand the present conditions. During the planning stage, the information gained from the assessment is used to determine strategies and select therapeutic techniques to address specific conditions found during the assessment. The performance is the actual application of the selected techniques. The evaluation examines the outcome of the session in regard to the effectiveness of the selected procedure for the condition.
19. The therapeutic process can be implemented for long-range goal setting, covering several sessions, short-range planning, covering a single session and during an actual massage session.
20. Three parts of the assessment are taking a client history, observation, and examination.
21. When testing range of motion, passive movement, active movement and restricted movement are examined.
22. According to Dr. James Cyriax, contractile tissues are the fibrous tissues that have tensions placed on them during muscular contractions and include muscle tissue, tendons, and the muscle attachments. Inert tissues are the tissues that are not contractile such as bone, ligament, bursae, blood vessels, nerves, nerve coverings, cartilage, etc. End feel refers to the quality of the sensation the therapist feels as he or she passively moves a joint to the full extent of its possible range.
23. Three classifications of normal end feel are hard end feel, soft end feel, and springy end feel.
24. Abnormal end feel is similar to normal end feel except that there is reduced movement or there is associated pain.
25. Therapeutic massage is like an intense conversation because the therapist listens, observes, and

examines the client to get an idea of the condition. Then the therapist's hands listen to the client's body and respond with manipulative touch. The body listens to the manipulations and responds. Hearing and feeling these responses, the therapist replies with the next movement.

26. The evaluation is important because:
- The client and therapist can gauge the effectiveness of the selected course of therapy according to the success in attaining the goals.
- It provides a rationale for applying similar therapies for similar conditions in the future.
- It is the grounds for altering portions or all of the process to better achieve desired results.
- It helps determine if goals have been met and if a referral to another professional is warranted.

CHAPTER 13 FACE AND SCALP MASSAGE

1. When the client does not want face massage or when there is some contraindication to face massage.
2. Cleansing the face.
3. In face massage, movements are very gentle. While movements such as hacking, twisting, or heavy strokes may be beneficial to parts of the body, they are not used on face.
4. Face massage increases circulation of the blood, which nourishes the tissues. Face massage also helps to tone muscles and keeps sebacious (oil) glands and sudoriferous (sweat) glands functioning properly.
5. Cleansing removes deeply embedded and surface soil. The cleansing procedure removes this debris and helps to prevent blackheads and infectious conditions.
6. Scalp massage stimulates the flow of blood to the tissues. Scalp massage soothes the nerves and is an aid to keeping the scalp healthy and hair lustrous.
7. When the client does not want it and when there are certain contraindications for scalp massage.
8. The massage practitioner gives face and scalp massage as an aid to relaxing and soothing the client, and as an aid to healthy functioning of the face and scalp tissues.

CHAPTER 14 HYDROTHERAPY

1. Electrical apparatus should be used by qualified persons with proper training. The practitioner must have sound knowledge of procedures involving electrical equipment and its benefits as well as any contraindications of its use. Always follow manufacturer's instructions.
2. The practitioner's main concern when advising a client about suntanning is that he or she acquires the suntan in the most safe and healthful manner. The practitioner must be concerned about his or her

own responsibility when operating or supervising suntanning equipment and should not allow the client to misuse equipment.
3. The application of heat causes an increase of circulation, pulse rate, and white blood cell count. A local application will cause local reddening, increased metabolism and leukocyte migration to the area, relaxation of local musculature and a slight analgesia.
4. Cryotherapy is the application of ice for therapeutic purposes.
5. The local application of ice acts as an analgesic to reduce pain and causes vasoconstriction to limit swelling. It is beneficial on painful, inflamed, and swollen areas.
6. In the acronym RICE, R.= rest, I.= ice, C.= compression and E.= elevation. RICE is the standard first-aid treatment when a soft tissue injury such as a sprain or strain occurs. It reduces swelling, pain, and the secondary tissue damage that results from excessive swelling.
7. A contrast bath is the alternating application of hot and cold baths to a portion of the body.
8. Contrast baths are one of the most effective methods of increasing local circulation by causing an alternating vasodilatation and vasoconstriction of the blood vessels in an area.
9. Hydrotherapy is the application of water in any of its three forms (ice, water, vapor) to the body for therapeutic purposes.
10. Water treatments are controlled by regulating the temperature, pressure and duration, of the treatment.
11. The qualities of water that make it an effective therapeutic tool are that it is readily available, relatively inexpensive to use, and has the ability to absorb and conduct heat.
12. The three classifications of effects of hydrotherapy on the body are thermal, mechanical, and chemical.
13. Water treatments that involve hot or cold applications should not be given when the client has cardiac impairment, diabetes, lung disease, kidney infection, extremely high or low blood pressure, or an infectious skin condition.
14. Cold applications are beneficial because they improve circulation, stimulate nerves, and increase the activity of body cells.
15. Cold applications are undesirable over prolonged periods as they may produce a depressing effect. If after a cold bath or shower the client comes out chilly, shivering, blue-lipped, or goose-fleshed, it indicates that his or her body reaction is not good.
16. Hot water applications improve skin functions by promoting perspiration and by increasing the circulation of blood to the surface of the skin.
17. The skin can safely tolerate 115 °F of hot water and approximately 140°F of steam vapor. Water at

110°F over a prolonged period of time would raise the body temperature to a dangerous level.

18. Two objectives of baths are external cleanliness and stimulation of bodily functions.
19. A warm bath is 95 to 100 °F, equal to 35 to 37.7°C. A hot bath is 100 to 115°F, equal to 37.7 to 43.3°C.
20. The average duration of a cold bath, shower or sitz bath is approximately three to five minutes.
21. The duration of a hot saline or sitz bath is approximately ten to twenty minutes.
22. A Swedish shampoo is a cleansing body bath applied with the aid of a brush or bath mitt and mild soap and warm water, followed by rinsing and drying the body.
23. A salt rub is usually given following a hot bath or cabinet bath, or it may be given as a separate treatment.
24. The purpose of a cabinet bath is to induce perspiration that contributes to a weight reduction, and to induce relaxation. It is also considered to be a cleansing procedure.
25. Safety precautions to observe during the operation of a bath cabinet include following the manufacturer's instructions for use of the cabinet, and observing the client's general reactions, state of health, and tolerance to temperature.
26. The main benefits of a whirlpool bath are increased blood circulation, the soothing of nerves, and relaxing of the muscles.
27. The Russian bath is a full-body steam bath for the purpose of causing perspiration. The primary benefits are cleansing, relaxation, and improved metabolism.

CHAPTER 15 MASSAGE FOR NURSING AND HEALTH CARE

1. To teach a patient to maintain his or her health and to live a healthy and productive life.
2. The general practitioner deals with healthy clients or those sent by a physician. The nurse deals with patients under a physician's care who are ill, injured, or recovering.
3. The Swedish method is made up of movements that have been recognized by the medical profession as being beneficial.
4. While massage may not affect a healthy person adversely, the same movements could be detrimental to someone who is ill or has been injured.
5. Active movements help to prevent loss of muscle strength and tone.
6. It is important to know the client's or the patient's physical condition in order to determine if massage will be beneficial or harmful. Also, the medical history form signed by the patient or client serves as protection for the massage practitioner or healthcare professional.

7. The alcohol rubdown refreshes the patient when a bath cannot be given. It tends to lower temperature when a fever is present, creates a soothing and cooling effect after applications of heat, and has a beneficial astringent effect on the skin.
8. The oil rubdown is particularly beneficial in relieving dry skin and skin sensitivity caused by the patient having to lie in bed for long periods of time.

CHAPTER 16 ATHLETIC/SPORTS MASSAGE

1. Athletic massage, also called sports massage, is the application of massage techniques that combine sound anatomical and physiological knowledge, an understanding of strength training and conditioning, and specific massage skills to enhance athletic performance.
2. The therapist must know the functions of the circulatory, skeletal, muscular, and nervous systems of the body.
3. The overload principle in conditioning refers to the necessity of applying stresses to the body greater than it is accustomed to in order to increase strength or endurance.
4. Negative effects of exercise include:
• Increased metabolic waste build-up in the tissues
• Strains in the muscle or connective tissue. These may range from microscopic microtrauma to major injury.
• Inflammation and associated fibrosis
• Spasms and pain that restrict movement.
5. Techniques commonly used in sports massage include those of Swedish massage plus compression, cross-fiber friction, deep pressure, and active joint movements.
6. The primary goal of compression is to create hyperemia in the muscle tissue.
7. In athletic massage, hyperemia refers to the increased amount of blood and other fluids in and moving through the muscle tissue.
8. In athletic massage, deep pressure is used to relieve stress points and deactivate trigger points.
9. Transverse friction massage was popularized by the British osteopath Dr. James Cyriax.
10. The objective of using cross-fiber friction in athletic massage is to reduce fibrosis, encourage the formation of strong, pliable scar tissue at the site of healing injuries, and prevent or soften adhesions in fibrous tissue.
11. The four basic applications for athletic massage are massage previous to an event, massage after an event, massage during training, and massage during injury rehabilitation.
12. The goal of pre-event massage is to increase circulation and flexibility in the areas of the body about to be used. The goal of post-event massage is to increase circulation to clear out metabolic wastes,

reduce muscle tension and spasm, and quiet the nervous system. The goal of massage during training is to allow the athlete to train at a higher level of intensity, more consistently, with less chance of injury, and to maintain muscles in the best possible state of nutrition, flexibility, and vitality. The goal of massage during rehabilitation is to get the athlete back into full performance as soon as possible with less chance of reinjury.

13. Massage is considered to be most beneficial to the athlete as a regular part of his or her scheduled training.

14. Stress points are areas of chronic stress or the site of microtrauma that are generally located at the ends of muscles or in taut bands of muscle tissue.

15. The therapist must be sure to apply proper techniques in order to avoid aggravating a condition or causing permanent damage to the area.

16. The best way to treat an athletic injury is to prevent it.

17. Rehabilitative massage:
- Shortens the time it takes for an injury to heal
- Maintains or increases range of motion
- Helps to reduce swelling and edema
- Helps to form strong, pliable scar tissue
- Eliminates splinting in associated muscle tissue
- Locates and deactivates trigger points that form as a result of the trauma
- Helps get the athlete back into training sooner with less chance of reinjury

18. Proper massage therapy improves circulation, enabling damaged tissue to be carried away while making rebuilding nutrients available so that healing time is reduced.

19. Massage for new or fresh injuries should only be given by properly trained therapists in conjunction with a physician's approval.

20. RICE is an acronym for rest, ice, compression and elevation. This represents proper first aid for soft tissue injuries.

21. Rehabilitative massage can be given at the rate of once or twice a day during the time the athlete is out of training and every other day or every third day until he or she is back to a full training schedule.

22. Acute injuries have a sudden and definite onset and are usually of relatively short duration. Chronic injuries have a gradual onset, tend to last for a long time, or reoccur often.

23. Massage is contraindicated at the site of fresh acute muscle injuries.

24. Strains involve the tearing of muscle tissue or tendons. Sprains involve ligaments.

25. Athlete massage is contraindicated in any abnormal condition, injury, illness, or disease except as advised by the athlete's physician.

CHAPTER 17 SPECIALIZED MASSAGE

1. Properly applied, prenatal massage can aid relaxation, benefit circulation, and soothe the nerves.

2. Correct lymph massage helps to stimulate the flow of lymph, which rids the body of toxins and waste materials. It promotes the balance of the body's internal chemistry, purifies and regenerates tissues, and helps to normalize the functions of all body organs and the immune system.

3. Lymphocytes (leukocytes) are white corpuscles are found in lymphatic tissue, blood, and lymph. They are active in the immune responses of the body and play a major part in healing wounds and fighting infections.

4. Lymph is the portion of the interstitial fluid that is absorbed into the lymph capillaries. It consists of water, proteins, cellular debris, bacteria, viruses, and other inorganic materials.

5. Deep tissue massage refers to various regimens or massage styles that affect the deeper tissue structures of the body. Deep tissue massage techniques affect the various layers of fascia that support muscle tissues and loosen bonds between the layers of connective tissues.

6. Structural integration attempts to bring the physical structure of the body into balance and alignment around a central axis.

7. Neurophysiological therapies recognize the importance of neurological feedback between the central nervous system and the musculo-skeletal system in maintaining proper tone and function. Alterations or disturbances in the neuromuscular relationship often result in dysfunction and pain. Neuro-physiological therapies utilize methods of assessing tissues and soft tissue manipulative techniques to normalize the tissues and reprogram the neurological loop in order to reduce pain and improve function.

8. A trigger point is a hyperirritable spot that is painful when compressed. When stimulated, active trigger points refer pain and tenderness to another area of the body. Latent trigger points only exhibit pain when compressed and do not refer pain.

9. Myofascial trigger points are found in muscle tissue or its associated fascia. They are located in a taut band of muscle fibers.

10. Procedures for deactivating trigger points include injections, stretch and spray, active stretching, and ischemic compression.

11. Neuromuscular therapy was developed in England in the 1930s by Dr. Stanley Lief. It has been popularized in the United States through the teachings of Paul St. John.

12. Abnormal tissue signs that indicate neuromuscular lesions include:
- Congestion in the tissues

- Contracted tissue or taut, fibrous bands
- Nodules or lumps
- Trigger points
- Restrictions between the skin and underlying tissues
- Variations in temperature (warmer or cooler than surrounding tissues)
- Swelling or edema
- General tenderness

Neuromuscular lesions are always hypersensitive to pressure and often associated with trigger points.

13. The primary treatment techniques used in neuro-muscular therapy include gliding, ischemic compression, skin rolling, and stretching.
14. The two basic inhibitory reflexes produced during MET manipulations are post-isometric relaxation and reciprocal inhibition.
15. The three active joint movements used in MET are contract-relax, antagonist-contract, and contract-relax-antagonist -contract.
16. Passive positioning techniques are perhaps the gentlest of soft tissue manipulations wherein joints associated with constricted muscles are passively placed into their preferred position of greatest comfort.
17. Three important considerations of passive position-ing techniques are:
    a. Gently moving a joint into its position of maximum comfort
    b. Holding that position for an adequate period of time
    c. Slowly and passively returning the joint to its neutral position.
18. Strain-counter-strain was developed by Dr. Lawrence Jones.
19. In strain-counter strain, the preferred position is determined by palpating and monitoring the sensitivity of the associated tender points while positioning the joint. When the client indicates that the pain in the point is reduced and there is a noticeable "letting go" in the palpated tissues, the pain or discomfort in the joint is also reduced, and the client is in a comfortable position, the correct position has been established.
20. The primary techniques used in Structural Muscu-lar Balancing include precision muscle testing, passive positioning, directional massage, and deep pressure.
21. Precision muscle testing is a type of specialized kinesiology that is used to evaluate energetic imbalances in the body and determine exactly what remedies will work best for the individual at that particular time.
22. Acupuncture is said to have originated in China more than 5000 years ago.
23. Yin and yang are the two parts that contrast or exist as opposites of the same phenomenon.

24. Acupressure techniques include rubbing, touching, and pressing of pressure points.
25. The Japanese word shiatsu (shi, finger; and atsu, pressure) means pressure of the fingers.
26. Doctors often recommend massage for the relief of tension, anxiety, and stress.
27. Reflexology is used to stimulate the body's own healing forces through the stimulation of reflex points on the hands, feet, or other areas of the body.

CHAPTER 18 THERAPEUTIC EXERCISE

1. Individuals should consult with a physician to determine if there are any health reasons for restricting an exercise program. They should consult an exercise specialist before beginning an exercise program in order to develop an exercise program to best fit their needs and interests.
2. The major benefits of exercise include:
    Improvement in appearance
    Improvement in body functions
    Maintenance of normal weight
    Relief of tension and stress
    Prevention of fatigue
    Improvement of coordination
    Increased mental alertness
    Increased strength
    Increased endurance
    Improved posture
    Enhanced sense of well-being.
3. Therapeutic exercise is any exercise done with the intent of improving some physical condition.
4. The goal of therapeutic exercise is to regain, improve, or maintain the function of the body or a part of the body regarding strength, endurance, mobility, flexibility, coordination, and relaxation.
5. A consultation with the client helps in determining the correct exercise program, gives insight into the client's health condition, and helps to prevent legal problems for the place of business and its employ-ees.
6. The overload principle maintains that when trying to increase strength, endurance, or flexibility the individual must apply stresses to the body that are greater that what the body is accustomed to.
7. Strength is the ability of a muscle or muscle group to contract and produce tension with a resultant maximum force exerted on some resistance. Strength is usually measured as the ability of a muscle or group of muscles to exert a maximum force one time.
8. Two main factors that determine relative strength include muscle size and the number of motor units involved in the contraction.
9. Hypertrophy refers to the increased bulk of a muscle that is the result of an increase in the

thickness of myofibrils (actin and myosin filaments) in the muscle fiber and an increase in the density of the capillary bed within the muscle.

10. An isometric contraction is when the force of the contraction is equal to the resistance, there is no perceivable movement, and the muscle length remains the same.

11. An isotonic contraction is when the force of resistance is different from the force of the contraction, the muscle changes length, and there is movement.

12. An eccentric contraction is an isotonic contraction in which the resistance is greater than the force of the contraction and the muscle lengthens.

13. A concentric contraction is an isotonic contraction in which the resistance is less than the force of the contraction and the muscle shortens.

14. As a muscle contracts through its available range of motion, the force it generates varies. When exercising against a constant weight the muscle exerts maximum force at only a very small portion of its available range. When a variable resistance is used to provide maximum load at several points during the muscle contraction, the exercise is much more effective.

15. Six methods of providing resistance for strength training exercises include manual resistance, free weights, pulley weights, body weight, variable resistance equipment, and elastic bands.

16. A muscle or muscle group is said to have endurance when it can hold a contraction for an extended period of time or perform a great number of contractions without becoming fatigued.

17. Cardiorespiratory endurance is the ability of an individual to continue a general exercise over an extended period of time. Cardiorespiratory fitness is the ability of the cardiovascular and cardiopulmonary systems to deliver an adequate supply of oxygen to the exercising muscles and the muscles' ability to efficiently extract and convert the oxygen to energy.

18. Factors that determine the effectiveness of an aerobic exercise program are the type of exercise, and the duration, frequency and intensity of that exercise.

19. Two methods for monitoring the intensity of an aerobic workout are determining the target heart rate and the talk test.

20. The components of an aerobic workout are the warm-up, the primary activity, and the cool-down.

21. The purpose of the warm-up exercise is to gradually increase the heart rate, blood pressure, and elasticity of the muscles.

22. Cooling-down exercises bring body functions back to normal and help to prevent soreness and stiffness in muscles and joints.

23. Flexibility refers to the ability of a joint to move freely and painlessly through its range of motion.

24. A contracture is a reduction of joint mobility that is the result of decreased extensibility of muscle or other tissues crossing the joint.

25. Elasticity refers to the tissue's ability to return to normal resting length when a stress that has been placed on it is removed.

26. Plasticity refers to the tissue's ability to adapt to ongoing stresses and conditions.

27. Range of motion exercises are carried out by moving the affected segment of the body through its available movement but do not challenge limitations of movement in order to increase ROM. Stretching exercises travel beyond movement limits in order to increase ROM.

28. Ballistic movements tend to fire the myotatic reflex, causing muscle contraction, and may force connective tissue structures beyond their elastic limits. The firing of the stretch reflex actually increases muscle tension and increases the possibility of injury to the muscle. Moving beyond the elastic limits of the connective tissue may result in injury to tendons, ligaments, or fascia.

29. Exercises that use repetition and positive reinforcement tend to improve coordination and skill.

30. Hatha yoga is a form of exercise that combines mental concentration, muscular control, breathing, and relaxation in the performance of a series of postures and body positions.

31. Yoga improves the posture, relaxes and tones the muscles, and relieves mental and physiological stress. It increases stamina and imparts a sense of physical and mental balance.

32. Lordosis is a form of swayback; kyphosis affects the shoulders and is associated with humpback; scoliosis is a lateral deviation of the spine.

CHAPTER 19 BUSINESS PRACTICES

1. A positive attitude and good self-image are reflected in the enthusiasm and quality exhibited in your work. They are the foundation for creating a good public image. A good public image along with good business practices breeds success.

2. A sole proprietorship is a business owned and operated by an individual. In a partnership, two or more people combine resources to operate a business. In both a sole proprietorship and a partnership, the owners are responsible for the obligations and liabilities of the business and take the profits. A corporation is managed by a board of directors, the owners are not directly liable, and the profits are shared by the stock holders.

3. Start-up costs of a massage business may include rent or lease, equipment, supplies, furniture and decorating costs, printing and advertising, license, insurance, and other miscellaneous expenses.

4. The location for a massage business should accommodate your business needs, be pleasing to

your clients, fit your image, be properly zoned, and be within your budget. The office location must be easy to locate, with the address clearly visible from the street. It should be easily accessible and relatively quiet. An ideal space would have one or more massage rooms, a reception/waiting area, an office, and bathroom facilities with a shower.

5. Permits and licenses necessary to operate a massage business may include fictitious name statement; business license; massage license, sales tax permit; planning and zoning permits; building safety permit; employer's identification number (EIN).

6. The types of insurance a massage business owner should carry to protect his or her business include liability insurance; malpractice liability insurance; automobile insurance; fire and theft insurance; medical health insurance; worker's compensation insurance.

7. Keeping accurate records is necessary in a successful business in that it records the progress of the business, especially the cost of doing business in relation to income. Business records are also necessary to meet the requirements of local, state, and federal laws pertaining to taxes and employees.

8. The major ingredients of a basic bookkeeping system are a checking account with an updated ledger; income and disbursement ledgers; accounts receivable and accounts payable files; bank statements and reconciliations; filed business receipts; an inventory system; an assets and depreciation file; a mileage log.

9. Marketing is the business activity done to promote and increase your business. Marketing is an educational process of getting yourself and what you do known. It is the enticement that encourages an individual to seek your services.

10. Marketing activities commonly used in the massage industry include advertising, promotion, public relations, referrals and client retention.

11. A target market is a segment of the population with certain characteristics that make them good prospec-tive consumers of a particular product or service.

12. The three R's of referrals are:
Request: Request the referral.
Reward: Acknowledge and reward the person who sends the referral.
Reciprocate: Use the services of or send referrals back to those who send you referrals.

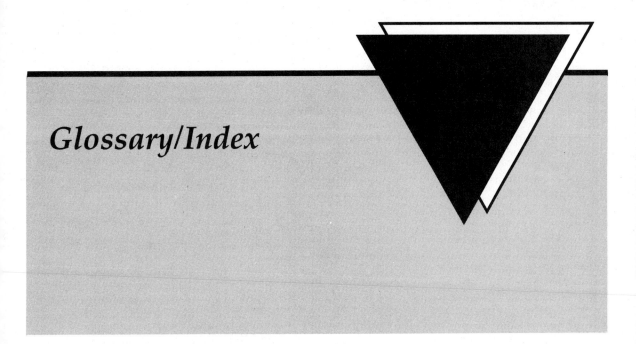

Glossary/Index

Muscle fibers, are the functional contractile unit of muscle tissue, 108-109
  neuromuscular connection, 109, 111
  organization of, 108-109
  structure of, 109, 110
Muscles
  of abdominal area, 148
  characteristics of muscles, 106
  of the eye, 159
  of facial expression, 157-158
  of the fingers, 132-133, 135-137
  of the foot, 145-147
  of the forearm, 129-130
  of the hyoid, 156
  of the lower leg, 142
  of mastication, 157
  of the neck, 152-155
  of respiration, 149-150
  of the scapula, 124-125
  of the spine, 151
  structure of, 106-111
  of the thigh, 138-141, 143-144
  types of, 105-106
  of the upper arm, 126-128
  of the wrist and hand, 131
Muscle spasm, is a sudden involuntary contraction of a muscle or group of muscles, 120
Muscle spindle cells, 202, 594
Muscle strains, are torn or pulled muscles, 120, 123
  grades of, 120
Muscle testing
  precision muscle testing, 560-561
  use of resisted movement in, 438
Muscle tissue
  cardiac muscle, 60, 61, 106-107
  composition of, 106-107
  function of, 60
  smooth muscle, 105
  striated muscle, 60, 61, 105
Muscle tone, is a type of muscle contraction present in healthy muscles when they are at rest, 113
Muscular dystrophy, is a progressive degeneration of the voluntary muscle system, 123
Muscular system, is made up of voluntary and involuntary muscles that are necessary for

movement and that shapes and supports the skeleton, 70, 105-159
  anterior view of, 121
  connective tissue, 107
  functions of, 105
  massage, effects on, 248-249, 294
  muscle interaction, 115-119
  muscular contraction, 111-114
  posterior view of, 122
  terms related to, 120
Muscular system dysfunctions
  atrophy, 123
  dystrophy, 123
  fibrosis, 123
  hypertrophy, 123
  muscle spasms, 120
  muscle strains, 120, 123
  myofibrosis, 123
Myocardium, is the cardiac muscle and is responsible for the muscular pumping of the heart, 164
Myofibrils, are muscle fibers containing filaments that give muscles their contractile ability, 109
Myofibrosis, is the replacement of muscle with fibrous connective tissue, 123
Myosin, is a muscular filament that plays a role in giving muscle its contractile ability, 109

N

Naevus, is a discoloration of the skin commonly known as a birthmark, 84-85
Nails, composition of, 78
Neck
  arteries of, 176-178
  athletic massage, 536-537
  athletic massage, 531-533
  bones of, 96
  massage procedure, 381-382, 393-396
  muscles of, 152-155
  nerves of, 206
  veins of, 180, 181
Nerve cell, 190
Nerve fibers, 190
  types of, 190

Nerves, are bundles of nerve fibers extending from the central nervous system to the tissue the neurons enervate, 191
  of abdomen, 208
  of arms/legs, 209
  of back, 208
  of chest, 206
  cranial nerves, 193-194, 195
  of head/face, 207
  of neck, 206
  spinal nerves, 194
  types of, 191
Nerve tissue, initiates, coordinates, and controls body's adaption to environment, 60, 61
Nervous system, is composed of the brain, spinal cord, and nerves; it collects sensory information and processes it to initiate appropriate responses in the body, 70, 190
  autonomic nervous system, 196, 198
  central nervous system, 191-193
  cranial nerves, 193-194
  functions of, 190
  massage, effects of, 249-250
  neurons, 190-191
  peripheral nervous system, 193
  proprioception, 202-203
  reflexes, 201-202
  spinal nerves, 194, 196
Nervous system disorders
  encephalitis, 205
  epilepsy, 204
  meningitis, 205
  multiple sclerosis, 204
  neuritis, 205
  Parkinson's disease, 204
  poliomyelitis, 204-205
  shingles, 205
  stroke, 204
Neuralgia, 205
Neuritis, is an inflammation of a nerve, 205
Neurological pathway, 201
Neuromuscular junction, is the site where a muscle fiber and nerve fiber meet, 109
Neuromuscular therapy, identifies soft tissue abnormalities

Phlebitis, is an inflammation of a vein, 170
  as contraindications to massage, 256-257
Physiology, is the study of vital processes, mechanisms, and functions of organs or systems of organs, 35, 48
Pia mater, 191
Pigmentation, of skin, 84-85
Pituitary gland
  disorders of, 219
  hormones of, 217, 219
  structure of, 217
Pivot joints, 98, 99
Planes of body, 64
Plantar flexion movement, 117
Plasma, is the fluid part of the blood, 173
  composition of, 173, 174
Plasticity, 592
Platelets. See Thrombocytes
Pneumocystis carinii pneumonia, and AIDS, 263
Polarity therapy, uses massage, exercises, and thinking practices to balance the body physically and energetically, 16
Poliomyelitis, is a disease affecting the motor neurons and resulting in paralysis of the related muscle tissue, 204-205
Pons, 193
Popliteal region, 67, 68
Positional release, 561-562
Posture
  observation of, 435
  varieties of, 436, 606
Posture improvement program, 606-613
  exercises in, 607-613
Powder for massage, 276
Precision muscle testing, 560-561
Prenatal massage, 242-243, 259-261, 539-541
  contraindications for, 540-541
Pressure deep pressure, 509-510, 562
  in massage, 308-310, 329
Pressure points, 568-572
  anterior view, 568-570
  posterior view, 570-572

Prime mover, muscle as, 115
Progesterone, 222, 241
Prolactin, 217
Pronation movement, 119
Prophase, is a stage in cell division, 51
Proprioception, is a system of nerve activity that provides information as to the position and rate of movement of parts of the body, 202
Proprioceptive neuromuscular facilitation, 514-515
Proprioceptors, 202, 203
Prostate gland, 239
Protoplasm, is the substance that is the composition of all living matter, 48
Protraction movement, 119
Psoriasis, is a chronic skin disease of dry round patches with silvery scales that are found on scalp, elbows, knees, chest and lower back, 81
Pulmonary circulation, is circulation of blood from the heart to the lungs and back to the heart, 168-169
Pulmonary semilunar valve, of the heart directs the blood to flow from the right ventricle into the pulmonary arteries as it travels to the lungs, 165
Pulse, taking pulse, 303
Pustule, is an elevation of the skin containing pus, 79
Pyloric sphincter, 230

Q
Quadriplegia, 204
Quaternary ammonium compounds, 285, 286

R
Range of motion, is the action of a joint through the entire extent of its movement, 435
  assessment of, 435-439
  end feel, 327
  restrictions to, 327
Range of motion exercises, 594
Records, 295-302
  body diagrams, 296, 298-300

information card, 300-301
intake forms, 296, 297
  updating, 302
Red bone marrow, 87-88
Red corpuscles. See Erythrocytes
Reduction, means realigning the bone that is dislocated, 99
Referrals, sources of, 646-647
Reflex arc, 201
Reflexes, 201-202
  nature of, 201
Reflexology, is based on the idea that stimulation of specific points on the body affects other areas or organs, 17, 572-573
Regions of body
  anterior view, 67, 68
  posterior view, 67, 68
Rehabilitative massage, 519-521
  effects of, 520
  guidelines for, 520-521
Relaxation program, 601-604
  relaxation exercise, 602
  stress-reduction exercises, 602-603
  yoga, 603-604
Renaissance, history of massage in, 9
Renin, 234
Reproductive system
  female, 240-242
  male, 239-240
  pregnancy, 242-243
Respiration, is the exchange of carbon dioxide and oxygen in the body, 71, 225-227
  muscles of, 149-150
  process of, 225, 227
Respiratory system, components of, 225, 226
Reticular layer of skin, 74
Reticular tissue, forms the framework of the liver and lymphoid organs, 58-59, 62
Retraction movement, 119
Rhazes, was an Islamic Persian physician who advocated diet/exercise/massage in the treatment of disease, 9
Rheumatoid arthritis, is a chronic inflammatory disease in which the articular cartilage of joints erodes causing the